Disorders of the Liver, Exocrine Pancreas, and Gastrointestinal Tract in Dogs and Cats

Disorders of the Liver, Exocrine Pancreas, and Gastrointestinal Tract in Dogs and Cats

Edited by

Harry Cridge

Aarti Kathrani

Andrea N. Johnston

WILEY

Published by John Wiley & Sons, Inc., Hoboken, New Jersey.

For general information on our other products and services or for technical support, please contact our Customer Care Department within the United States at (800) 762-2974, outside the United States at (317) 572-3993 or fax (317) 572-4002.

Wiley also publishes its books in a variety of electronic formats. Some content that appears in print may not be available in electronic formats. For more information about Wiley products, visit our web site at www.wiley.com.

Library of Congress Cataloging-in-Publication Data has been applied for:

Print ISBN: 9781394306695
ePDF ISBN: 9781394306718
ePUB ISBN: 9781394306701
oBook ISBN: 9781394306725

Cover Design: Wiley
Cover Images: Courtesy of Harry Cridge, Courtesy of Aarti Kathrani, Courtesy of Andrea Johnston, Courtesy of Shannon Dehghanpir

Printed in Singapore
M132393160126

Contents

39a Disorders of the Esophagus – Megaesophagus 323

Jillian M. Haines

39b Disorders of the Esophagus (Excluding Megaesophagus) 331

Dan Batchelor

List of Contributors

Frederik William Scott Allan
North Downs Specialist Referrals
Bletchingley
United Kingdom

Yuvani Bandara
Department of Clinical Sciences, College of Veterinary Medicine & Biomedical Sciences
Colorado State University
Fort Collins
CO
USA

Patrick C. Barko
Department of Veterinary Clinical Medicine, College of Veterinary Medicine
University of Illinois at Urbana-Champaign
Urbana-Champaign
IL
USA

Dan Batchelor
Department of Veterinary Clinical Sciences, School of Veterinary Science
University of Liverpool
Neston
UK

Nick Bexfield
Department of Veterinary Medicine, The Queen's Veterinary School Hospital
University of Cambridge
Cambridge
United Kingdom

Melissa Bucknoff
Department of Small Animal Clinical Sciences, College of Veterinary Medicine
University of Florida
Gainesville
FL
USA

Agostino Buono
Department of Veterinary Clinical Sciences, School of Veterinary Medicine
Louisiana State University
Baton Rouge
LA
USA

Sharon A. Center
Department of Clinical Sciences and Biomedical Sciences
College of Veterinary Medicine
Cornell University
Ithaca
NY
USA

Betty Chow
VCA Animal Specialty and Emergency Center
Los Angeles
CA
USA

Francisco O. Conrado
Department of Comparative Pathobiology
Cummings School of Veterinary Medicine
Tufts University
North Grafton
MA
USA

Harry Cridge
Department of Small Animal Clinical Sciences, College of Veterinary Medicine
Michigan State University
East Lansing
MI
USA

Julien R.S. Dandrieux
Royal (Dick) School of Veterinary Studies
University of Edinburgh
Easter Bush
United Kingdom

Shannon D. Dehghanpir
Department of Veterinary Clinical Sciences, Veterinary Clinical Pathology
School of Veterinary Medicine
Louisiana State University
Baton Rouge
LA
USA

Autumn Dutelle
Department of Veterinary Clinical Sciences, School of Veterinary Medicine
Louisiana State University
Baton Rouge
LA
USA

Marnin Forman
Cornell University Veterinary Specialists
Stamford
CT
USA

Jillian M. Haines
Department of Veterinary Clinical Sciences
College of Veterinary Medicine
Washington State University
Pullman
WA
USA

Edward Hall
Bristol Veterinary School
University of Bristol
Langford
Bristol
UK

Romy M. Heilmann
Department of Small Animal Medicine, College of Veterinary Medicine
University of Leipzig
Leipzig
Saxony
Germany

Anke Hendricks
Department of Clinical Sciences & Services
Royal Veterinary College
Hatfield
Hertfordshire
UK

Séamus Hoey
School of Veterinary Medicine
University College Dublin
Ireland
Vet CT
Cambridge
UK
School of Veterinary Medicine
University of Wisconsin-Madison
USA

Sara Jablonski
Department of Small Animal Clinical Sciences, College of Veterinary Medicine
Michigan State University
East Lansing
MI
USA

Jared A. Jaffey
Chief of Small Animal Internal Medicine
Midwestern University College of Veterinary Medicine
Glendale
AZ
USA

Andrea N. Johnston
Departments of Pathobiology and Diagnostic Investigation/Small Animal Clinical Sciences, College of Veterinary Medicine
Michigan State University
East Lansing
MI
USA

Aarti Kathrani
Department of Clinical Sciences & Services
Royal Veterinary College
Hatfield
Hertfordshire
UK

Andrew Kent
Blaise Veterinary Referral Hospital
Rednal, Birmingham
UK

Jessica Kerley
Department of Clinical Sciences & Advanced Medicine, School of Veterinary Medicine
University of Pennsylvania School of Veterinary Medicine
Philadelphia
PA
USA

Daniel K. Langlois
Department of Small Animal Clinical Sciences, College of Veterinary Medicine
Michigan State University
East Lansing
MI
USA

Rommaneeya Leela-arporn
Department of Clinical Sciences, College of Veterinary Medicine and Biomedical Sciences
Colorado State University
Fort Collins
CO
USA

Jonathan A. Lidbury
Department of Small Animal Clinical Sciences, College of Veterinary Medicine & Biomedical Sciences
Texas A&M University
College Station
TX
USA

Sue Yee Lim
Department of Small Animal Clinical Sciences, College of Veterinary Medicine & Biomedical Sciences
Texas A&M University
College Station
TX
USA

Vicky Lipscomb
Department of Clinical Sciences & Services
Royal Veterinary College
Hatfield
Hertfordshire
UK

Sarah Long
Bristol Veterinary School
University of Bristol
Langford
Bristol
UK

Bruna Correa Lopes
Gastrointestinal Laboratory, Department of Small Animal Clinical Sciences, College of Veterinary Medicine
Texas A&M University
College Station
TX
USA

Alison C. Manchester
Department of Clinical Sciences, College of Veterinary Medicine
Cornell University
Ithaca
USA

Angela Marolf
Department Veterinary Clinical Sciences
College of Veterinary Medicine
The Ohio State University
Columbus
OH
USA

Emma J. O'Neill
School of Veterinary Medicine
University College Dublin
Belfield
Dublin
Ireland

Rachel Pilla
Department of Veterinary Medicine and Animal Sciences
University of Milan
Milan
Italy
Gastrointestinal Laboratory, Department of Small Animal Clinical Sciences, College of Veterinary Medicine
Texas A&M University
College Station
TX
USA

Simon L. Priestnall
Department of Pathobiology and Population Sciences
Royal Veterinary College
London
United Kingdom

Fabio Procoli
Anicura Ospedale Veterinario I Portoni Rossi
Zola Predosa
BO
Italy

Beatrice Ruggerone
Anicura Ospedale Veterinario I Portoni Rossi
Zola Predosa
BO
Italy

Silke Salavati Schmitz
Royal (Dick) School of Veterinary Studies
University of Edinburgh
Easter Bush
United Kingdom

Leslie C. Sharkey
Department of Clinical Sciences
Cummings School of Veterinary Medicine
Tufts University
North Grafton
MA
United States

Eimear Shorten
Department of Equine Studies, Anaesthesia and Diagnostic Imaging, School of Veterinary Medicine
University College Dublin
Dublin
Belfield
Ireland

Sarah Shropshire
Department of Clinical Sciences, College of Veterinary Medicine and Biomedical Sciences
Colorado State University
Fort Collins
CO
USA

Rebecca Smedley
Veterinary Diagnostic Laboratory
Michigan State University
Lansing
MI
USA

Joshua Sparago
Le Centre Hospitalier Universitaire Vétérinaire – Faculté de Médecine Vétérinaire
Université de Montréal
Saint-Hyacinthe
QC
CA

Jörg Steiner
Gastrointestinal Laboratory, Department of Small Animal Clinical Sciences, School of Veterinary Medicine and Biomedical Sciences
Texas A&M University
College Station
TX
USA

Jonathan Stockman
Department of Molecular Biosciences
School of Veterinary Medicine
University of California Davis
Davis
California
USA

Alejandro Suarez Bonnet
Department of Pathobiology and Population Sciences
Royal Veterinary College
London
United Kingdom

Sarah Tayler
Department of Clinical Sciences & Services
Royal Veterinary College
Hatfield
Hertfordshire
UK

Vincent Thawley
Department of Clinical Sciences & Advanced Medicine, School of Veterinary Medicine
University of Pennsylvania
Philadelphia
PA
USA

Mickey Tivers
Paragon Veterinary Referrals
Paragon point
Wakefield
West Yorkshire
UK

Cecilia Villaverde
Expert Pet Nutrition
Fermoy
County Cork
Ireland

Mandy L. Wallace
Department of Small Animal Medicine and Surgery, College of Veterinary Medicine
University of Georgia
Athens
GA
USA

Penny Watson
Emeritus Fellow – Emmanuel College
University of Cambridge
Cambridge
UK

Victoria Watson
Department of Pathobiology & Diagnostic Investigations, College of Veterinary Medicine
Michigan State University
East Lansing
MI
USA

Cynthia R. L. Webster
Department of Clinical Sciences, Cummings School of Veterinary Medicine
Tufts University
North Grafton
MA
USA

David A. Williams
Department of Veterinary Clinical Medicine, University of Illinois
Urbana
IL
USA

Panagiotis G. Xenoulis
Faculty of Veterinary Science
University of Thessaly
Volos
Greece

Preface

Disorders of the liver, exocrine pancreas, and gastrointestinal tract are common in small animal practice and can present diagnostic and therapeutic challenges. Over the last decade, advances in clinical research, diagnostic techniques, and therapeutic approaches have transformed our understanding of these conditions. Yet, for many clinicians, particularly those in general practice, staying up-to-date with these latest developments while managing a busy caseload can be difficult.

This textbook was developed to address this challenge. Our goal is to provide a single, practical reference that brings together current knowledge on the pathogenesis, diagnosis, and management of disorders affecting the liver, exocrine pancreas, and gastrointestinal tract in dogs and cats.

To support rapid access to recent developments, we have included clearly marked "key points" boxes within most chapters. These highlight key changes in our understanding or management strategies over the past decade, allowing readers to quickly identify clinically relevant advances. In addition, the use of charts and tables, where appropriate, is intended to enhance the book's utility in a clinical setting.

While many existing references focus heavily on gastrointestinal disease, this text also gives expanded attention to hepatic and exocrine pancreatic disorders – areas that are often underrepresented in alimentary disorders despite their clinical importance. The content reflects a balance of depth and practicality, suited to both the general practitioner and those preparing for further specialization.

The editorial team brings together expertise from both sides of the Atlantic, encompassing diverse training backgrounds, clinical experience, and academic perspectives. We share a common goal of providing veterinarians with the tools to deliver informed, confident, and effective care.

It is our hope that this book will serve not only as a valuable day-to-day reference but also as a foundation for continued learning and professional growth.

Harry Cridge
Aarti Kathrani
Andrea N. Johnston

List of Abbreviations

AA: atresia ani
a1-PI: alpha 1 proteinase inhibitor
Ach: acetylcholine
ACTH: adrenocorticotropic hormone
ACVIM: American College of Veterinary Internal Medicine
AD: aerodigestive disorder
AGASAC: apocrine gland anal sac adenocarcinoma
AHDS: acute hemorrhagic diarrhea syndrome
AHI: acute hepatic injury
AIEC: adherent invasive *E. coli*
AIP: autoimmune pancreatitis
AKI: acute kidney injury
AL: amyloid
ALF: acute liver failure
ALI: acute lung injury
ALP: alkaline phosphatase
ALT: alanine aminotransferase
AP: acute pancreatitis
APN: acute pancreatic necrosis
ARDS: acute respiratory distress syndrome
ARE: antimicrobial responsive enteropathy
ARF: adverse reaction to food
AVDC: American Veterinary Dental College
BA: bile acids
BAL: bronchoalveolar lavage
BCS: body condition score
BE-tube: balloon-dilation esophagostomy tube
BOAS: brachycephalic obstructive airway syndrome
BT-PABA: N-benzoyl-L-tyrosyl p-aminobenzoic acid
CAPC: Companion Animal Parasite Council
CBC: complete blood count
CCK: cholecystokinin
CCUS: canine chronic ulcerative stomatitis
CDV: canine distemper virus
CE: chronic enteropathy
CH: chronic hepatitis
CIE: chronic inflammatory enteropathy
CKD: chronic kidney disease
CMO: craniomandibular osteopathy
CN: cranial nerve
CNS: central nervous system
CP: chronic pancreatitis
CRP: C reactive protein
CRTZ: chemoreceptor trigger zone
CT: computed tomography
CUPS: chronic ulcerative paradental stomatitis

CVE: colonic vascular ectasia
DGGR: 1,2-o-dilauryl-rac-glycero3-glutaric acid-(6'-methylresorufin) ester
DIC: disseminated intravascular coagulation
DM: diabetes mellitus
DRE: digital rectal exam
DSH: domestic short hair
ECG: electrocardiography
ECGS: E.coli associated granulomatous colitis
ECS: English Cocker Spaniel
ECLs: enterochromaffin-like cells
EHBDO: extra hepatic bile duct obstruction
ELISA: enzyme linked immunosorbent assay
EMD: enteric microbiota dysbiosis
ENS: enteric nervous system
EPI: Exocrine pancreatic insufficiency
FB: foreign body
FCGS: feline chronic gingivostomatitis
FCoV: feline coronavirus
FCV: feline calicivirus
FDA: Food and Drug Administration
fDI: fecal dysbiosis index
FECV: feline enteric coronavirus
FEGC: feline eosinophilic granuloma complex
FeLV: feline leukemia virus
FEPLO: fibromatous epulis of periodontal ligament origin
FHV: feline herpesvirus
FIAD: fecal incontinence associated dermatitis
FIP: feline infectious peritonitis
FISH: fluorescent in situ hybridization
FIV: feline immunodeficiency virus
FMT: fecal microbiota transplantation
FNA: fine-needle aspirate
FORLs: feline resorptive lesions
fPL: feline pancreatic lipase
FRE: food responsive enteropathy
fT4: free thyroxine
GA: general anaesthetic
GER: gastroesophageal reflux
GERD: gastroesophageal reflux disease
GESF: gastrointestinal eosinophilic sclerosing fibroplasia
GI: gastrointestinal
GIST: gastrointestinal stromal tumor
GMS: Gomori methenamine silver
GSD: German Shepherd Dog
HD: high definition
HE: hematoxylin and eosin
HH: hiatal hernia
HGAL: high-grade alimentary lymphoma
HL: hepatic lipidosis
HSCR: Hirschsprung's
IBD: inflammatory bowel disease
ICC: interstitial cells of Cajal
IFA: indirect fluorescent antibody
Ig: immunoglobulin

IGAL: intermediate-grade alimentary lymphoma
IGF: insulin growth factor
IHC: immunohistochemistry
IL: intestinal lymphangiectasia
IRE: immunosuppressant responsive enteropathy
IV: intravenous
IVFT: intravenous fluid therapy
KCS: keratoconjunctivitis sicca
LCL: large cell lymphoma
LES-AS: lower esophageal sphincter achalasia-like syndrome
LES: lower esophageal sphincter
LGITL: low grade intestinal T cell lymphoma
LGL: large granular lymphoma
LPE: lymphoplasmacytic enteritis
MCLE: mucocutaneous lupus erythematosus
MCT: medium chain triglycerides
MDR: multidrug resistant
ME: megaesophagus
MER: maintenance energy requirement
MG: myasthenia gravis
MLDB: minimum laboratory database
MMA: methylmalonic acid
MMC: migrating motor complexes
MODS: multi organ dysfunction syndrome
MRI: magnetic resonance imaging
MrMRE: microbiota-related modulation-responsive enteropathy
MST: median survival time
MVD: microvascular dysplasia
N:C: nuclear-to-cytoplasmic ratio
NNASD: non neoplastic anal sac disease
NO: nitric oxide
NRE: non-responsive enteropathies
NSAID: non-steroidal anti-inflammatory drug
PAA: pancreatic acinar atrophy
PARR: PCR for antigen receptor rearrangement
PAS: periodic-acid Schiff
PCR: polymerase chain reaction
PCV: packed cell volume
PEG: percutaneous endoscopic gastrostomy tube
PERT: pancreatic enzyme replacement therapy
PLE: protein losing enteropathy
PLI: pancreatic lipase immunoreactivity
PLN: protein losing nephropathy
PMPs: pacemaker potentials
PN: parenteral nutrition
PO: per os
POCT: point-of-care test
POF: peripheral odontogenic fibromas
PPI: proton pump inhibitor
PPP: pancreatitis, panniculitis, and polyarthritis
PRAA: persistent right aortic arch
PTE: pulmonary thromboembolism
PVH: portal vein hypoplasia
PVT: portal vein thrombosis

qPCR: quantitative PCR
RER: resting energy requirement
RI: reference interval
RIA: radioimmunoassay
RVF: rectovaginal fistula
SBS: short bowel syndrome
SCC: squamous cell carcinoma
SCL: small cell lymphoma
SI: small intestine
SIBO: small intestinal bacterial overgrowth
SIRS: systemic inflammatory response syndrome
SRE: steroid responsive enteropathy
T-FOCUS: thoracic focal point of care ultrasound
TLI: trypsin-like immunoreactivity
TMJ: temporomandibular joint
tT4: total thyroxine
UES: upper esophageal sphincter
UPC: urine protein creatinine ratio
USG: urine specific gravity
VFSS: videofluoroscopic swallow study
VH: vacuolar hepatopathy
WSAVA: world small animal veterinary association

About the Companion Website

This book is accompanied by a companion website:

www.wiley.com/go/cridge/disorders

- Videos of chapter 35

Liver Enzymes and Liver Function Testing

CHAPTER 1

Nick Bexfield

Department of Veterinary Medicine, The Queen's Veterinary School Hospital, University of Cambridge, Cambridge, United Kingdom

KEY POINTS

- Liver enzymes are sensitive indicators of hepatic insult but lack specificity for liver function.
- Reduced albumin, urea, cholesterol, glucose, or elevated bilirubin can indicate impaired hepatic function in advanced disease. Although bilirubin can be elevated for pre- or post-hepatic causes.
- Total serum bile acids are the most reliable routine marker for detecting hepatic dysfunction although they are not interpretable in patients with hyperbilirubinemia due to hepatic or post-hepatic cholestasis.

LIVER ENZYMES

INTRODUCTION

Liver enzymes are typically categorized based on their origin and function into hepatocellular (or leakage) enzymes and biliary (or inducible) enzymes. This classification helps guide the interpretation of laboratory findings in veterinary patients. Alanine aminotransferase (ALT) and aspartate aminotransferase (AST) are key markers of hepatocellular injury, while alkaline phosphatase (ALP) and gamma-glutamyl transferase (GGT) are markers of biliary tract disease or enzyme induction. Understanding the origin, behavior, and species-specific differences in these enzymes is essential for accurate clinical interpretation.

HEPATOCELLULAR ENZYMES: ALT AND AST

ALT is a cytosolic enzyme predominantly found in hepatocytes. When hepatocyte membrane integrity is compromised, as seen with inflammation or necrosis, ALT is released into the bloodstream. It is considered a sensitive and relatively liver-specific enzyme in both dogs and cats. While ALT is also present in skeletal muscle and kidney tissue, elevations due to these sources are usually minor unless there is significant muscle damage. The half-life of ALT in dogs varies in the literature but ranges from 6 hours to 2.5 days. In cats, the half-life is much shorter, which means that even mild ALT elevations are more clinically significant in this species (Stockham and Scott 2020).

ALT elevations can occur rapidly, within 24–48 hours, following hepatic injury, with peak values around day five. These elevations may be dramatic, sometimes exceeding 10 times the reference range. In cases of acute injury, a decline in ALT by 50% every 2–3 days is generally considered a positive prognostic sign. Chronic liver diseases, such as canine chronic hepatitis, are often present with persistent ALT elevations. Importantly, ALT can also rise in response to cholestasis or hepatotoxic drugs like corticosteroids and phenobarbital, though the pattern and degree of increase vary. Interpretation of ALT must be contextual and include assessment of other diagnostic findings, patient history, and breed-specific considerations.

AST is another marker of hepatocellular damage. Like ALT, it is found in hepatocytes, but also in skeletal and cardiac muscle. Approximately 30% of AST in the liver is located in mitochondria, making it a marker of more severe injury when elevated. The half-life of AST is shorter than ALT, about 4–20 hours in dogs and approximately 1 hour in cats. In liver disease, AST usually increases in parallel with ALT but normalizes more quickly due to its shorter half-life. Persistent AST elevation may suggest ongoing hepatocellular necrosis and may carry a poorer prognosis (Center 2007). As AST is present in muscle tissue, it should be interpreted alongside creatine kinase (CK) to differentiate between hepatic and muscular sources, especially if ALT is not elevated.

CHOLESTATIC OR INDUCIBLE ENZYMES: ALP AND GGT

ALP is a membrane-bound enzyme found in liver, bone, kidney, and intestinal tissues. It has higher sensitivity but poorer specificity for hepatobiliary disease in dogs. In contrast, ALP has lower sensitivity but higher specificity for hepatic disease in cats. This reflects differences in ALP isoenzyme production and clearance between species. Dogs express several isoenzymes including liver ALP (L-ALP), bone ALP (B-ALP), and glucocorticoid-induced ALP (G-ALP), while cats mainly produce L-ALP and B-ALP. The lack of G-ALP in cats contributes to their more specific ALP responses in liver disease, particularly hepatic lipidosis.

ALP elevations in dogs can result from cholestasis, induction of synthesis by drugs or endogenous corticosteroids, bone growth in young animals, or bone lesions such as osteosarcoma. In cats, ALP has a much shorter half-life, around six hours, meaning that elevations tend to be modest but often more clinically meaningful. In dogs, values may rise four to five times the reference range with relatively benign causes, while cats with liver disease may only show two- to threefold increases.

ALP activity increases in dogs with cholestasis and corticosteroid exposure. While corticosteroids are known to induce ALP synthesis via glucocorticoid-responsive elements, the role of bile acids in transcriptional induction remains unproven in dogs, and increases may instead reflect cholangiocellular membrane injury or altered enzyme clearance. Corticosteroid induction occurs within 24–48 hours and may persist for weeks after exposure ends. This can obscure interpretation, particularly in dogs receiving chronic medications or topical corticosteroids. G-ALP increases are not specific to corticosteroid use; they also occur in diabetes mellitus, liver disease, and chronic illnesses. Thus, isoenzyme analysis has limited utility in clinical practice.

Persistent ALP elevation is generally more concerning than a single abnormal result. A study involving 270 dogs with confirmed liver disease found that the highest ALP increases occurred with cholestasis (median tenfold), followed by steroid hepatopathy, chronic hepatitis, and hepatic necrosis (Center et al. 2012). ALP levels did not reliably correlate with disease severity or prognosis. Other conditions that may increase ALP include endocrine disorders such as hyperadrenocorticism, chronic drug administration (e.g. corticosteroids), and some extrahepatic diseases such as pancreatitis.

GGT, another membrane-bound enzyme, originates primarily from biliary epithelial cells. Like ALP, its serum levels increase with cholestasis and enzyme induction. GGT is more liver-specific than ALP, as it lacks bone isoforms. Although it may also be induced by corticosteroids, GGT is less responsive to phenobarbital. GGT and ALP often rise in parallel and comparing both enzymes can help clarify the nature of liver injury, particularly in dogs where multiple isoenzymes may be present. GGT is also helpful in distinguishing hepatic from bone causes of ALP elevation.

CONCLUSION AND CLINICAL RELEVANCE

In summary, liver enzymes are valuable tools in detecting liver injuries but have limitations in specificity and prognostic value. ALT and AST provide information about hepatocellular integrity, while ALP and GGT reflect cholestasis, bile duct epithelial injury, or enzyme induction. Interpretation must always be integrated with the patient's clinical picture, history, and results from other diagnostic modalities. Serial monitoring enhances clinical insight, as patterns over time can help differentiate transient insults from chronic liver disease. Ultimately, careful interpretation of enzyme data contributes significantly to diagnosing and managing liver disorders in both dogs and cats.

LIVER FUNCTION TESTING

INTRODUCTION

Assessing liver function involves evaluating parameters that reflect the liver's synthetic and excretory capacity. Due to its significant functional reserve, signs of hepatic impairment often do not become apparent until around 75% of liver mass is lost. In acute hepatocyte loss, functional deficits can occur more rapidly, whereas chronic diseases may allow time for compensation by remaining hepatocytes.

Several liver function tests are commonly included in standard biochemical profiles, such as albumin, blood urea nitrogen (BUN), cholesterol, and glucose, but these are not particularly sensitive or specific. More useful tests include total serum bile acids (TSBAs), plasma ammonia, bilirubin, and coagulation proteins. These can often help to differentiate primary hepatic disease from secondary or reactive hepatopathies. However, in cats, reduced liver function is not always observed even with primary liver disease. While portal and bridging fibrosis are commonly seen in conditions such as lymphocytic and chronic cholangitis, progression to cirrhosis and hepatic failure appears to be relatively uncommon in this species.

ALBUMIN

Albumin is synthesized solely by the liver, and serum levels are regulated by the balance between production and degradation. Hypoalbuminemia may suggest reduced hepatic function or liver hypoperfusion, but is not liver-specific, as it may also result from protein-losing nephropathy, enteropathy, or inflammation.

Due to albumin's relatively long half-life (8–10 days in dogs and cats) and the liver's synthetic reserve, hypoalbuminemia generally indicates chronic, advanced liver disease. An exception is acute hepatic inflammation, where albumin may fall due to a negative acute-phase response, though this tends to be mild. Serum protein electrophoresis can help differentiate hypoalbuminemia due to liver dysfunction from that related to inflammation. Studies have shown that low albumin levels combined with low acute-phase protein concentrations suggest a poor prognosis in liver failure, whereas low albumin with normal or elevated acute-phase proteins suggests a better outlook (Gagne et al. 1999).

BLOOD UREA NITROGEN

The liver converts ammonia to urea, which is then excreted by the kidneys. Reduced liver function may lead to decreased BUN, but this is only seen in advanced disease and is not specific, as many non-hepatic conditions can also lower BUN. Therefore, it is a poor standalone marker for liver function.

CHOLESTEROL

The liver plays a central role in lipid metabolism, including the synthesis and breakdown of cholesterol. While advanced liver disease can cause hypocholesterolemia, this finding is inconsistent and nonspecific as it can also occur with systemic diseases such as protein-losing enteropathy, sepsis, or endocrine disorders. Hence, changes in cholesterol concentration should be interpreted alongside other markers.

GLUCOSE

The liver contributes to glucose homeostasis through gluconeogenesis, glycogen storage, glycogenolysis, and insulin degradation. Hypoglycemia can occur with severe hepatic dysfunction due to reduced glucose production and impaired insulin clearance. When present, it is more often associated with acute hepatic injury (AHI) or fulminant liver failure. However, it remains uncommon in dogs and is rarely seen in cats, even in advanced liver disease, due to the liver's substantial compensatory capacity.

TOTAL SERUM BILE ACIDS

TSBAs are among the most sensitive markers of hepatic function. Bile acids are synthesized from cholesterol in the liver, conjugated, and stored in the gallbladder. After a meal, cholecystokinin stimulates bile release into the intestine, where bile acids aid fat digestion and are then reabsorbed in the ileum and returned to the liver through enterohepatic circulation, which is over 95% efficient.

In liver dysfunction, portosystemic shunting, or cholestasis, this circulation is disrupted, causing elevated TSBAs. A paired test, with measurements taken after a 12-hour fast and 2 hours post-meal, provides greater sensitivity. In normal animals, postprandial values may be three to four times higher than fasting values. Elevated fasting or postprandial TSBAs indicate impaired bile acid clearance, but elevations in jaundiced animals reflect cholestasis rather than functional loss and thus add little diagnostic value in that context.

Cutoff values for diagnosis vary. In dogs, fasting values over 15 μmol/L and postprandial levels over 25 μmol/L are highly specific for hepatobiliary disease (Pena-Ramos et al. 2021). In cats, similar cutoffs show specificities of 96 and 100%, respectively. Sensitivity ranges from 54 to 74%, though values up to 100% have been reported in cirrhotic dogs (Johnson et al. 1995).

Clinicians should remember that secondary hepatopathies, including extrahepatic causes of cholestasis such as pancreatitis or bile duct obstruction, and gastrointestinal conditions like small intestinal bacterial overgrowth (SIBO), may also affect bile acid metabolism. In SIBO, bacterial deconjugation can increase levels of unconjugated bile acids in the intestine, although whether this leads to a quantifiable increase in TSBA concentrations in dogs or cats has not been clearly established (Simpson 2004). Levels above 50 μmol/L are more suggestive of primary hepatic disease and may warrant further investigation such as liver biopsy. However, overlap exists, and significantly elevated TSBAs can occasionally occur in secondary disease (Pena-Ramos et al. 2021).

Test interpretation can be affected by several factors. There is no standardized test meal, and variables such as gallbladder contraction timing, gastric emptying, and intestinal motility can influence results. Occasionally, fasting values may exceed postprandial values, possibly due to spontaneous gallbladder contraction. In these cases, the higher of the two values should be used. Lipemia and hemolysis may also falsely elevate results.

AMMONIA

Ammonia is produced in the gastrointestinal tract from protein metabolism and enters the portal circulation. A healthy liver extracts nearly all of it and converts it to urea. In liver dysfunction or portosystemic shunting, this process is impaired, resulting in hyperammonemia.

Because of the liver's reserve capacity, fasting ammonia levels are relatively insensitive indicators of liver failure (Center 2007). Ammonia tolerance testing was once used to improve diagnostic sensitivity, but oral or rectal administration of ammonium salts can trigger hepatic encephalopathy and is now discouraged.

Sample handling is critical. Ammonia samples must be collected in heparinized tubes on ice, centrifuged quickly, and plasma separated and analyzed within 30 minutes. Hemolysis, delays, or poor handling can cause spurious results. While conventional lab testing is cumbersome, newer point-of-care analyzers have improved the feasibility and accuracy of in-clinic testing.

TOTAL SERUM BILIRUBIN

Bilirubin is produced during red blood cell breakdown and circulates bound to albumin. In the liver, it is conjugated and excreted into bile. Hyperbilirubinemia can arise from hemolysis, hepatocellular dysfunction, or biliary obstruction.

In liver disease, hyperbilirubinemia reflects impaired uptake, conjugation, or excretion, referred to as intrahepatic cholestasis. However, significant liver dysfunction must be present for bilirubin to rise, making it an insensitive marker of early disease. Measuring conjugated versus unconjugated bilirubin is not generally clinically helpful in dogs or cats, although a predominance of unconjugated bilirubin may be seen in cases of sepsis (Odunayo et al. 2010).

COAGULATION PROTEINS

The liver synthesizes most coagulation factors and also contributes to vitamin K metabolism. Reduced hepatic function may alter coagulation parameters, though these changes are neither sensitive nor specific. Changes may include prolonged prothrombin time (PT) or activated partial thromboplastin time (aPTT), and reduced levels of fibrinogen, protein C, or vitamin K-dependent proteins.

CONCLUSIONS AND CLINICAL RELEVANCE

While routine biochemical tests offer some insight into liver function, they lack sensitivity and specificity. More informative functional assessments include TSBAs and, to a lesser extent, ammonia, bilirubin, and coagulation parameters. TSBAs remain the most practical and reliable functional test for both dogs and cats, provided that sample handling and interpretation consider physiological and pathological variables.

REFERENCES

Center, S.A. (2007). Interpretation of liver enzymes. *Veterinary Clinics of North America: Small Animal Practice* 37 (2): 297–333. https://doi.org/10.1016/j.cvsm.2006.09.006.

Center, S.A., Warner, K.L., Corbin, J.E. et al. (2012). Evaluation of 270 dogs with clinical hepatobiliary disease: retrospective study from 1983 to 1998. *Journal of Veterinary Internal Medicine* 26 (4): 844–854. https://doi.org/10.1111/j.1939-1676.2012.00944.x.

Gagne, J.M., Weiss, D.J., Armstrong, P.J. et al. (1999). Acute phase protein concentration and hepatic function in dogs with chronic hepatitis. *Journal of Veterinary Internal Medicine* 13 (6): 606–609. https://doi.org/10.1111/j.1939-1676.1999.tb01482.

Johnson, S.E., Center, S.A., McDonough, S.P. et al. (1995). Resting and postprandial serum bile acid concentrations in dogs with liver disease. *Journal of the American Veterinary Medical Association* 207 (4): 456–460.

Odunayo, A., Tobias, K.M., and Sharp, C.R. (2010). Hyperbilirubinemia in critically ill dogs: prevalence, causes and diagnostic approach. *Journal of Veterinary Emergency and Critical Care* 20 (6): 576–585. https://doi.org/10.1111/j.1476-4431.2010.00596.

Pena-Ramos, J., Barker, L., Saiz, R. et al. (2021). Resting and postprandial serum bile acid concentrations in dogs with liver disease. *Journal of Veterinary Internal Medicine* 35 (3): 1333–1341. https://doi.org/10.1111/jvim.16134.

Simpson, K.W. (2004). Bacterial flora of the gastrointestinal tract. *The Veterinary Clinics of North America. Small Animal Practice* 34 (2): 341–355. https://doi.org/10.1016/j.cvsm.2003.10.003.

Stockham, S.L. and Scott, M.A. (2020). *Fundamentals of Veterinary Clinical Pathology*, 3e. Ames, IA: Wiley-Blackwell.

Webster, C.R.L., Center, S.A., Cullen, J.M. et al. (2019). ACVIM consensus statement on the diagnosis and treatment of chronic hepatitis in dogs. *Journal of Veterinary Internal Medicine* 33 (4): 1173–1200. https://doi.org/10.1111/jvim.15475.

CHAPTER 2

Diagnostic Imaging of the Hepatobiliary System

Angela Marolf

Department of Veterinary Clinical Sciences, College of Veterinary Medicine, The Ohio State University, Columbus, OH, USA

KEY POINTS

- Ultrasound is a common first-line imaging modality to evaluate the liver and biliary tract in dogs and cats.
- The use of intravenous contrast with computed tomography (CT) and magnetic resonance (MR) provides additional information that can aid in distinguishing different disease processes.
- For CT and MR, the lack of superimposition of adjacent stomach and bowel gas as well as decreased operator dependence of these imaging modalities leads to more accurate assessments of the cranial abdomen.

INTRODUCTION

Ultrasound has been utilized in dogs and cats for evaluation of liver and biliary abnormalities for many years in veterinary medicine. Abdominal ultrasound is readily available and can be performed on awake or sedated patients. Ultrasound imaging is very sensitive at identifying liver and biliary abnormalities but often lacks specificity, and cytology or histology are required for definitive diagnosis.

Computed Tomography (CT) and Magnetic Resonance (MR) imaging are becoming more available for diagnosis of abdominal diseases in dogs and cats. The ability to image veterinary patients without superimposition of other organs or bowel gas as well as to perform a complete assessment of the biliary tree and liver offer distinct advantages. Both CT and MR imaging utilize intravenous contrast to better evaluate the blood flow to organs and adjacent tissues with CT imaging utilizing iodinated contrast agents and MR imaging utilizing gadolinium contrast agents.

NORMAL ULTRASOUND OF THE LIVER AND BILIARY SYSTEM

On ultrasound imaging, the normal liver parenchyma is of medium echogenicity and is hypoechoic compared to the spleen and falciform fat. Internally, the liver has hyperechoic portal veins that have bright walls and help differentiate the liver from other parenchymal organs. The gallbladder is ovoid in shape and located between the right medial and quadrate liver lobes. Normal thickness for the gallbladder wall is less than 1 mm in cats and less than 2 mm in dogs (Hittmair et al. 2001; Kealy et al. 2011). Bilobed gallbladders are a normal variant in cats (Spain et al. 2022). The normal intrahepatic biliary tract in not visible on ultrasound. The normal extrahepatic common bile duct may not be identified; when identified, it should be less than 4 mm in diameter for cats and less than 3 mm in diameter for dogs (Leveille et al. 1996; Mattoon and Nyland 2015). The common bile duct empties into the duodenum through the major duodenal papilla for both dogs and cats.

Disorders of the Liver, Exocrine Pancreas, and Gastrointestinal Tract in Dogs and Cats, First Edition. Edited by Harry Cridge et al. Published 2026 by John Wiley & Sons, Inc. Companion Website: www.wiley.com/go/cridge/disorders

MR AND CT OF THE NORMAL LIVER AND BILIARY SYSTEM

On MR imaging, the normal liver is uniformly hypointense relative to the spleen on T1 and T2 weighted sequences with homogeneous contrast enhancement of the parenchyma. The gallbladder and common bile duct are homogenously hyperintense on T2 weighted images and hypointense on T1 weighted images.

On CT imaging, the normal liver is isoattenuating to the spleen with uniformly contrast enhancing parenchyma and a hypoattenuating gallbladder due to storage of bile. Normal size for the common bile duct in dogs based on weight has been established ranging from approximately 2–3.5 mm at the mid-level of the duct (Kim et al. 2023). To specifically evaluate the hepatic arteries, hepatic and portal veins, CT angiography, which is a timed bolus of intravenous contrast followed by multiple specifically timed scans to capture the arterial, venous, and delayed phases of contrast passage through an organ (three phase angiogram), must be performed (Caceres et al. 2006; Makara et al. 2015). CT angiography is typically performed via installed software that determines timing of the phases based on the contrast medium bolus tracer placed over the aorta at a specific site for best effect. Arterial phase images are acquired first followed by venous phase and delayed phase (acquired approximately 1.5–2 minutes after contrast injection). This technique can be especially advantageous in evaluating the vascular system in dogs with suspected portosystemic shunts (Zwingenberger 2009).

ABNORMAL CONDITIONS OF THE LIVER AND BILIARY SYSTEM

NEOPLASIA OF THE LIVER AND BILIARY TRACT

Primary liver and gallbladder neoplasia is relatively uncommon in dogs and cats; metastatic liver nodules and masses from other organ neoplasia are more common (Strombeck 1978). In cats, bile duct adenoma/cystadenoma and bile duct carcinoma/cystadenocarcinoma are more common than in dogs (Lawrence et al. 1994). Ultrasound is usually performed for initial imaging of the liver and biliary tract; however, there is overlap in the appearance of different neoplastic, benign, and inflammatory processes (Feeney et al. 2008). With ultrasound imaging, focal masses, nodules, or parenchymal echogenicity changes can be identified; however, these are usually non-specific to tumor type.

Further characterization of liver masses, staging, and surgical planning are reasons to perform cross-sectional imaging with either CT or MR for suspected liver masses based on abdominal ultrasound. CT can provide further information regarding involvement of the portal vein and other vasculatures relative to the tumor and assist with surgical approach based on origin of the mass. Size, shape, and margination of masses and nodules should be noted; however, these characteristics cannot definitively differentiate tumor types. Several studies in dogs have looked at the CT characteristics of liver masses with hepatocellular carcinoma having central and marginal enhancement in the arterial phase and becoming hypoattenuating in the delayed phase. Nodular hyperplasia often has diffuse enhancement in the arterial phase and is isoattenuating to normal liver parenchyma in the delayed phase (Fukushima et al. 2012; Kutara et al. 2014).

MR imaging of the liver and liver masses has also been performed in dogs and cats. MR imaging of hepatic lesions utilizing standard gadolinium contrast has shown good sensitivity and specificity for differentiating malignant from benign lesions (Clifford et al. 2004). Newer MR contrast agents which target the hepatobiliary system have been evaluated in dogs and have shown increased conspicuity of liver metastatic lesions (Yonetomi et al. 2012) (Figure 2.1).

INFLAMMATION OF THE LIVER AND BILIARY TRACT

Inflammation of the biliary tract or gallbladder is more common in cats than in dogs. This may be due to the unique ductal anatomy of cats in which the common bile duct and pancreatic duct both open onto the major duodenal papilla (Smallwood 1993). One of the challenges with ultrasound is the overlap in sonographic changes that can occur with different disease processes; histology is still recommended for definitive diagnosis (Warren-Smith et al. 2012; Kemp et al. 2013).

Acute or chronic forms of hepatitis/cholangitis as well as cholecystitis and hepatic abscesses can be identified. With all imaging modalities, liver size, margination, and parenchymal changes can be used to assess the liver. In chronic forms of hepatitis/cholangitis, the liver may be small, irregularly marginated, and have a heterogeneous parenchyma. With acute hepatitis/cholangitis, the liver may be of normal size or enlarged and have a normal or abnormal parenchymal appearance. Biliary tract and gallbladder inflammation may manifest as thickening of the gallbladder wall, gallbladder intraluminal contents such as debris or cholelithiasis, and/or dilation of the biliary tract. Changes in hepatic parenchymal echogenicity or contrast enhancement along with enhancement of the gallbladder wall may be identified with CT or MR imaging (Figure 2.2a, b).

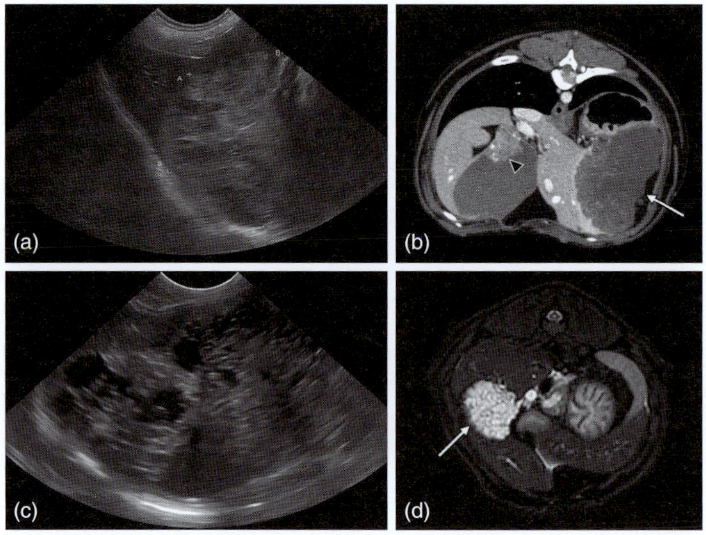

FIGURE 2.1 (a) Sagittal plane ultrasound image of a dog with a mixed echoic left liver mass (within calipers). (b) Transverse CT image venous phase of the same dog with a liver and gallbladder mass. Note the minimal contrast enhancement in the hypoattenuating liver mass (arrow) and strong enhancement in the gallbladder mass (arrowhead). Gallbladder mass was biopsied and diagnosed as a benign polyp and the liver mass was a carcinoma. (c) Transverse ultrasound image of biliary cystadenoma with multiple internal fluid regions. (d) Transverse T2-weighted MR image of same cat with a biliary cystadenoma. Note the bright mass (arrow) on T2-weighted imaging, indicative of fluid-filled masses

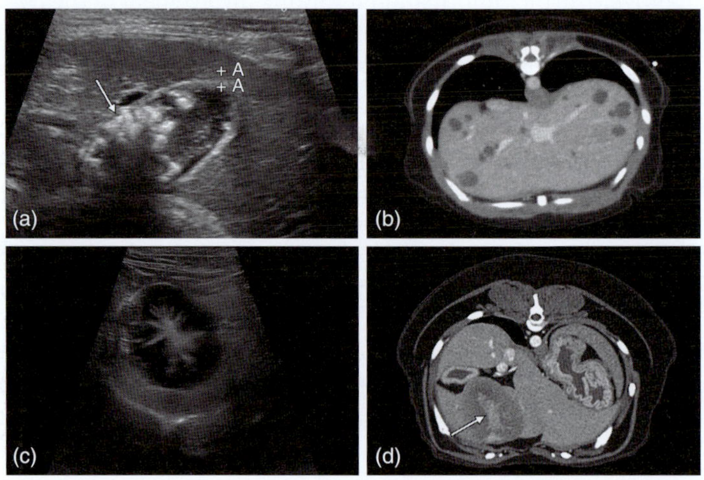

FIGURE 2.2 (a) Oblique ultrasound image of a cat with cholelithiasis and cholecystitis. Note the thickened gallbladder wall (calipers) and hyperechoic calculi with shadowing (arrow). (b) Transverse CT image venous phase of a dog with neutrophilic cholangitis. Note the multiple hypoattenuating nodules in the liver (cystic changes). (c) Transverse ultrasound image of a gallbladder mucocele. Note the classic kiwi pattern of the intraluminal contents. (d) CT image of the same gallbladder mucocele. Note the central mineralization (arrows)

A unique MR sequence named MR cholangiography (MRCP) highlights fluid within the biliary tract and pancreatic ducts to diagnose intra- and extra-hepatic biliary tract inflammation or obstruction (Vitellas et al. 2000). In normal dogs and in post-mortem studies, MRCP has been studied and deemed feasible (Rahmani et al. 2024; Heo et al. 2012). MR has been used to assess liver, biliary and pancreatic inflammation in cats (Marolf et al. 2013). Generally, ultrasound should be utilized as a first line diagnostic imaging examination. MRI is more helpful in diagnosing pancreatitis than cholangitis in cats and should be reserved for more complicated cases.

GALLBLADDER MUCOCELES

In addition to intraluminal debris and cholelithiasis, gallbladder mucoceles are another intraluminal gallbladder disease. Gallbladder mucoceles often have recognizable sonographic features including a stellate or kiwi like pattern (Choi et al. 2014; Besso et al. 2000). With CT imaging, gallbladder mucoceles are characterized by central mineralization and increased CT attenuation values (Fuerst and Hostnik 2019) (Figure 2.2c, d).

EXTRAHEPATIC BILIARY OBSTRUCTION

With ultrasound, CT, and MR imaging, the extrahepatic portion of the common bile duct can be evaluated for evidence of obstruction and dilation. Causes can include surrounding organ neoplasia, pancreatitis, and cholelithiasis. Cholelithiasis and choledocholithiasis are readily identified with ultrasound, CT, and MR imaging. Common bile duct dilation greater than 5 mm has been associated with obstruction in cats (Leveille et al. 1996). Evaluation of the duodenal papilla for masses, thickening, or distal calculi is important (Figure 2.3a, b).

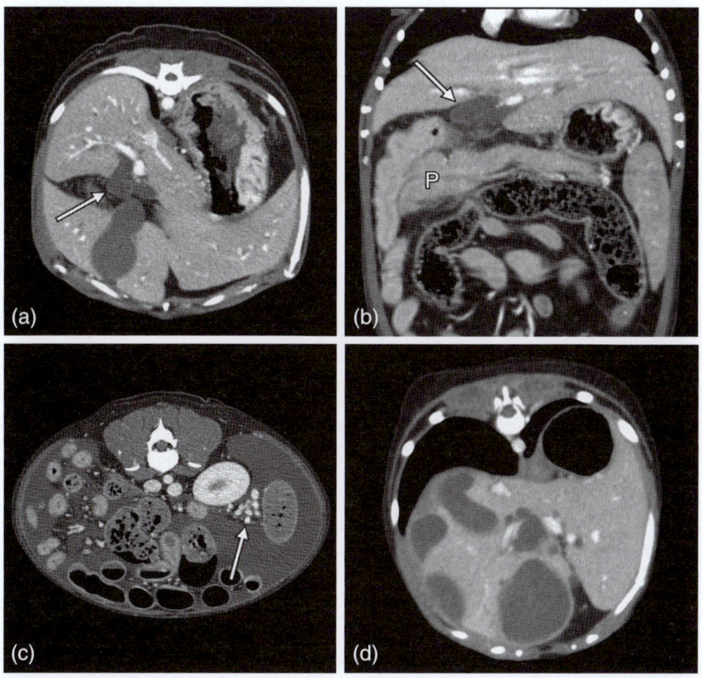

FIGURE 2.3 (a) Transverse CT image in venous phase of a dog showing extrahepatic biliary obstruction. This dog had acute pancreatitis. Note the dilated common bile duct (arrow). (b) Dorsal CT image in venous phase of same dog. Note the dilated common bile duct (arrow) and enlarged pancreas (P) indicative of pancreatitis. (c) Transverse CT image venous phase of a dog with multiple acquired shunts adjacent to left kidney (arrow) with a large amount of peritoneal fluid consistent with portal hypertension. (d) Transverse CT image venous phase of a dog with Caroli's disease. Note the multiple dilated biliary tracts and cystic changes in the liver

VASCULAR AND DUCTAL PLATE ANOMALIES

Portosystemic shunts are a group of congenital or acquired diseases that can result in abnormal shunting of blood. Portosystemic shunts are grouped into intrahepatic, extrahepatic, and acquired forms and arterioportal fistulae. Ductal plate anomalies are a congenital group of diseases that can cause dilation of the biliary tract and include biliary cystadenomas, Caroli's disease or syndrome, and congenital hepatic fibrosis (Lawrence et al. 1994; Watson 2017; King et al. 2023). Ultrasound can be utilized in the diagnosis of these conditions; however, CT (three phase angiography) is ideal for making these diagnoses and identifying portal hypertension, including acquired shunts and varices, portal vein thrombosis, and free fluid, if present (Zwingenberger 2009; Brancatelli et al. 2005) (Figure 2.3c, d).

SUMMARY

Ultrasound, MR, and CT imaging are often utilized in the diagnosis of hepatobiliary disorders in dogs and cats. CT and MR imaging provide additional information for dogs and cats with hepatobiliary diseases due to lack of superimposition of structures, operator dependence, and through intravenous contrast administration. Diagnostic imaging can assist clinicians by aiding diagnosis, prognostication, and surgical planning.

REFERENCES

Besso, J.G., Wrigley, R., Gliatto, J. et al. (2000). Ultrasonographic appearance and clinical findings in 14 dogs with gallbladder mucocele. *Veterinary Radiology & Ultrasound* 41 (3): 261–271.

Brancatelli, G., Federle, M., Vilgrain, V. et al. (2005). Fibropolycystic liver disease: CT and MR imaging findings. *Radiographics* 2 (3): 659–670.

Caceres, A.V., Zwingenberger, A., Hardam, E. et al. (2006). Helical computed tomographic angiography of the normal canine pancreas. *Veterinary Radiology & Ultrasound* 47 (3): 270–278.

Choi, J., Kim, A., Keh, S. et al. (2014). Comparison between ultrasonographic and clinical findings in 43 dogs with gallbladder mucoceles. *Veterinary Radiology & Ultrasound* 55 (2): 202–207.

Clifford, C.A., Pretorius, E., Weisse, C. et al. (2004). Magnetic resonance imaging of focal splenic and hepatic lesions in the dog. *Journal of Veterinary Internal Medicine* 18 (3): 330–338.

Feeney, D.A., Anderson, K., Ziegler, L. et al. (2008). Statistical relevance of ultrasonographic criteria in the assessment of diffuse liver disease in dogs and cats. *American Journal of Veterinary Research* 69 (2): 212–221.

Fuerst, J.A. and Hostnik, E.T. (2019). CT attenuation values and mineral distribution can be sued to differentiate dogs with and without gallbladder mucoceles. *Veterinary Radiology & Ultrasound* 60 (6): 689–695.

Fukushima, K., Kanemoto, H., Ohno, K. et al. (2012). CT characteristics of primary hepatic mass lesions in dogs. *Veterinary Radiology & Ultrasound* 53 (3): 252–257.

Heo, J., Constable, P., Naughton, J. (2012). Dynamic secretin-enhanced magnetic resonance cholangiopancreatography and pancreatic ultrasonography in normal dogs. *Veterinary Radiology and Ultrasound*. 53 (6): 681.

Hittmair, K.M., Vielgrader, J., and Loupal, G. (2001). Ultrasonographic evaluation of gallbladder wall thickness in cats. *Veterinary Radiology & Ultrasound* 42 (2): 149–155.

Kealy, J.K., McAllister, H., Graham, J.P. (eds.) (2011). *Diagnostic Radiology and Ultrasonography of the Dog and Cat*, 5e, 49. St. Louis: Saunders.

Kemp, S.D., Panciera, D., Larson, M. et al. (2013). A comparison of hepatic sonographic features and histopathologic diagnosis in canine liver disease: 138 cases. *Journal of Veterinary Internal Medicine* 27 (4): 806–813.

Kim, Y., Kim, S., Kwon, D. et al. (2023). Computed tomographic quantitative evaluation of common bile duct size in normal dogs: a reference range study considering body weight. *Frontiers in Veterinary Science* 10. https://doi.org/10.3389/fvets.2023.1137400.

King, E.M., Pappano, M., Lorbach, S. et al. (2023). Severe polycystic liver disease in a cat. *Journal of Feline Medicine and Surgery Open Reports* 9 (2): 20551169231216859. https://doi.org/10.1177/20551169231216859.

Kutara, K., Seki, M., Ishikawa, C. et al. (2014). Triple-phase helical computed tomography in dogs with hepatic masses. *Veterinary Radiology & Ultrasound* 55 (1): 7–15.

Lawrence, H.J., Erb, H.N., and Harvey, H.J. (1994). Nonlymphomatous hepatobiliary masses in cats: 41 cases (1972 to 1991). *Veterinary Surgery* 23 (5): 365–368.

Leveille, R., Biller, D., and Shiroma, J. (1996). Sonographic evaluation of the common bile duct in cats. *Journal of Veterinary Internal Medicine* 10 (5): 296–299.

Makara, M., Chau, J., Hall, E., et al. (2015). Effects of two contrast injection protocols on feline aortic and hepatic enhancement using dynamic computed tomography. *Veterinary Radiology & Ultrasound* 56 (4): 367–373.

Marolf, A.J., Kraft, S., Dunphy, T. et al. (2013). Magnetic resonance (MR) imaging and MR cholangiopancreatography findings in cats with cholangitis and pancreatitis. *Journal of Feline Medicine and Surgery* 15 (4): 285–294.

Mattoon, J.S. and Nyland, T.G. (eds.) (2015). *Small Animal Diagnostic Ultrasound*, 3e, 332–399. St. Louis: Elsevier.

Rahmani, V., Peltonen, J., Hmelnikov, D. et al. (2024). Three-dimensional magnetic resonance cholangiography is superior to two-dimensional single-shot magnetic resonance cholangiography for visualization and image quality of the feline and canine biliary tract: a postmortem study. *Veterinary Radiology & Ultrasound* 54 (4): 377–384.

Smallwood, J.E. (1993). Atlas of feline anatomy for veterinarians. In: *Digestive System* (ed. L. Hudson and W. Hamilton), 166–167. Philadelphia: Saunders, W.B.

Spain, H.N., Penninkc, D., Thelen, M., et al. (2022). Ultrasonographic prevalence and proposed morphologic classification of bilobed gallbladder in cats. *Journal of Feline Medicine and Surgery* 24 (10): 986–993.

Strombeck, D.R. (1978). Clinicopathologic features of primary and metastatic neoplastic disease of theliver in dogs. *Journal of the American Veterinary Medical Association* 173 (3): 267–269.

Vitellas, K.M., Keogan, M.T., and Freed, K.S. (2000). Radiologic manifestations of sclerosing cholangitis with emphasis on MR cholangiopancreatography. *Radiographics* 20: 959–975.

Warren-Smith, C.M., Andrew, S., Mantis, P. et al. (2012). Lack of associations between ultrasonographic appearance of parenchymal lesions of the canine liver and histological diagnosis. *Journal of Small Animal Practice* 53 (3): 168–173.

Watson, P. (2017). Canine breed-specific hepatopathies. *Veterinary Clinics: Small Animal Practice* 47 (3): 665–682.

Yonetomi, D., Kadosawa, T., Miyoshi, K. et al. (2012). Contrast agent Gd-EOB-DTPA (EOB.Primovist®) for low-field magnetic resonance imaging of canine focal liver lesions. *Veterinary Radiology & Ultrasound* 53 (4): 371–380.

Zwingenberger, A. (2009). CT diagnosis of portosystemic shunts. *The Veterinary Clinics of North America. Small Animal Practice* 39 (4): 783–792.

CHAPTER 3 Hepatic Cytology

Shannon D. Dehghanpir

Department of Veterinary Clinical Sciences, Veterinary Clinical Pathology, School of Veterinary Medicine, Louisiana State University, Baton Rouge, LA, USA

KEY POINTS

- Hepatic cytology is a useful diagnostic tool to guide clinical decision-making.
- Certain diseases of the liver – including several non-hepatobiliary neoplasms, poorly differentiated hepatocellular carcinomas, various infections, hepatic lipidosis, and amyloidosis – can be definitively diagnosed using cytopathology.
- While histopathologic assessment of the liver is required for disease distribution and grading of inflammation, copper accumulation, and fibrosis, the presence of these changes can be documented using cytopathology to facilitate case management.

INTRODUCTION

Fine-needle sampling of the liver is often performed to investigate abnormal biochemical or ultrasonographic findings and stage cancer. While the diagnostic accuracy of hepatic cytology ranges between 30.3 and 80% (Wang et al. 2004; Roth 2001), there are several abnormalities and definitive diagnoses that can be ascertained by the competent cytopathologist. As instructions for sample acquisition and cytologic descriptions of common abnormalities of hepatic cytology are detailed extensively elsewhere (Amy and Rick 2019), this chapter will focus on indications for performing hepatic cytology and report interpretation.

INDICATIONS AND LIMITATIONS

Sampling of the liver for cytologic evaluation is indicated when there are persistent, unexplainable hepatobiliary biochemical abnormalities (e.g., persistent increase in ALT activity), hepatic imaging abnormalities (e.g., hepatomegaly, focal or disseminated nodules, heterogeneous echotexture), or cancer staging. In some instances, such as staging of mast cell neoplasm or lymphoma, the liver should be sampled regardless of imaging findings, as it may appear ultrasonographically unremarkable with metastatic disease (Book et al. 2011; Crabtree et al. 2010). The major limitation of hepatic cytology is the inability to assess lobular architecture, and therefore, portal tracts and disease distribution (Cullen 2009). However, some specific diagnoses or preliminary information that would guide case management can be gained with hepatic cytology. While post-sampling hepatic hemorrhage is a complication to consider, there are conflicting reports in the literature regarding the use of platelet concentration and blood clotting times to assess bleeding risk (Reece et al. 2020).

Disorders of the Liver, Exocrine Pancreas, and Gastrointestinal Tract in Dogs and Cats, First Edition. Edited by Harry Cridge et al. Published 2026 by John Wiley & Sons, Inc. Companion Website: www.wiley.com/go/cridge/disorders

SAMPLE SUBMISSION

Prior to submission to a cytopathologist, it is recommended to stain at least one smear with a rapid aqueous Romanowsky stain (e.g., Diff-Quik) to confirm adequate sample cellularity and preservation. A diagnostic hepatic cytology smear usually contains numerous hepatocytes that are easily observed on low-power evaluation (i.e., 10× objective). Well-differentiated hepatocytes are arranged in organized cohesive clusters and exhibit mild-to-moderate anisokaryosis, occasional binucleation, and low to moderate nuclear: cytoplasmic ratios. They have round central nuclei with coarse chromatin, 1–3 small round nucleoli, and moderate to abundant amounts of amphophilic textured cytoplasm with blue-green lipofuscin granules and possible vacuoles (Figure 3.1a). Smears of low diagnostic quality often exhibit marked blood contamination with few to no hepatocytes, while smears with poor cellular preservation may contain mostly ruptured cells or abundant necrosis. If poor cellularity or preservation is noted upon screening a quick-stained smear, the quality of the remaining smears should be assessed, and resampling should occur if necessary.

A thorough but pertinent patient history on the specimen submission form is essential and should include an overview of clinical signs and the indication for fine-needle sampling of the liver. Clinicopathologic abnormalities, such as liver enzyme activities, should be reported as the specific numerical result, rather than vague descriptors such as "increased." The ultrasonographic, laparoscopic, or gross (surgical) appearance of the liver with distribution of disease should also be provided. If multiple areas of the liver were sampled, the smears should be labeled separately, with the sites clearly stated on the submission form (e.g., hepatic nodule and ultrasonographically unremarkable hepatic parenchyma). Finally, inclusion of previous cytopathologic and/or histopathologic results and information on whether a concurrent tissue biopsy sample was collected is helpful.

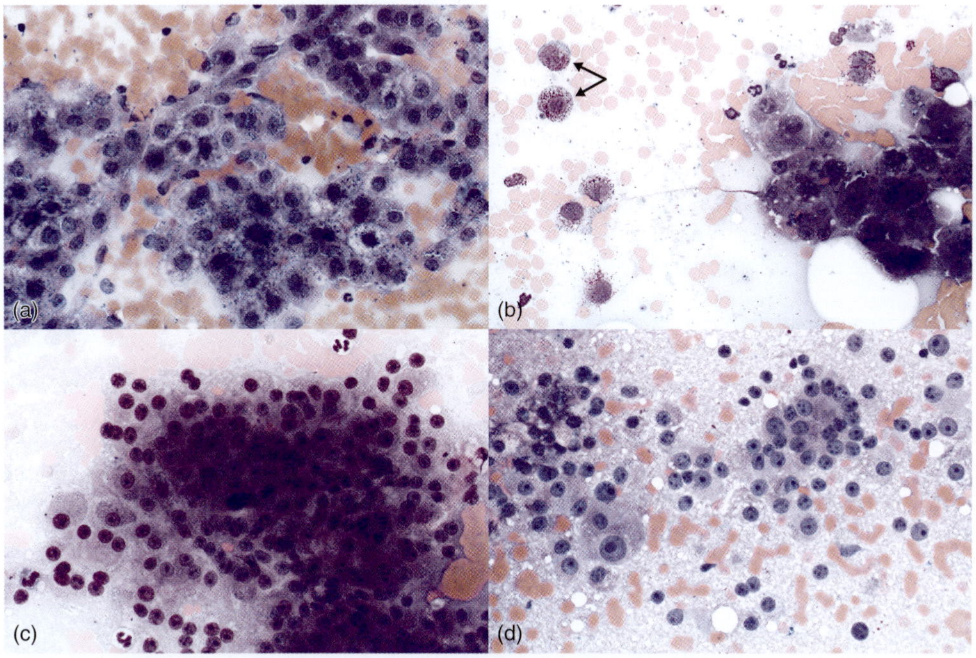

FIGURE 3.1 Photomicrographs of canine hepatic aspirate smears, detailing: (a) well-differentiated hepatocytes. (b) Metastatic mast cell neoplasm (arrows). (c) Well-differentiated hepatocellular neoplasm. (d) Poorly differentiated hepatocellular carcinoma (Wright Giemsa)

HEPATOBILIARY NEOPLASIA

Several primary and metastatic lesions within the liver can be readily cytologically diagnosed with varying degrees of confidence, presuming that they are exfoliative. Common metastatic or non-hepatobiliary neoplasms that can be definitively cytopathologically diagnosed include intermediate-to-large cell lymphoma, mast cell neoplasm (Figure 3.1b), sarcoma (e.g., histiocytic sarcoma, hemangiosarcoma), carcinoma (e.g., exocrine pancreatic adenocarcinoma), and many others (Bahr et al. 2013). The reported sensitivities for these neoplasms are relatively high (Bahr et al. 2013); therefore, a cytologic diagnosis can be trusted if a definitive interpretation is provided by the cytopathologist.

Well-differentiated primary hepatobiliary neoplasms, including well-differentiated hepatocellular and cholangiocellular neoplasms, can be challenging to cytologically diagnose and differentiate into adenoma or carcinoma. The reported diagnostic accuracy of the cytologic diagnosis of hepatocellular carcinoma ranges from 18.9 to 65.6% (Moyer et al. 2021; Cray et al. 2023; Suarez-Rodriguez et al. 2023). This wide range can be attributed to the subtle cytomorphologic changes observed in well-differentiated hepatocellular carcinoma as well as the presumption that hepatocellular carcinomas have been histopathologically overdiagnosed (Cullen 2016). The cytopathologic findings of well-differentiated hepatocellular neoplasms include hepatocytes with minimal nuclear atypia, decreased lipofuscin pigment, and crowded clustering, as well as the presence of increased capillaries, fibrosis, and necrosis (Figure 3.1c) (Cullen 2016; Masserdotti and Drigo 2012). As the false negative rate is moderately high (Suarez-Rodriguez et al. 2023), histopathology and correlation with clinical and imaging findings are recommended when a cytology report states concern for a well-differentiated hepatocellular carcinoma. In contrast, poorly differentiated hepatocellular carcinomas can be diagnosed with more confidence, as these hepatocytes have marked nuclear atypia and pleomorphism (Figure 3.1d).

Cholangiocellular neoplasms arise from the biliary epithelium and are often intrahepatic, cystic lesions (Cullen 2009). Biliary epithelial cells are cuboidal to columnar in shape with minimal nuclear atypia and high nuclear: cytoplasmic ratios, while cystic fluid appears pale basophilic with occasional macrophages. As cholangiocellular neoplasms are often intrahepatic, well-differentiated hepatocytes may also be present on aspirate smears from these lesions. The differentiation between biliary cyst, cholangiocellular adenoma, and well-differentiated cholangiocarcinoma is a diagnostic challenge cytologically. Imaging to screen for other cystic lesions (e.g., renal cysts in cats) or metastatic disease as well as histopathology are recommended to follow up a cytologic diagnosis of a cystic biliary lesion.

While primary hepatic neuroendocrine neoplasms of the liver exist, they are rare (Patnaik et al. 2005). A cytologic interpretation of neuroendocrine neoplasm within the liver should be presumed metastatic (e.g., insulinoma). The origin of neuroendocrine neoplasms often cannot be determined cytologically. Clinical and biochemical abnormalities (e.g., hypoglycemia) as well as other imaging findings are used to prioritize the diagnosis of the primary neoplasm.

NODULAR HYPERPLASIA AND REGENERATION

Nodular hyperplasia is a proliferative lesion of hepatocytes that is common in older dogs. Cytologically, the hepatocytes appear well-differentiated with or without cytoplasmic vacuolation. These nodules cannot be reliably differentiated from hepatocellular adenoma even with histopathology, as normal lobular architecture is retained (Cullen 2016). Serial ultrasonographic monitoring of nodule size or histopathology is recommended when nodular hyperplasia is suspected on cytologic aspirate smears.

In contrast, regenerative nodules occur secondarily to chronic hepatic injury in dogs without an age correlation. On histopathology, there is loss of lobular architecture and presence of fibrosis, along with possible other changes like inflammation (Cullen 2016). While regenerative hepatocytes often have increased nuclear atypia (moderate anisokaryosis, multinucleation), nuclear: cytoplasmic ratios, and cytoplasmic basophilia on cytology smears, they may also sometimes appear cytologically unremarkable. Additionally, the cytologic documentation of the associated findings of inflammation and fibrosis has inherent challenges. Thus, histopathology is recommended when a cytologic diagnosis of regenerative nodule is proposed.

INFLAMMATION

Hepatic cytology has low diagnostic sensitivity for the documentation of inflammation (Wang et al. 2004; Roth 2001; Bahr et al. 2013), particularly in diseases with mild severity or patchy distribution of inflammation. Hepatic aspirate smears also have significant blood contamination, with contribution of blood neutrophils or lymphocytes that may confound interpretation if neutrophilia or lymphocytosis is present. However, the number, type, and arrangement of inflammatory cells within hepatic cytology samples can aid in diagnosis. A more confident cytologic diagnosis can be made when infectious organisms are identified. Ultimately, histopathology may be needed to determine the distribution (e.g., centrilobular, periportal) and severity of inflammatory diseases, as well as the cause.

Neutrophilic inflammation is diagnosed when degenerate or non-degenerate neutrophils are increased in number, arranged in aggregates adjacent to hepatocytes, or embedded within the hepatocyte clusters (Figure 3.2a). Observation of numerous degenerate neutrophils warrants screening for intracellular bacteria (e.g., as observed with hepatic abscess). Otherwise, neutrophilic inflammation may be secondary to hepatocellular necrosis (e.g., as observed with hypoxia or toxic insult) or with neutrophilic cholangitis/cholangiohepatitis (Amy and Rick 2019; Cullen 2009).

Lymphoplasmacytic inflammation is diagnosed when there are increased numbers of small lymphocytes and plasma cells in close association with the hepatocytes; this pattern of inflammation may occur in isolation or along with neutrophils and macrophages. In cats, chronic cholangitis/cholangiohepatitis is the primary differential (Cullen 2009). If abundant small lymphocytes are present, then small cell lymphoma should be excluded via histopathology or molecular diagnostics (e.g., PARR) (Cullen 2009).

The presence of epithelioid macrophages along with small lymphocytes, plasma cells, and possibly neutrophils warrants a diagnosis of granulomatous to pyogranulomatous inflammation, which is often secondary to infectious disease. Careful screening for bacteria (e.g., *Mycobacterium* spp.), fungi (e.g., hyalohyphomycosis), oomycetes, algae (e.g., *Prototheca* spp.), flukes (e.g., *Heterobilharzia americana*), protozoa (e.g., *Toxoplasma gondii*), and cestodes (e.g., *Echinococcus* spp.) is recommended. In cats, this pattern of hepatic inflammation may be observed secondary to feline infectious peritonitis (FIP) (Amy and Rick 2019).

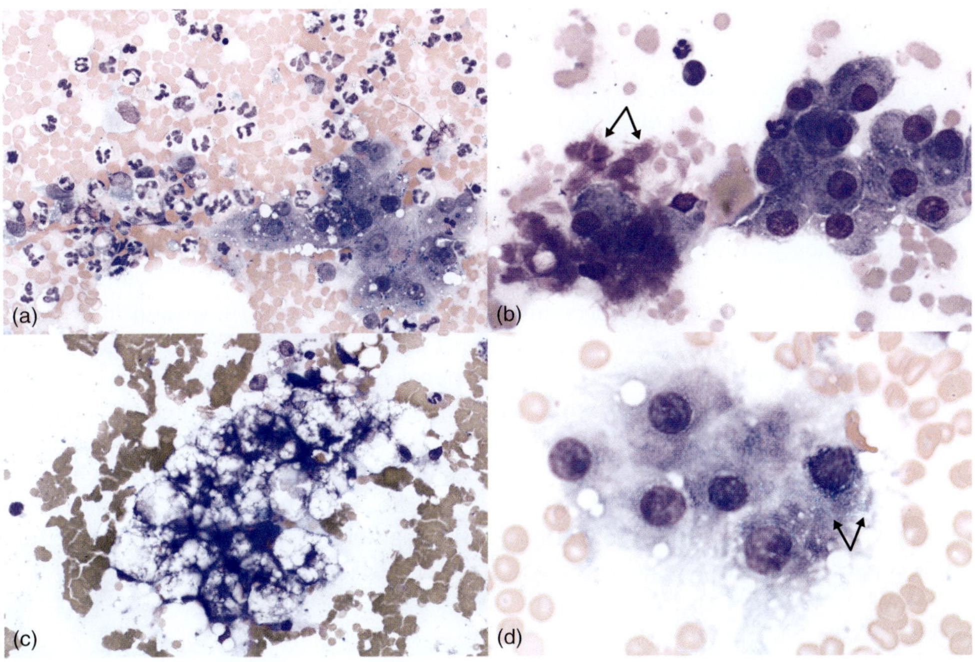

FIGURE 3.2 Photomicrographs of canine (a, d) and feline (b, c) hepatic aspirate smears, detailing: (a) neutrophilic inflammation, (b) amyloidosis (arrows), (c) hepatic lipidosis, and (d) copper (arrows) accumulation (Wright Giemsa)

FIBROSIS

Hepatic fibrosis is a secondary change, often from chronic inflammation, which requires histopathologic assessment of lobular distribution for diagnosis and grading. The cytologic diagnosis of fibrosis is suspected when increased numbers of fibroblasts (often admixed with eosinophilic matrix), mast cells, and/or eosinophils occur in close association with hepatocytes (Masserdotti and Bertazzolo 2016). When hepatic fibrosis is suspected cytologically, histopathology is recommended for confirmation and grading.

AMYLOIDOSIS

Reactive or familial amyloidosis is the pathologic accumulation of serum amyloid A protein in various organs, including the liver. Amyloid deposition most often occurs secondary to chronic antigenic stimulation. Familial amyloidosis is observed in Chinese Shar Pei dogs as well as Abyssinian, Siamese, and Oriental cats. Amyloid appears cytologically as fibrillar eosinophilic material that is present either extracellularly, associated with hepatocyte clusters, or intracellularly within macrophages (Figure 3.2b). This material can be readily diagnosed on cytology and confirmed with Congo red cytochemical staining of stained or unstained aspirate smears (Amy and Rick 2019).

METABOLIC DISEASE

Hepatocellular vacuolation is often a nonspecific finding secondary to metabolic disease or cellular injury. Cytoplasmic vacuolation of hepatocytes can be subdivided into indistinct rarefied vacuoles or discrete lipid vacuoles. Hepatocellular rarefaction is common in dogs and occurs secondary to glycogen accumulation or water accumulation. The latter is termed "hydropic degeneration" and is a nonspecific sign of hepatocellular injury. Dogs with increased endogenous or exogenous glucocorticoids will also develop hepatocellular rarefaction due to the accumulation of glycogen. Cytology cannot differentiate between glycogen and water accumulation within hepatocytes, and diagnosis of hepatocellular rarefaction outside of clinical and biochemical evidence of hyperadrenocorticism or glucocorticoid therapy is considered a nonspecific finding.

Discrete lipid vacuolation most often occurs secondary to triglyceride accumulation in states of excess lipid mobilization (e.g., diabetes mellitus); however, this change may also be observed with nonspecific liver injury. A cytologic diagnosis of feline hepatic lipidosis can be made when >80% of hepatocytes are markedly discretely vacuolated (Figure 3.2c) (Center 2005). The cytopathologist should screen for secondary causes of hepatic lipidosis, including evidence of inflammation or neoplasia (particularly lymphoma) within the hepatic aspirate smears.

Copper is a trace mineral that may accumulate in the hepatocytes of dogs and rarely cats. Certain breeds of dog have a higher risk of developing excessive hepatic copper accumulation, and dietary intake is also presumed to play a role. While copper pigment granules can appear cytologically as faint seafoam green inclusions within the hepatocyte cytoplasm, its presence is often missed with routine staining (Figure 3.2d) (Moore et al. 2019). Application of a cytochemical stain for copper (e.g., rhodanine) to aspirate smears can be used to confirm its presence within hepatocytes (Moore et al. 2019). When a cytologic report suspects hepatocellular copper accumulation, confirmation with cytochemical staining and ultimately histopathology to assess distribution, grade, and severity of copper deposition is recommended.

Hemosiderosis is the excessive accumulation of iron pigment secondary to increased iron turnover or decreased iron utilization. Disease conditions associated with hepatic hemosiderosis include hemolytic anemia, precursor-targeted immune-mediated anemia, recent blood transfusion, chronic inflammation, or iron-containing/erythropoiesis-stimulating therapeutics (Amy and Rick 2019). Hemosiderin appears as blue-green, pale-blue, or golden pigment granules, which can be confused for lipofuscin and possibly copper. Cytochemical staining for iron (e.g., Prussian blue) on aspirate smears can be used to confirm its presence.

SUMMARY

Fine-needle sampling of the liver is a practical and minimally invasive tool for the diagnosis of hepatobiliary disorders. While the major limitation to hepatic cytology is the inability to assess lobular architecture, certain diseases can be definitively diagnosed or preliminary information can be obtained that will guide case management.

REFERENCES

Amy, C.V. and Rick, L.C. (2019). *Cowell and Tyler's Diagnostic Cytology and Hematology of the Dog and Cat - E-Book*, 5th ed. Philadelphia: Mosby.

Bahr, K.L., Sharkey, L.C., Murakami, T. et al. (2013). Accuracy of US-guided FNA of focal liver lesions in dogs: 140 cases (2005–2008). *Journal of the American Animal Hospital Association* 49: 190–196.

Book, A.P., Fidel, J., Wills, T. et al. (2011). Correlation of ultrasound findings, liver and spleen cytology, and prognosis in the clinical staging of high metastatic risk canine mast cell tumors. *Veterinary Radiology & Ultrasound* 52: 548–554.

Center, S.A. (2005). Feline hepatic lipidosis. *Veterinary Clinics: Small Animal Practice* 35: 225–269.

Crabtree, A.C., Spangler, E., Beard, D. et al. (2010). Diagnostic accuracy of gray-scale ultrasonography for the detection of hepatic and splenic lymphoma in dogs. *Veterinary Radiology & Ultrasound* 51: 661–664.

Cray, M., Hokamp, J., Abrams, B. et al. (2023). Clinical utility of cytology from preoperative percutaneous fine needle aspirates of solitary liver masses in 220 dogs: a retrospective study (2009–2019). *Journal of the American Animal Hospital Association* 59: 12–19.

Cullen, J.M. (2009). Summary of the World Small Animal Veterinary Association standardization committee guide to classification of liver disease in dogs and cats. *The Veterinary Clinics of North America. Small Animal Practice* 39: 395–418.

Cullen, J.M. (2016). Tumors of the Liver and Gallbladder. In: *Tumors in Domestic Animals* (ed. D.J. Meuten), 602–631. John Wiley & Sons.

Masserdotti, C. and Bertazzolo, W. (2016). Cytologic features of hepatic fibrosis in dogs: a retrospective study on 22 cases. *Veterinary Clinical Pathology* 45: 361–367.

Masserdotti, C. and Drigo, M. (2012). Retrospective study of cytologic features of well-differentiated hepatocellular carcinoma in dogs. *Veterinary Clinical Pathology* 41: 382–390.

Moore, A.R., Medrano, E., Coffey, E. et al. (2019). Clinicopathological correlation and prevalence of increased copper in canine hepatic cytology. *Journal of the American Animal Hospital Association* 55: 8–13.

Moyer, J., Lopez, D.J., Balkman, C.E. et al. (2021). Factors associated with survival in dogs with a histopathological diagnosis of hepatocellular carcinoma: 94 cases (2007–2018). *Open Veterinary Journal* 11: 144–153.

Roth, L. (2001). Comparison of liver cytology and biopsy diagnoses in dogs and cats: 56 cases. *Veterinary Clinical Pathology* 30: 35–38.

Suarez-Rodriguez, J.I., Liu, C.C., Dehghanpir, S. et al. (2023). Lymphopenia predicts reduced survival in canine hepatocellular carcinoma. *Journal of Veterinary Science* 24: e36.

Wang, K.Y., Panciera, D.L., Al-Rukibat, R.K. et al. (2004). Accuracy of ultrasound-guided fine-needle aspiration of the liver and cytologic findings in dogs and cats: 97 cases (1990–2000). *Journal of the American Veterinary Medical Association* 224: 75–78.

CHAPTER 4 Histopathology of the Liver

Rebecca Smedley

Veterinary Diagnostic Laboratory, Michigan State University, Lansing, MI, USA

KEY POINTS

- Communication between the clinician and pathologist before and after biopsy is the key.
- Every liver biopsy should be stained with Hematoxylin and Eosin (HE) in addition to a number of special stains and/or immunohistochemical markers based on the HE findings.
  - Copper staining should be performed in most canine cases.
  - Staining for fibrous connective tissue is important in many cases.
  - Reticulin staining is helpful for identifying subtle structural changes.
- Hepatic biopsy interpretation should include a scored/graded evaluation of type and degree of inflammation/degeneration, fibrosis/nodularity, and location and degree of copper accumulation.
- Feline lymphocytic portal infiltrates can be difficult to classify as inflammatory or lymphoma, and final interpretation must take into account histopathologic findings, results of immunophenotyping, and polymerase chain reaction (PCR) results (Sebastian et al. 2023).

INTRODUCTION

Histopathologic evaluation of the liver is a crucial tool for the diagnosis of liver diseases that is often underutilized. A team approach that includes communication among clinicians and pathologists will ensure the best results for diagnosis and patient management. The clinician should not hesitate to call the pathologist to discuss a case before sample submission or after the report is received. Verbal discussions are often more informative than interpretations of a submitted history form or a received biopsy report.

This chapter will discuss recommendations for liver sampling, normal hepatic histology, trimming of liver biopsy specimens; histopathologic evaluation of special stains, immunohistochemical (IHC) markers, and sample quality; and histopathologic lesions of some common liver diseases.

RECOMMENDATIONS FOR LIVER SAMPLING

- Ideally, a minimum of three laparoscopic or surgical biopsy specimens from at least two liver lobes should be obtained for histopathology and placed in formalin (see below). The diagnostic accuracy of liver biopsies increases with the size of the biopsy specimens and the number of lobes sampled. Peripheral wedge biopsies should be 1–2 cm deep to account for changes caused by capsular fibrosis at the edge. If punch biopsy samples are taken, they should be obtained from the center rather than the edge of the lobe, as the periphery of the lobe may be affected by fibrosis. In addition, if indicated, obtain one fresh sample for aerobic and anaerobic culture and one fresh sample for quantitative copper analysis.

Disorders of the Liver, Exocrine Pancreas, and Gastrointestinal Tract in Dogs and Cats, First Edition. Edited by Harry Cridge et al. Published 2026 by John Wiley & Sons, Inc. Companion Website: www.wiley.com/go/cridge/disorders

  - For histopathology samples, if there are gross differences in the areas sampled, submit each in a different container labeled with the location.
- If laparoscopic or surgically obtained biopsies are not possible, needle biopsies, Tru-Cut or Menghini, can be performed.
  - Obtain at least five samples for histopathology, one for bacterial culture if indicated (can be a very small one or a portion of a needle biopsy), and at least two for mineral analysis (see below).
  - Medium- and large-sized dogs → use a 14G needle.
  - Smaller dogs and cats → use a 16G needle.
  - Needle biopsy specimens should be at least 1 cm long, but ideally 2 cm, to ensure adequate sampling depth.
  - If the samples obtained are not ideal, submit anyway.
- If there is a focal lesion, sample from the periphery and the center.
- Be careful not to crush samples with forceps.
- Do not set specimens on paper, cloth, or tongue depressors.
- Needle biopsies should be placed in mesh cassettes to prevent fragmentation; non-compressive sponges can be used in the cassettes if they do not compress or perforate the biopsy specimens.
- If a liver lobectomy is performed to remove a mass, submit the entire lobe. Inking the surgical margin is very helpful before placing the lobe in formalin. To help the fixative penetrate the specimen, slices can be made throughout the lobe as long as they are **NOT** made through a surgical margin and the lobe is kept intact.
- Place samples for histopathology into **10% neutral buffered formalin immediately at a ratio of 10:1 formalin to tissue**; make sure the container is filled completely with formalin to decrease stirring which can lead to fragmentation; ideally, samples should be less than 1 cm to ensure adequate fixation.
- If mineral analysis is desired (e.g., concern for copper associated hepatopathy):
  - Sample the most normal-appearing areas to avoid regions of fibrosis and nodular regeneration.
  - Submit liver biopsy(ies) in an empty metal-free and rubber-free glass or plastic tube (rubber can cause zinc contamination); microcentrifuge tubes work well.
  - A minimum mass of 50 mg is recommended for mineral analysis.
    - Approximate wet tissue masses collected from selected surgical biopsy instruments are:
      - Stryker Double Action Biopsy Clamp (5.0 mm diameter): 100–200 mg.
      - Acu Punch (6 mm): 90–180 mg (dependent on depth of punch).
      - TruCut (14G): 20–25 mg (This is the amount collected if the notch in the instrument is full. Thus, two samples are required for optimal sample size, if the notch is full, more if it is only partially full). Note: when ultrasound-guided needle biopsies are submitted directly for mineral analysis, they may contain other tissues such as skeletal muscle, which can result in a falsely low copper value. Fibrotic or regenerative areas can also result in low copper values.
  - Refrigerate or freeze sample until shipment. Ship with a cold pack.
  - Note: mineral analysis can be performed on fresh, formalin-fixed, or formalin-fixed paraffin embedded samples by some laboratories (check with the laboratory to see which sample type is preferred).

- **Note: mineral analysis should always be performed in conjunction with assessment/grading of copper staining on histopathology samples.**

- If bacterial infection is of concern, submit one liver sample in a red top tube with 0.5 ml of sterile saline for culture. The specimen should be kept moist but not saturated. Bile can also be collected in a red top tube for culture. Culture swabs may be submitted as well. Refrigerate the sample until shipment. Ship the specimen that day with a cold pack for overnight delivery.
- Clearly label all samples and submit together with a submittal form that includes a thorough, but relevant, history including clinicopathologic and gross findings and where the samples were taken.

NORMAL HEPATIC HISTOLOGY

The main components of the liver are the hepatocytes, sinusoids, portal tracts, and central (terminal) hepatic veins. These components form hexagon-shaped lobules with the central vein at the center and multiple portal tracts at the periphery. Alternatively, the arrangement has been described as having an acinar shape with the portal arterioles and veins radiating from the portal tract and forming the center of the acinus while the central veins are at the periphery of the acinus. The three main components of portal tracts, also called portal triads, are bile ducts, hepatic arteries, and portal veins, which are all supported by collagenous connective tissue (Figure 4.1d). Additionally, lymphatic vessels and small nerves are present in portal tracts. In dogs, central veins have a smooth muscle wall that is not present in cats (Figure 4.1c).

Hepatocytes are arranged in cords/plates that are usually one cell thick. Hepatic cords radiate out from central veins in a regular pattern (Figure 4.1a–c). Further away from the central veins, they lose their radiating pattern and are not quite as organized (Figure 4.1d). The hepatocytes furthest away from the central veins abut the limiting plate of the portal tract, which separates the hepatocytes from the stroma of the portal tract. The zone of hepatic cords around the central veins is called the centrilobular area (acinar zone 3), the zone around the portal tracts is called the periportal area (acinar zone 1), and the zone in between these regions is called the midzonal area (acinar zone 2) (Figure 4.1b).

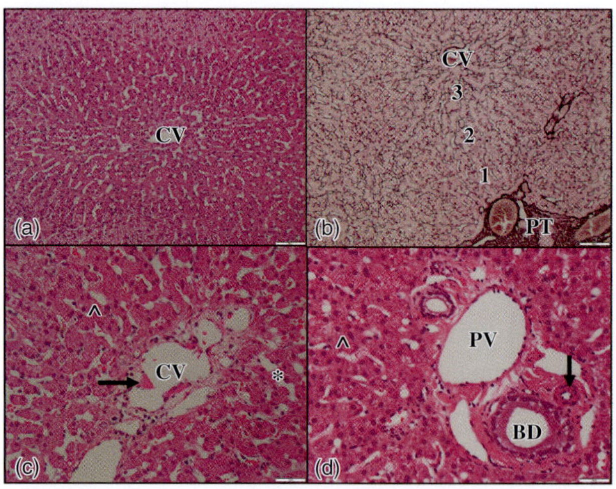

FIGURE 4.1 Normal liver from a dog. (a) The central vein (CV) is in the center with radiating cords of hepatocytes extending away from it. Hematoxylin and eosin (HE). (b) Black reticulin fibers highlight the radiating pattern of the hepatic cords extending away from the CV. There is a portal tract (PT) in the lower right corner. Reticulin. (c) In dogs there is smooth muscle (horizontal arrow) in the wall of the CV. Hepatocytes (^) arranged in cords radiate out from the central vein and are separated by sinusoids (*). HE. (d) PTs contain a portal vein (PV), bile ducts (BD), and arterioles (vertical arrow). Hepatocytes (^) are arranged in slightly less regular cords around the PT

Sinusoids are between the hepatic cords, are lined by fenestrated endothelium, and contain circulating red blood cells (Figure 4.1c). A reticulin support network is also present between hepatic cords and can be visualized with a reticulin stain, such as Gordon and Sweet, that highlights the radiating nature of the cord architecture (Figure 4.1b). Kupffer cells are resident hepatic macrophages that extend to the lumen of the sinusoids. When they are not active, they are very small with scant to no apparent cytoplasm and small round hyperchromatic nuclei, resembling small lymphocytes. When active, they are plump and may contain brown to yellow pigment.

The space of Disse is between the sinusoids and the hepatocytes and cannot be visualized microscopically in biopsy specimens unless it is abnormally distended by some material, such as amyloid. In postmortem samples it may be seen artifactually, as sinusoidal endothelium appears to separate from the hepatocytes. Ito cells, also referred to as hepatic stellate cells or fat storing cells, are present in the space of Disse. They usually appear as single cells with a large cytoplasmic lipid vacuole.

Bile canaliculi are narrow channels in between secretory hepatocytes that are sealed off by tight junctions between adjacent hepatocytes. They cannot be visualized microscopically unless they are abnormally distended with bile due to cholestasis. Bile canaliculi in portal areas drain into cholangioles/terminal ductules referred to as canals of Hering, which are lined by ductal epithelial cells (cholangiocytes) and hepatocytes. These ductules extend through the limiting plate of small portal tracts and join to form interlobular bile ducts lined by cuboidal epithelium. The interlobular ducts unite to form larger intrahepatic bile ducts lined by tall columnar epithelium and basally located nuclei. These larger intrahepatic bile ducts join to form the main hepatic ducts that finally unite to form the common bile duct. The common bile duct empties into the duodenum at Vater's papilla (major duodenal papilla). The gall bladder communicates with the main hepatic ducts and the common bile duct via the cystic duct (Rothuizen et al. 2006).

The surface of the liver is covered by a capsule, known as Glisson's capsule. There are mesothelial cells along the surface that are only visible microscopically when they are reactive due to some type of pathology in the abdominal cavity (e.g., free fluid, peritonitis, adjacent pancreatitis, etc.)

TRIMMING OF LIVER BIOPSIES

If the samples submitted in formalin are small, particularly needle biopsies, they should be completely embedded for histologic evaluation. Punch biopsies may be bisected and completely embedded, or half may be embedded and the other half retained for the possibility of mineral analysis or special staining (e.g., Oil red O for lipid). This latter method ensures that the area evaluated histologically is very close to the area submitted for mineral analysis, which should improve correlation between copper staining and mineral analysis results. For entire liver lobes submitted for mass evaluation, 2–3 representative sections through the mass, including the center and the edge, one section from the mass to the margin, and tangential sections taken through the proximal surgical margin, should be evaluated so that accurate margin evaluation is possible. The pathologist should state in the biopsy report how the specimens were trimmed. Some laboratories provide gross images of the received specimen that are annotated to indicate where the sections were taken (Figure 4.2).

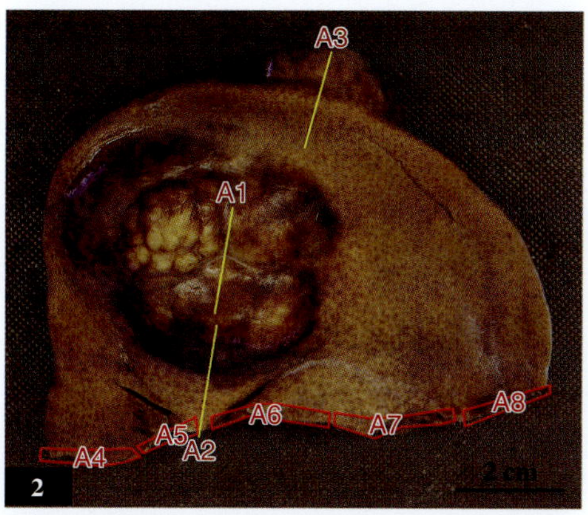

FIGURE 4.2 Annotated image of trimming of a combined hepatocellular carcinoma and cholangiocellular carcinoma (hepatocholangiocellular carcinoma) in a dog. The yellow sections (A1–A3) are representative sections through the two masses and section A2 extends from the mass to the surgical margin, allowing for a numeric margin to be provided. The red sections (A4–A8) represent tangential sections taken through the surgical margin

HISTOPATHOLOGIC EVALUATION

STAINING AND IMMUNOHISTOCHEMISTRY

Biopsy samples are routinely stained with HE. Many diseases/lesions can be identified with this staining technique, but additional stains are often necessary for better assessment of lobular architecture and degree of fibrosis, identifying pigments such as copper and iron, screening for vascular anomalies and ductal plate malformations, and differentiating neoplasms. There are many different types of stains that can be used for these purposes, but only the most common ones are briefly described in Table 4.1. Most special stains and IHC markers can be performed on formalin-fixed paraffin embedded tissues. An example of a section of liver stained with a rhodanine stain for copper is shown in Figure 4.3.

IHC markers are helpful in cases of suspected vascular anomalies or ductal plate malformations, for differentiating between different neoplastic processes, and for detecting certain types of infectious agents. Labeling for CD31 helps to identify increases in the number of small arterioles within portal tracts or between hepatic cords. Labeling for cytokeratin (CK) 19 or CK7 is useful for identifying bile ductule proliferation. While CK19 and CK7 are not specific for biliary epithelium, they can be used to differentiate between a cholangiocarcinoma, a hepatocholangiocellular carcinoma, and a poorly differentiated hepatocellular carcinoma (HCC). HepPar-1 is a marker that is used to confirm hepatocellular origin of a neoplasm. Some IHC markers may be used to attempt to

Table 4.1 Common Special Stains Used for Liver Biopsies

Substance detected	Examples of stains	Use
Reticulin fibers	e.g., Gordon and Sweet stain; automated options	Assess cord architecture, identify areas of lobular collapse or atrophy (increased density of staining) and areas of hepatocellular proliferation (decreased density of staining)
Fibrosis	e.g., Masson's trichrome	Detect fibrosis and allow for grading
Copper	e.g., Rhodanine, rubeanic acid	Identifies copper in hepatocytes, Kupffer cells, and macrophages, and allows for grading
Iron (hemosiderin)	e.g., Perl's stain, Prussian blue	Detects iron in hepatocytes, Kupffer cells, and macrophages
Glycogen	Periodic acid-Schiff (PAS) and PAS with diastase	If glycogen is not washed-out during processing it will stain pink with PAS and will be digested with PAS with diastase so that it will not stain; helps to confirm steroid hepatopathy
Lipid	e.g., Oil red O, Sudan IV	Stains lipid but can only be performed on fresh frozen or formalin-fixed tissues that are NOT paraffin-embedded
Amyloid	e.g., Congo red	Stains amyloid that can be found in the space of Disse in cases of amyloidosis
Bile	e.g., Hall's bilirubin stain	Stains bile in canaliculi or bile ducts
Infectious agents	e.g., PAS, Grocott–Gömöri's methenamine silver (GMS), acid-fast bacteria, gram	PAS and GMS can detect fungal organisms; Acid-fast stain detects acid-fast bacteria; Gram identifies bacteria as gram + or gram –

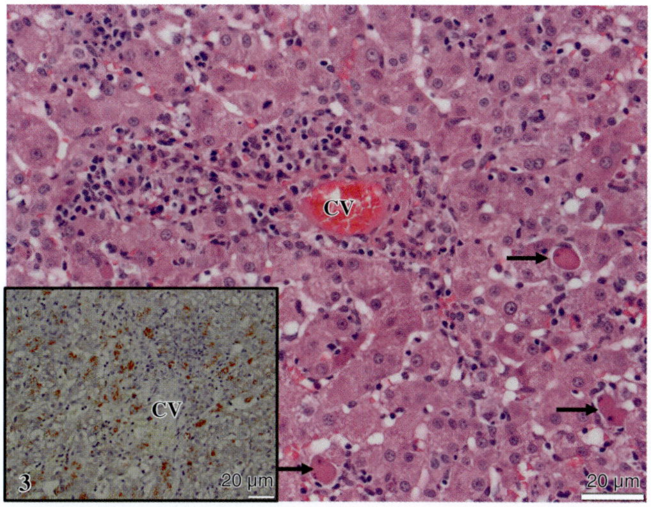

FIGURE 4.3 Liver from a dog with chronic copper associated hepatitis. The central vein (CV) is surrounded by a mixed inflammatory cell infiltrate and there are scattered acidophil bodies (arrows) characterized by hypereosinophilic cytoplasm and pyknotic nuclei. (HE). Inset: Centrilobular copper accumulation stains dark orange with a rhodanine stain

predict prognosis of HCCs (e.g., CK19, HepPar-1, arginase-1, P-glycoprotein, pSTAT3) but may not be available at all diagnostic laboratories (Kim et al. 2021; Shin et al. 2024; van Sprundel et al. 2010). Several other markers can be used to diagnose suspected metastatic neoplasms in the liver.

SAMPLE QUALITY

Sample quality is greatest when surgically obtained liver biopsies are submitted because it is easier for surgeons to identify any gross lesions; the specimens are larger, contain more portal tracts and central veins, and are less likely to fragment upon processing; and because more tissue is available for special stains and mineral analysis. Larger specimens significantly improve the likelihood of an accurate diagnosis, but they must be weighed against the clinical challenges, risks, and costs of surgery versus laparoscopic or ultrasound guided liver biopsies. For needle biopsies, the pathologist should indicate in the report whether or not the sample is considered to be a diagnostic sample. Ideally, 12–15 portal triads should be present in histologic sections for the specimens to be considered diagnostic samples (Webster et al. 2019). However, one reference found that if the needle biopsy specimens contain at least 3–12 portal triads, histopathologic interpretation in the dog is unlikely to vary (Kemp et al. 2015). Also, liver samples from dogs with vacuolar hepatopathy are more likely to fragment, making it more difficult to obtain a diagnostic sample via needle biopsy. Clinicians should be aware of the lower diagnostic accuracy of these types of biopsies.

HISTOPATHOLOGIC LESIONS OF COMMON LIVER DISEASES

Hepatic lesions can be grouped into parenchymal disorders, biliary tract disorders, vascular disorders, and neoplastic diseases. Types of hepatocellular degeneration are described in Table 4.2. Common grading schemes for histologic hepatic lesions are provided in Tables 4.3 and 4.4. For a more detailed and comprehensive description of hepatic histopathologic lesions in dogs and cats the reader is referred to Rothuizen et al. (2006).

Table 4.2 Three Types of Hepatocellular Vacuolar Degeneration

Type of vacuolar degeneration	Cause(s)	Substance that accumulates	Histologic findings
Hydropic degeneration	Inability of cells to maintain ionic and fluid balance due to cell membrane damage from ischemia, cholestasis, or toxins	Excess water, Na+, glucose	None detectable; if mild (need EM); if more severe hepatocytes are markedly swollen and cytoplasm has thin wispy pale eosinophilic strands or indiscrete clear vacuoles; nuclei is usually not displaced; ballooning degeneration in severe cases can lead to cell death
Glycogen-type degeneration	Secondary to exogenous steroid administration or excessive endogenous steroid production (hyperadrenocorticism) either pituitary-dependent or due to adrenocortical tumors	Excess glycogen	Indistinguishable from hydropic degeneration above; may start midzonally and extend to periportal hepatocytes or be random and patchy; graded on a scale of 0–3 (see Table 4.3); hypersegmented neutrophils in sinusoids are often present due to the effect of cortisol; extramedullary hematopoiesis (EMH) may be present; PAS stains glycogen bright pink (when glycogen is not washed out during processing) and PAS with diastase digests the glycogen resulting in clear staining hepatocytes
Lipidosis (aka steatosis, fatty liver, and fatty change)	Five potential causes: Excessive transport of fatty acids into liver from dietary intake or from mobilization of triglycerides from adipose tissue (starvation, diabetes mellitus); Abnormal hepatocyte function with decreased energy for oxidation of fatty acids (hypoxia) or toxic damage to mitochondria (e.g., tetracycline); Increased esterification of fatty acids to triglycerides in response to increased amounts of glucose and insulin (hyperadrenocorticism); Decreased apoprotein synthesis (dietary deficiency, hepatotoxins, and toxic drugs); Impaired secretion of lipoproteins from liver caused by secretory defects (hepatotoxins and toxic drugs)	Triglycerides (triacylglycerol)	Clear discrete intracytoplasmic vacuoles in hepatocyte differentiates lipidosis from hydropic or glycogen-type degeneration; may be small (microvesicular) or large (macrovesicular) vacuoles or both; need to differentiate macrovesicular lipid accumulation from Ito cells; Oil red O or Sudan IV stains can be performed on frozen unfixed or formalin-fixed, non-paraffin-embedded liver to identify the lipid

EM: electron microscopy.

Table 4.3 Grading Scales for Liver Biopsies

Category	Grade 0	Grade 1	Grade 2	Grade 3	Grade 4
Steroid hepatopathy	Absent	Mild = solitary hepatocytes or few small groups of hepatocytes with ballooning	Moderate = multiple groups of hepatocytes or moderate sized areas of hepatocytes with ballooning	Marked = extensive presence or diffuse ballooning of hepatocytes	—
Interface hepatitis (piecemeal necrosis)	Absent	Focal alteration of periportal plate in some portal tracts	Diffuse alteration of periportal plate in some portal tracts or focal lesions around all portal tracts	Diffuse alteration of periportal plate in all portal tracts	—
Centrilobular inflammation	Absent	Presence of mononuclear aggregates in some centrilobular areas	Mononuclear aggregates in all centrilobular areas	Large and dense mononuclear aggregates in all centrilobular areas	—
Lobular necrosis	Less than one necro-inflammatory focus per lobule	At least one necro-inflammatory focus per lobule	Several necro-inflammatory foci per lobule or confluent or bridging necrosis	—	—
Portal inflammation	Absent	Presence of mononuclear aggregates in some portal tracts	Mononuclear aggregates in all portal tracts	Large and dense mononuclear aggregates in all portal tracts	—
Fibrosis	Absent	Portal fibrosis without septae	Portal fibrosis with rare septae	Numerous septae without cirrhosis	Cirrhosis
Activity score	PMN0+LN0=A0	PMN0+LN1=A1	PMN0+LN2=A2	PMN3+LN1=A3	
		PMN1+LN0=A1	PMN1+LN2=A2	PMN3+LN1=A3	
		PMN1+LN1=A1	PMN2+LN0=A2	PMN3+LN2=A3	
			PMN2+LN1=A2		

Source: Adapted from Bedossa and Poynard (1996); Ishak (2000); Raghu et al. (2018).

Table 4.4 Qualitative Copper Scores

Grade 0	Copper not detected, care taken to avoid confusing lipofuscin or hemosiderin with copper granules
Grade 1	Variable copper granules in an occasional hepatocyte (<2 hepatocytes/10× field)
Grade 2	Obvious small to moderate numbers of copper granules in <50% of zone 3 hepatocytes (or <4 clusters/10× field)
Grade 3	All lobules contain groups of hepatocytes (>50% but <75%) predominantly in zone 3 with moderate to large numbers of copper granules); Macrophages with copper granules may also be present
Grade 4	Most (>75%) zone 3 hepatocytes contain moderate to large numbers of copper granules; Macrophages with copper granules may also be present.
Grade 5	Panlobular presence of large numbers of copper granules in hepatocytes, usually associated with copper-containing macrophages; Tissue remodeling may obscure lobular zones

Source: Center et al. (2013)/American Veterinary Medical Association.

REFERENCES

Bedossa, P. and Poynard, T. (1996). An algorithm for the grading of activity in chronic hepatitis C. The METAVIR Cooperative Study Group. *Hepatology* 24 (2): 289–293. https://doi.org/10.1002/hep.510240201.

Center, S.A., McDonough, S.P., and Bogdanovic, L. (2013). Digital image analysis of rhodanine-stained liver biopsy specimens for calculation of hepatic copper concentrations in dogs. *American Journal of Veterinary Research* 74 (12): 1474–1480. https://doi.org/10.2460/ajvr.74.12.1474.

Ishak, K.G. (2000). Pathologic features of chronic hepatitis. A review and update. *American Journal of Clinical Pathology* 113 (1): 40–55. https://doi.org/10.1309/42D6-W7PL-FX0A-LBXF.

Kemp, S.D., Zimmerman, K.L., Panciera, D.L. et al. (2015). A comparison of liver sampling techniques in dogs. *Journal of Veterinary Internal Medicine* 29 (1): 51–57. https://doi.org/10.1111/jvim.12508.

Kim, S.H., Seung, B.J., Cho, S.H. et al. (2021). Arginase-1 and P-glycoprotein are downregulated in canine hepatocellular carcinoma. *Journal of Veterinary Science* 22 (5): e61. https://doi.org/10.4142/jvs.2021.22.e61.

Raghu, C., Ekena, J., Cullen, J.M. et al. (2018). Evaluation of potential serum biomarkers of hepatic fibrosis and necroinflammatory activity in dogs with liver disease. *Journal of Veterinary Internal Medicine* 32 (3): 1009–1018. https://doi.org/10.1111/jvim.15064.

Rothuizen, J., Bunch, S.E., Charles, J.A. et al. (eds.) (2006). *Standards for Clinical and Histological Diagnosis of Canine and Feline Liver Diseases. WSAVA Liver Standardization Group*, 15–39. Philadelphia, PA: Saunders Elsevier.

Sebastian, K., Smedley, R.C., Bartel, A. et al. (2023). Patterns of lymphocytic infiltrates can differentiate feline hepatic lymphoma from lymphocytic portal hepatitis. *Veterinary Sciences* 10 (2): 127. https://doi.org/10.3390/vetsci10020127.

Shin, H.K., Chung, H.J., and Kim, W.H. (2024). Overactivation of signal transducer and activator of transcription 3 in canine hepatocellular carcinoma and its prognostic significance. *Veterinary and Comparative Oncology* 22 (4): 490–499. https://doi.org/10.1111/vco.12998.

van Sprundel, R.G., van den Ingh, T.S., Desmet, V.J. et al. (2010). Keratin 19 marks poor differentiation and a more aggressive behaviour in canine and human hepatocellular tumours. *Comparative Hepatology* 9 (1): 4. https://doi.org/10.1186/1476-5926-9-4.

Webster, C.R.L., Center, S.A., Cullen, J.M. et al. (2019). ACVIM consensus statement on the diagnosis and treatment of chronic hepatitis in dogs. *Journal of Veterinary Internal Medicine* 33 (3): 1173–1200. https://doi.org/10.1111/jvim.15467.

Other Liver Diagnostic Tests

CHAPTER 5

Agostino Buono

Department of Veterinary Clinical Sciences, School of Veterinary Medicine, Louisiana State University, Baton Rouge, LA, USA

KEY POINTS

- Patients with hepatobiliary disease may be hypo- and/ or hypercoagulable.
- Risk of bleeding should be assessed prior to performing invasive procedures. A minimum coagulation database includes platelet count, PT/aPTT, and fibrinogen concentration.
- While coagulation tests can help clinicians assess the risk of hemorrhage prior to invasive procedures, no single test consistently predicts bleeding complications in cats and dogs with hepatobiliary disease.
- Protein C activity is a valuable biomarker to differentiate between macroscopic portovascular anomalies and hepatic microvascular anomalies, or to assess portosystemic shunt ligation when compared to a baseline value.

COAGULATION TESTING

Coagulation abnormalities are prevalent in dogs and cats with liver disease, impacting up to 82% of cats and 57% of dogs (Prins et al. 2010; Lisciandro et al. 1998). The liver synthesizes the majority of the coagulation, anticoagulation, and fibrinolysis factors (Webster 2017). Cats and dogs have a "rebalanced hemostasis" that is more fragile than that of healthy animals, and if disrupted, it can result in either thrombosis or bleeding (Lisman et al. 2021). While spontaneous bleeding is uncommon in clinically stable animals with hepatobiliary disease, the risk of bleeding increases with invasive procedures (e.g., liver biopsy). Therefore, assessing bleeding risks is necessary before fine-needle aspirates and liver biopsies. Coagulation testing assesses primary and secondary hemostasis as well as fibrinolysis.

PRIMARY HEMOSTASIS

Testing begins with a platelet count. What constitutes a safe platelet count varies among internists; the author recommends that greater than 60 000 platelets is a minimum value for invasive diagnostics. When platelet count is within the normal reference interval, platelet function testing is also a consideration. In breeds predisposed to von Willebrand Disease (e.g., Type I: Bernese Mountain dogs, Doberman Pinscher, Irish Setters, Poodles, West Highland white terriers; Type II: German Wirehaired Pointers, Shorthaired Pointers; Type III: Scottish terriers, Shetland Sheepdogs, Chesapeake Bay retrievers), von Willebrand factor (vWF) activity should also be assessed before elective procedures. If vWF concentration is subnormal, cryoprecipitate or fresh frozen plasma can be preemptively administered to reduce the risk of bleeding during procedures. A buccal mucosal bleeding time (BMBT) can be performed in the clinic to assess qualitative platelet disorders (i.e., thrombocytopathia or vWF deficiency). In normal patients, a clot is formed within 4–5 minutes. In academic settings, platelet function may also be measured by platelet aggregometry (e.g., platelet function analyzers, multiplate platelet aggregometry) (Kalbantner et al. 2011; Wilkinson et al. 2022; Shropshire et al. 2022).

Disorders of the Liver, Exocrine Pancreas, and Gastrointestinal Tract in Dogs and Cats, First Edition. Edited by Harry Cridge et al. Published 2026 by John Wiley & Sons, Inc. Companion Website: www.wiley.com/go/cridge/disorders

SECONDARY HEMOSTASIS

PROTHROMBIN TIME AND ACTIVATED PARTIAL THROMBOPLASTIN TIME

Secondary hemostasis is evaluated by measuring prothrombin time (PT), activated partial thromboplastin time (aPTT), and fibrinogen. If these are within normal limits or less than 1.5× the upper limit of normal (ULN), an invasive procedure can be performed without preemptive administration of clotting factors. PT and aPTT are widely used; they reflect the functions of the extrinsic (factor VII) and intrinsic (factors VIII, IX, XI, and XII) coagulation pathways, respectively, in addition to the common pathway (factors II, V, and X). Many point-of-care assays can rapidly measure PT and aPTT (Hyatt and Brainard 2016), which is useful especially in emergency situations. However, these assays have variable sensitivity and specificity when compared to reference laboratory assays, which remain the gold standard. Results from different analyzers should not be used interchangeably.

FIBRINOGEN/FDPs

Patients with liver disease may exhibit hypofibrinolysis or hyperfibrinolysis, which can lead to thrombosis or consumptive coagulopathy, respectively. To assess the fibrinolytic system in dogs and cats, available tests include fibrinogen, fibrin degradation products (FDPs), and a specific type of FDP, D-dimers. In small animals with hepatic disease, D-dimer concentrations can be high due to impaired hepatic clearance of FDPs and enhanced fibrinolysis caused by an impaired synthesis of fibrinolysis inhibitors and delayed clearance of tissue plasminogen activation, rather than being secondary to increased fibrin formation.

VISCOELASTIC TESTING

There are two main laboratory viscoelastic tests available, thromboelastography (TEG) and rotational thromboelastometry (ROTEM). Although the results from these two methodologies cannot be directly interchanged (Wikkelsø et al. 2016), both are whole-blood-based assays that dynamically evaluate the speed of clot formation, clot strength, and clot lysis. As a result, these viscoelastic testing can provide information about all aspects of the hemostatic process (Whitton and Healy 2023). Here, we will discuss TEG since it is the one that has been more widely used in small animals with hepatobiliary disease. To perform TEG, blood is collected in a 1:9 ratio of citrate-to-blood. Maintaining the citrate-blood ratio is crucial for the accuracy of test results. The values generated by TEG include reaction time (R), kinetic time (K), alpha angle (α-angle), maximum amplitude (MA), lysis at 30 minutes (Ly30), and G value (Figure 5.1). Prolongation of R is due to abnormalities in the coagulation factors or the presence of anticoagulants. Reduced α-angle and increased K can be caused by a reduced platelet count, platelet dysfunction, or fibrinogen deficiency. Decreased MA can occur secondary to severe platelet deficiency, abnormal coagulation factors, or fibrin formation. The G value is mathematically derived from MA and indicates the overall clot strength, which is commonly used to indicate the overall coagulation status. A point-of-care coagulation monitor (VCM-Vet) has also been used to detect hemostatic abnormalities in pets (Hennink et al. 2023; Buriko et al. 2023). Based on comparative studies, results from VCM-Vet to TEG or ROTEM cannot be used interchangeably. VCM can be used to identify hypocoagulable states, but it is not a reliable method to identify hypercoagulable states (Hennink et al. 2023; Buriko et al. 2023). Therefore, in the context of canine and feline hepatobiliary diseases, VCM may help identify patients at risk of bleeding prior to invasive procedures, but this test cannot accurately assess risk of thrombosis.

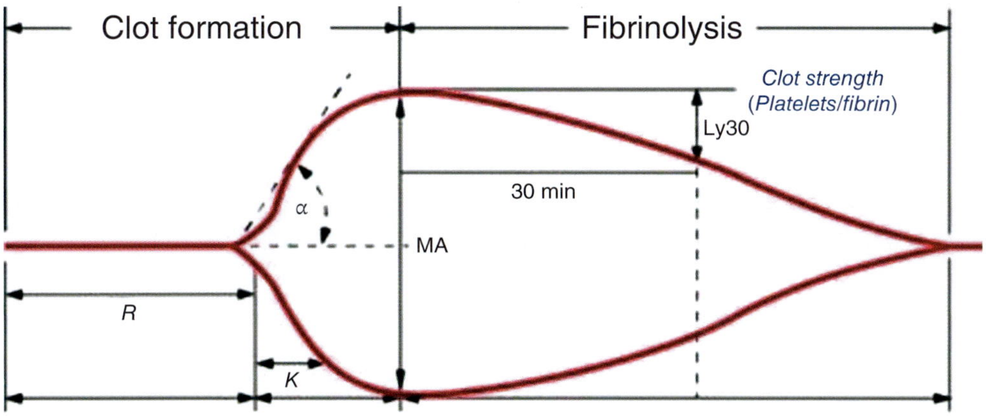

FIGURE 5.1 Thromboelastogram. *R* is the measure of the time from the start of the assay to the point where the clot strength reaches 2 mm of amplitude. *R* estimates the time from activation of the coagulation cascade to the generation of fibrin and clot propagation. *K* represents the time from *R* to the point where the clot reaches a strength of 20 mm. The α-angle is determined by the *x*-axis and the tangent to curve made by *K*. *K* and α-angle are measures of the coagulation cascade, formation of fibrinogen into fibrin, and cross-linking. MA is the maximum value of clot strength. MA and α-angle depend on platelet number and function, and fibrinogen levels. Ly30 is the percent of clot lysis 30 minutes after maximum amplitude is reached. An increased Ly30 reveals hyperfibrinolysis. Abbreviations: *R*, reaction time; *K*, kinetic time; α, alpha angle; MA, maximum amplitude; Ly30, lysis at 30 minutes. *Source*: Dias et al. 2017/College of American Pathologist

COAGULATION SCREENING SUMMARY

While coagulation tests can help clinicians to assess the risks of bleeding in patients with hepatobiliary disease prior to invasive procedures (Table 5.1), it is important to recognize that no single test consistently predicts bleeding complications in these patients (Webster et al. 2019). A comprehensive approach and clinical judgement are required, as coagulation testing in animals with liver conditions can be complex, difficult to predict, and sometimes inconclusive.

Table 5.1 Coagulation Screening Results That Suggest a High Risk of Bleeding with Invasive Procedures

Coagulation screening tests	High risk of bleeding
PCV	<30%
Platelet count	<50,000/µL
PT/aPTT	1.5–2× ULN
Fibrinogen	<100 µg/dL
BMBT	>5 minutes
vWF antigen assay	Abnormal vWF:Ag
TEG	Low G; high Ly30 – hyperfibrinolytic

PCV, packed cell volume; PT, prothrombin time; aPTT, activated partial thromboplastin time; BMBT, buccal mucosal bleeding time; vWF, von Willebrand Factor; TEG, thromboelastography.

COMMON FINDINGS IN DOGS AND CATS WITH HEPATOBILIARY DISEASE

Thrombocytopenia, which may result from decreased thrombopoietin production or increased consumption, is a common finding in animals with hepatobiliary disease ranging from mild to severe dependent on the underlying disease (Webster 2017).

ACUTE LIVER INJURY

Dogs with acute liver injury (ALI) are more often hypocoagulable and hyperfibrinolytic, demonstrated by prolonged PT and aPTT, decreased fibrinogen, and antithrombin concentrations (Webster 2017). Dogs with ALI present multiple coagulation profiles on TEG but are more commonly hypocoagulable and hyperfibrinolytic (Kelley et al. 2015; Webster 2017). When hyperfibrinolytic, these patients have usually normal D-dimer concentrations, attributing the hyperfibrinolysis to a reduction of the inhibitors of fibrinolysis (e.g., plasminogen activator inhibitor-1) (Birkbeck et al. 2019).

CANINE CHRONIC HEPATITIS

A variety of TEG profiles are common in dogs with chronic hepatitis. One study revealed that 43% of dogs with chronic hepatitis are normocoagulable despite prolonged PT/aPTT and low antithrombin (Fry et al. 2017). However, dogs with advanced liver disease are more commonly hypocoagulable on TEG with concomitant low fibrinogen, platelet count, as well as coagulation factors (Prins et al. 2010; Fry et al. 2017). In addition, secondary hyperfibrinolysis can also be present in dogs with late-stage liver disease.

CHOLESTATIC DISEASE

In patients with cholestatic disease, the concentration of vitamin K is decreased secondary to reduced bile acid-mediated lipid saponification and intestinal malabsorption of fat-soluble vitamins. Vitamin K promotes activation of prothrombin, protein C, protein S, and factors II, VII, IX, and X. Cholestatic hepatopathies predispose patients, particularly cats, to coagulopathies.

CONGENITAL PORTOSYSTEMIC SHUNTS

Mildly prolonged PT, aPTT, subnormal platelet counts, and deficiencies in procoagulant factors are observed in dogs with portosystemic shunts (PSS) (Prins et al. 2010). In contrast, reduced antithrombin and protein C activity, along with increased factor VIII activity, increased vWF, and hypercoagulable TEG profile have also been identified (Webster 2017; Toulza et al. 2006). Yet, dogs with congenital PSS rarely have clinically significant coagulopathies (Kelley et al. 2013).

FELINE HEPATOBILIARY DISEASE

In cats with hepatic lipidosis and cholangitis, vitamin K deficiency is common, resulting in reduced factors II, VII, and X activities (Lisciandro et al. 1998; Dircks et al. 2012; Center et al. 2000). In addition, cats with cholestatic disease that have been supplemented with vitamin K have a variety of coagulation profiles on TEG (Webster 2017; Kakar et al. 2021). TEG detected coagulation abnormalities more commonly than conventional methods (i.e., PT, aPTT, and platelet count) (Kakar et al. 2021). Administration of vitamin K (0.5–1.0 mg/kg SQ, *maximum of 3 doses to avoid oxidant injury to red blood cells*) is advisable prior to and after invasive sampling in cats with hepatobiliary disease.

PROTEIN C

Protein C is a vitamin K-dependent anticoagulant glycoprotein produced by the liver. Although protein C activity diminishes in several canine hepatobiliary diseases (Kelley et al. 2013), protein C is not a reliable marker of coagulation status. Rather, its diagnostic utility is in distinguishing vascular anomalies, such as PSS and microvascular anomalies (Toulza et al. 2006). Ninety-five percent of dogs with microscopic primary portal vein hypoplasia (microvascular dysplasia) maintain protein C activity >70%. This distinction makes protein C a useful marker for differentiating portal vein hypoplasia from PSS. While values of protein C activity below 70% strongly support PSS (or hepatic failure), values above this threshold do not categorically exclude PSS, especially if they fall in the "grey zone" (70–100%). Therefore, computed tomography angiography is still recommended in those dogs with clinical signs and biochemical parameters consistent with PSS, regardless of protein C activity. In cats, protein C activity is not used as a biomarker of PSS; however, it decreases in various liver diseases, including hepatic lipidosis and inflammatory liver diseases (Dircks et al. 2012).

MICRORNAS

MicroRNAs (miR), short non-coding RNAs, are emerging as promising disease biomarkers for a wide variety of diseases in humans as well as in dogs and cats (Colaianni et al. 2024), due to their organ-specificity and stability in biological matrices. Among these, miR-122 is a hepatocyte-specific microRNA. In dogs, serum miR-122 concentrations are increased in those patients with liver disease, with a significant correlation with serum ALT activity. However, serum miR-122 did not differentiate the subtypes of liver disease (Oosthuyzen et al. 2018). In a small cohort of Labrador retrievers, miR-122 proved to be a more sensitive marker of hepatocellular injury than ALT (Dirksen et al. 2016). However, studies aimed at evaluating whether miR-122 can serve as an earlier marker of hepatocellular injury than ALT need to be conducted prospectively. Serum miR-122 concentrations are also increased in cats with concurrent elevated serum ALT activity (Armstrong et al. 2022). But no prospective study has evaluated this biomarker in cats with hepatobiliary disease. In addition to miR-122, other miR have also been found to be dysregulated in dogs with hepatobiliary diseases. For example, a more recent study reported that serum miR-30b is increased in Labradors with copper hepatopathy (Roelen et al. 2025). Despite progress in microRNA research, currently, serum microRNA testing does not differentiate types of hepatobiliary disease or provide information beyond standard ALT measurements. Further, microRNA testing is not commercially available for routine use in veterinary medicine.

URINE ISOPROSTANES

Urinary isoprostanes, particularly F2-isoprostanes, are biomarkers of oxidative stress and lipid peroxidation (Phillips et al. 2023). Few studies have evaluated urinary F2-isoprostane in dogs with liver diseases and showed a variable degree of oxidative stress in dogs with hepatobiliary disease, but interestingly, this biomarker did not seem to be affected by antioxidant therapies (e.g., S-adenosylmethionine, milk thistle extract, or vitamin E) (Phillips et al. 2023). At this time, urinary F2-isoprostane measurement is not recommended as a reliable diagnostic or monitoring tool for dogs with hepatobiliary disease. While some studies have evaluated urinary isoprostanes in cats with chronic kidney and metabolic diseases, no studies have investigated this biomarker in cats with liver disease.

REFERENCES

Armstrong, S.K., Oosthuyzen, W., Gow, A.G. et al. (2022). Investigation of a relationship between serum concentrations of microRNA-122 and alanine aminotransferase activity in hospitalised cats. *Journal of Feline Medicine & Surgery* 24: e289–e294.

Birkbeck, R., Humm, K., and Cortellini, S. (2019). A review of hyperfibrinolysis in cats and dogs. *Journal of Small Animal Practice* 60: 641–655.

Buriko, Y., Chalifoux, N.V., Clarkin-Breslin, R. et al. (2023). Comparison of a viscoelastic point-of-care coagulation monitor with thromboelastography in sick dogs with hemostatic abnormalities. *Veterinary Clinical Pathology* 52: 217–227.

Center, S. A., Warner, K., Corbett, J. et al. (2000). Proteins invoked by vitamin K absence and clotting times in clinically ill cats. *Journal of Veterinary Internal Medicine* 14: 292–297.

Colaianni, F., Zelli, V., Compagnoni, C. et al. (2024). Role of circulating microRNAs in liver disease and HCC: focus on miR-122. *Genes* 15: 1313.

Dias, J. D., Haney, E. I., Mathew, B. A.et al. (2017). New-generation thromboelastography: comprehensive evaluation of citrated and heparinized blood sample storage effect on clot-forming variables. *Archives of Pathology & Laboratory Medicine* 141(4): 569–577.

Dircks, B., Nolte, I., and Mischke, R. (2012). Haemostatic abnormalities in cats with naturally occurring liver diseases. *The Veterinary Journal* 193: 103–108.

Dirksen, K., Verzijl, T., van den Ingh, T.S.G.A.M. et al. (2016). Hepatocyte-derived microRNAs as sensitive serum biomarkers of hepatocellular injury in labrador retrievers. *The Veterinary Journal* 211: 75–81.

Fry, W., Lester, C., Etedali, N.M. et al. (2017). Thromboelastography in dogs with chronic hepatopathies. *Journal of Veterinary Internal Medicine* 31: 419–426.

Hennink, I., Peters, L., van Geest, G. et al. (2023). Evaluation of a viscoelastic coagulation monitoring system (VCM Vet®) and its correlation with thromboelastometry (ROTEM®) in diseased and healthy dogs. *Animals (Basel)* 13: 405

Hyatt, C.E. and Brainard, B.M. (2016). Point of care assessment of coagulation. *Topics in Companion Animal Medicine* 31: 11–17.

Kakar, N., Daniel, G., Fellman, C. et al. (2021). Thromboelastography in cats with cholestatic liver disease. *Journal of Feline Medicine and Surgery* 23: 160–167.

Kalbantner, K., Meyer-Lindenberg, A., and Mischke, R. (2011). Platelet function in dogs with congenital portosystemic shunt. *The Veterinary Journal* 188: 189–192.

Kelley, D., Lester, C., DeLaforcade, A. et al. (2013). Thromboelastographic evaluation of dogs with congenital portosystemic shunts. *Journal of Veterinary Internal Medicine* 27 (5): 1262–1267. https://doi.org/doi:10.1111/jvim.12130.

Kelley, D., Lester, C., Shaw, S. et al. (2015). Thromboelastographic evaluation of dogs with acute liver disease. *Journal of Veterinary Internal Medicine* 29: 1053–1062.

Lisciandro, S.C., Hohenhaus, A., and Brooks, M. (1998). Coagulation abnormalities in 22 cats with naturally occurring liver disease. *Journal of Veterinary Internal Medicine* 12: 71–75.

Lisman, T., Hernandez-Gea, V., Magnusson, M. et al. (2021). The concept of rebalanced hemostasis in patients with liver disease: communication from the ISTH SSC working group on hemostatic management of patients with liver disease. *Journal of Thrombosis and Haemostasis* 19: 1116–1122.

Oosthuyzen, W., Ten Berg, P.W.L., Francis, B. et al. (2018). Sensitivity and specificity of microRNA-122 for liver disease in dogs. *Journal of Veterinary Internal Medicine* 32: 1637–1644.

Phillips, R.K., Steiner, J.M., Suchodolski, J.S. et al. (2023). Urinary 15-F2t-isoprostane concentrations in dogs with liver disease. *Veterinary Sciences* 10: 82.

Prins, M., Schellens, C.J.M.M., van Leeuwen, M.W. et al. (2010). Coagulation disorders in dogs with hepatic disease. *The Veterinary Journal* 185: 163–168.

Roelen, Y.S., Spee, B., van Wolferen, M.E. et al. (2025). Serum miR-30b is increased in Labrador Retrievers with elevated hepatic copper levels. *The Veterinary Journal* 311: 106335.

Shropshire, S.B., Olver, C.S., Twedt, D.C. et al. (2022). Multiplate platelet aggregometry in dogs undergoing laparoscopic liver biopsy for diagnosis of chronic hepatopathy. *Journal of Small Animal Practice* 63: 389–396.

Toulza, O., Center, S.A., Brooks, M.B. et al. (2006). Evaluation of plasma protein C activity for detection of hepatobiliary disease and portosystemic shunting in dogs. *Journal of the American Veterinary Medical Association* 229 (11): 1761–1771. https://doi.org/10.2460/javma.229.11.1761.

Webster, C.R.L. (2017). Hemostatic disorders associated with hepatobiliary disease. *Veterinary Clinics of North America: Small Animal Practice* 47: 601–615.

Webster, C.R.L., Center, S.A., Cullen, J.M. et al. (2019). ACVIM consensus statement on the diagnosis and treatment of chronic hepatitis in dogs. *Journal of Veterinary Internal Medicine* 33: 1173–1200.

Whitton, T. and Healy, W. (2023). Review of thromboelastography (TEG): medical and surgical applications. *Therapeutic Advances in Pulmonary and Critical Care Medicine* 18: 29768675231208426.

Wikkelsø, A., Wetterslev, J., Møller, A.M. et al. (2016). Thromboelastography (TEG) or thromboelastometry (ROTEM) to monitor haemostatic treatment versus usual care in adults or children with bleeding. *Cochrane Database of Systematic Reviews* 2016: CD007871.

Wilkinson, A., Panciera, D., DeMonaco, S. et al. (2022). Platelet function in dogs with chronic liver disease. *Journal of Small Animal Practice* 63: 120–127.

Congenital Portosystemic Shunts

CHAPTER 6

Mandy L. Wallace

Department of Small Animal Medicine and Surgery, College of Veterinary Medicine, University of Georgia, Athens, GA, USA

KEY POINTS

- Diagnosis of a congenital portosystemic shunt is based on a combination of clinical signs and clinical-laboratory findings, with definitive diagnosis confirmed by diagnostic imaging, specifically computed tomography angiography (CTA), or visualization during surgery.
- Medical management of congenital portosystemic shunts (cPSS) can result in significant improvement in clinical signs; however, surgical attenuation of the abnormal vessel results in the best long-term outcomes.
- Minimally invasive treatment of intrahepatic portosystemic shunts via percutaneous transvenous coil embolization (PTCE) has a low complication rate and results in excellent long-term outcomes in the majority of dogs.
- Cats with extrahepatic portosystemic shunts can have excellent long-term outcomes with surgical attenuation of their shunting vessel; however, continued shunting through the vessel after surgery occurs at rates higher than their canine counterparts.

INTRODUCTION

Congenital portosystemic shunts (cPSS) are vascular anomalies that allow venous blood from the gastrointestinal tract to bypass the liver, moving directly into the systemic circulation. This results in decreased growth factors being delivered to the liver, and increased endogenous waste products in the systemic circulation, leading to a variety of clinical signs in affected dogs and cats. cPSS are separated into two main categories: extrahepatic cPSS, which occur outside of the hepatic parenchyma, and intrahepatic cPSS, which occur within the hepatic parenchyma.

ANATOMY

The portal vein is formed by the confluence of the cranial and caudal mesenteric veins. The left gastric vein joins the splenic vein prior to connection of the splenic vein to the portal vein. Cranially, the gastroduodenal vein joins the portal vein to complete the extrahepatic portal system. The portal vein splits into left and right portal branches cranial to the entrance of the gastroduodenal vein. The right portal vein supplies the right lateral liver lobe and the caudate process of the caudate liver lobe. The left portal vein is the larger of the two branches, and the central portal vein splits off of the left portal vein. The central portal vein supplies the right medial liver lobe and the papillary process of the caudate liver lobe. The remainder of the left portal vein supplies the quadrate, left medial, and left lateral liver lobes. The portal system provides the venous drainage to the entire gastrointestinal tract except for the caudal rectum and anal canal. The hepatic artery and portal vein supply all the blood to the liver, with the portal vein supplying 50% of the oxygen supply and 75–80% of the blood volume.

Disorders of the Liver, Exocrine Pancreas, and Gastrointestinal Tract in Dogs and Cats, First Edition. Edited by Harry Cridge et al. Published 2026 by John Wiley & Sons, Inc. Companion Website: www.wiley.com/go/cridge/disorders

PATHOPHYSIOLOGY

Extrahepatic cPSS develop secondary to errors in embryologic development of the cardinal and vitelline systems. This produces abnormal connections between the portal system and the systemic circulation, specifically the caudal vena cava or azygos vein. For intrahepatic cPSS, left-sided shunts are typically the result of a patent ductus venosus. The ductus venosus develops from the portal sinus and terminates dorsally on the ampulla, which is the dilation occurring where the left phrenic vein, hepatic vein, and ductus venosus join. The ductus venosus should close functionally between days two and six after birth, with structural closure occurring at around three weeks of age. Central intrahepatic cPSS may result from developmental abnormalities in the vitelline system or from malformation in the hepatic sinusoids.

SIGNALMENT

Extrahepatic cPSS most commonly occur in small breed dogs, with Yorkshire terriers being 36 times more likely to develop this condition than any other breed. Other breeds that are overrepresented for extrahepatic cPSS are Maltese, Pugs, Dandie Dinmont terriers, Havanese, and Miniature Schnauzers. Extrahepatic cPSS is known to be or considered likely to be heritable in Maltese, Yorkshire terriers, and Cairn terriers. Diagnosis of cPSS typically occurs around 6–12 months of age; however, diagnosis can occur at any age and may occur later in animals with certain shunt configurations, such as portoazygos extrahepatic cPSS. Additionally, Miniature Schnauzers may be more likely to be diagnosed at an older age. Cats are more likely to have extrahepatic cPSS when compared to intrahepatic cPSS, though both may occur. Domestic shorthair, Persian, Siamese, Burmese, and Himalayan cats are the most commonly reported cat breeds with cPSS.

Intrahepatic cPSS are more commonly seen in large to giant breed dogs, with the Irish Wolfhound, Golden retriever, Labrador retriever, Australian shepherd, and Australian Cattle dog predisposed. Shunt configurations vary with breed in dogs with intrahepatic cPSS, with Irish wolfhounds predisposed to left divisional intrahepatic cPSS and Australian Cattle dogs being more likely to develop right divisional intrahepatic cPSS.

CLINICAL SIGNS

Dogs and cats with cPSS can be asymptomatic; however, the majority of animals will have clinical signs that fall into one of three main categories: neurologic, gastrointestinal, or urinary. Neurologic signs are related to hepatic encephalopathy (please see Chapter 8). Gastrointestinal signs are nonspecific and include vomiting, diarrhea, anorexia, and failure to maintain or reach an appropriate weight. In cats, ptyalism may also be seen. Urinary signs are often related to the presence of ammonium urate cystoliths and include stranguria, hematuria, pollakiuria, and difficulty house training. Ammonium urate urolithiasis has been reported in 19.3–36% of dogs with cPSS (Walton-Clark et al. 2025). Dogs with extrahepatic cPSS were affected more commonly than dogs with intrahepatic cPSS, and older dogs and neutered male dogs were more likely to have urolithiasis in one study (Walton-Clark et al. 2025). Another clinical sign seen specifically in cats is the presence of copper irises that are inappropriate for the breed or color of the cat (Figure 6.1).

DIAGNOSIS

cPSS are often suspected based on a combination of signalment, clinical signs, and abnormal values on complete blood count and biochemistry profiles. On complete blood count, a microcytic, normochromic non-regenerative anemia and neutrophilia may be present. On the biochemistry profile,

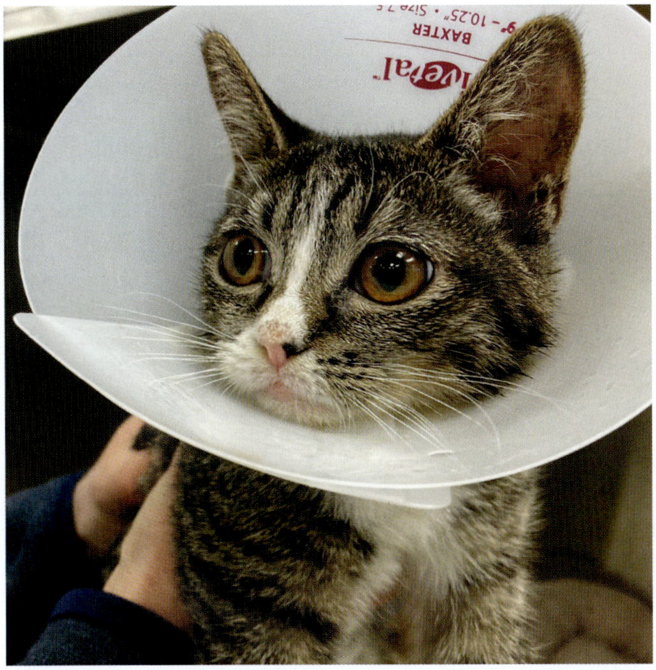

FIGURE 6.1 A domestic shorthair cat with an extrahepatic cPSS and copper irises that are unexpected for the coat color

abnormalities are often present in the values that are indicative of hepatic hypoperfusion, including a low blood urea nitrogen value, hypocholesterolemia, hypoalbuminemia, and hypoglycemia. Liver enzyme activities, such as ALT or ALP, are often normal to slightly elevated. Coagulation profiles can be performed and may reveal prolongation of PT or aPTT; however, despite these abnormalities, spontaneous bleeding or hemorrhage during surgery is rare.

Hepatic function tests are often performed once a cPSS is suspected. Pre- and post-prandial serum bile acid values are stable in serum during transport to a commercial laboratory. Bile acids are released by the gallbladder into the duodenum after gallbladder contraction secondary to eating or smelling food, and are subsequently resorbed in the terminal ileum, recirculated through the portal system, and cleared by the liver. In an animal with hepatic dysfunction or a portal vascular anomaly, bile acids are not immediately cleared and recirculate in the systemic circulation, leading to increases in serum bile acid concentrations. Elevations in either pre- and/or post-prandial bile acids are consistent with hepatic hypoperfusion but do not definitively diagnose a cPSS. Baseline ammonia levels can also be performed; however, ammonia is not stable for transport and can be falsely elevated if not tested quickly. Point-of-care ammonia testing is available in the form of a benchtop dry chemistry analyzer and a handheld analyzer in veterinary medicine and has been found to be accurate for determining normal or high ammonia levels, though the actual values may be less accurate with the point-of-care machines. Increased fasting serum bile acid concentrations are very sensitive for cPSS (98%) on their own; however, the specificity increases when combined with fasting ammonia levels (97%) in one study (van Straten et al. 2015). Protein C measurement has been evaluated to differentiate cPSS from microvascular dysplasia-portal vein hypoplasia. One study found that 88% of dogs with cPSS had a protein C level below 70%, whereas dogs with microvascular dysplasia-portal vein hypoplasia had levels above 70% in 95% of cases (Toulza et al. 2006). This test cannot be used alone for evaluation of cPSS, though it may be beneficial as a preliminary test in some cases. Presence of ammonium urate crystalluria should raise suspicion for cPSS, especially in breeds that are not known to have other predispositions toward ammonium urate urolith or crystal formation. In one study, almost 40% of dogs with cPSS had crystalluria, including 45% of dogs with intrahepatic cPSS and 38% with extrahepatic cPSS. The crystals in those dogs were predominantly ammonium urate (Walton-Clark et al. 2025).

Abdominal radiographs can be performed and may show renal enlargement, microhepatica, and potentially uroliths. As ammonium urate uroliths are the most common urolith in animals with cPSS, these are more radiolucent than other uroliths and may be challenging or impossible to see on radiographs. Definitive diagnosis of cPSS is via diagnostic imaging or visualization in surgery during an exploratory laparotomy. Abdominal ultrasonography, computed tomography angiography (CTA), and nuclear scintigraphy have all been described for diagnosis of cPSS. With abdominal ultrasonography, the operator is looking for any abnormal vessel going from the portal system to the systemic circulation. This can be challenging to identify, particularly with portoazygos or portophrenic cPSS configurations. If an abnormal vessel is not identified, a portal vein to aorta ratio can also be measured and may indicate that a cPSS is likely present. If the portal vein to aorta ratio is <0.7, the suspicion for cPSS is higher. Ultrasonography is also used to detect radiolucent uroliths that may be present. Use of abdominal ultrasonography for diagnosis of cPSS is operator dependent with a sensitivity of 80.8% and specificity of 90% in a recent study (Devriendt et al. 2022). Nuclear scintigraphy is another option for diagnostic imaging for diagnosis of cPSS. With this modality, a radionuclide (technetium pertechnetate or technetium mebrofenin) is administered either via injection into the spleen (transsplenic) or via rectal catheter into the colon (transcolonic). Transsplenic injection results in less radionuclide being used and provides a better study. With this method, after the radionuclide is administered, the radioisotope will be seen in the heart first if the patient has a cPSS. If they do not have a cPSS, the radioisotope is seen in the liver first, then the heart, yet it does not show the specific location of the cPSS or whether the cPSS is intrahepatic or extrahepatic, which makes it less useful for surgical planning. Additionally, the patient must be isolated until the radioisotope has cleared (30 minutes to 24 hours after the procedure). CTA has a higher sensitivity and specificity than abdominal ultrasonography and does not use radioactive material. For these reasons, CTA has gained favor for use in surgical planning for extrahepatic and intrahepatic cPSS (Figure 6.2). With CTA, intravenous contrast material is injected, and three phases are captured: arterial, portal, and venous. This modality provides an excellent view of the abnormal vasculature, making it an excellent choice for surgical planning. It is also useful for detecting if a second cPSS is present. CTA does require that the patient be heavily sedated or anesthetized; however, adverse effects associated

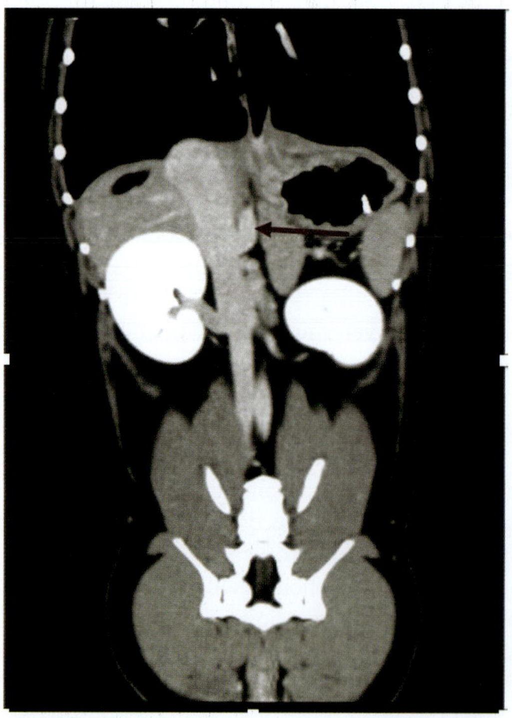

FIGURE 6.2 A CT angiogram of the abdomen of a dog with an extrahepatic cPSS. The arrow indicates the cPSS.

with this are not often reported. Dosages of pre-medications for general anesthesia or sedatives may need to be lowered due to slower hepatic clearance of these medications. Please see Chapter 2 for a detailed summary of Hepatobiliary Diagnostic Imaging.

TREATMENT

MEDICAL MANAGEMENT

Please see Chapter 8 for a detailed summary of medical management for hepatic encephalopathy.

Levetiracetam has been suggested as a preoperative medical management option to decrease the risk of post-attenuation seizures (PAS) in dogs undergoing surgery for cPSS. However, studies evaluating this association found no difference in PAS occurrence with or without preoperative levetiracetam administration (Mullins et al. 2019; Strickland et al. 2018). Based on these studies, there is likely no benefit of levetiracetam administration in the majority of cPSS patients; however, there is no evidence to indicate that administration of levetiracetam is harmful and may be considered on a case-by-case basis. For intrahepatic cPSS, omeprazole is also recommended in addition to the other medical treatments for cPSS. This is due to a perceived increased incidence of gastric ulceration in dogs with intrahepatic cPSS before and after surgical attenuation (Pascarella et al. 2025; Weisse et al. 2014).

A new possibility for medical management in dogs with cPSS with hepatic encephalopathy refractory to traditional medical management options is therapeutic plasma exchange. This has been shown to improve neurologic status within 24 hours in a dog with worsening hepatic encephalopathy after undergoing general anesthesia for diagnostic imaging. This dog was able to undergo surgical shunt attenuation five days after receiving therapeutic plasma exchange and was free of clinical signs at 100 days after surgery (Culler et al. 2020). Further research is needed to determine if there are certain cPSS patients that would have significant benefit from this treatment.

SURGICAL TREATMENT

Surgical attenuation of cPSS can be accomplished via two main methods: ligation or gradual attenuation of the shunt vessel. Complete or partial ligation can be utilized for both types of cPSS but generally may be more successful for intrahepatic cPSS than extrahepatic cPSS. With complete or partial ligation, it is recommended to measure portal pressures before ligation and after temporary occlusion of the shunt vessel to determine if complete ligation is feasible in that patient or will result in portal hypertension. Portal pressures should not exceed 12.5–17.6 mmHg and should not change more than 6.6–7.4 mmHg after ligation to prevent portal hypertension. Portal pressures are ideally measured with a water manometer; however, other devices, such as arterial pressure transducers, are also considered to be accurate. Additionally, visual evaluation of the gastrointestinal tract for hypermotility and the pancreas for a change in color to blue/purple may also indicate evidence of portal hypertension. If complete ligation is not tolerated, partial ligation can be considered; however, it is important to note that up to 40–60% of dogs undergoing partial ligation of extrahepatic cPSS require continued medical management to control clinical signs and may require a second surgery. In dogs with intrahepatic cPSS, good to excellent outcomes were achieved with suture ligation in 76–100% of dogs that survived the perioperative period.

Gradual occlusion devices include the ameroid constrictor and thin film banding. The purpose of these devices is to close the shunting vessel gradually to allow for a slower increase in blood flow through the portal system, which decreases the risk of portal hypertension and allows more time for portal system hypertrophy. The ameroid constrictor works in two ways. (Figure 6.3) First, the casein portion of the device absorbs some fluid from the abdominal cavity, leading to partial closure of the inner portion of the device and some direct physical attenuation of the shunt vessel after 6–9 weeks (Hunt et al. 2014). Second, as casein is a foreign protein within the peritoneal cavity, inflammation and fibrosis occur around the device, which ideally completes the closure of the shunt

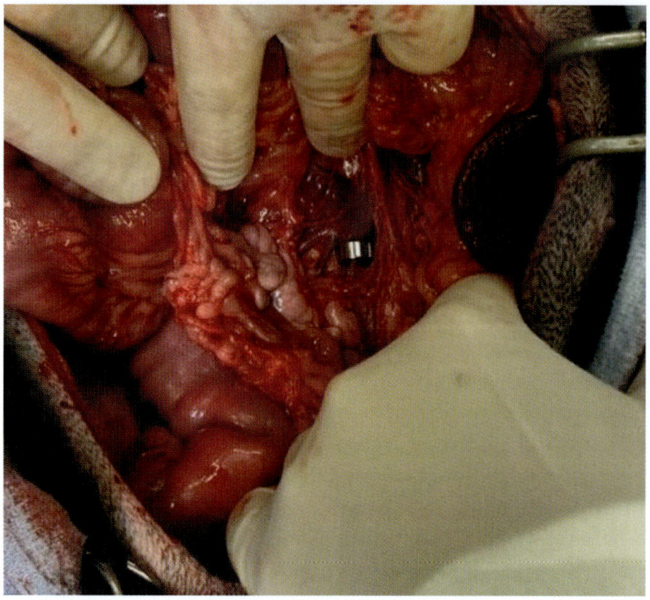

FIGURE 6.3 An ameroid constrictor placed around an extrahepatic cPSS vessel in the abdomen of a dog

vessel (Hunt et al. 2014). Thrombosis within the shunt vessel may also occur after ameroid constrictor placement, often in the first 3–14 days after surgery. This is likely due to damage to the vessel during vessel isolation and placement of the ameroid constrictor. Similarly, thin film banding, which was initially known as cellophane banding, results in shunt closure by eliciting a foreign body reaction with closure of the vessel occurring completely through inflammation and fibrosis. While it was initially thought that all thin films being used for this purpose were cellophane, a spectroscopic and mechanical study of thin films found that most of the thin films being used were not truly cellophane, resulting in variation in the foreign body reaction with each different type of thin film and therefore, variability in shunt vessel closure across studies and in individual patients. Thin film bands are usually folded to a three-layer band and are secured with four hemoclips placed in an alternating fashion. Outcomes following surgical attenuation for extrahepatic cPSS are good to excellent overall, with most patients requiring minimal to no medical management following surgery and having long survival times. When comparing outcomes between dogs that underwent surgical attenuation with an ameroid constrictor compared to a thin film band, no differences have been found in postoperative complications, postoperative mortality, or long-term outcome overall (Matiasovic et al. 2020). In cats, excellent long-term outcomes can be achieved with both the ameroid constrictor and thin film banding. Postoperative complications across devices range from 22 to 77%, with a postoperative mortality rate of 0–22%. Excellent outcomes were achieved in 44–89% of cats across studies, though a high rate of persistent shunting was present, ranging from 11–57% (Janas et al. 2024; Valiente et al. 2020). Interestingly, it has been noted that cats can experience recanalization of their shunt vessel after confirmation of complete closure following thin film banding, and that inconsistent closure of intra-abdominal vessels may occur after thin film band placement in cats. Despite these reports, outcomes in clinical studies with thin film banding in cats have shown good to excellent outcomes. This variability in results in cats may also be related to the different compositions of the thin films used in individual patients. As the composition of different thin films used in this procedure is variable, the inflammatory response is also variable. Additionally, each individual patient will have a variable inflammatory response to the foreign object within the abdomen, leading to differences in vessel closure times and closure completeness.

Minimally invasive surgical shunt attenuation can be performed for both extrahepatic and intrahepatic cPSS. For extrahepatic cPSS, minimally invasive attenuation using thin film bands or suture ligation via laparoscopy has been reported in 36 dogs, with a postoperative mortality rate of 5.6% and no portal hypertension or residual shunting in the attenuated vessels present at 1–2 months after surgery (Shigemoto et al. 2024). However, minimally invasive treatment for extrahepatic cPSS is not routinely performed. Minimally invasive treatment for intrahepatic cPSS via PTCE is well-established and often performed for this condition. With this procedure, a vascular stent is placed in the caudal vena cava with access via the right jugular vein and placement occurring under fluoroscopic guidance. Thrombogenic coils are inserted through the vascular stent via a catheter into the shunt vessel. Portal pressures are obtained before and after stent placement and after insertion of each coil into the shunt vessel to ensure that the portal pressures do not rise above 16 mmHg and that there is an adequate change in portal pressures (around 6–7 mmHg), indicating that enough coils have been placed within the shunt to cause gradual closure of the vessel. In a study of 100 dogs undergoing this procedure, median survival time was 2,204 days with excellent outcomes in 66% of dogs. Intraoperative complications occurred in 3% of dogs and included severe portal hypertension and gastrointestinal hemorrhage. Postoperative complications occurred in 13%, most of which were dogs having PAS or post-attenuation neurologic signs (PANS) (Weisse et al. 2014). When compared to thin film banding, dogs undergoing PTCE had shorter hospitalization times and fewer postoperative complications than dogs undergoing thin film banding for intrahepatic cPSS. The survival rates were similar at one, two, and five years between the two procedures. This procedure appears to be safe and effective for the treatment of intrahepatic cPSS.

Other procedures may be performed during the same surgical episode, including cystotomy if cystoliths are present, sterilization procedures, liver biopsy, and any other necessary procedures. The decision to perform these procedures often depends on patient stability under general anesthesia. The risks and benefits of any added procedure should be evaluated on a case-by-case basis.

MEDICAL VERSUS SURGICAL TREATMENT OUTCOMES

Given the risk of perioperative mortality associated with cPSS attenuation, it is important to determine whether the potential benefits of surgery justify the risk. Surgical attenuation of cPSS has been shown to reduce clinical signs, increase postoperative liver volume, enhance portal vasculature, and lower C-reactive protein levels.

In long-term outcome studies, 89% of dogs with extrahepatic cPSS managed medically either died or were euthanized during the study period (MST 836 days), compared to only 21% of dogs who underwent surgery (MST not reached) (Greenhalgh et al. 2014). Similarly, among 351 dogs diagnosed with EHPSS at five years of age or older, those treated surgically had significantly longer survival (estimated at 10.9 years) compared to those receiving only medical management (3.4 years) (Wallace et al. 2022). These findings underscore the value of surgical attenuation in improving outcomes for dogs with cPSS.

POSTOPERATIVE MANAGEMENT

Management of animals undergoing surgical attenuation of cPSS includes appropriate pain management, continuation of medical management therapies, and monitoring for signs of PAS or neurologic signs. Administration of local anesthetic blocks, such as incisional blocks and transverse abdominal plane blocks, can be beneficial to decrease the amount of systemic opiate pain medications required postoperatively. As these animals are slow to metabolize medications due to their decreased hepatic function, prolonged effects of general anesthesia and from opiate administration can be seen; therefore, any option for local pain control may be beneficial to decrease those effects during hospitalization. Prior to hospital discharge and in the days following hospital discharge, animals are closely monitored for changes in neurologic status and signs of seizure activity. Supportive care via intravenous fluid therapy, antiemetic drugs, and other therapies is initiated as needed based on examination of the patient. Medical management therapies, such as lactulose, antibiotics, and therapeutic hepatic diets, are continued after surgery and can be slowly tapered, one at a time, in the weeks and months following surgery. Patients that were receiving anti-seizure medications prior to surgery due to previous seizure activity should continue to receive those medications after the procedure. The decision to taper those medications should be made on a case-by-case basis. For dogs with intrahepatic cPSS, omeprazole should also be tapered, and patients monitored carefully for signs of melena, hematemesis, anemia, or other signs consistent with gastric ulceration.

If gastric ulceration is confirmed or highly suspected, omeprazole may need to be administered for a longer course. Some animals may require all or a portion of their prior medical management therapies after surgery for the rest of their lives to reduce or eliminate clinical signs. This is due to a variety of reasons, including continued shunting through the primary shunt vessel, development of acquired shunt vessels due to portal hypertension, or presence of other hepatic disorders leading to decreased hepatic function, which can occur concurrently with cPSS. Please see Chapter 9 for a detailed discussion of etiology.

POSTOPERATIVE COMPLICATIONS

Complications associated with cPSS surgery include portal hypertension, hemorrhage, hypoglycemia, gastric ulceration (particularly with intrahepatic cPSS (Pascarella et al. 2025)), central blindness (notably in cats), failure of shunt closure, sudden death, and PANS. Portal hypertension may be acute or chronic in nature. Signs of acute portal hypertension include abdominal pain, abdominal distension, hematochezia or melena, vomiting, diarrhea, ascites, and signs associated with hypovolemic shock. With chronic portal hypertension, ascites may appear and resolve spontaneously within days to weeks. These patients typically go on to form multiple acquired shunt vessels and may require lifelong medical management to address associated clinical signs.

PAS occur in approximately 5–8% of patients (Mullins et al. 2020; Weisse et al. 2014). One study found that 11% of dogs developed PANS after shunt attenuation, with 5% specifically experiencing PAS (Strickland et al. 2018). Risk factors for PANS include preoperative hepatic encephalopathy and older age (Strickland et al. 2018). Additionally, certain breeds, such as Pugs, may be more susceptible. The prognosis for dogs that develop PAS is poor, with only 32.3% surviving to 30 days postoperatively in one study (Mullins et al. 2020). However, survival was more likely in dogs with a history of seizures prior to surgery and in those that developed only focal seizures after surgery (Mullins et al. 2020). Unfortunately, no consistent preoperative or intraoperative method has been shown to reliably prevent PAS. Dogs that develop PANS and survive the initial postoperative period are reported to have a high quality of life; however, seizures are likely to recur in those that develop PAS as well.

Shunt closure failure is another significant concern. Recent reports indicate failure in up to 18% of dogs with ameroid constrictor placement and 35% with thin film banding (Hunt et al. 2014; Nelson and Nelson 2016). In one study, dogs undergoing thin film banding were more likely to undergo revision surgery for persistent shunting than dogs undergoing ameroid constrictor placement (Matiasovic et al. 2020). Despite this, most dogs with incomplete shunt attenuation remain asymptomatic, suggesting that mild residual blood flow may not always be clinically significant.

Diagnosing residual flow postoperatively typically requires advanced imaging or nuclear scintigraphy, as commonly used tests, such as paired serum bile acids or fasting ammonia, are unreliable for determining complete shunt closure. Several blood-based tests, including the lidocaine/MEGX test, serum hyaluronic acid, protein C, and serum insulin-like growth factor, have shown potential in assessing postoperative shunt attenuation. However, these tests remain less accurate than advanced imaging, are not widely available in general practice, and require further research to validate their clinical utility.

REFERENCES

Culler, C.A., Reinhardt, A., and Vigani, A. (2020). Successful management of clinical signs associated with hepatic encephalopathy with manual therapeutic plasma exchange in a dog. *Journal of Veterinary Emergency and Critical Care* 30 (3): 312–317. https://doi.org/10.1111/VEC.12940.

Devriendt N., Serrano G., Stock E., et al. (2022). Diagnostic value of liver function tests and ultrasonography in dogs with suspected congenital portosystemic shunts. *Veterinary Record* 190 (10): e1381. https://doi.org/10.1002/vetr.1381.

Greenhalgh, S.N., Reeve, J.A., Johnstone, T. et al. (2014). Long-term survival and quality of life in dogs with clinical signs associated with a congenital portosystemic shunt after surgical or medical treatment. *Journal of the American Veterinary Medical Association* 245 (5): 527–533. https://doi.org/10.2460/JAVMA.245.5.527.

Hunt, G.B., Culp, W.T.N., Mayhew, K.N. et al. (2014). Evaluation of in vivo behavior of ameroid ring constrictors in dogs with congenital extrahepatic portosystemic shunts using computed tomography.

Veterinary Surgery 43 (7): 834–842. https://doi.org/10.1111/j.1532-950X.2014.12196.x.

Janas, K.E.A., Tobias, K.M., and Aisa, J. (2024). Clinical outcomes for 20 cats with congenital extrahepatic portosystemic shunts treated with ameroid constrictor ring attenuation (2002–2020). *Veterinary Surgery* 53 (2): 243–253. https://doi.org/10.1111/VSU.14066.

Matiasovic, M., Chanoit, G.P.A., Meakin, L.B. et al. (2020). Outcomes of dogs treated for extrahepatic congenital portosystemic shunts with thin film banding or ameroid ring constrictor. *Veterinary Surgery* 49 (1): 160–171. https://doi.org/10.1111/VSU.13273.

Mullins, R.A., Sanchez Villamil, C., de Rooster, H. et al. (2019). Effect of prophylactic treatment with levetiracetam on the incidence of postattenuation seizures in dogs undergoing surgical management of single congenital extrahepatic portosystemic shunts. *Veterinary Surgery* 48 (2): 164–172. https://doi.org/10.1111/vsu.13141.

Mullins, R.A., Sanchez Villamil, C., Selmic, L.E. et al. (2020). Prognostic factors for short-term survival of dogs that experience postattenuation seizures after surgical correction of single congenital extrahepatic portosystemic shunts: 93 cases (2005–2018). *Veterinary Surgery* 49 (5): 958–970. https://doi.org/10.1111/VSU.13422.

Nelson, N.C. and Nelson, L.L. (2016). Imaging and clinical outcomes in 20 dogs treated with thin film banding for extrahepatic portosystemic shunts. *Veterinary Surgery* 45 (6): 736–745. https://doi.org/10.1111/VSU.12509.

Pascarella, J.M., Gibson, E.A., Rondeau, M.P. et al. (2025). Gastroduodenal ulceration and erosion occurs in dogs with intrahepatic portosystemic shunts prior to and following percutaneous transvenous coil embolization. *Journal of the American Veterinary Medical Association* 263 (6): 1–8. https://doi.org/10.2460/JAVMA.24.11.0744.

Shigemoto, J., Kaneko, Y., Kawazu, M. et al. (2024). Laparoscopic treatment of congenital portosystemic shunts with portal pressure measurement and portal angiography in 36 dogs. *Frontiers in Veterinary Science* 11: 1291006. https://doi.org/10.3389/FVETS.2024.1291006.

Strickland, R., Tivers, M.S., Adamantos, S.E. et al. (2018). Incidence and risk factors for neurological signs after attenuation of single congenital portosystemic shunts in 253 dogs. *Veterinary Surgery* 47 (6); 745–755. https://doi.org/10.1111/VSU.12925.

Toulza, O., Center, S.A., and Brooks, M.B. (2006). Evaluation of plasma protein C activity for detection of hepatobiliary disease and portosystemic shunting in dogs. *Journal of the American Veterinary Medical Association* 229 (11): 1761–1771. https://doi.org/10.2460/JAVMA.229.11.1761.

Valiente, P., Trehy, M., and White, R. (2020). Complications and outcome of cats with congenital extrahepatic portosystemic shunts treated with thin film: thirty-four cases (2008–2017). *Journal of Veterinary Internal Medicine* 34 (1): 117–124. https://doi.org/10.1111/JVIM.15649.

van Straten, G., Spee, B., Rothuizen, J. et al. (2015). Diagnostic value of the rectal ammonia tolerance test, fasting plasma ammonia and fasting plasma bile acids for canine portosystemic shunting. *Veterinary Journal* 204 (3): 282–286. https://doi.org/10.1016/j.tvjl.2015.04.020.

Wallace, M.L., Grimes, J.A., Edwards, L. et al. (2022). Dogs ≥ five years of age at the time of congenital extrahepatic portosystemic shunt diagnosis have better long-term outcomes with surgical attenuation than with medical management alone. *Journal of the American Veterinary Medical Association* 260 (7): 758–764. https://doi.org/10.2460/JAVMA.21.09.0417.

Walton-Clark, M., Travail, V., Sparks, T. et al. (2025). Retrospective analysis of the incidence and clinicopathological findings associated with ammonium urate urolithiasis in dogs with congenital portosystemic shunts: 363 cases (2010–2023). *Journal of Small Animal Practice* 66 (4): 248–257. https://doi.org/10.1111/jsap.13821.

Weisse, C., Berent, A.C., Todd, K. et al. (2014). Endovascular evaluation and treatment of intrahepatic portosystemic shunts in dogs: 100 cases (2001–2011). *Journal of the American Veterinary Medical Association* 244 (1): 78–94. https://doi.org/10.2460/JAVMA.244.1.78.

CHAPTER 7

Microvascular Dysplasia/Portal Vein Hypoplasia

Andrew Kent

Blaise Veterinary Referral Hospital, Rednal, Birmingham, UK

KEY POINTS

- Primary portal vein hypoplasia (PVH) is a common cause of increased serum bile acids but is typically clinically insignificant.
- Given the overlap of presentation and clinicopathological changes, exclusion of a macroscopic portosystemic shunt by diagnostic imaging is an important component of investigation.
- PVH with portal hypertension is a comparatively rare presentation, but it is much more likely to cause clinical signs and can have a variable prognosis.

INTRODUCTION

Microvascular dysplasia/primary portal vein hypoplasia (MVD/PVH) is a congenital hepatic vascular abnormality. It can be further divided into PVH without portal hypertension and PVH with portal hypertension (Weisse and Berent 2024).

PVH without portal hypertension (PH) is a microscopic malformation of the hepatic vasculature, which is characterized by small/absent intrahepatic portal venules with arteriolar proliferation (**a pattern seen with any cause of portal hypoperfusion**). This allows communication between the intrahepatic portal and systemic circulation at a microscopic level. The condition can be present in isolation or in combination with macroscopic portosystemic shunting. When it exists alone, clinical signs are often minimal to absent with a good long-term prognosis.

PVH with PH is a rare presentation that occurs when smaller portal vein branches are incompletely developed leading to PH without the presence of necroinflammatory or advanced liver disease. This tends to lead to multiple acquired portosystemic shunts (PSSs) and consequent clinical signs of hepatic encephalopathy (HE). This is a complex, and poorly understood, group of conditions and there is a lack of consensus in this area. Many of these patients may previously have been classified as non-cirrhotic portal hypertension (NCPH) or may have had conditions which were under recognized (such as ductal plate malformation). The reader is referred to Chapters 9 and 10.

SIGNALMENT

There is significant overlap in the signalment between PVH and macroscopic portosystemic shunting. Predisposed breeds include the Maltese, Cairn terrier, and Yorkshire terrier (Schermerhorn et al. 1996). The age of diagnosis is typically greater than PSSs due to the lack of clinical signs (Christiansen et al. 1995); there is no clear sex predisposition.

Disorders of the Liver, Exocrine Pancreas, and Gastrointestinal Tract in Dogs and Cats, First Edition. Edited by Harry Cridge et al. Published 2026 by John Wiley & Sons, Inc. Companion Website: www.wiley.com/go/cridge/disorders

CLINICAL SIGNS

The majority (>90%) of dogs with PVH without PH are diagnosed incidentally and do not have any significant clinical signs (Christiansen et al. 1995). However, some will show clinical signs of HE. HE can present as a wide spectrum of clinical signs ranging from mild to severe. Classical signs include gastrointestinal (vomiting, diarrhea, inappetence), urinary (polydipsia and polyuria), and neurological signs (behavior changes, ataxia, pacing, circling, seizures). Please see Chapter 8. In the author's hospital, PVH is commonly suspected when increased bile acids are identified incidentally or during investigation of an unrelated condition.

PVH with PH is typically quiescent in the early stages but can progress. In that event, dogs will present once obvious ascites develop as a sequel to PH or when multiple acquired PSSs develop, leading to signs of HE as described above.

DIAGNOSIS

PVH is ultimately diagnosed based on identifying consistent features on hepatic histology, as detailed below, although many patients will have a presumptive diagnosis based on the lack of clinical signs, supportive laboratory tests, and diagnostic imaging (Figure 7.1). It is important to note that liver histopathology cannot exclude the presence of a macroscopic PSS, and diagnostic imaging is therefore a vital component and should be performed prior to considering biopsy. PVH with PH is diagnosed when intra-abdominal PH is demonstrated with a normal to small portal vein without other histologically evident causes of hepatic PH.

LABORATORY TESTING

- Hematology is typically normal in PVH. Derangements may be seen in PVH with PH once acquired shunts develop, potentially associated with gastrointestinal bleeding.
- Serum biochemistry – While some of the biochemical changes associated with PSS may be present, frequently the biochemistry may be normal or only minimally abnormal.

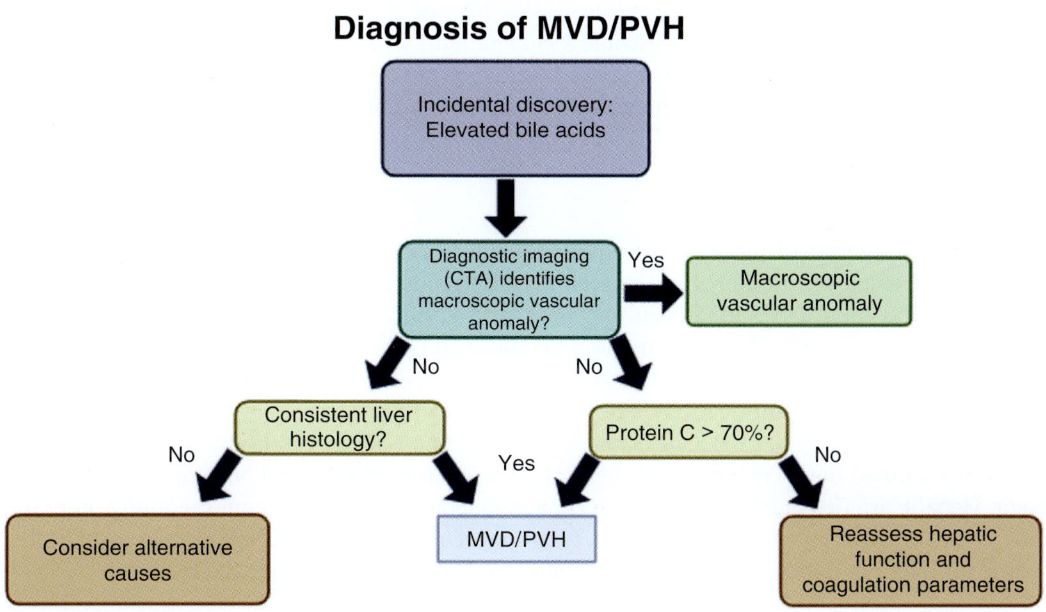

FIGURE 7.1 Diagnostic scheme for MVD/PVH. Image created in BioRender

- Dynamic bile acid testing – Bile acids are frequently utilized in the diagnosis of hepatic vascular disease although they are relatively nonspecific, so interpretation can be challenging. Bile acids continuously undergo enterohepatic recirculation meaning all the stages of this process can impact bile acid concentrations (i.e., gastrointestinal disease, gallbladder, or biliary tract disease etc.). Typically, bile acids will be measured following a 12-hour fast and then 2 hours post-prandially. PVH will lead to increased fasting and/or post-prandial bile acid levels. Anecdotally, bile acid concentrations will be less than with macroscopic portosystemic shunting. This finding is also very nonspecific. Some authors report that indeterminate bile acid increases can be seen in certain breeds (Maltese) and with cholestasis, glucocorticoid administration, and gastrointestinal disease among others (Stockham and Scott 2008).
- Blood ammonia – Ammonia is also used in the investigation of PSS. Ammonia is converted to urea in the liver, and this process is likely to be less efficient in the presence of liver disease and hypoperfusion. Ammonia is very labile and requires rapid analysis, which makes this test less practical. Readers are referred to Chapter 1 for a complete discussion of ammonia.
- Protein C – Protein C (an anticoagulant protein) has garnered significant interest over the last few years as a noninvasive tool for differentiating PVH from PSS. In general, dogs with macroscopic PSS will have protein C levels below 70% (Toulza et al. 2006). It is expected to be above this level with PVH. See Chapter 5. However, access to this test remains variable depending on location.

*Please see Chapter 9 for a discussion of the sequelae of PH.

DIAGNOSTIC IMAGING

While various abnormalities can be seen on imaging. In this presentation, the primary aim is to exclude a macroscopic PSS. Please see Chapter 2.

- Abdominal radiographs – Often normal in PVH, although a small liver may be seen. The presence of abdominal effusion may be detected in PVH with PH.
- Abdominal ultrasound – often normal in PVH. The identification of PSS by ultrasound is operator dependent so other modalities may be preferable unless this expertise is available. In PVH with PH, ascites may be seen along with variable liver size, acquired PSSs might be identified.
- Computed Tomographic Angiography (CTA) – CTA is considered the optimal modality for evaluating the portal venous system, given its availability and the ability for remote reporting. CTA allows confident exclusion of macroscopic PSS in patients with PVH. A degree of expertise is still required to optimize the post-contrast scans to enhance the diagnostic potential. In PVH with PH the presence of ascites with or without acquired portosystemic shunting will be seen.

HISTOPATHOLOGY

The definitive diagnosis of these conditions requires histopathology. The author typically obtains these samples using laparoscopy, but laparotomy or tru-cut biopsy is also acceptable. Whatever biopsy method is chosen, it is important to collect several samples from across the liver to obtain a representative sample and achieve a confident diagnosis. It is good practice to also culture the liver, sample the bile for culture and cytology, and consider freezing some fresh liver tissue in case further testing (such as copper quantification) is required.

The histopathology in PVH is the same as that seen in any other condition causing inadequate portal venous blood flow. The profile of the portal vein in the portal tracts becomes diminished or absent. Hepatic arteries increase their blood flow in response, leading to them becoming more tortuous, with arteriolar proliferation and/or hypertrophy. Other changes include lobular atrophy, the presence of lipogranulomas, and sinusoidal dilatation (Figure 7.2) (Cullen et al. 2006).

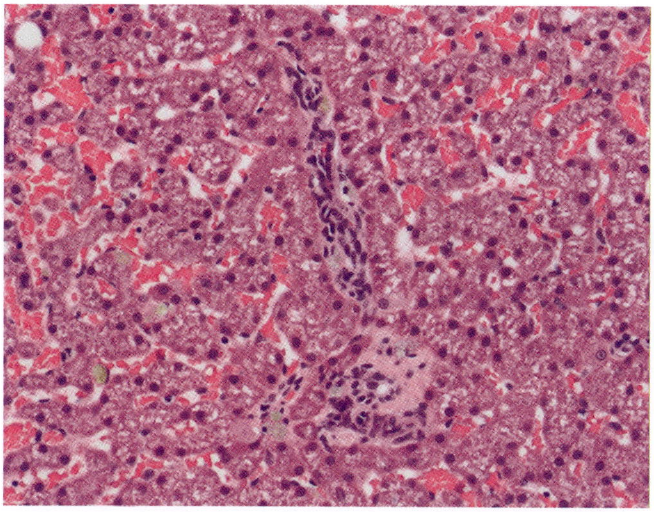

Photo by Dr. Rebecca Smedley

FIGURE 7.2 H&E liver histology from a dog with MVD/PVH. Small portal tract with inapparent portal venous profiles, arteriolar proliferation, and small lipogranulomas adjacent to the portal adventitia

PVH with PH shares the above histopathological pattern of portal vein hypoperfusion; however, in addition, a variable amount of fibrosis is likely to be present. It is important that appropriate staining techniques are utilized to demonstrate fibrosis (Masson's trichrome or picrosirius red). See Chapter 4.

TREATMENT

The aim of treatment is to control the clinical signs. Given that these are often absent in PVH, it is possible that many of these patients **do not require any treatment**. If HE is present (either in PVH or PVH with PH), this should be managed as would be the case in a macroscopic PSS (see Chapter 8). Acutely this might involve fluid therapy, monitoring and addressing electrolyte imbalance, lactulose enemas, and potentially antimicrobials. Chronically, this typically involves nutritional therapy and lactulose with or without antimicrobials.

NUTRITION

In asymptomatic dogs, no dietary modification is necessary but in patients with clinical signs, nutrition is a critical component of management. Please see Chapter 20.

ANTIFIBROTICS

Given that fibrosis may be a feature of PVH with PH, there is interest in whether antifibrotics might be a useful component of therapy. Options include spironolactone, telmisartan (or other angiotensin receptor blockers), and ursodeoxycholic acid. The benefit of these is currently unknown and some carry an adverse effects profile, which could have a negative impact. Colchicine is no longer recommended for use in small animals due to risk of adverse effects.

HEPATOPROTECTIVE THERAPIES

A number of supportive treatments are frequently utilized in liver disease including silybin, S-adenosyl-L-methionine (SAMe), vitamin E, and ursodeoxycholic acid. The benefit of these in PVH or PVH with PH is unknown; however, they are unlikely to have a negative impact.

Overall, several possible avenues of therapy are available to clinicians managing PVH and PVH with PH. The optimal approach should be individualized to each patient based on the presenting signs, age, and presence of other comorbidities. In many cases that may mean that no therapy is necessary.

MONITORING

Optimal monitoring is likely dependent on the presentation and severity of clinical signs. Many patients may require minimal monitoring. If clinical signs have been present then the author would suggest periodic monitoring of hematology, serum albumin, and liver enzymes. Other testing would be dictated by clinical progression.

PROGNOSIS

PVH carries an excellent prognosis, with >90% of dogs having excellent long-term survival or dying of unrelated causes.

PVH with PH may be more variable although survival studies with modern diagnostic and therapeutic strategies are lacking. Most patients will initially have a good response to medical management; however, once acquired PSSs develop, progressive clinical signs may be life limiting (Bunch et al. 2001).

REFERENCES

Bunch, S.E., Johnson, S.E., and Cullen, J.M. (2001). Idiopathic noncirrhotic portal hypertension in dogs: 33 cases (1982-1998). *Journal of the American Veterinary Medical Association* 218 (3): 392–399.

Christiansen, J.S., Hottinger, H.A., Allen, L. et al. (1995). Hepatic microvascular dysplasia in dogs: a retrospective study of 24 cases (1987-1995). *Journal of the American Veterinary Medical Association* 36: 385–389.

Cullen, J., van den Ingh, T.S.G.A.M., Bunch, S.E. et al. (2006). Morphological classification of circulatory disorders of the canine and feline liver. In: *WSAVA Standards for Clinical and Histological Diagnosis of Canine and Feline Liver Diseases* (ed. J. Rothuizen, S.E. Bunch, J. Charles, et al.). Elsevier.

Schermerhorn, T., Center, S.A., Dykes, N.L. et al. (1996). Characterization of hepatoportal microvascular dysplasia in a kindred of cairn terriers. *Journal of Veterinary Internal Medicine* 10 (4): 219–230.

Stockham, S.L. and Scott, M.A. (2008). Liver Function. In: *Fundamentals of Veterinary Clinical Pathology*, 2e, 675–706. Blackwell Publishing.

Toulza, O., Center, S.A., Brooks, M.B. et al. (2006). Evaluation of plasma protein C activity for detection of hepatobiliary disease and portosystemic shunting in dogs. *Journal of the American Veterinary Medical Association* 229 (11): 1761–1771.

Weisse, C. and Berent, A.C. (2024). Congenital vascular liver diseases. In: *Textbook of Veterinary Internal Medicine*, 9e (ed. E. Côté, S.J. Ettinger, and E.C. Feldman), 1782–1800. Elsevier Inc.

Hepatic Encephalopathy

CHAPTER 8

Mickey Tivers[1] *and Vicky Lipscomb*[2]

[1] *Paragon Veterinary Referrals, Paragon point, Wakefield, West Yorkshire, UK*
[2] *Department of Clinical Sciences & Services, Royal Veterinary College, Hatfield, Hertfordshire, UK*

KEY POINTS

- Ammonia is the most important factor in hepatic encephalopathy (HE) in dogs and cats. However, there is increasing evidence that other factors such as inflammation, manganese, and neurosteroids play important roles.
- The most common cause of HE in small animals is congenital portosystemic shunts (CPSS) (Type B), with hepatocellular disease associated with portal hypertension and multiple acquired shunts (MAS) (Type C) being the second most common. Acute liver failure (Type A) is rare.
- Typically, antimicrobials are not required for management of chronic HE and should be reserved for animals that do not respond to dietary adjustments and lactulose.
- New therapies used in people (rifaximin, L-ornithine-L-aspartate, L-carnitine, prebiotics, probiotics) or described in veterinary case reports (therapeutic plasma exchange, intravenous lipid emulsion) could represent novel treatments, but further research is needed, and logistical or financial factors may prohibit their use.

INTRODUCTION

Hepatic encephalopathy (HE) is a complex neurological syndrome seen in dogs and cats with impaired liver function. It is most common in animals with congenital portosystemic shunts (CPSS) but can occur with severe liver disease due to various causes. The pathogenesis of HE is poorly understood, and multiple substances are implicated. Ammonia is a key factor, but it is not the sole cause. It is likely that several factors act synergistically in each animal, and this may explain the variation in signs between individuals. Much of what we know about HE is extrapolated from experimental studies and clinical studies in people.

PATHOPHYSIOLOGY

AMMONIA

Ammonia is a by-product of protein digestion in the small intestine. Glutamine is converted into glutamate in enterocytes, producing ammonia. This is the main source of ammonia, but it is also produced by urease-producing bacteria and the degradation of bacterial proteins.

Ammonia produced in the intestine is transported, via the portal vein, directly to the liver where it is metabolized. Ammonia is converted into urea in the periportal hepatocytes via the urea cycle. Urea is then excreted by the kidneys. Ammonia is also consumed in the conversion of glutamate to glutamine in the perivenous hepatocytes. The liver is extremely efficient in processing ammonia, and therefore systemic blood has very low concentrations. Indeed, there is significant

Disorders of the Liver, Exocrine Pancreas, and Gastrointestinal Tract in Dogs and Cats, First Edition. Edited by Harry Cridge et al. Published 2026 by John Wiley & Sons, Inc. Companion Website: www.wiley.com/go/cridge/disorders

reserve capacity meaning that hyperammonemia is only seen with marked hepatic impairment or significantly reduced portal blood flow. This can occur due to acute liver failure, advanced liver disease with or without multiple acquired shunts (MAS), or in CPSS.

The kidneys play an important role in ammonia metabolism, and they can metabolize and synthesize glutamine. They can therefore excrete ammonia in response to hyperammonemia. Significantly, alkalosis and hypokalemia decrease ammonia secretion and increase renal ammonia production, respectively, making HE worse. Skeletal muscle also plays a role in ammonia metabolism. Myocytes can remove ammonia from the circulation by converting it to glutamine. This allows the temporary buffering of hyperammonemia, but this effect can be mitigated by glutamine release into the circulation. Ammonia can pass freely across the blood brain barrier, where it is metabolized by the astrocytes, resulting in increased glutamine and lactate and ultimately astrocyte swelling.

In dogs and cats with CPSS, ammonia is typically increased and decreases following surgical shunt attenuation. Plasma ammonia concentration is predictive of the presence of HE in dogs with CPSS, although dogs with HE can have normal ammonia (Tivers et al. 2014). This suggests that in some animals, other factors, in addition to ammonia, are important in the pathophysiology of HE. Alternatively, if an animal has evidence of apparent HE but ammonia is normal, then the clinical signs could be due to a non-hepatic cause (i.e., not HE), and this should be considered and investigated as appropriate.

INFLAMMATION

It is well recognized in human medicine that inflammation and infection play an important role in the pathophysiology of HE. Inflammatory mediators contribute to HE by potentiating the effect of ammonia on the brain. Indeed, severe HE in people is associated with systemic inflammation rather than ammonia. Inflammation drives HE by increasing cerebral blood flow and increasing the permeability of the blood brain barrier to ammonia.

In dogs, both systemic inflammatory response syndrome (SIRS) and C-reactive protein have been associated with HE (Lidbury et al. 2016; Gow 2017). In dogs with increased ammonia, SIRS was a risk factor for the development of clinical HE (Tivers et al. 2014). In dogs or cats with chronic HE a focus of inflammation/infection can cause a deterioration of clinical signs. These data support the role of inflammation in HE in companion animals.

MANGANESE

Manganese (Mn) in high concentrations can be neurotoxic. Mn is absorbed from the intestine, filtered by the liver, and excreted in the bile. Liver disease is associated with increased circulating Mn, which accumulates in astrocytes, causing similar lesions as ammonia (Alzheimer type II astrocytes). It is believed that Mn acts synergistically with ammonia to increase the production of neurosteroids. There is an increase in Mn blood concentrations in dogs with CPSS and liver disease, and MRI brain lesions, similar to those identified in people, in dogs and cats with CPSS (Lidbury et al. 2016; Gow 2017). These findings support a similar role of Mn in HE in dogs and cats.

NEUROSTEROIDS

Neurosteroids (e.g., allopregnanolone and tetrahydrodeoxycorticosterone) are gamma-aminobutyric acid (GABA) receptor ligands and are significantly increased in people with HE (Lidbury et al. 2016; Gow 2017). Ammonia and Mn are thought to increase the synthesis of neurosteroids by activating the peripheral type benzodiazepine receptor (PTBR) (Lidbury et al. 2016; Gow 2017). Data supports that increased GABAergic tone is associated with HE in dogs (Lidbury et al. 2016).

FALSE NEUROTRANSMITTERS

In people with cirrhosis, the ratio of aromatic amino acids is significantly increased compared to branched chain amino acids. Experimental evidence suggests that increased concentrations of aromatic amino acids in the brain cause the production of false neurotransmitters, reducing neural excitation (Lidbury et al. 2016). However, treatment with branched chain amino acids in people is not considered effective in reducing signs of HE (Lidbury et al. 2016).

Historically, several substances including aromatic amino acids (phenylalanine, tyrosine, tryptophan, and methionine), central nervous system inhibitors (GABA and GABA receptors), mercaptans, and short-chain fatty acids have been associated with HE in small animals. However, based on the human literature, these may be less important. Nevertheless, a recent study in dogs with various liver diseases showed similar changes in amino acid profiles to those seen in people (Imbery et al. 2022), and another study demonstrated that total aromatic amino acids were significantly increased in CPSS dogs (Phillips et al. 2025).

OTHER FACTORS

In people, hyponatremia, hypokalemia, and alkalosis are associated with HE.

Hypokalemia causes increased renal ammonia production and reduced excretion. Also, movement of potassium out of cells can trap intracellular ammonium. Hyponatremia increases cerebral edema and astrocyte swelling. Alkalosis causes a shift from ammonium to ammonia, which can pass through cell membranes.

Other precipitating factors include gastrointestinal hemorrhage, constipation, diarrhea, infection, and excessive dietary protein.

It is assumed that these derangements will have a similar effect in dogs and cats. However, a study investigating potential precipitating factors for HE in dogs did not confirm this (Lidbury et al. 2015). Nevertheless, consideration should still be given to treating these factors in animals with HE (see below).

ASTROCYTES, ACUTE AND CHRONIC HE

One of the key changes in HE is astrocyte swelling. As outlined above, many factors contribute to this, including ammonia (through the action of glutamine), Mn, inflammatory cytokines, and hyponatremia.

In acute HE, the astrocyte swelling is severe, resulting in cerebral edema and increased intracranial pressure, which is exacerbated by increased cerebral blood flow. In severe cases, this can lead to herniation, brainstem compression, and death.

In chronic HE, astrocyte swelling is less severe and results in Alzheimer type II astrocytes. Alzheimer type II astrocytes are a characteristic pathological cell type characteristic of hyperammonemia. Other factors play a more significant role in chronic HE, and ammonia is less directly correlated. Chronic HE is more common in dogs and cats due to the types of disorders seen. A histopathological study of the brains of dogs with HE and CPSS confirmed Alzheimer type II astrocytes, consistent with changes seen in people with HE (Williams et al. 2020).

CAUSES OF HE

In humans, HE is classified into three types based on etiology:

- Type A: acute liver failure in the absence of preexisting liver disease
- Type B: portosystemic bypass with no intrinsic hepatic disease (i.e., a CPSS)
- Type C: associated with cirrhosis, portal hypertension, and MAS.

Unlike people, CPSS (Type B) represents the most common cause of HE in dogs and cats. In dogs and cats, Type C would be better defined as "associated with all types of hepatocellular disease, portal hypertension, and MAS." Acute liver failure (Type A) is the least common in companion animals. Thus, primary hepatopathies, such as acute hepatitis, advanced chronic hepatitis in dogs, and cholangitis or hepatic lipidosis in cats, may also manifest with HE, although other signs such as jaundice and/or ascites are often present. In addition, although uncommon, dogs and cats can have increased ammonia and HE because of congenital abnormalities of their urea cycle.

In one study investigating increased ammonia in 90 dogs, ultrasound diagnosed CPSS in 68% and MAS (including hepatic arteriovenous malformation) in 19% (Szatmari et al. 2004). A more recent study found that of 102 dogs with HE and complete diagnostic information, 72% were Type B and 28% were Type C (with no Type A) (Lidbury et al. 2015).

In a study of 49 dogs with acute liver failure, 57% showed signs of HE during hospitalization (Lester et al. 2016). The signs of HE developed or persisted despite appropriate medical treatment, although the specific details of this were not included in the study.

It is important to note that, overall, the treatment for HE remains the same, regardless of the cause. However, the underlying condition should also be managed, and this will be dictated by the disease process. In addition, any exacerbating factors (such as electrolyte disturbances) must also be addressed.

CLINICAL SIGNS

Clinical signs associated with HE can be relatively mild, such as subtle changes in behavior, to very severe, such as stupor or seizures.

A modification of a human grading scale has been suggested for dogs and cats.

HE grade	Clinical signs
0	Asymptomatic
I	Mild decrease in mobility, apathy, or both
II	Severe apathy, mild ataxia
III	Combination of hypersalivation, severe ataxia, head pressing, blindness, circling
IV	Stupor/coma, seizures

Source: Gow, 2017/with permission of Elsevier.

Clinical signs can be relatively subtle and can wax and wane. Some animals may appear "normal." In human patients with liver disease a syndrome of minimal HE or covert HE is recognized. People appear normal but demonstrate significant abnormalities on psychometric testing and in neurophysiological performance. It is unknown whether this occurs in dogs or cats. However, if this does happen then it could lead to under-recognition and/or undertreatment of affected individuals.

HE can be acute or chronic and this can also affect the clinical signs. Chronic HE is commonly seen in dogs and cats with CPSS or MAS due to severe, chronic liver disease. Some animals may experience acute deterioration of chronic HE associated with another disease process that "destabilizes" their condition, such as a urinary tract infection or gastroenteritis.

Acute HE is seen in severe liver disease/failure. The signs are severe (grades III or IV) and rapidly progressive. In these animals, HE is typically complicated by other contributing factors such as electrolyte derangements.

DIAGNOSIS

HE is suspected based on history and appropriate clinical signs. The index of suspicion should be very high in animals known to have a CPSS or significant liver disease. Typically, dogs and cats with HE will have increased plasma ammonia concentrations. Ammonia can be difficult to measure in practice, as false positives can occur if approved protocols are not followed, as ammonia can increase in vitro due to release by red blood cells. Animals should be fasted for 12 hours prior to sampling to avoid lipemia, which can interfere with the test. Samples are collected in a heparin or ethylenediaminetetraacetic acid (EDTA) tube, which must be completely filled, well mixed, and the lid kept closed until the test is run. The sample must be placed on ice immediately and the plasma must be separated within 15 minutes. The sample should be run as soon as possible (within 30 minutes). In-house dry chemistry analyzers are too inaccurate to be recommended. Nevertheless, ammonia is the most useful biochemical marker of HE. In addition to ammonia, one study found that a high SIRS score was also predictive of HE and this may be useful to assess, particularly if ammonia measurement is not available (Tivers et al. 2014).

Routine hematology and biochemistry should be performed in animals with a suspicion of HE to check for liver disease and to identify any exacerbating factors that might need to be addressed (e.g., electrolyte disturbances). Diagnostic imaging and appropriate sampling should also be performed to obtain further information regarding liver disease or CPSS.

MEDICAL TREATMENT (ACUTE AND CHRONIC)

Medical management involves the emergency treatment of acute HE or flare-ups of chronic HE and the long-term management of chronic HE. Importantly, consideration must also be given to treatment of the underlying cause (e.g., CPSS attenuation).

Medical management treats the clinical signs of HE, primarily by modifying the gut environment to reduce the production and absorption of ammonia and other compounds. However, medical management does not treat the underlying cause.

Medical management involves treating with one or more of dietary modification, lactulose, and antibacterials (Table 8.1). For the management of chronic HE, it is best practice to start with dietary modification and to add lactulose and then antibacterials to the treatment regimen as necessary. Medication should be tailored to reach the minimum effective treatment. Animals with CPSS should be stabilized with medical management for a minimum of 2–4 weeks prior to surgery. The authors will routinely treat animals with CPSS with diet and lactulose but do not routinely use antimicrobials.

DIET

Bacterial metabolism of dietary protein, particularly protein in red meats that is rich in aromatic amino acids (e.g., tyrosine, tryptophan, phenylalanine), is a source of ammonia. Therefore, modification of dietary protein content is extremely important in moderating HE. However, severe protein restriction is not recommended as it can lead to malnutrition, reduced serum albumin concentration, and a potentially poorer prognosis. There are a variety of commercially available hepatic diets, which may be suitable for animals with HE. A hydrolyzed soy protein diet is recommended for

Table 8.1 Recommended Medical Management for Animals with Chronic Hepatic Encephalopathy

Medical treatment	Recommended dose and frequency
Lactulose	Dogs: 0.5–1.0 mL/kg orally q8–12h (ideally two to three soft stools per day)
	Cats: 0.5–5.0 mL orally q8–12h (ideally two to three soft stools per day)
Antibiotics*	
Ampicillin	10–20 mg/kg orally q8h
Potentiated amoxycillin	12.5 mg/kg orally q12h
Metronidazole	7.5–10 mg/kg orally q12h
Neomycin†	20 mg/kg orally q8–12h

*Antimicrobials not required in many instances and should be reserved for animals nonresponsive to diet and lactulose.
†Contraindicated if concurrent intestinal disease, as it may be absorbed and cause nephrotoxicity and/or ototoxicity.

young, growing animals, as this has a high-quality protein content and thus limits ammonia production, while not restricting the protein available for growth. The author prefers a hydrolyzed soya diet (e.g., Purina Pro Plan Veterinary Diet HA Canine and Feline), particularly in puppies and kittens, as it is suitable for growth. Please see Chapter 20 for further information on diet in animals with HE.

LACTULOSE

Successful management of HE often requires the administration of lactulose in addition to dietary modification. However, its mechanism of action and benefit is still debated. Lactulose is used in combination with antimicrobials and can be synergistic.

Lactulose is a non-absorbable, synthetic disaccharide (fructose-galactose) that passes through the small intestine without being absorbed or metabolized. It is hydrolyzed by colonic bacteria (primarily *Bacteroides* spp.) to lactic, acetic, and formic acids. These organic acids reduce the pH of the colonic contents trapping fee ammonia (NH3) as ammonium (NH4+) ions. Ammonia diffuses freely across the mucosa whereas ammonium does not. Hence, acidification reduces the amount of ammonia absorbed and therefore increases fecal ammonia and nitrogen excretion.

In addition, lactulose is an osmotic laxative and therefore may act, in part, by decreasing intestinal transit time, reducing the production and absorption of ammonia and other toxins.

Lactulose also increases fecal nitrogen content via the incorporation of ammonia into bacterial proteins.

The effect of lactulose on fecal consistency is quite variable, and the recommended initial dose should be adjusted empirically until an individual animal is producing two to three soft stools a day. Both too little lactulose, with continued fecal retention, and too much, with consequent diarrhea, can worsen HE. In animals with severe HE causing stupor or coma, a lactulose retention enema may be given.

A recent study found good evidence that lactulose modified the fecal microbiota in healthy dogs, supporting its use for the management of HE (Ferreira et al. 2019).

ANTIMICROBIALS

These are used to reduce the urease-positive gut bacteria implicated in the production of ammonia and can therefore ameliorate the signs of HE. Ideally these antimicrobials should not be absorbed in the intestine and should be effective against ammonia producing bacteria. Ampicillin, amoxicillin, amoxicillin clavulanate, neomycin, and metronidazole have all been used to treat HE in dogs and cats. However, the chronic administration of antibacterials is a potential public health risk because of the selection of antibiotic resistance, and their use should be kept to a minimum. Antibacterials are therefore reserved for those animals where dietary modification and lactulose produce inadequate control of signs.

A recent study showed that antimicrobials are not essential for managing HE in dogs with CPSS, reporting a relatively good long-term outcome with dietary modification with or without lactulose and no antibiotics (Favier et al. 2020). Another study found that lactulose and diet alone was sufficient for the stabilization of dogs with CPSS prior to surgery, with hepatic diet alone or in combination with metronidazole not resulting in a significant improvement in clinical signs (Serrano et al. 2022).

EMERGENCY MEDICAL MANAGEMENT

Animals can be presented collapsed, comatose, or in status epilepticus due to severe HE. On occasion this may have been precipitated by an anesthetic episode or other insult in an animal with chronic HE. A variety of factors have been implicated in worsening HE or precipitating it in a previously stable animal, although specific evidence is lacking (Lidbury et al. 2015). Dehydration, hypokalemia, and metabolic alkalosis, either because of diarrhea or overzealous furosemide administration, or portal hypertension in animals with chronic liver disease, should be corrected with intravenous fluid therapy and potassium supplementation. If diuresis is necessary, spironolactone should be used instead of furosemide.

Other potential risk factors include hypovolemia, GI hemorrhage, constipation, and azotemia, and these should be addressed when present.

A minimum database (including blood glucose and serum electrolytes) should be performed to rule out other potential causes of seizure or collapse and to identify any complicating factors. Animals should be given intravenous fluid therapy with appropriate supplementation to correct any hypoperfusion, dehydration, or metabolic abnormalities. Medical therapy should be started as described above with lactulose and antimicrobials, although in a comatose or seizuring animal it will not be possible to administer drugs orally. Parenteral antimicrobials can be given, although they are likely to be less effective than oral antimicrobials in managing HE. Alternatively, neomycin can be given rectally. Antimicrobials will be particularly important in an animal with a documented infection or sepsis contributing to HE. Lactulose can be administered as a retention enema. The lactulose is diluted in a 3:7 ratio with warm water and administered at a dose of 10 mL/kg, retained for 30 minutes. A warm water cleansing enema should be given prior to medicated enemas as this will remove feces and hence reduce ammonia absorption from the colon. These are typically given at a dose of 10 mL/kg every 4–6 hours.

Diazepam is often given as a first line treatment for seizures. However, there is some controversy over the use of diazepam in animals with HE due to concerns over increased GABA and GABA receptors. Individuals which do not respond to diazepam should ideally be treated with levetiracetam intravenously. Phenobarbital is hepatically metabolized so it should be avoided or used with caution in animals with liver disease. Once the animal is stabilized, oral medication can be started, and antimicrobials are withdrawn if possible (see above). Rarely, it may be necessary to treat with propofol or alfaxalone, either by bolus or infusion to control the seizures.

In animals with severe HE, cerebral edema can develop and may contribute to neurologic signs. A single bolus of mannitol can be given as a therapeutic trial, though mannitol should not be used in severely dehydrated or hypoperfused animals. Monitoring progression and response to therapy of severely encephalopathic animals may be facilitated by use of the modified Glasgow Coma Scale.

OTHER MEDICATIONS

Rifaximin is an antimicrobial used for the management of HE in people and is well tolerated and effective either alone or in combination with lactulose (Lidbury et al. 2016). However, it is very expensive, and this is likely to be prohibitive for use in cats and dogs.

Therapeutic plasma exchange (TPE) and continuous renal replacement therapy (CRRT) have been used to improve signs of HE in people and there is a case report suggesting that TPE could have potential in dogs (Culler et al. 2020). This involves removing the plasma component of blood and replacing it with donated plasma or a substitute (crystalloids and colloids). Therefore, TPE removes ammonia and other toxins associated with HE. The case report describes a dog with a CPSS and significant signs of HE associated with hyperammonemia, which did not respond to standard medical management (Culler et al. 2020). There was a significant reduction in ammonia and an improvement in HE signs, suggesting a beneficial effect for TPE. TPE has potential but is not widely available in veterinary practice.

A case report described the successful use of intravenous lipid emulsion (ILE) therapy for the management of signs of severe HE associated with marked hyperammonemia in a dog with a CPSS (Spillane et al. 2021). ILE was initially given due to a suspicion of naproxen intoxication, that was subsequently ruled out. Ammonia is a lipophilic compound, and it is hypothesized that ILE drew the ammonia from the brain and into the lipid partition in the intravascular space. There was a rapid resolution of clinical signs, and blood ammonia concentration was dramatically reduced within 24 hours (with additional lactulose treatment). Further research is needed to assess this treatment further.

A study investigated the efficacy of oral sodium benzoate and sodium phenylbutyrate for the treatment of HE in dogs with CPSS (van Straten et al. 2019). These treatments are used in people with urea cycle deficiencies and lower blood ammonia concentration through alternative pathways (van Straten et al. 2019). However, the study did not find any benefit of these drugs on ammonia levels or clinical signs, and they were not considered to be effective treatment options.

In people, several other treatments have been used for the management of HE. Flumazenil is a benzodiazepine receptor antagonist and has been used for the short-term management of overt HE in people (Lidbury et al. 2016). It may be particularly useful when managing HE associated with the use of benzodiazepines. However, experimental data in dogs suggests that flumazenil does not improve signs of HE (Meyer et al. 1998). L-ornithine-L-aspartate is believed to increase the detoxification of ammonia through acting on the urea cycle and the conversion of ammonia to glutamine. It is effective in treating people with mild-to-moderate HE (Lidbury et al. 2016). Treatment of HE with L-carnitine to prevent glutamate mediated neurotoxicity has shown promise in reducing ammonia concentrations and improving neurophysiological performance in people (Lidbury et al. 2016). In addition, modification of the microbiota of the gastrointestinal tract toward non-urease producing bacteria has been proposed through the use of prebiotics, probiotics, and synbiotics (Lidbury et al. 2016). However, the evidence is variable, and the efficacy of these treatments remain controversial. To the authors' knowledge there is no evidence for the use of these treatments in small animals.

CONCLUSION

HE is complex and our understanding of its pathophysiology and treatment in dogs and cats is limited. Ammonia remains the most important factor in terms of monitoring and treatment, but consideration must be given to other compounds and predisposing factors. Further research might concentrate on validating novel treatments, optimizing dietary modifications, and improving short- and long-term outcomes for our patients.

REFERENCES

Culler, C.A., Reinhardt, A., and Vigani, A. (2020). Successful management of clinical signs associated with hepatic encephalopathy with manual therapeutic plasma exchange in a dog. *Journal of Veterinary Emergency and Critical Care (San Antonio)* 30 (3): 312–317.

Favier, R.P., de Graaf, E., Corbee, R.J. et al. (2020). Outcome of non-surgical dietary treatment with or without lactulose in dogs with congenital portosystemic shunts. *Veterinary Quarterly* 40 (1): 108–114.

Ferreira, M.D.F., Salavati Schmitz, S., Schoenebeck, J.J. et al. (2019). Lactulose drives a reversible reduction and qualitative modulation of the faecal microbiota diversity in healthy dogs. *Scientific Reports* 9 (1): 13350.

Gow, A.G. (2017). Hepatic encephalopathy. *Veterinary Clinics of North America: Small Animal Practice* 47 (3): 585–599.

Imbery, C.A., Dieterle, F., Ottka, C. et al. (2022). Metabolomic serum abnormalities in dogs with hepatopathies. *Scientific Reports* 12 (1): 5329.

Lester, C., Cooper, J., Peters, R.M. et al. (2016). Retrospective evaluation of acute liver failure in dogs (1995-2012): 49 cases. *Journal of Veterinary Emergency and Critical Care (San Antonio)* 26 (4): 559–567.

Lidbury, J.A., Cook, A.K., and Steiner, J.M. (2016). Hepatic encephalopathy in dogs and cats. *Journal of Veterinary Emergency and Critical Care (San Antonio)* 26 (4): 471–487.

Lidbury, J.A., Ivanek. R., Suchodolski, J.S. et al. (2015). Putative precipitating factors for hepatic encephalopathy in dogs: 118 cases (1991-2014). *Journal of the American Veterinary Medical Association* 247 (2): 176–183.

Meyer, H.P., Legemate, D.A., van den Brom, W. et al. (1998). Improvement of chronic hepatic encephalopathy in dogs by the benzodiazepine-receptor partial inverse agonist sarmazenil, but not by the antagonist flumazenil. *Metabolic Brain Disease* 13 (3): 241–251.

Phillips, R.K., Blake, A.B., Tivers, M.S. et al. (2025). Serum amino acid profiles in dogs with a congenital portosystemic shunt. *Metabolites* 15 (4): 258.

Serrano, G., Devriendt, N., de Rooster, H. et al. (2022). Comparison of diet, lactulose, and metronidazole combinations in the control of pre-surgical clinical signs in dogs with congenital extrahepatic portosystemic shunts. *Journal of Veterinary Internal Medicine* 36 (4): 1258–1266.

Spillane, A.M., Haraschak, J.L., and McMichael, M.A. (2021). Resolution of severe neurologic signs following intravenous lipid emulsion therapy in a young dog with a portosystemic shunt: case report. *Frontiers in Veterinary Science* 8: 798198.

Szatmari, V., Rothuizen, J., van den Ingh, T.S. et al. (2004). Ultrasonographic findings in dogs with hyperammonemia: 90 cases (2000-2002). *Journal of the American Veterinary Medical Association* 224 (5): 717–727.

Tivers, M.S., Handel, I., Gow, A.G. et al. (2014). Hyperammonemia and systemic inflammatory response syndrome predicts presence of hepatic encephalopathy in dogs with congenital portosystemic shunts. *PLoS One* 9 (1): e82303.

van Straten, G., van Dalen, D., Mesu, S.J. et al. (2019). Efficacy of orally administered sodium benzoate and sodium phenylbutyrate in dogs with congenital portosystemic shunts. *Journal of Veterinary Internal Medicine* 33 (3): 1331–1335.

Williams, A., Gow, A., Kilpatrick, S. et al. (2020). Astrocyte lesions in cerebral cortex and cerebellum of dogs with congenital ortosystemic shunting. *Journal of Veterinary Science* 21 (3): e44.

CHAPTER 9

Portal Hypertension and Acquired Portosystemic Shunts

Joshua Sparago[1] *and Andrea N. Johnston*[2]

[1] *Le Centre Hospitalier Universitaire Vétérinaire – Faculté de Médecine Vétérinaire, Université de Montréal, Saint-Hyacinthe, QC, Canada*
[2] *Departments of Pathobiology and Diagnostic Investigation/Small Animal Clinical Sciences, College of Veterinary Medicine, Michigan State University, East Lansing, MI, USA*

KEY POINTS

- Portal hypertension (PH) is classified based on anatomic location of increased resistance or impedance of portal blood flow relative to the liver (e.g., prehepatic, intrahepatic, or posthepatic).
- Diagnosis of PH in clinical veterinary medicine is inferred based on physical exam findings and diagnostic imaging that reveal sequelae of PH (e.g., acquired portosystemic shunts).
- Treatment of PH focuses on correction of the underlying cause, if possible, and management of secondary complications.
- Prognosis in patients with portal hypertension and acquired portosystemic shunts is variable, but some dogs can survive for years with minimal supportive care.

HEPATIC BLOOD FLOW

The portal venous circulation begins in the abdomen at the confluence of the cranial and caudal mesenteric veins, receiving venous blood from the gastrointestinal tract, pancreas, and spleen. The portal vein merges with the hepatic circulation at the porta, sequentially arborizing on its path to the hepatic lobules. Nutrient rich portal venous blood mixes with oxygenated arterial blood as it traverses the hepatic sinusoids to the hepatic venules. Hepatic venous blood exits the liver into the vena cava *en route* to the right atrium. Portal venous blood contributes ~70–80% of the hepatic blood flow and under basal conditions maintains a perfusion pressure of ~5–9 mmHg in dogs and cats. The hepatic sinusoids are essential for preserving this low portal pressure due to their high capacitance, low resistance, and ability to release vasoactive substances that regulate sinusoidal blood flow (Buob et al. 2011; Johnston 2023).

PORTAL HYPERTENSION

Portal hypertension (PH) is an increase in portal venous pressure (Dogs: >11 mmHg, Cats: >12 mmHg) subsequent to increased resistance or impedance of flow within the portal circulation (Johnston 2023). The increased pressure gradient may occur at multiple anatomic locations relative to the liver; thus, PH is classified based on its locus: prehepatic (portal vein), intrahepatic (pre-sinusoidal, sinusoidal, post-sinusoidal), and posthepatic (right atrium, caudal vena cava [CVC], hepatic veins, Table 9.1).

Prehepatic PH is associated with conditions that impede portal circulation at the level of the extrahepatic portal vein by intraluminal obstruction, extraluminal compression, or derangements of blood flow as with congenital or acquired mesenteric arteriovenous malformations.

Table 9.1 Examples of Portal Hypertension Etiology (*List Is Not Exhaustive*)

Location	Etiology
Prehepatic (portal vein)	Congenital portal vein aplasia, atresia, or macroscopic hypoplasia
	Increased venous pressure gradient (mesenteric AV malformation, complication of congenital portosystemic shunt attenuation)
	Intraluminal obstruction
	• *Thrombus, neoplasm, thrombophlebitis, stenosis/stricture*
	Extraluminal compression
	• *Neoplasm, lymphadenomegaly, granuloma, abscess*
Intrahepatic (liver)	Pre-sinusoidal
	• Hepatic arteriovenous malformation
	• Cholangitis (neutrophilic, lymphoplasmacytic)
	• Trematode infestation (e.g., *Heterobilharzia americana, Platynosomum concinnum, Metorchis orientalis, Metorchis conjunctus*)
	• Fibropolycystic liver disease (e.g., *congenital hepatic fibrosis*)
	• Nodular regenerative hyperplasia
	Sinusoidal
	• Chronic hepatitis
	• Sinusoidal fibrosis or cirrhosis (uncommon in dogs and cats)
	• Cholangiohepatitis
	• Ductal plate malformations (e.g., *polycystic liver disease)*
	Post-sinusoidal
	• Obliterative or occlusive venopathy – *idiopathic, NSAIDs, toxins, severe copper hepatopathy, thrombosis, degeneration, compression by lipogranulomas or extramedullary hematopoiesis*
Posthepatic (hepatic veins, caudal vena cava, heart)	Obstructive hepatic venous outflow (*Budd–Chiari syndrome*)
	• *Thrombosis, neoplasia, caval syndrome (heartworm-associated), congenital fibrous webs or acquired kinking, liver lobe entrapment*
	Right heart failure
	• *Congestive, pericardial disease, intracardiac neoplasm, pulmonary hypertension*

Intrahepatic PH results from impedance of blood flow through the macroscopic or microscopic hepatic circulation. Intrahepatic PH is also spatially defined relative to venous vascular flow through the hepatic sinusoids (pre-sinusoidal [e.g., cholangitis], sinusoidal [e.g., chronic hepatitis], and post-sinusoidal [e.g., veno-occlusive disease]).

Posthepatic PH is caused by attenuation or obstruction of hepatic venous outflow at the level of the larger hepatic veins, posthepatic CVC, or right atrium due to intraluminal obstruction, extraluminal compression, or stenosis of the larger hepatic veins or posthepatic CVC (sometimes referred to as Budd–Chiari syndrome) (Bayraktar et al. 2007).

COMPLICATIONS OF PH

PERITONEAL EFFUSION

Peritoneal effusion results from disruptions in Starling's forces, where elevated portal vein hydrostatic pressure and its associated sequelae drive fluid out of the vascular space. Activation of the renin–angiotensin–aldosterone system, sympathetic neurons, and non-osmotic release of anti-diuretic hormone (ADH) result in volume expansion and further increases in vascular hydrostatic pressure (Buob et al. 2011; Leiva et al. 2007). Peritoneal effusion may be exacerbated if concurrent hypoalbuminemia (all causes) is present due to decreased intravascular oncotic pressure (Buob et al. 2011).

MULTIPLE ACQUIRED PORTOSYSTEMIC SHUNTS

As PH progresses, luminal distension of the remnant embryonic splanchnic vasculature in conjunction with *de novo* vasculogenesis leads to the development of multiple acquired portosystemic shunts (MAPSSs). These collateral vessels divert portal blood directly into systemic circulation (Fernandez et al. 2009). MAPSSs can be a consequence of prehepatic or intrahepatic PH, and in experimental canine models, MAPSS have been shown to form over a period of 5–14 weeks (Bosch et al. 1983; Howe et al. 2000). Unlike humans, esophageal varices (MAPSSs that develop between the portal vein and the submucosal esophageal vessels) and associated rupture and hemorrhage are uncommon in dogs and cats (Johnston 2023).

HEPATIC ENCEPHALOPATHY

Hepatic encephalopathy (HE) is a syndrome of diminished cerebral function caused by the accumulation of neurotoxic substances secondary to failed hepatic clearance (Buob et al. 2011). In cases of PH, HE may develop secondary to advanced primary hepatic disease or the development of MAPSS, which bypass the hepatic sinusoidal blood flow. Several neurotoxins have been implicated in the development and perpetuation of HE, including ammonia, glutamate, and manganese. When left unchecked, these substances induce mitochondrial dysfunction, neurotransmission impairment, and cellular swelling of astrocytes, which are the primary site of ammonia detoxification, glutamate metabolism, and manganese accumulation. Additionally, excess ammonia can stimulate the release of proinflammatory cytokines and generation of reactive oxygen species, contributing to inflammation and oxidative damage in the brain. Please see Chapter 8 for a complete discussion on HE.

COAGULOPATHY

Hemostatic balance is precarious in PH. Turbulent portal blood flow and hepatic hypoperfusion can modulate platelet synthesis through diminished thrombopoietin synthesis and deranged platelet activation. Further, the liver synthesizes and clears most procoagulant, anticoagulant, and fibrinolytic factors. The liver is also required for activation of vitamin K-dependent clotting factors II, VII, IX, and X, as well as anticoagulant protein C. In dogs and cats with PH, the balance of hemostasis can shift toward either hypocoagulability or hypercoagulability, increasing their susceptibility to bleeding or thrombosis, respectively (Webster 2017).

PORTAL HYPERTENSIVE GASTROPATHY

Portal hypertensive gastropathy leading to gastrointestinal hemorrhage is a well-described complication in humans with PH but has been poorly documented in dogs (Tan 2024). The pathogenesis of portal hypertensive gastropathy is related to venous congestion, reduced arterial perfusion, and abnormal mucosal function but not erosive ulceration as seen in gastritis. Ultrastructural studies have shown that bleeding occurs through extravasation of red blood cells.

DIAGNOSIS OF PH AND MAPSS

Historically, definitive diagnosis of PH required direct or indirect techniques to measure the portal venous pressure, but this is impractical in clinical settings. Typically, the presence of portal hypertension is reliant upon definitive (MAPSS) and supportive (abdominal effusion) markers of PH sequelae and other correlative vascular imaging findings (Please see Chapter 2). As shear wave elastography and magnetic resonance elastography are used more commonly at veterinary referral institutions, it is hoped that additional noninvasive metrics of PH detection will become common place in dogs and cats, as with human patients.

CLINICAL SIGNS AND PHYSICAL EXAMINATION FINDINGS

The clinical presentation of PH and MAPSSs may include abdominal distension secondary to peritoneal effusion and episodic neurological signs secondary to HE (ranging from apathy, mental obtundation, and ptyalism to stupor, coma, and even seizures). Melena or hematemesis may be seen secondary to gastrointestinal bleeding, and acute abdominal pain can be present with portal vein thrombosis (Respess et al. 2012; Rogers et al. 2008). Nonspecific signs are more commonly observed and include lethargy, anorexia, weight loss, vomiting, and polyuria/polydipsia.

CLINICAL PATHOLOGY

The minimum database for all patients suspected of having PH includes a complete blood count (CBC), biochemistry, urinalysis, ± assessment of coagulation status, ± serum total bile acid concentrations or, if unavailable, arterial ammonia levels.

Complete Blood Count

The CBC may reveal microcytosis (low mean corpuscular volume) in dogs with MAPSSs. This is presumed to be associated with a currently unidentified defect in mobilization of iron stores rather than a true state of iron deficiency (Simpson et al. 1997). Some dogs with PH may also have thrombocytopenia, anemia, and poikilocytosis associated with microangiopathic red blood cell injury.

Serum Biochemistry

Serum liver enzyme activity may be normal or increased, dependent on the underlying cause of PH. Patients with prehepatic PH may have completely normal liver enzymes to mild elevations. Mild to moderate increases are usually caused by posthepatic PH, while moderate to marked increases are typically seen with intrahepatic PH associated with necroinflammatory disorders (Buob et al. 2011).

Urinalysis

Urine specific gravity in PH patients is variable. The urinalysis may reveal proteinuria, which can contribute to hypoalbuminemia. Protein-losing nephropathy is associated with hypercoagulability in dogs and weakly in cats, predisposing them to the development of thromboembolic complications such as portal vein thrombosis (Respess et al. 2012; deLaforcade et al. 2022).

Ammonia or ammonium biurate crystals may be present in cats and dogs with MAPSS or advanced liver disease. Inflammatory cells and bacteria may be correlated with systemic or hepatobiliary infections. Rarely, acquired collateral vessels can develop in the bladder wall and rupture may cause hematuria.

Coagulation

If invasive procedures such as liver biopsy are planned, a platelet count, prothrombin time (PT), and activated partial thromboplastin time (aPTT) should be assessed and addressed (Center et al. 2000). Since PT and aPTT do not reflect the entire state of coagulation, additional parameters to consider include fibrinogen, antithrombin (AT), protein C, D-dimers, and fibrin degradation products (FDPs). Decreased serum concentrations of fibrinogen, AT, and protein C are associated with the presence of PH in dogs (Buob et al. 2011). Prior to invasive procedures, the authors perform a blood smear to confirm that the platelet count is ≥100 000 platelets/μL, PT, and aPTT. If thrombocytopathia is possible, buccal mucosal bleeding time and/or von Willebrand factor (vWF) are also assessed. Vitamin K_1 is administered to hyperbilirubinemic patients (0.5–1 mg/kg SQ or IM, every 12 hours for 3 doses prior to tissue sampling). If the patient has documented coagulation abnormalities and hepatic sampling is deemed diagnostically necessary, appropriate blood products are transfused prior to and during sampling.

LIVER FUNCTION

Increases in blood ammonia or total serum bile acid concentrations may be observed with PH due to synthetic dysfunction or reduced hepatic clearance but also result from hepatic hypoperfusion secondary to acquired shunts. Synthesis of albumin, cholesterol, BUN, and glucose can also be deranged due to true hepatic dysfunction or hypofunction secondary to hypoperfusion. Results must be interpreted cautiously due to the clinical overlap in PH and MAPSS. Bilirubin may be a more helpful biomarker when trying to distinguish hepatic function abnormalities from liver hypoperfusion. Hepatocellular uptake and efflux of bilirubin is unaffected by reduced liver perfusion except in cases of prehepatic (hemolytic) hyperbilirubinemia.

Fluid Analysis

Peritoneal effusion in PH may be a low, moderate, or high protein effusion. The effusion typically has a low cell count ($< 5.0 \times 10^3/\mu L$), but the presence of inflammatory or atypical cells should prompt a search for an infectious or neoplastic etiology. In early disease, the protein concentration of the effusion correlates with the anatomic location of PH. Prehepatic and pre-sinusoidal PH increases intestinal lymph formation. The ascitic fluid has a low protein concentration (<2.5 g/dL). Posthepatic, post-sinusoidal, and sinusoidal intrahepatic PH increase hepatic lymph formation, leading to a moderate or high protein effusion (>2.5 g/dL) through the porous sinusoidal endothelium. Yet, over time, intrahepatic sinusoidal PH can result in sinusoidal capillarization (loss of sinusoidal permeability) and synthetic failure, thus the protein content of the abdominal effusion will reduce.

DIAGNOSTIC IMAGING

Radiography

Radiography is often performed due to its wide availability and may provide useful information when evaluating dogs and cats with suspected PH. Thoracic radiographs may reveal changes supportive of an intrathoracic cause of posthepatic PH, such as cardiomegaly, prominent pulmonary vasculature, or alterations of the caudal vena cava. Abdominal radiographs can enable assessment of liver size and reveal a loss of serosal detail consistent with the presence of effusion, but these findings alone lack specificity for PH and more advanced imaging modalities, such as ultrasound, computed tomographic angiography (CTA), or magnetic resonance imaging should be used when available.

Abdominal Ultrasound and CTA

Ultrasound and CTA can reveal minimal peritoneal effusion and facilitate diagnostic abdominocentesis. Ultrasound and CTA can also help identify the underlying cause of PH by screening for abnormalities associated with the liver, biliary tract, heart, thoracic cavity, or abdominal vasculature. MAPSS may develop anywhere in the abdomen but are most easily visualized using color flow doppler ultrasonography immediately adjacent to the left kidney and usually occur as a nest of vessels with turbulent blood flow. In some instances, macroscopic MAPSS can be challenging to identify during imaging studies, as they can be present without abdominal effusion. If MAPSS are clinically suspected, a preemptive request to search for anomalous vessels should be included in the diagnostic imaging request.

For a more comprehensive overview of diagnostic imaging for dogs and cats, please refer to Chapter 2.

LIVER HISTOPATHOLOGY

Histopathology can provide identification of and differentiation between most of the underlying causes of intrahepatic PH. Once MAPSS are present, caution must be exercised when interpreting the finding of "primary hypoplasia of the portal vein" on liver histology. While this may be a congenital abnormality, the same histologic appearance occurs secondary to portal venous hypoperfusion from portosystemic shunting. Microscopic "primary hypoplasia of the portal vein" is an unlikely cause of PH.

Please refer to Chapter 4 for a review of liver histology findings.

TREATMENT OF PH

Treatment strategies for dogs and cats with PH consist of correcting the underlying cause, if possible, and managing secondary complications. In humans with intrahepatic PH, directly lowering the portal pressure is achievable with the use of nonselective beta-blockers. However, the administration of propranolol to dogs with intrahepatic PH has been shown to exhibit only minimal effects on hepatic circulation while imposing significant effects on systemic hemodynamics. Anecdotally, one of the authors (ANJ) has used the angiotensin II receptor blocker, losartan (begin at 0.125 mg/kg/d PO titrate to maximum dose of 0.5 mg/kg/d), to treat pre-sinusoidal and sinusoidal PH with subjective clinical improvement. Unlike telmisartan, losartan does not potentiate systemic hypotension and is considered a safer alternative, but serum creatinine and potassium are monitored 5–10 days after drug initiation and following dose increases. Additional research is required to provide definitive diagnostic recommendations.

MANAGING COMPLICATIONS

Peritoneal Effusion

Strategies for controlling peritoneal effusion center around establishing natriuresis through dietary sodium restriction and enhanced sodium excretion. A diet with a sodium content of <0.05 g/100 kcal is recommended (Johnston 2023). Many diets formulated for cardiovascular disease meet this requirement. Cumming's School of Veterinary Medicine maintains a list of low sodium diets for dogs on their Heart Disease - Nutrition website (heartsmart.vet.tufts.edu). If dietary sodium restriction is inadequate or proves challenging in patients with unreliable appetite, diuretics should be added. The initial diuretic strategy is a combination of spironolactone (1–2 mg/kg/d) and low-dose furosemide (0.5–1 mg/kg/d). Spironolactone can be gradually increased every 3–5 days to a total dose of 4 mg/kg/d divided twice daily, but a full response may take up to 14 days. Furosemide can also be increased to a total dose of 4 mg/kg/d divided twice daily if suboptimal response is seen with initial doses. Once the effusion is stabilized, the diuretic dosages are tapered to the lowest effect dose beginning with furosemide. Ideally, a maintenance regimen with spironolactone alone will be achieved. While receiving diuretics, weight and abdominal girth should be assessed daily, with a fluid reduction goal of 0.5% of body weight per day. Monitoring should also include hematocrit, creatinine, and electrolytes. If hyponatremia, hypokalemia, azotemia (increase in serum creatinine concentration ≥30% of the baseline concentration), or signs of HE worsen, diuretic dosages should be reduced or discontinued altogether.

Therapeutic abdominocentesis should be performed in patients exhibiting inadequate cardiac output, respiratory difficulty, discomfort, or inappetence as a consequence of tense abdominal distention. This may be necessary during the initial stabilization alone or may be intermittently required depending on the patient's response to management. The goals of abdominocentesis are to remove enough fluid to improve comfort, renal perfusion, cardiac output, ventilation, and enhance response to diuretics. *Fluid removal should be limited to 20–50% of ascitic volume to minimize the risk of decreased renal function or circulatory collapse.* Because rapid intravascular fluid shifts may occur in PH patients, intravenous administration of a balanced crystalloid equilibrated to the patient's serum or plasma sodium level should be administered concurrently. Abdominocentesis should be performed at the lateral body wall rather than ventrally to avoid persistent dripping of effusion and subdermal fluid accumulation. The sight of aspiration should be sterilely prepared and maintained to prevent bacterial peritonitis.

Hepatic Encephalopathy

Please refer to Chapter 8 for management of HE.

Coagulopathy

Hypocoagulable Patients: If invasive procedures such as fine needle aspiration, cholecystocentesis, or biopsy are planned, supplementation of Vitamin K_1 (0.5–1 mg/kg SQ q12h, 3 doses) may be empirically administered prior to sampling. Exceeding the recommended dosage or frequency can cause Heinz body hemolysis particularly in cats. For patients that are actively bleeding or demonstrate prolongation of PT or aPTT greater than 1.5× the upper limit of the reference interval prior to an invasive procedure, administration of clotting factors ± blood products, as needed, is recommended (Fresh frozen plasma – contains all coagulation factors and plasma proteins, cryoprecipitate – contains fibrinogen and factors VIII, vWF, and XIII).

Hypercoagulable Patients: For hypercoagulable patients with PH, treatment options are not clearly defined. The pharmacokinetics of most available anticoagulants, such as clopidogrel, a platelet aggregation inhibitor, or rivaroxaban, a coagulation factor Xa inhibitor, are unpredictable in the presence of hepatic hypoperfusion due to their reliance on hepatic activation, metabolism, or elimination. However, in patients with PH secondary to portal vein thrombosis, the use of anticoagulants, such as low-molecular-weight heparin or rivaroxaban, may increase survival.

Gastropathy

Management of suspected portal hypertensive gastropathy in dogs and cats with PH should be targeted toward maintenance of enteral alimentation through administration of antiemetics, appetite stimulants, and, if required, feeding tubes. Gastric acid inhibition is unlikely to be effective in the management of portal hypertensive gastropathy. Proton pump inhibitors should be avoided due to the risk if exacerbating HE (Ma et al. 2019).

MAPSS

There are no specific treatments for patients with MAPSSs. Because these shunts develop as a compensatory mechanism secondary to PH, surgical ligation is not recommended.

PROGNOSIS

The prognosis for dogs and cats with PH is dependent on the underlying cause. Studies on long-term outcome are limited. Further, the available survival data are difficult to interpret due to elective euthanasia; however, prolonged survival (e.g., years) is reported (Anglin et al. 2021; Calleja et al. 2023). Treatment of the underlying disease and PH sequelae should be considered before recommending euthanasia at the time of diagnosis.

REFERENCES

Anglin, E.V., Lux, C.N., Sun, X. et al. (2021). Clinical characteristics of, prognostic factors for, and long-term outcome of dogs with multiple acquired portosystemic shunts: 72 cases (2008-2018). *Journal of the American Veterinary Medical Association* 260: S30–S39.

Bayraktar, U.D., Seren, S., and Bayraktar, Y. (2007). Hepatic venous outflow obstruction: three similar syndromes. *World Journal of Gastroenterology* 13: 1912–1927.

Bosch, J., Enriquez, R., Groszmann, R.J. et al. (1983). Chronic bile duct ligation in the dog: hemodynamic characterization of a portal hypertensive model. *Hepatology* 3: 1002–1007.

Buob, S., Johnston, A.N., and Webster, C.R. (2011). Portal hypertension: pathophysiology, diagnosis, and treatment. *Journal of Veterinary Internal Medicine* 25: 169–186.

Calleja, S., Shiel, R., Bree, L. et al. (2023). Prognostic indicators in dogs with intra-hepatic portal hypertension. *Canadian Veterinary Journal* 64: 174–180.

Center, S.A., Warner, K., Corbett, J. et al. (2000). Proteins invoked by vitamin K absence and clotting times in clinically ill cats. *Journal of Veterinary Internal Medicine* 14: 292–297.

deLaforcade, A., Bacek, L., Blais, M.C. et al. (2022). 2022 Update of the consensus on the rational use of antithrombotics and thrombolytics in veterinary critical care (CURATIVE) domain 1-defining populations at risk. *Journal of Veterinary Emergency and Critical Care* 32: 289–314.

Fernandez, M., Semela, D., Bruix, J. et al. (2009). Angiogenesis in liver disease. *Journal of Hepatology* 50: 604–620.

Howe, L.M., Boothe, Jr, H.W., Miller, M.W. et al. (2000). A canine model of multiple portosystemic shunting. *Journal of Investigative Surgery* 13: 45–57.

Johnston, A.N. (2023). Portal hypertension. In: *Small Animal Critical Care Medicine*, 3e (ed. D.C. Silverstein and K. Hopper), 668–673. St. Louis, MO: Elsevier.

Leiva, J.G., Salgado, J.M., Estradas, J. et al. (2007). Pathophysiology of ascites and dilutional hyponatremia: contemporary use of aquaretic agents. *Annals of Hepatology* 6: 214–221.

Ma, Y.J., Cao, Z.X., Li, Y. et al. (2019). Proton pump inhibitor use increases hepatic encephalopathy risk: a systematic review and meta-analysis. *World Journal of Gastroenterology* 25: 2675–2682

Respess, M., O'Toole, T.E., Taeymans, O. et al. (2012). Portal vein thrombosis in 33 dogs: 1998-2011. *Journal of Veterinary Internal Medicine* 26: 230–237.

Rogers, C.L., Keating, J.H., Penninck, D.G. et al. (2008). Portal vein thrombosis in cats: 6 cases (2001-2006). *Journal of Veterinary Internal Medicine* 22: 282–287.

Simpson, K.W., Meyer, D.J., Boswood, A. et al. (1997). Iron status and erythrocyte volume in dogs with congenital portosystemic vascular anomalies. *Journal of Veterinary Internal Medicine* 11: 14–19.

Tan, S. (2024). Molecular mechanism of portal hypertensive gastropathy: an update. *Clinics and Research in Hepatology and Gastroenterology* 48: 102423.

Webster, C.R.L. (2017). Hemostatic disorders associated with hepatobiliary disease. *Veterinary Clinics of North America: Small Animal Practice* 47: 601–615.

CHAPTER 10 Ductal Plate Malformations

Sarah Shropshire

Department of Clinical Sciences, College of Veterinary Medicine and Biomedical Sciences, Colorado State University, Fort Collins, CO, USA

KEY POINTS

- A ductal plate malformation (DPM) should be considered in a young, otherwise healthy dog (often between six months and two years of age) with a severely elevated alanine aminotransferase (ALT) and aspartate aminotransferase (AST).
- A DPM should be considered in a young puppy or kitten with moderate to severely elevated hepatocellular enzymes (i.e., ALT, AST), ascites, and suspected or documented acquired portosystemic shunts (PSS).
- A DPM can have a highly variable prognosis with some dogs and cats succumbing to complications within a year of diagnosis while many (even with ascites) can live for multiple years with a good quality of life.
- Complications of DPMs can include portal hypertension (PH) with acquired shunts, ascites, gastrointestinal bleeding, and hepatic encephalopathy (HE). Other complications can include cholelithiasis, hepatobiliary tract infections, and urolithiasis.

INTRODUCTION

The condition ductal plate malformation (DPM) is becoming more commonly diagnosed in liver pathology reports, which can create confusion for veterinarians that are unfamiliar with this term. There are case series and case reports (more in dogs than cats) for veterinarians to read, but management and prognosis can still appear somewhat elusive (Pillai et al. 2016; Watson 2017; Roberts et al. 2018; King et al. 2023). Indeed, when presented with a patient with evidence of synthetic liver dysfunction (e.g., decreased blood urea nitrogen [BUN], albumin, cholesterol) and ascites, the prognosis is often thought to be poor to grave. One study, however, showed that dogs lived for many years even with acquired portosystemic shunts (PSS), demonstrating that veterinarians should not prematurely recommend euthanasia (Pillai et al. 2016). So, what is a DPM? In general, it is defined as a congenital biliary tract disorder that starts with the embryonic structure called the ductal plate that surrounds the future hepatic portal triad which, in health, undergoes developmental changes that result in the final development of biliary ducts.

This process can go awry and result in failure of the typical involution of embryonal ducts leading to too many biliary ducts within the portal triad or throughout the liver (without any associated portal triad) and diminished or absent portal vein profiles. Bile ducts can be small with a narrow or absent lumen, cystic, or sacculated. Portal to portal bridging fibrosis characterized by fibrous septa containing numerous abnormal bile ducts is typical. The malformation can affect different segments of the biliary tree. For example, von Meyenburg complex, also termed bile duct hamartoma, describes an abnormality limited to the smallest branches of the biliary tree leading to a small (<3 mm) subcapsular focus of expanded extracellular matrix studded with abnormal bile ducts. Abnormalities affecting larger branches of the biliary tree can have several appearances. Small-duct phenotype refers to forms in which only small-diameter bile ducts populate the portal tracts and bridging fibrous septa (Figure 10.1). When there is a large component of fibrosis, particularly bridging fibrosis with associated increased biliary ducts throughout, the term "congenital hepatic fibrosis" is reported (Cullen and Stalker 2016). Other variants may be characterized by cystic

Disorders of the Liver, Exocrine Pancreas, and Gastrointestinal Tract in Dogs and Cats, First Edition. Edited by Harry Cridge et al. Published 2026 by John Wiley & Sons, Inc. Companion Website: www.wiley.com/go/cridge/disorders

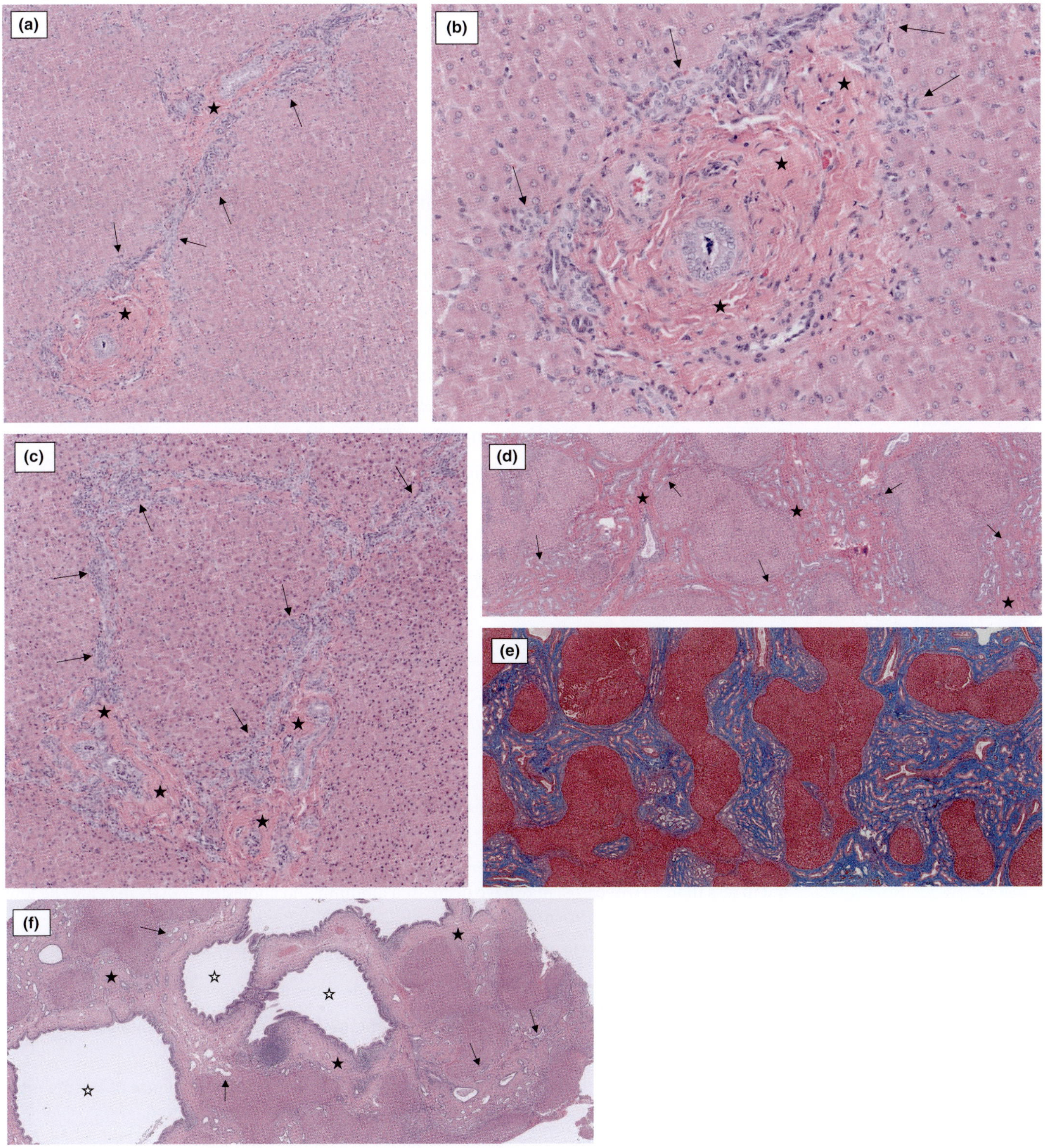

FIGURE 10.1 (a–c): Example of "small duct" ductal plate malformation with evidence of lack of inflammatory infiltrate, persistent biliary structures (arrows), excessive extracellular matrix (stars), and small diameter bile ducts proliferating in a bridging pattern. (d, e) Example of "congenital hepatic fibrosis" ductal plate malformation with persistent biliary structures, excessive extracellular matrix (fibrosis) in large bridging patterns most noticeable on Masson's trichrome stain (e). (f) Example of "Caroli malformation" ductal plate malformation with sacculated or cystic biliary duct profiles (affecting large intrahepatic ducts) (open stars), persistent biliary structures, excessive extracellular matrix (fibrosis), and bile ducts proliferating in a bridging pattern

or sacculated ducts. For example, when the larger intrahepatic bile ducts are affected, the term "polycystic" or "Caroli malformation" may be applied (Figure 10.1). A common finding in all these scenarios is the absence of normal portal vein morphology seen either as diminutive or absent portal vein profiles. Note: It is also important to consider an obstructive process within the biliary system so the patient should always be concurrently assessed for biliary outflow tract obstruction.

These general guidelines for diagnostic terminology are not agreed upon by all pathologists however as some feel that the term DPM should only be used unless there are cystic or sacculated biliary ducts (personal communication with Dr. April Choi, DACVP). Portal vein hypoplasia (microvascular dysplasia) is characterized histologically by the absence or reduction of portal vein profiles and may have mild increases in fibrosis and bile duct profiles leading to potential overlap in the histologic appearance of these two conditions. Rather than diagnosing a DPM, some pathologists may instead diagnose portal vein hypoplasia (PVH) with ductular reaction. Note: Ductular reaction is an acquired condition versus a congenital proliferation of biliary ducts such as occurs in DPM. From a clinical standpoint, however, these patients can behave similarly (ranging from minimal to no clinical signs to polydipsia/polyuria to signs of hepatic encephalopathy [HE] due to the development of acquired shunts) so the differentiation may not always be clinically relevant. Other common histologic features of DPM include:

- Lack of regenerative nodules. If present, other differentials should be considered.
- No evidence of inflammation histologically (exceptions would be a concurrent bacterial hepatobiliary tract infection).

Note: In the author's experience, cats seem to more commonly have the cystic and sacculated forms, but this could be a limitation of how many cats are biopsied compared to dogs.

CLINICAL SIGNS

A general rule of thumb is that most dogs will be diagnosed after investigating elevated hepatocellular liver enzyme activities noted on spay/neuter or routine blood work. Most dogs present with the following diagnostic flow:

- Clinically asymptomatic moderate-to-severe elevation of alanine aminotransferase (ALT) alone or ALT and aspartate aminotransferase (AST) (ALT > AST). ALT activities tend to range from 300 to 3000 IU/L.
- Commonly have normal synthetic liver function parameters (glucose, albumin, and cholesterol) but in less than 15% of cases, may have decreased albumin and cholesterol. BUN may also be low if concurrent PU/PD is present.
- Total bilirubin is commonly normal unless there is a concurrent infection.
- Bile acid testing is normal unless acquired PSS have developed from portal hypertension (PH).
- Urinalysis is normal unless acquired PSS are present, in which case ammonium biurate crystals may be observed.
- Ultrasound commonly reveals a small to normal appearing liver with no evidence of a congenital extrahepatic PSS. A heterogeneous, irregular liver with nodules is not observed.
- Cholelithiasis (intrahepatic, within the gall bladder, or within the common bile duct) can be observed.

In a minority of cases, dogs can present initially with complications from their DPM which are typically hepatobiliary infections (that may or may not be due to cholelithiasis) or complications from PH such as ascites, gastrointestinal bleeding, HE, etc. Additionally, some dogs may be diagnosed late in life and DPM should still be considered as a differential if the histology is consistent with this condition.

In contrast to dogs, cats seem to present either as kittens/young cats or as adults (>10 years of age). In general, cats can present with the following diagnostic flow:

- Abrupt development of ascites in kittens can mimic feline infectious peritonitis (FIP), as FIP can also be associated with ascites, +/− elevated liver values, and +/− icterus (elevated total bilirubin). A key difference between DPM and FIP is that DPM cats often have one or many cystic structures within the liver in addition to cystic abnormalities associated with the biliary tree (e.g., common bile duct).
- Palpation of a large "mass" in the abdomen in an older cat with probable concurrent gastrointestinal signs (decreased appetite and vomiting), which can mimic neoplasia. Aspirates often show biliary epithelial proliferation or is consistent with bile.
- Mild-to-moderate elevations in ALT (150–500 IU/L) and AST.

  If the cysts become very large and compressive, ALP elevations (often less than 3000 IU/L) and total bilirubin elevations (3–15 mg/dL) can be observed. This pattern can also occur if there is a concurrent hepatobiliary tract infection (Center et al. 2022).

DIAGNOSIS

In cases suspected to have DPM, liver histopathology is required for a definitive diagnosis. When performing liver biopsies, it is imperative to get samples from multiple lobes. This goes for any type of liver disease in general, in which one lobe can look dramatically different from another lobe, so it is vital to have representative samples. It is also highly important to communicate signalment, clinical, and imaging findings in the submitted report to help the pathologist formulate differentials.

TREATMENT

The management of DPM in dogs and cats has not been rigorously studied, however in the author's experience, there are several key features to consider for management. The most important aspect is to ensure individualized tailored treatment; this means one size does not fit all. And less is more; this is a lifelong disease, so starting 5–8 supplements/medications can be intimating to clients (and typically unnecessary). Many veterinarians might reach for antioxidant therapy due to the elevated liver values, a formulated "liver diet", lactulose if there are elevated bile acids, and +/− an antimicrobial for management of possible HE. In the author's opinion, there is no evidence that antioxidant therapy is important for management of this disease; however, the use of a choleretic such as ursodiol could be considered. Because of the abnormal biliary ducts, particularly in cases where the ducts are cystic or sacculated, this could put a patient at risk for infection, biliary stone formation, or cholestasis. The use of a choleretic has been shown to be beneficial in some human studies, so ursodiol is a therapy that the author will often consider (Kriegermeier and Green 2020; Yuan et al. 2024).

With regards to diet, this is also highly variable as many of these patients over time will struggle with gastrointestinal signs such as weight loss and diarrhea. The author rarely places patients on a therapeutic liver diet but focuses more on targeting what the patient likely needs (e.g., highly digestible). The times when the author implements a therapeutic liver diet may include when protein restriction is needed to help control HE signs or when a lower copper composition is desired. As many veterinarians know, increased copper in the liver is becoming an increasingly recognized issue, particularly in dogs (Center et al. 2021). However, elevated bile acids are not an indication to start a liver diet, unless there are signs of protein intolerance, such as HE or urate urolithiasis.

Lactulose and an antimicrobial are often part of management of HE, most commonly when considering congenital extrahepatic PSS. The author will only implement the use of lactulose if the patient appears to be suffering from signs of HE and although this is not traditional, in the author's experience, many owners of dogs with DPM comment that even the lowest dosages of lactulose cause significant diarrhea. As a result, the author utilizes lactulose on a case-by-case basis versus as a mainstay of therapy. The author does not use any antimicrobial therapy for HE unless clinically indicated (i.e., infection). Because these patients can be at risk for hepatobiliary tract infections, having them on chronic antimicrobial therapy promotes resistance and could limit antimicrobial choices should an infection occur.

One therapy that the author implements when there is evidence of PH (e.g., ascites, acquired shunts, significantly elevated bile acids, etc.) is telmisartan, an angiotensin receptor blocker (Buob et al. 2011). The author has used this medication for this purpose in many dogs but not in cats, thus far. One very important consideration for telmisartan in this clinical scenario is that the author recommends low dosages due to the potential for reduced hepatic metabolism and observed risk for acute kidney injury. The author typically starts at 0.2–0.5 mg/kg/day telmisartan and monitors blood pressure, kidney values, and electrolytes as is standardly recommended. In addition to telmisartan, when ascites is present, the author will also start spironolactone therapy (dose range 1–4 mg/kg/day). The author and colleagues are currently conducting a prospective life-long longitudinal study in dogs and cats, so it is currently unknown how robust the response is to these medications for the control of PH. At the time of this writing, the institution of these two medications resulted in the resolution of ascites and improvement to the resolution of synthetic liver dysfunction in multiple clinical trial dogs for over four years and counting, so preliminary data appears promising.

For long-term management, it is important for veterinarians to understand that many of these dogs will never have normal liver values, and they can fluctuate dramatically over time. An example is of one clinical trial dog that had an ALT of 230 IU/L, one month later; 654 IU/L, two months later; 898 IU/L, and three months later; 215 IU/L. No therapy was instituted as the patient was feeling clinically well. Thus, these fluctuations can occur and be clinically insignificant, but it is important to consider how the patient is doing clinically in addition to monitoring their total bilirubin. The total bilirubin is more likely to be elevated in true hepatobiliary tract infections. How often to monitor these patients can be very patient dependent but if they are doing well and medications are not being adjusted, the author recommends once to twice yearly assessments. It is unknown if it is beneficial to start telmisartan prior to the development of PH but the author recommends at least once to twice yearly monitoring for PH (bile acid testing, POCUS of the abdomen for fluid, hepatobiliary ultrasounds, etc.).

For cats specifically, the degree of liver enzyme fluctuation does not seem to be as prevalent as in dogs, and long-term management is focused on monitoring for hepatobiliary infections and progression of the cystic structures within the hepatobiliary system. If progression occurs, it depends on where the cysts are or how numerous they are, but surgical interventions may be warranted and should be evaluated on a case-by-case basis.

PROGNOSIS

The prognosis for DPM in general appears to be fair to good with multiple years of good quality of life but there are some exceptions to that statement. Clinical situations where a worse prognosis is anticipated would be in dogs with severe icterus and a probable hepatobiliary tract infection with concurrent PH with melena, HE, and anorexia. For cats, the same could be said when there are tense ascites and massive cysts throughout the liver as that process can be highly difficult to control and results in significant quality of life concerns.

CONCLUSIONS

It is suspected that the term DPM will evolve in veterinary medicine over time to include more specific histologic criteria and clinical characteristics. Nonetheless, this differential is important to be aware of and understand that the prognosis for this disease can be good for some patients with years of excellent quality of life.

REFERENCES

Buob, S., Johnston, A.N., and Webster, C.R.L. (2011). Portal hypertension: pathophysiology, diagnosis, and treatment. *Journal of Veterinary Internal Medicine* 25 (2): 169–186.

Center, S.A., Richter, K.P., Twedt, D.C. et al. (2021). Is it time to reconsider current guidelines for copper content in commercial dog foods? *Journal of the American Veterinary Medical Association* 258 (4): 357–364.

Center, S.A., Randolph, J.F., Warner, K.L. et al. (2022). Clinical features, concurrent disorders, and survival time in cats with suppurative cholangitis-cholangiohepatitis syndrome. *Journal of the American Veterinary Medical Association* 260 (2): 212–227.

Cullen, J. and Stalker, M. (2016) *Jubb, Kennedy & Palmer's Pathology of Domestic Animal Sixth Edition,* Volume 2, *Liver and Biliary System*. St. Louis: Elsevier.

King, E.M., Pappano, M., Lorbach, S.K. et al. (2023). Severe polycystic liver disease in a cat. *Journal of Feline Medicine and Surgery Open Reports* 9 (2): 20551169231216859. https://doi.org/10.1177/20551169231216859.

Kriegermeier, A. and Green, R. (2020). Pediatric cholestatic liver disease: review of bile acid metabolism and discussion of current and emerging therapies. *Frontiers in Medicine (Lausanne)* 7: 149. https://doi.org/10.3389/fmed.2020.00149.

Pillai, S., Center, S.A., McDonough, S.P. et al. (2016). Ductal plate malformation in the liver of boxer dogs: clinical and histological features. *Veterinary Pathology* 53 (3): 602–613.

Roberts, M., Rine, S., and Lam, A. (2018). Caroli's type ductal plate malformation and a PSS in a 4-month-old kitten. *Journal of Feline Medicine and Surgery Open Reports* 4 (2): 2055116918812329. https://doi.org/10.1177/2055116918812329.

Watson, P. (2017). Canine breed-specific hepatopathies. *Veterinary Clinics: Small Animal Practice* 47: 665–682.

Yuan, W., Zhang, Z., Pan, Q. et al. (2024). Risk factors for recurrence of common bile duct stones after surgical treatment and effect of ursodeoxycholic acid intervention. *World Journal of Gastrointestinal Surgery* 16 (1): 103–112.

CHAPTER 11 Acute Liver Injury

Jessica Kerley and Vincent Thawley

Department of Clinical Sciences & Advanced Medicine, School of Veterinary Medicine, University of Pennsylvania, Philadelphia, PA, USA

KEY POINTS

- Acute Liver Injury (ALI) and Acute Liver Failure (ALF) are serious conditions characterized by rapid liver dysfunction, leading to complications such as coagulopathy, encephalopathy, and multi-organ failure. ALF represents the more severe form, with a significantly worse prognosis.
- Broad diagnostic testing (i.e., laboratory testing, imaging, and tissue sampling) is essential to determine the underlying cause of ALI/ALF and guide treatment decisions. Toxicologic screening and infectious disease testing may also be considered.
- Management is largely supportive, with key components including IV fluid therapy, management of hepatic encephalopathy (HE) (lactulose, antibiotics), and nutritional support. Hepatoprotective agents (NAC, SAMe) may be used, and therapeutic interventions like plasma exchange, continuous renal replacement therapy, or intermittent hemodialysis can be considered in severe cases.
- The prognosis for ALI varies. When ALF occurs, the outcome is generally poor with survival rates as low as 14%. The response to therapy and reversibility of the inciting cause are key factors in determining prognosis.

INTRODUCTION

Acute liver injury (ALI) and acute liver failure (ALF) are serious, and potentially life-threatening, clinical syndromes in the dog and cat. The liver is a vital organ responsible for detoxification, metabolic and immune regulation, protein synthesis, and bile production and secretion. Prior to the development of liver transplantation techniques, the survival rate in humans with ALF was less than 20% but has since increased to approximately 70% (Pievsky et al. 2018). In veterinary medicine, the prognosis varies depending on etiology but is generally poor when ALF occurs.

Despite the importance of prompt recognition and management of these syndromes, they lack clear definitions throughout the veterinary and human literature. Numerous definitions have been used for ALF in the human literature, most of which involve the acute onset (within 2–8 weeks) of clinical signs as well as the presence of icterus, HE, coagulopathy, and lack of previously existing liver disease (Wlodzimirow et al. 2012). In contrast, ALI involves hepatocellular damage and necrosis without the loss of hepatic function where if the causative factor is removed, recovery may occur without progression to more severe liver damage.

The definitions of ALI and ALF in humans provide important context for understanding these conditions in veterinary patients. While similar mechanisms of injury are at play in dogs and cats, the manifestation, progression, and treatment of hepatic disease in these species can differ. This chapter provides an in-depth overview of ALI and ALF in dogs and cats, with a focus on understanding disease pathophysiology as well as integrating current recommendations for diagnostic approaches and treatment strategies.

Disorders of the Liver, Exocrine Pancreas, and Gastrointestinal Tract in Dogs and Cats, First Edition. Edited by Harry Cridge et al. Published 2026 by John Wiley & Sons, Inc. Companion Website: www.wiley.com/go/cridge/disorders

ETIOLOGY

A variety of insults can disrupt the liver's structural and functional integrity, resulting in ALI/ALF (Rabinowich and Bernal, 2022). In veterinary patients, general causes of ALI/ALF include toxic exposures, drug reactions, infectious and inflammatory diseases, metabolic disorders, neoplasia, ischemic injury, and idiopathic. The most common causes in veterinary medicine are listed in Table 11.1. A comprehensive discussion of these causes is beyond the scope of this chapter and can be found elsewhere (Weingarten and Sande, 2015). In a retrospective study of 49 dogs, neoplasia was the most common cause of ALF; however, the identifying cause was only confirmed in 37% of cases (Lester et al. 2016).

PATHOPHYSIOLOGY

The hepatic acinus is considered the functional unit of the liver. It consists of hepatocytes oriented around the portal triad, which contains the portal vein, the hepatic artery, and the bile duct. Portal venous and arterial blood flows centripetally, toward the central vein. The portal vein carries nutrient-rich, oxygen-poor blood from the gastrointestinal tract and spleen, while the hepatic artery supplies oxygenated blood from the heart. The bile duct, which flows centrifugally, away from the central vein, collects bile acids and other bile constituents produced by hepatocytes and transports them from the hepatocytes to the gallbladder.

The surrounding hepatocytes are divided into three distinct zones based on proximity to blood flow. A clear understanding of this hepatic zonal structure is essential for recognizing the varying susceptibilities of hepatocytes in different zones to specific types of injury. Zone 1 hepatocytes, located closest to the portal triads, receive the blood richest in oxygen as well as other substances such as hormones (e.g., insulin and glucagon) and metabolites. These hepatocytes also receive blood with the highest concentration of toxins delivered via portal blood flow from the gastrointestinal tract. Due to their proximity to the blood supply, hepatocytes located in this zone are less vulnerable

Table 11.1 Common Causes of Acute Liver Injury/Acute Liver Failure in Dogs and Cats

Toxins	Drugs	Infectious	Idiopathic	Neoplasia
Xylitol Blue-green algae Cycads (Sago palms) Amanita mushrooms Aflatoxins	*Anti-inflammatory and immunosuppressive* Acetaminophen Carprofen Azathioprine *Anticonvulsants* Diazepam Phenobarbital Zonisamide *Antimicrobials* Sulfonamides Tetracyclines Azole antifungals *Chemotherapeutics* Lomustine (CCNU) Mitotane *Miscellaneous* Methimazole Manganese (joint supplements)	*Bacterial* Leptospirosis *Viral* Adenovirus (canine infectious hepatitis) Coronavirus (feline infectious peritonitis) *Fungal* Histoplasmosis Coccidioidomycosis *Protozoal* Toxoplasmosis *Parasitic* Liver flukes	Feline hepatic lipidosis	*Round cell neoplasia* Lymphoma Malignant histiocytosis Systemic mastocytosis *Other* Hepatocellular carcinoma

to hypoxic injury but more vulnerable to injury from directly acting toxins than hepatocytes in other zones. Zone 2 hepatocytes lie in the intermediate area between zones 1 and 3 and represent a transitional zone. Zone 3 hepatocytes, which reside at the periphery of the acinus closest to the central vein, receive the most oxygen-poor blood and are thus the most susceptible to hypoxic injury. Although zone 3 hepatocytes are less susceptible to injury resulting from directly acting toxins than those in zones 1 and 2, they are at higher risk of injury from toxic metabolites of the cytochrome P450 system, as these biotransformation pathways are most active in zone 3.

The pathophysiology of ALF depends somewhat on etiology. Insult may occur directly via the destruction of liver tissue or indirectly via disruption of normal liver function. In most cases, there is evidence of hepatocyte death via apoptosis and/or necrosis, regardless of the cause. In dogs with ALF, diffuse hepatic necrosis is the most consistent histopathologic finding. If hepatocyte injury and death are limited, hepatic regeneration is possible; however, the rate of hepatocyte death may exceed regenerative capacity, at which point the liver's structural and functional integrity becomes compromised. The clinical syndrome of ALF ensues when greater than 70% of functional hepatic mass is lost.

HEPATIC ENCEPHALOPATHY

HE is a neuropsychiatric syndrome that is considered a hallmark feature in defining ALI and ALF in humans. It is divided into three types, depending on etiology of the disorder, with ALF being associated with type A HE (Lidbury et al. 2016). The pathophysiology of HE is multifactorial and involves complex metabolic disturbances, immune dysregulation, accumulation of neurotoxic substances, and development of cerebral edema. Ammonia, a neurotoxin produced in, and normally detoxified by, the liver via the urea cycle, is one such neurotoxic substance that is believed to play a key role in the development of HE. In the setting of liver failure, the liver's ability to metabolize ammonia is significantly impaired, leading to its accumulation in systemic circulation and subsequent penetration of the blood–brain barrier and conversion to glutamine by astrocytes. Accumulation of glutamine triggers mitochondrial damage, oxidative stress, and osmotic swelling of astrocytes, ultimately resulting in astrocyte dysfunction and worsening cerebral edema. Neuroinflammation and metabolic imbalances such as hypoglycemia, hyponatremia, and hypokalemia further complicate HE pathophysiology. For a more comprehensive review on HE, please refer to Chapter 8.

INITIAL EVALUATION OF PHYSICAL EXAM

On initial arrival, a primary survey is conducted to identify imminently life-threatening problems related to the respiratory, cardiovascular, or neurologic systems. Signs of respiratory compromise can include tachypnea, dyspnea, orthopnea, and dull or diminished lung sounds, and may be the result of aspiration pneumonia, pleural effusion resulting from hypoalbuminemia and low intravascular osmotic pressure, or atelectasis. Less commonly, respiratory compromise may be the result of pulmonary hemorrhage or thromboembolism, acute respiratory distress syndrome, or neurogenic pulmonary edema. Pulse oximetry or arterial blood gas analysis may be useful in determining the severity of hypoxemia; when in doubt, however, supplemental oxygen therapy should be provided and thoracic imaging pursued to determine the cause. Thoracocentesis is indicated if pleural effusion is present and causing respiratory distress.

Signs of cardiovascular compromise can include tachycardia, abnormal mentation, altered mucous membrane color and capillary refill time, abnormal pulse quality, and cool extremities. These signs of abnormal tissue perfusion may be the result of increased fluid losses (vomiting, diarrhea, polyuria, third-spacing due to hypoalbuminemia, and hemorrhage), abnormal vascular tone resulting from systemic inflammation or sepsis, or a combination, often coupled with reduced oral fluid intake. When signs of abnormal perfusion are present, bolus fluid therapy is indicated and typically begins with administration of an isotonic crystalloid in aliquots (10–15 mL/kg in dogs,

5–10 mL/kg in cats) given to effect. Synthetic colloids such as hydroxyethyl starch (3–5 mL/kg) may be considered in hypoproteinemic patients; however, there is evidence to suggest that use of these fluids has been associated with the development of coagulopathy and acute kidney injury (Byers 2025). In severely hypoalbuminemic patients, albumin replacement with either canine or human serum albumin may be considered, although there is some risk of acute and delayed hypersensitivity reaction, particularly with the use of human products (Mazzaferro and Edwards 2020). Blood products are typically reserved for resuscitation in patients with hemorrhagic shock or coagulopathy resulting in hemorrhage. Patients with continued signs of poor perfusion despite adequate intravascular volume resuscitation may require vasopressor therapy.

Signs of neurological compromise can include lethargy, altered mentation, head pressing, blindness, circling, tremors or seizures. In the ALI/ALF patient, these signs may be the result of circulatory shock and poor cerebral perfusion, hypoglycemia, or HE. Patients presenting with an abnormal mentation should have measurement of whole blood or plasma glucose; when symptomatic hypoglycemia is identified, a bolus of dextrose (0.5–1 g/kg) is indicated, followed by dextrose supplementation in the intravenous fluids. Further discussion of management of HE is found below.

Once immediate threats to life are identified and appropriate stabilization is underway, a full physical exam is performed. Common findings include icterus, pain on abdominal palpation, cranial organomegaly, or abdominal distension, especially in the presence of ascites. Melena or hematochezia may be found on rectal exam. Assessment of the body condition and lean muscle mass may help to determine the chronicity of the underlying disease process. Findings on physical exam, however, are commonly nonspecific for the cause of liver injury.

DIAGNOSTIC APPROACH

There is no single test to directly evaluate liver function in veterinary patients. Furthermore, the laboratory findings that accompany ALI/ALF are not specific to an underlying etiology; rather, they are suggestive of the disruption of one or more functions specific to hepatic tissue. Therefore, the diagnostic approach to ALI or ALF usually includes a combination of blood tests, infectious disease testing (e.g., Leptospirosis), imaging studies, and potentially obtaining liver tissue for cytologic and/or histopathologic evaluation.

SERUM BIOCHEMISTRY PANEL

One of the most specific biochemical findings with ALI/ALF is an increase in liver enzymes. There are two general types of liver enzymes: transaminases and cholestatic or inducible enzymes. The transaminases consist of alanine aminotransferase (ALT) and aspartate aminotransferase (AST). These enzymes, which are stored in hepatocyte cytosol, are released into circulation upon injury to the hepatocyte membrane. When found in elevated serum levels, they are considered markers of hepatocyte injury and death. AST is also found in large amounts in extrahepatic tissue, most notably in the cytosol of skeletal muscle, making it a less sensitive marker of hepatocyte injury than ALT. Additionally, AST is present in the mitochondria of hepatocytes in higher concentrations than are found in the cytosol. Therefore, when of hepatic origin, AST may serve as a marker of more severe hepatocellular necrosis than ALT.

Because ALT is more liver-specific, it is often considered the gold-standard marker of hepatocyte injury, and the magnitude of increase in serum ALT may be useful in providing insight as to the degree of hepatocyte injury. ALT may increase up to 100-fold approximately 24–48 hours after the initial insult and is thought to peak at around 5 days (Weingarten and Sande 2015). If the insult is removed, it will then begin to gradually decline and a falling ALT level may be indicative of hepatic recovery; however, the half-life of ALT is debated, most commonly cited as 40–60 hours in dogs and 3–4 hours in the cats (Chapman and Hostutler 2013; Lawrence and Steiner 2017), and so the timeline of this decline is variable. Because ALT is produced by the hepatocytes, a decline in ALT may also suggest such extensive hepatic damage that the cells are no longer able to generate the enzyme.

It is important to note that the pattern and degree of increase in transaminases is generally not reflective of a specific underlying etiology. Generally, toxic insults to the liver will lead to more rapid peaks in ALT than will a viral insult; however, as different toxins exert distinct effects on hepatocyte function, there are exceptions to this trend. For example, microcystins produced by *Cyanobacteria* (blue-green algae) impair hepatocyte synthesis of ALT, blunting the serum increase of the enzyme following hepatocellular damage (Thawley 2017).

The cholestatic/inducible enzymes consist of alkaline phosphatase (ALP), a metalloprotein, and gamma-glutamyl transpeptidase (GGT), a glycoprotein. They are associated with the hepatocyte membrane and must be cleaved by endogenous phospholipases to become soluble and appear in serum concentrations. Serum levels of these enzymes tend to increase with cholestatic disease, where phospholipase activity is enhanced in the presence of bile acids. In the face of ALI/ALF, cholestasis is usually intrahepatic in origin, where hepatocyte dysfunction leads to impairment in the uptake, conjugation, and excretion of bilirubin. Accordingly, increases in ALP and GGT are often accompanied by an increase in serum total bilirubin (Thawley 2017).

Hyperammonemia is another common finding with ALI/ALF. As described previously, the liver plays a central role in the detoxification of ammonia via its conversion to urea in the urea cycle. Secondary to hepatic dysfunction, ammonia levels will begin to rise in circulation. The degree of hyperammonemia may or may not be associated with the severity of clinical signs of HE.

When liver function is severely compromised, a decrease in the liver function parameters may be noted. This consists of hypoglycemia, hypocholesterolemia, hypoalbuminemia, and decreased serum blood urea nitrogen. Hypoglycemia occurs due to impairment of the liver's crucial role in both gluconeogenesis and glycogen storage. Albumin, cholesterol, and blood urea nitrogen may decrease due to impairment of hepatic synthesis. Albumin, which is synthesized solely by the liver, begins to decrease when greater than 60–80% of hepatocyte function is lost.

Other common biochemical findings with ALI/ALF include electrolyte disturbances such as hypokalemia, hyperkalemia, hyponatremia, hypernatremia, hypophosphatemia, and hyperphosphatemia, as well as increases in serum creatinine and lactate. These findings are nonspecific and are often sequelae of the clinical signs associated with ALI/ALF, rather than a direct result of hepatocellular injury. Hypophosphatemia, which occurs due to intracellular shifting of phosphate during hepatocellular regeneration, may serve as a positive prognostic indicator (Schmidt and Dalhoff 2002).

In a retrospective study of 49 dogs with ALF, common abnormalities on the serum biochemistry panel included increases in transaminases and inducible enzymes and hypoalbuminemia. The most common electrolyte abnormality noted was hypokalemia. Hyperlactatemia was also common. While blood ammonia was only measured in 11 dogs, it was increased in 7 of those dogs. Hyperbilirubinemia was a criterion for inclusion and was therefore present in all 49 dogs (Lester et al. 2016).

COMPLETE BLOOD COUNT

Abnormalities in the complete blood count are less consistent and often more subtle than the serum biochemistry panel. Hemoconcentration often occurs as a sequela of the clinical signs of ALI/ALF. Microcytic, non-regenerative anemia may be noted with chronic liver disease. A regenerative anemia, as well as consumptive thrombocytopenia, may result from blood loss secondary to coagulopathy or gastroduodenal ulceration. Thrombocytopenia may also occur due to impaired hepatic synthesis of thrombopoietin (Prins et al. 2010). With infectious or inflammatory causes of ALI/ALF, a leukocytosis or leukopenia may be present.

URINALYSIS

Urinalysis with sediment evaluation is an essential part of the diagnostic workup in any sick animal. In dogs and cats with hepatic disease, urinalysis may be unremarkable. The most noted abnormality in cases of ALI/ALF is bilirubinuria, reflecting the liver's inability to properly metabolize or excrete bilirubin. It is important to note that in dogs, bilirubinuria can occur in healthy animals due to their unique ability to produce and conjugate bilirubin within renal tubules; however, it is often considered a pathologic finding, especially in the context of liver disease. In contrast, cats do not normally excrete bilirubin in the urine, and bilirubinuria should, therefore, always be considered a pathologic finding. Ammonium biurate or urate crystals may also be noted on sediment exam due to increased ammonia levels in the urine secondary to decreased hepatic conversion of ammonia to urea.

COAGULATION TESTING

In addition to its role in platelet production, the liver is crucial to the maintenance of functional hemostasis due to its critical role in both production and clearance of clotting factors. This includes factors II, V, VII, IX, X, XI, and XIII, as well as fibrinogen. The liver is also responsible for the production of proteins important for both anticoagulant function and regulation of fibrinolysis, such as protein C. Additionally, the liver acts as the site of the vitamin K cycle, which is essential to the function of factors II, VII, IX, X, and protein C. Thus, abnormalities in coagulation testing are common with ALF.

Historically, prothrombin time (PT) and activated partial thromboplastin time (aPTT) have been used to evaluate coagulation and assess bleeding risk in patients with ALF. Prolongation in PT and aPTT is common in dogs with ALF (Lester et al. 2016); however, studies in human patients have found that spontaneous hemorrhage is rare in patients with ALF (Stravitz et al. 2018). Thus, relying on PT and aPTT may overestimate the need for targeted therapy, such as fresh frozen plasma. A more recent veterinary study evaluated the findings of thromboelastography (TEG) in 21 dogs with ALF. This study found that severity of hepatic impairment was correlated with hypocoagulability; however, multiple dogs with PT/aPTT findings consistent with hypocoagulability were normocoagulable on TEG (Kelley et al. 2015).

In dogs with ALF, fibrinogen levels may be reduced due to impaired hepatic synthetic function. In the previously referenced study evaluating coagulation parameters in dogs with ALF via TEG, hypocoagulable dogs with ALF had lower fibrinogen levels than those with TEG findings suggestive of normo- or hypercoagulability (Kelley et al. 2015). This suggests that measurement of fibrinogen, specifically a finding of hypofibrinogenemia, may be a useful tool in identifying patients at higher risk of hemorrhage.

DIAGNOSTIC IMAGING

In the emergency setting, focused assessment with sonography for trauma (FAST) is a rapid and effective tool for assessing free fluid within the abdominal, pleural, or pericardial cavities, especially in patients with unstable cardiovascular status. For patients exhibiting signs of shock, respiratory distress, abdominal distention, or pain, abdominal and thoracic FAST scans should be routinely employed to identify any potential issues requiring emergency intervention.

Abdominal radiographs may reveal hepatomegaly or a lack of serosal detail, potentially indicating peritoneal effusion. For patients with respiratory distress, thoracic radiography is also recommended to assess for pleural effusion, alveolar infiltrates, or possible underlying neoplasia. While survey radiographs can provide basic information about liver size, detect conditions such as cholelithiasis, and highlight poor serosal detail to alert the clinician to possible peritoneal effusion, radiographs are subjective, nonspecific, and provide limited information. Therefore, the use of complete abdominal ultrasonography may prove more valuable. Ultrasound enables evaluation of liver size and parenchymal assessment of structural changes as well as the detection of secondary conditions like pancreatitis or gastrointestinal ulcers. Additionally, ultrasound offers a more sensitive evaluation of the biliary system and associated vascular structures. In dogs with ALF, ultrasound findings can vary, with some showing hepatomegaly and changes in hepatic parenchymal echogenicity, while others may present with normal sonographic findings. Unfortunately, the ability of ultrasound to differentiate diffuse hepatic diseases such as neoplasia, fatty infiltration, or toxic hepatopathy is limited. In one study, the diagnostic accuracy in differentiating causes of diffuse hepatic disease was less than 40% in dogs and less than 60% of cats (Feeney et al. 2008). This makes it necessary to combine sonographic findings with clinical history, physical exam, and laboratory results. Ultrasonography is also a useful tool for the guidance of tissue sampling for cytologic and histopathologic evaluation, the results of which may greatly improve diagnostic accuracy. This is described in more detail below.

Although less commonly used in veterinary practice, computed tomography (CT) and magnetic resonance imaging (MRI) are valuable tools in human medicine for evaluating liver morphology. The use of these advanced imaging techniques in veterinary medicine is limited by the need for sedation or anesthesia, cost, and the availability of experienced personnel for interpretation. However, their diagnostic value may increase with greater experience and expertise.

CYTOLOGY AND HISTOPATHOLOGY

Tissue sampling of the liver allows for the assessment of both parenchymal and vascular structures, enables evaluation of the scope of disease distribution as well as chronicity of the condition, and can aid in obtaining a definitive diagnosis for the underlying etiology of ALI/ALF. Before any tissue sampling is conducted, a thorough coagulation screening (platelet count, PT, and aPTT) is recommended to assess the risk of hemorrhage. The thresholds at which abnormal coagulation parameters become contraindications for liver biopsy are still debated. One study showed that an increased risk of bleeding may be associated with a platelet count $<80 \times 10^9$/L, aPTT >1.5 times the upper limit of the reference range in cats, and prolonged PT (above the reference range) in dogs (Bigge et al. 2001). In cases where there is significant concern for clotting abnormalities, the administration of fresh frozen plasma should be considered prior to sampling to minimize complications.

Fine needle aspirate (FNA), usually via ultrasound guidance, is a less invasive and more cost-effective sampling technique. However, this method has several limitations, including the retrieval of only small tissue samples, which may compromise diagnostic accuracy, and the inability to assess the liver's overall architecture. Additionally, FNA may not be suitable for all liver diseases. It is most effective for diagnosing certain diffuse conditions, such as hepatic lipidosis and diffuse neoplastic disease. On the other hand, liver biopsy—whether performed percutaneously under ultrasound guidance or via laparoscopy or laparotomy—can yield larger tissue samples, but carries a higher risk of hemorrhage. Because it allows for a more detailed assessment of cellular morphology and tissue architecture, histopathology via liver biopsy may be necessary for achieving a definitive diagnosis. Additionally, histopathology can provide information regarding the severity of inflammation, as well as the chronicity of the condition via assessment of the degree of fibrosis. In cases where hemorrhage is a concern, laparoscopic biopsies may be preferred over percutaneous approaches, as laparoscopy allows for direct visualization and better control of potential bleeding.

THERAPEUTIC APPROACH

The clinical management of an ALI/ALF patient is largely supportive in nature, as there is often no definitive therapy for most causes of liver dysfunction. These patients are commonly critically ill and may require vigilant monitoring and aggressive supportive care to optimize outcomes.

IV fluid therapy is a cornerstone in the management of the ALI/ALF patient, as a means of restoring and ensuring optimal tissue perfusion, correcting hydration deficits, and maintaining euhydration, particularly if oral fluid intake is diminished. Balanced electrolyte solutions are commonly used in this setting, although fluids containing lactate should be avoided, as patients with hepatic dysfunction may not be able to effectively metabolize lactate to bicarbonate. Although it is an acidifying fluid, 0.9% NaCl may be considered in patients with HE, as the increased osmolality, compared to other isotonic crystalloids, may help to prevent the development of cerebral edema. Excessive volumes of an isotonic crystalloid can lead to interstitial edema, pleural effusion, or ascites, particularly in patients with hypoalbuminemia or systemic inflammation and increased capillary permeability; thus, careful attention to fluid balance and frequent reassessment of the fluid prescription are warranted. As discussed previously, synthetic or natural colloids may be considered in hypoalbuminemic patients requiring ongoing fluid support. Whole blood or packed red blood cell transfusion may be required in patients with moderate or severe anemia; however, the concentration of ammonia increases with time in stored blood, and this may be deleterious in patients with abnormal liver function. While coagulopathy is common in patients with ALI/ALF, spontaneous hemorrhage appears to be rare in this patient population, and the authors generally recommend reserving plasma products for patients with a documented coagulopathy and active hemorrhage or before an invasive procedure.

When severe signs of HE are present, a warm water cleansing enema (10 mL/kg) is recommended to reduce the number of urease-producing bacteria within the gastrointestinal tract. This is followed by a lactulose retention enema (2 mL/10 kg lactulose, diluted 1:1 in warm water). Lactulose is a nonabsorbable disaccharide that acts as both an osmotic laxative and by reducing the pH of the colonic lumen, which limits systemic uptake of ammonia produced by bacteria within the gastrointestinal tract. Metronidazole (7.5 mg/kg IV or PO every 12 hours) is administered to reduce urease-producing bacterial populations within the gastrointestinal tract. As cerebral edema may result from HE, mannitol (0.5–1 g/kg IV over 15–20 minutes) may be considered in patients with severe neurologic compromise. Once the patient is more neurologically stable and able to be transitioned to oral medications, metronidazole and lactulose are continued orally. Oral lactulose (1–3 mL/10 kg every 6–8 hours) is titrated to create soft, but not watery, feces.

Other supportive measures include the use of antiemetics, prokinetics in the event of gastrointestinal ileus, and antacids. Gastroduodenal ulceration is a common complication of liver disease, and bleeding into the gastrointestinal tract may precipitate HE. A proton-pump inhibitor (pantoprazole or omeprazole, 1 mg/kg IV or PO every 12–24 hours), or histamine-2 receptor antagonist (famotidine, 1 mg/kg IV loading dose, followed by 8 mg/kg/day CRI) could be considered. Vitamin K_1 deficiency is common, resulting from reduced oral intake, cholestasis and reduced uptake from the gastrointestinal tract, and the use of systemic antimicrobials, which may disrupt normal gastrointestinal flora that synthesize vitamin K_2. As vitamin K is necessary for the function of coagulation factors II, VII, IX, and X, supplementation at 1 mg/kg SQ once daily is recommended. Prophylactic administration of antimicrobials is generally only recommended for patients with fluid- and vasopressor-refractory hypotension, evidence of sepsis, or progressive HE, or as directed by a positive bacterial culture. Empiric antimicrobial therapy is typically initiated with broad-spectrum coverage but, ideally, narrowed based on culture/susceptibility data when available.

A variety of hepatoprotectant medications have been suggested in the treatment of liver disease, although there is limited evidence of efficacy available in the published literature. N-acetylcysteine (NAC) (140 mg/kg IV or PO loading dose, followed by 70 mg/kg IV or PO every 6 hours for at least 7 doses) has anti-inflammatory and antioxidant properties, may improve hepatic blood flow via vasodilation, and is a source of glutathione. NAC is considered the antidote of choice in acetaminophen intoxication, although it may be considered more broadly in liver injury of other causes. If given IV, it should be diluted to 5% and given slowly over 15 minutes using a 0.2-micron filter. NAC is very unpalatable, so mixing it with fruit juice may help with oral administration. S-adenosylmethionine (17–22 mg/kg PO once daily) may help to stabilize hepatic cell membranes and increase the availability of glutathione. Silymarin (10–20 mg/kg/day PO, divided every 8 hours), derived from the milk thistle plant *Silybum marianum*, may reduce hepatic oxidative stress. Vitamin E (15 IU/kg/day PO) may reduce hepatic oxidative stress via inhibition of lipid peroxidation of cell membranes.

HE should be considered in any patient with hepatic dysfunction and concurrent signs of central nervous system dysfunction or hyperexcitability. Precipitating factors of HE, including electrolyte disturbances and gastrointestinal hemorrhage, should be identified and treated as necessary. A blood ammonia level can be measured to identify the presence of hyperammonemia; however, a normal blood ammonia level does not preclude the possibility of HE. For patients with HE experiencing seizures, levetiracetam (20–60 mg/kg IV loading dose, followed by 20 mg/kg IV every 8 hours) is recommended over the use of benzodiazepines, as there is some evidence to suggest that the presence of endogenous benzodiazepine receptor ligands may play a role in the development of HE.

Early nutritional support is indicated in patients who are not voluntarily consuming sufficient calories, and, when possible, enteral nutrition is preferred over parenteral. Antiemetics, prokinetics, and antacids may improve tolerance of enteral nutrition, although support via a feeding tube may be necessary for patients who are tolerant of enteral nutrition but not consuming sufficient calories voluntarily. The resting energy requirement (RER) is calculated as $70 \times \text{BW (kg)}^{0.75}$ = kilocalories per day, and patients are generally prescribed 25% of their RER divided over several meals on the first day of nutritional support to assess tolerance. The amount of delivered calories is increased daily, pending patient tolerance, with a goal of reaching 100% RER by day 3 or 4. For diet selection, milk and vegetable proteins are preferable for patients with a predisposition to HE, as animal proteins are more likely to precipitate HE.

Where available, therapeutic plasma exchange (TPE) may be considered for patients with ALF. TPE is an extracorporeal treatment involving processing of a patient's blood through an apheresis machine, where the plasma portion is separated, discarded, and replaced with a combination of crystalloids, colloids, and donor plasma. In the setting of ALF, TPE may help to remove protein-bound toxins, bilirubin, inflammatory mediators, ammonia, and other mediators of HE, and also provides a source of clotting factors via donor plasma. Hemodialysis can effectively reduce plasma ammonia concentration and could be considered for patients with severe or refractory hyperammonemia.

PROGNOSIS

The prognosis for ALI is variable and depends on the reversibility of the inciting cause as well as the response to therapy. Once ALF develops, the prognosis is generally thought to be poor, with only a 14% survival to discharge reported in a recent study (Lester et al. 2016).

REFERENCES

Bigge, L.A., Brown, D.J., and Penninck, D.G. (2001). Correlation between coagulation profile findings and bleeding complications after ultrasound-guided biopsies: 434 cases (1993–1996). *Journal of the American Animal Hospital Association* 37 (3): 228–233.

Byers, C.G. (2025). Crystalloids versus Colloids: same controversy, new information. *Veterinary Clinics North America: Small Animal Practice* 55 (3): 363–377. https://doi.org/10.1016/j.cvsm.2025.02.001.

Chapman, S.E. and Hostutler, R.A. (2015). A laboratory diagnostic approach to hepatobiliary disease in small animals. *Clinics in Laboratory Medicine* 35 (3): 503–519.

Feeney, D.A., Anderson, K.L., Ziegler, L.E. et al. (2008). Statistical relevance of ultrasonographic criteria in the assessment of diffuse liver disease in dogs and cats. *American Journal of Veterinary Research* 69 (2): 212–221.

Kelley, D., Lester, C., Shaw, S. et al. (2015). Thromboelastographic evaluation of dogs with acute liver disease. *Journal of Veterinary Internal Medicine* 29 (4): 1053–1062.

Lawrence, Y.A. and Steiner, J.M. (2017). Laboratory evaluation of the liver. *Veterinary Clinics North America: Small Animal Practice* 47 (3): 539–553.

Lester, C., Cooper, J., Peters, R.M. et al. (2016). Retrospective evaluation of acute liver failure in dogs (1995–2012): 49 cases. *Journal of Veterinary Emergency and Critical Care* 26 (4): 559–567. https://doi.org/10.1111/vec.12482.

Lidbury, J.A., Cook, A.K., and Steiner, J.M. (2016). Hepatic encephalopathy in dogs and cats. *Journal of Veterinary Emergency and Critical Care* 26 (4): 471–487.

Mazzaferro, E.M. and Edwards, T. (2020). Update on albumin therapy in critical illness. *Veterinary Clinics North America: Small Animal Practice* 50 (6): 1289–1305.

Pievsky, D., Rustgi, N., and Pyrsopoulos, N.T. (2018). Classification and epidemiologic aspects of acute liver failure. *Clinics in Liver Disease* 22 (2): 229–241.

Prins, M., Schellens, C.J.M.M., and Van Leeuwen, M.W. et al. (2010). Coagulation disorders in dogs with hepatic disease. *The Veterinary Journal* 185 (2): 163–168.

Rabinowich, L. and Bernal, W. (2022). Epidemiology of acute liver failure. In: *Textbook of Liver Transplantation* (ed. P. Burra). Cham: Springer. https://doi.org/10.1007/978-3-030-82930-8_26.

Schmidt, L.E. and Dalhoff, K. (2002). Serum phosphate is an early predictor of outcome in severe acetaminophen-induced hepatotoxicity. *Hepatology* 36 (3): 659–665.

Stravitz, R.T., Ellerbe, C., and Durkalski, V. et al. (2018). Bleeding complications in acute liver failure. *Hepatology* 67 (5): 1931–1942.

Thawley, V. (2017). Acute liver injury and failure. *Veterinary Clinics North America: Small Animal Practice* 47 (3): 617–630.

Weingarten, M.A. and Sande, A.A. (2015). Acute liver failure in dogs and cats. *Journal of Veterinary Emergency and Critical Care* 25 (4): 455–473.

Wlodzimirow, K.A., Eslami, S., Abu-Hanna, A. et al. (2012). Systematic review: acute liver failure - one disease, more than 40 definitions. *Alimentary Pharmacology & Therapeutics* 35 (11): 1245–1256. https://doi.org/10.1111/j.1365-2036.2012.05097.x.

Chronic Hepatitis

CHAPTER 12

Jonathan A. Lidbury

Department of Small Animal Clinical Sciences, College of Veterinary Medicine & Biomedical Sciences, Texas A&M University College Station, TX, USA

KEY POINTS

- Before immunomodulatory therapy is started for presumptive immune-mediated chronic hepatitis, other causes of chronic hepatitis (i.e., drugs, toxins, infectious agents, and copper) should be ruled out.
- Treatment with modified cyclosporine (or other immunomodulatory drugs) can lead to remission in dogs with immune-mediated chronic hepatitis.
- When granulomatous or pyogranulomatous hepatitis is diagnosed by biopsy, testing for geographically relevant infectious diseases should be performed.
- Long-term severe protein restriction is no longer recommended for dogs with hepatic encephalopathy, as it can lead to protein malnutrition and potentially worsen neurological signs.

INTRODUCTION

Chronic hepatitis (CH) is a significant cause of morbidity and mortality in dogs. For example, in a first-opinion practice necropsy-based study of dogs, 12% of all livers examined were found to have CH (Watson et al. 2010). CH is uncommonly reported in cats; cholangitis, where inflammation is centered around the bile ducts, is more common in this species (Chapter 16). If left untreated, CH can progress to cirrhosis/end-stage liver disease and lead to death or euthanasia. CH can present a diagnostic challenge, as in its early stages, dogs may not have any clinical signs, or they may only have nonspecific clinical signs, such as lethargy or dysrexia. Additionally, although laboratory testing and diagnostic imaging are helpful to identify patients that may have CH, definitive diagnosis requires histological examination of a liver biopsy specimen, a relatively expensive and invasive diagnostic test. There are several possible etiologies of CH, and therapy should ideally be biopsy-guided. Even then it can be hard to discern which dogs should be treated for copper-associated CH and which should be treated for immune-mediated CH. However, patients can have a good prognosis with early accurate diagnosis and appropriate therapy.

ETIOLOGY

DRUGS AND TOXINS

The liver plays a central role in the metabolism of xenobiotics (foreign chemical substances). Phase I biotransformation reactions, which occur mainly in zone three hepatocytes, may generate indeterminate metabolites that are more toxic than the parent compound. Therefore, many drugs and toxins can cause liver injury. It should be noted that drugs/toxins typically result in acute liver injury, and the most common outcomes are recovery or fulminant liver failure and death rather than progression to CH. However, some drugs/toxins have the potential to lead to CH. Drugs that can lead to CH include phenobarbital, lomustine (CCNU), primidone, phenytoin, carprofen, amiodarone, and oxibendazole. Toxins that can lead to CH include cycasin (from Sago palms) and aflatoxin. Nutritional supplements, including herbal remedies (e.g., herbal teas, pennyroyal oil, and comfrey), are a common cause of liver injury in humans (Navarro and Seeff 2013). Consequently, clients should be asked specifically if they are giving their pet any supplements.

Disorders of the Liver, Exocrine Pancreas, and Gastrointestinal Tract in Dogs and Cats, First Edition. Edited by Harry Cridge et al. Published 2026 by John Wiley & Sons, Inc. Companion Website: www.wiley.com/go/cridge/disorders

INFECTIOUS AGENTS

Many infectious agents can affect the liver and potentially lead to CH, including *Leishmania* sp., *Histoplasma capsulatum, Heterobilharzia americana, Leptospira* sp., *Mycobacteria* sp., *Neospora caninum, Toxoplasma gondii,* and *Sarcocystis* sp. However, these infections are often multisystemic, so affected patients don't present in a similar way to typical CH patients. In these multisystemic infections, hepatic inflammation is often characterized as being granulomatous or pyogranulomatous. Bacterial culture of liver or bile from dogs with CH is usually negative. Viruses are a common cause of CH in humans, but to date, they have not been found to be an important cause of CH in dogs. Interestingly, domestic cat hepadnavirus appears to be associated with hepatocellular carcinoma and CH (specifically, interface hepatitis) in cats (Pesavento et al. 2019).

COPPER

Copper is an essential trace element and is also a major cause of CH in dogs. Copper is absorbed from the GI tract and stored in the liver. When the capacity of the hepatocyte copper-binding proteins is saturated, free copper ions are released. These lead to the formation of hydroxyl radicals, which can subsequently cause oxidative damage. The following breeds are proven or suspected to have a predisposition: Bedlington terrier, Labrador retriever, Doberman pinscher, Dalmatian, West Highland white terrier, and Cavalier King Charles Spaniel. Copper-associated CH is discussed in Chapter 13.

IMMUNE-MEDIATED INJURY

In a study of dogs with biopsy-confirmed primary hepatitis (acute and chronic), the cause of liver injury was not identified despite a thorough diagnostic investigation in about 60% of the cases (Poldervaart et al. 2009). Dogs may be classified as having idiopathic CH where other causes of CH have been ruled out. Some dogs with idiopathic CH are likely have immune-mediated disease. Evidence supporting this includes a female predisposition in some breeds, an association with specific major histocompatibility haplotypes in Doberman pinschers and English Springer Spaniels, positive titers for autoantibodies that target hepatic proteins in Doberman pinschers, and a positive response to immunomodulatory drugs in some dogs (Bexfield et al. 2012; Andersson and Sevelius 1992; Dyggve et al. 2017; Ullal et al. 2019).

PATHOGENESIS

Regardless of the underlying cause of hepatocellular damage, CH is a syndrome histologically characterized by hepatocellular necrosis or apoptosis, a mononuclear or mixed inflammatory infiltrate, regeneration, and fibrosis (Figure 12.1a, b; van den Ingh et al. 2006). Due to its role in the metabolism of xenobiotics, its location between the splanchnic and systemic circulation, and its large

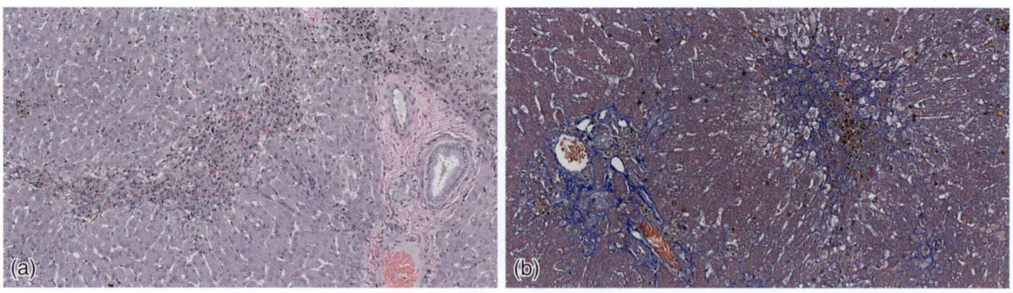

FIGURE 12.1 Liver from a dog with chronic hepatitis. (a) Areas of centrilobular collapse with replacement of hepatocytes by a mixture of hemosiderin and lipofuscin-laden macrophages and lymphocytes. Hepatocytes around the area of injury have cytoplasmic rarefaction and vacuolation consistent with degeneration.
(b) Centrilobular areas contain moderate amounts of pale to dark blue strands of collagen that replace injured hepatocytes. Masson's trichrome stain. Courtesy of Dr. Joao Cavasin

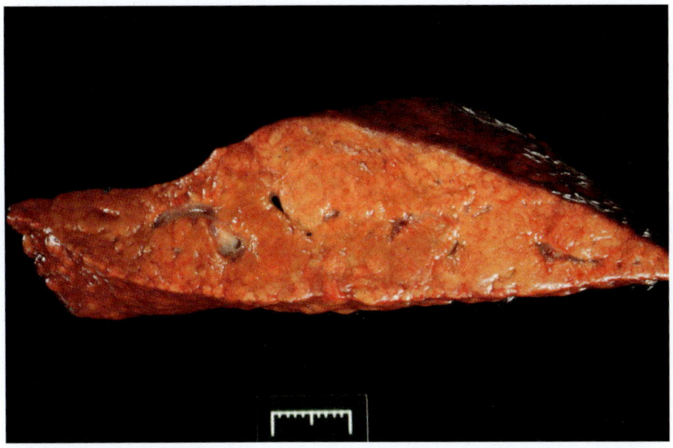

FIGURE 12.2 Liver from a dog with micronodular cirrhosis. Cross-section of a liver from a dog with micronodular cirrhosis. Courtesy of Dr. Randi Gold

population of resident macrophages, the liver is susceptible to oxidative stress. Oxidative stress has been documented in several canine liver diseases and can perpetuate liver injury.

Chronic inflammation of the liver leads to the activation of myofibroblasts, including hepatic stellate cells and portal fibroblasts. This results in excess deposition of extracellular matrix and hepatic fibrosis, the end stage of which is cirrhosis (Figure 12.2). Hepatic fibrosis can diminish liver function as fibroblasts and extracellular matrix replace hepatocytes. As the liver has a large functional reserve capacity, loss of liver function is detected relatively late during CH. Fibrosis can also contribute to the development of portal hypertension as the resistance to blood flow in the hepatic sinusoids increases.

In advanced disease, sinusoidal portal hypertension can lead to the formation of ascites (typically a high-protein transudate). Hypoalbuminemia may be present and this reduces oncotic pressure, which also contributes to imbalances in Starling forces. The development of ascites is an adverse prognostic factor (Raffan et al. 2009).

As the portal pressure increases, multiple vestigial vessels connecting the portal vasculature and caudal vena cava become patent. These acquired portosystemic collaterals (acquired portosystemic shunts) lead to the shunting of ammonia-rich blood from the splanchnic circulation into the systemic circulation bypassing the liver (Buob et al. 2011). Increased ammonia concentrations in the cerebrum contribute to the development of hepatic encephalopathy. Other factors, such as inflammatory cytokines, manganese, oxidative stress, and neurosteroids, play a coactive role.

The liver synthesizes thrombopoietin, nearly all the coagulant and anticoagulant factors, and the factors that regulate fibrinolysis. Additionally, it is responsible for the clearance of many of these factors and vitamin K-dependent activation of factors II, VII, IX, X, protein C, and protein S (Webster 2017). Patients with severe liver disease were traditionally believed to be at increased risk of bleeding, but this seldom occurs spontaneously. Because both the coagulant and anticoagulant systems are affected, patients with liver disease are often in an altered but balanced hemostatic state. However, this balance is more fragile than that of a healthy patient, and if it is disrupted, bleeding or thrombosis can occur. Portal vein thrombosis has been associated with CH in dogs and may lead to prehepatic portal hypertension (Respess et al. 2012).

SIGNALMENT AND CLINICAL FINDINGS

The breeds predisposed to copper-associated and immune-mediated CH are listed above. Notably, Doberman pinschers are predisposed to both (Mandigers et al. 2004). This can create a challenge during therapeutic planning. It is imperative to note that CH can also occur in mixed or non-predisposed breeds of dog and that any age or sex of dog can be affected.

In 384 dogs, from several studies, the most common clinical signs of CH were (in decreasing frequency) decreased appetite, lethargy/depression, icterus, ascites, polyuria/polydipsia, vomiting, diarrhea, hepatic encephalopathy, and melena (Webster et al. 2019). With increased recognition of the importance of pestilently increased serum alanine aminotransferase (ALT) concentrations, especially in predisposed breeds, many dogs are diagnosed before they develop any clinical signs. The earliest signs of CH are often nonspecific (e.g., dysrexia, lethargy), while more liver-specific signs (e.g., ascites, icterus, and hepatic encephalopathy) tend to occur later in the course of the disease.

DIAGNOSIS

LABORATORY TESTING

The earliest and most consistent biochemical change in dogs with CH is an increased serum ALT activity. This is often mild-to-moderate magnitude (typically 180–600 U/L). Increases in alkaline phosphatase (ALP), aspartate aminotransferase (AST), and gamma glutamyl transpeptidase (GGT) activity can also occur but are less consistent and tend to be of a relatively lower magnitude. Increases in liver enzyme activities, especially ALT, often precede the development of clinical signs. Single values of liver enzyme activities are not prognostic, but repeated measurements can provide helpful information. Even then, these changes must be interpreted cautiously considering the clinical picture. For example, a decreasing ALT activity could indicate either improving hepatocellular damage or replacement of hepatocytes with fibrous tissue.

In late-stage disease, hepatic synthetic failure can lead to decreases (below or within the reference interval) of serum BUN, cholesterol, and albumin concentrations. Hypoglycemia can occur with fulminant liver failure or acute liver injury. Patients with late-stage liver disease may also have hyperbilirubinemia; this is an adverse prognostic factor (Gomez Selgas et al. 2014). Because of the liver's large functional reserve capacity, the absence of these changes does not rule out CH (or other liver diseases).

Measurement of paired preprandial and postprandial bile acids or plasma ammonia are relatively sensitive tests for portosystemic shunting. However, because of the hepatic functional reserve capacity, these tests are not sensitive for detecting hepatic insufficiency in the absence of shunting, and normal results do not rule out CH.

Some dogs with CH have mild-to-moderate thrombocytopenia (possibly due to decreased hepatic production of thrombopoietin). Mild anemia, which may be due to chronic disease or GI bleeding, is observed in some, and dogs with acquired portosystemic collaterals may have microcytosis.

ABDOMINAL ULTRASOUND

Ultrasound changes in dogs with CH are variable but include a diffusely hyperechoic liver (due to fibrosis and/or glycogen deposition) and with advanced liver disease/cirrhosis mixed echogenicity, subjective microhepatia, an irregular margin, or hypoechoic nodules (Gaschen 2009; Webster et al. 2019). It is also important to remember that these changes are not specific to CH and that dogs with CH may not have any changes on abdominal ultrasound examination. Ultrasound also allows the detection of reduced or reversed (hepatofugal) portal blood flow, which suggests portal hypertension. Acquired portosystemic collateral blood vessels may be visualized as multiple extrahepatic anomalous vessels often found caudal to the kidneys (Buob et al. 2011).

LIVER/HISTOPATHOLOGY

Definitive diagnosis of CH requires histopathological assessment of liver tissue (Figure 12.3). Histopathological assessment can also help determine the cause of CH and direct treatment. Before liver biopsy, the patient's bleeding risk should be assessed. This involves performing a hematocrit and platelet count, measuring prothrombin time (PT) and activated partial thromboplastin time (aPTT), where possible, measuring fibrinogen concentrations, and possibly measuring buccal mucosal bleeding time (Webster 2017). Liver tissue in dogs can be collected by ultrasound-guided

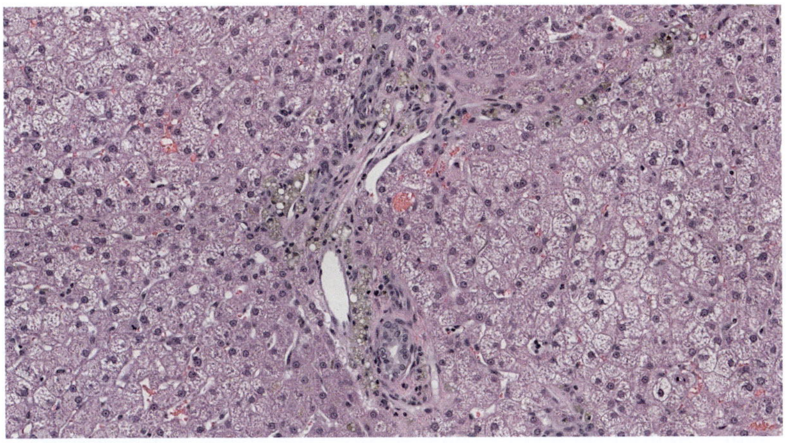

FIGURE 12.3 Liver from a dog with nonspecific reactive hepatitis. Portal tracts contain small numbers of macrophages containing a mixture of lipofuscin and lipid vacuoles interspersed by fewer lymphocytes. The infiltrate does not target bile ducts and does not breach the limiting plate. A similar infiltrate may also be present in central areas (not pictured). Courtesy of Dr. Joao Cavasin

Table 12.1 Advantages and Disadvantages of Different Liver Biopsy Techniques

Percutaneous needle biopsy	Laparoscopic biopsy	Surgical biopsy during laparotomy
Least invasive	Less invasive than surgical biopsy	Most invasive
General anesthesia or heavy sedation required	General anesthesia required	General anesthesia required
Small biopsy specimens 18-gauge Tru-cut needles do not provide adequate samples; 16-gauge recommended for small dogs, 14-gauge for larger dogs	Adequate biopsy specimens Closed cup biopsy forceps are used to collect multiple specimens	Adequate biopsy specimens Relatively large specimens can be collected with various techniques
Ultrasound can be used for guidance	Visualization with scope	Direct visualization
Not possible to directly observe hemorrhage	Hemorrhage can be observed Gel foam can be applied	Hemorrhage can be observed Various methods to achieve with hemostasis
Relatively simple to perform with commonly available equipment	Specialist equipment and training are needed	Simple to perform with common surgical equipment

percutaneous needle biopsy, laparoscopically using closed cup forceps, or during laparotomy using a variety of techniques. Each technique has advantages and disadvantages (Table 12.1). However, the latter two methods are preferred as the resulting biopsy specimens are better diagnostic quality. No matter the technique used, specimens should be collected from several different liver lobes. Several should be placed in a plastic cup with neutral buffered formalin and submitted for histopathological analysis.

Complete histological assessment encompasses examination of sections stained with hematoxylin and eosin, rhodanine or rubeanic acid (for copper), Masson's trichrome or picrosirius red (for connective tissue), Prussian blue or Perl's (for iron), Schmorl's (lipofuscin), and period Gordon and Sweet (for reticulin; Webster et al. 2019). The pathologist should be provided with a succinct medical history, including the patient's signalment, presenting complaint, past/current treatments, and pertinent laboratory testing and diagnostic imaging findings. Any specific clinical questions should also be recorded on the submission form. If there are localized liver lesions, biopsy specimens should be submitted separately.

CH is histologically characterized by hepatocellular necrosis or apoptosis, a mononuclear or mixed inflammatory infiltrate, and varying degrees of regeneration and fibrosis (Figure 12.2; van den Ingh et al. 2006). Sometimes the histomorphological diagnosis does not explicitly mention CH.

Therefore, it is helpful for clinicians to be familiar with the histological definition of CH and the terms used to describe histological findings of the liver. It is essential to differentiate CH from nonspecific reactive hepatitis. Hepatocyte apoptosis/necrosis and fibrosis are characteristic of the former but not the latter. It can be beneficial for the sections to be evaluated by a pathologist with expertise in hepatic pathology.

Another sample of liver should be submitted for aerobic/anaerobic bacterial culture and antimicrobial susceptibility testing. If bacterial infection is suspected, bile should also be collected and submitted for culture (Wagner et al. 2007). However, bacterial culture from the liver and bile of dogs with CH is usually negative.

An additional biopsy specimen (at least 20–40 mg of tissue) should be placed in a plastic container and either kept frozen pending histopathological assessment or directly submitted for copper quantification (preferably measured by flame atomic absorption spectroscopy on a dry weight basis). Regenerative nodules contain less copper than adjacent tissue, so biopsy specimens from nodules should not be submitted for copper quantification. If an additional specimen of liver is unavailable, it is possible to measure copper by deparaffinizing histologic blocks (Johnston et al. 2009); however, some pathology laboratories will not allow this. Alternatively, hepatic copper can be estimated by image analysis of copper-stained sections at Cornell University Animal Diagnostic Center. This technique has the advantage of allowing the assessment of copper in multiple specimens, reducing sampling error (Center et al. 2013).

MANAGEMENT

BIOPSY-GUIDED THERAPY

For dogs with a known history of exposure to drugs/toxins, future exposure should be prevented if possible. In some patients, this is not possible, in which case it should be reduced (e.g., reducing a phenobarbital dose based on drug levels), or steps should be taken to reduce hepatic injury (e.g., treating a dog receiving lomustine with S-adenosylmethionine and silymarin). Liver enzyme activities (especially that of ALT) and the dog's clinical condition can then be monitored while supportive care (see below) is provided.

The criteria for diagnosing copper-associated CH have evolved and are reviewed comprehensively in Chapter 13. Current guidelines state that chelation therapy should be initiated when hepatic concentrations are >1,000 μg/g and should be considered when copper concentrations are 600–1,000 μg/g, depending on the presence, grade, and localization of histological copper staining. (Webster et al. 2019) Occasionally, copper staining and copper quantification are discordant, in which case, additional liver biopsy specimens can be retrieved from the histologic paraffin-embedded block and submitted for quantification, or image-based estimation of the copper concentration can be performed (Center et al. 2013). Sometimes, copper can accumulate in the liver but not be the (primary) cause of liver injury. When copper is the primary cause, it accumulates in the centrilobular zones and colocalizes with inflammatory cells. However, in advanced disease, lobular collapse may make it hard to determine the distribution of copper staining. In some cases, trial chelation therapy is performed, and the dog's ALT activity is reassessed.

When granulomatous or pyogranulomatous hepatitis is confirmed, further testing for geographically relevant infectious diseases should be performed. Once infectious diseases have been ruled out, some dogs with granulomatous hepatitis respond to immunomodulatory therapy (Prentice et al. 2024).

In humans, autoimmune CH is diagnosed based on a scoring system that encompasses ruling out other causes, positive serology for hepatic-targeting autoantibodies, IgG levels, and compatible histopathological changes (Hennes et al. 2008). It is not possible to diagnose autoimmune hepatitis based on histopathology alone. There is currently no way to definitively diagnose immune-mediated CH in dogs, and hepatic-targeting autoantibody tests are not commercially available. Therefore, before immunomodulatory therapy is started for presumptive immune-mediated CH, other causes (i.e., drugs, toxins, infectious agents, and copper) should be ruled out. Some histological changes may be suggestive of immune-mediated CH in dogs: interface hepatitis (destruction of hepatocytes at the limiting plate), which can also be seen with drug reactions, and lymphocyte targeting of hepatocytes (especially if there is lymphocyte swarming). It should be noted that the association of these lesions with immune-mediated disease has not been proven and that not all pathologists are aware of their potential significance.

IMMUNOMODULATORY THERAPY

Once other causes of CH have been ruled out, it is reasonable to do a trial treatment with an immunomodulatory agent.

Prednisolone can be used to treat CH in dogs. Studies have shown beneficial effects, such as improved survival times in dogs with CH (Strombeck et al. 1988), decreased hepatic inflammation in some but not all dogs with idiopathic CH (Favier et al. 2013), and improved clinical and biochemical improvement in CH of English Springer Spaniels (Bayton et al. 2020). Typically, a dose of 1–2 mg/kg/day PO is given initially and this is tapered slowly. Prednisolone and other glucocorticoids can cause side effects, such as polyuria/polydipsia, polyphagia, panting, skin and hair coat changes, vacuolar hepatopathy, and hepatic oxidative stress. After starting treatment with prednisolone, serum liver enzyme activities may improve but do not often return to normal (Bayton et al. 2020).

An uncontrolled retrospective study of 48 dogs with CH treated with modified cyclosporine and hepatoprotective agents documented a 79% remission rate (defined as a return of ALT activity to the normal range). The median cyclosporine dose at remission was 7.9 mg/kg/day, the median time to remission was 2.5 months, and adverse events included GI signs (38% of dogs) and gingival hyperplasia (25% of dogs; Ullal et al. 2019). An advantage of cyclosporine is that it does not affect liver enzyme activities, so they can be used to monitor response to treatment. This drug is the author's first choice for treating dogs with suspected immune-mediated CH; however, it is costly in larger patients. Cyclosporine can predispose dogs to opportunistic fungal infections (and other infections), so owners should be instructed to check regularly for skin lesions. Mycophenolate mofetil (10 mg/kg PO q12 h) and azathioprine (2 mg/kg PO q48 h) have also been used to treat CH in dogs. It should be noted that azathioprine can cause hepatotoxicity in dogs, with one study reporting that 15% developing a >2-fold increase in serum ALT (Wallisch and Trepanier 2015).

CYTOPROTECTIVE AGENTS

Dogs with a variety of liver diseases were shown to have reduced concentrations of glutathione (the liver's main antioxidant). S-adenosylmethionine is a precursor that can increase hepatic glutathione concentrations in dogs. It has also been purported that S-adenosylmethionine has anti-inflammatory properties, modulates apoptosis, and is anti-carcinogenic. At the recommended dose of 20 mg/kg PO q12 h, S-adenosylmethionine rarely causes side effects in dogs other than occasional vomiting after dosing (Webster and Cooper 2009).

Vitamin E is a family of eight lipid-soluble vitamins, alpha-tocopherol being the most biologically active. It is an antioxidant, protecting phospholipids from oxidative injury by scavenging free radicals. Generally, vitamin E (alpha-tocopherol, 15 IU/kg PO, ideally with food q 24 h) is well tolerated in dogs (Webster and Cooper 2009).

Silymarin is extracted from the milk thistle plant. Silibinin is the most biologically active component. Silymarin is believed to have antioxidant effects by scavenging free radicals and reducing lipid peroxidation. It may also have anti-inflammatory and antifibrotic properties (Hackett et al. 2013).

Ursodeoxycholic acid is a hydrophilic bile acid believed to have multiple beneficial properties, including choleretic effects, displacement of other more toxic bile acids from the circulating pool, an antiapoptotic effect, and immunomodulatory effects. When used at a dose of 15 mg/kg/day PO, this drug has few side effects other than occasionally causing diarrhea. There is a rationale for using this drug in dogs with cholestasis (i.e., those with increased serum bilirubin), although use in animals with complete bile duct obstruction may be contraindicated; Webster and Cooper 2009).

It should be noted that no trials have been performed that evaluate the effects of these agents on the clinical outcome of dogs with CH. Therefore, their efficacy has not been proven (nor refuted). If using SAMe or silymarin supplements, it is essential to use products with adequate quality control and proven bioavailability in dogs.

MANAGING THE COMPLICATIONS OF LIVER DISEASE

Feeding a moderate sodium diet, such as a commercially available therapeutic diet for dogs with liver disease, is the first step in treating ascites due to CH. Diuretic therapy is often needed. The aldosterone receptor antagonist spironolactone should be used initially. If 1 mg/kg PO q24 h is ineffective, the dose may be slowly increased to 2 mg/kg q12 h. If this is ineffective, furosemide is added starting at a low dose of 1 mg/kg PO q12 h. The patient's general condition, hydration status, abdominal circumference, serum electrolytes, renal values, and serum protein concentration should be carefully monitored. Occasionally, in patients with compromise due to ascites, therapeutic abdominocentesis is needed. Usually, only about 20–50% of the ascitic fluid is removed at one time to reduce the risk of circulatory collapse. Administration of albumin or balanced crystalloid replacement fluids should be considered after therapeutic abdominocentesis. At a minimum, the patient should be carefully monitored for signs of hypovolemia (Bexfield 2014).

Long-term severe protein restriction is no longer recommended for dogs with hepatic encephalopathy, as it can lead to protein malnutrition and potentially worsening of neurological signs. Non-meat protein-based diets (e.g., soy-based diets) are sometimes recommended, as these protein sources may be less ammoniagenic (Proot et al. 2009). Once the signs of hepatic encephalopathy are controlled with a commercial therapeutic hepatic support diet (Hill's l/d or Royal Canin Hepatic Support), some clinicians add non-meat protein (e.g., cottage cheese) to the patient's diet to help prevent protein malnutrition. However, to avoid unbalancing the main diet, no more than 10% of the dog's total daily caloric intake should be from the supplemental protein source. Alternatively, a soy protein-based hydrolyzed diet can be fed (e.g., Purina HA Hydrolyzed Protein Vegetarian). Lactulose is a nonabsorbable disaccharide that decreases the absorption of ammonia from the GI tract. It is started at a dose of 1–3 mL per 10 kg of body weight PO q6–8 h. The dose is adjusted until the patient passes three to four soft stools daily. Metronidazole is an antimicrobial that is used for the treatment of hepatic encephalopathy in dogs if dietary management and lactulose are not sufficient to control the clinical signs. It is metabolized by the liver, and at higher doses, can cause neurotoxicity, signs of which could be confused with hepatic encephalopathy. Therefore, metronidazole should be given at a lower dose of 7.5 mg/kg PO q8–12 h in dogs with hepatic encephalopathy if needed. Ampicillin and amoxicillin are effective and generally well tolerated when used to treat hepatic encephalopathy. Neomycin is no longer recommended, as some patients develop ototoxicity or nephrotoxicity. Once a patient with hepatic encephalopathy has been stabilized, withdrawal of the antibiotic can be attempted (Serrano et al. 2022).

The prophylactic use of gastric acid-suppressing medications in dogs with CH is unwarranted. However, where GI bleeding is overt or is suspected (e.g., due to a decreasing hematocrit in the absence of other explanations), treatment with a gastric acid-suppressing drug is indicated. Proton pump inhibitors are more effective than histamine-2 receptor antagonists, especially when given twice daily (e.g., omeprazole or pantoprazole, 1 mg/kg PO q12 h; Tolbert et al. 2011). In dogs with liver disease that are actively vomiting or appear to be nauseated, antiemetic therapy is indicated. Maropitant (1 mg/kg SQ/IV/PO q24 h) and ondansetron (0.5 to 1 mg/kg IV/PO q12 h) are common choices.

PROGNOSIS

With early diagnosis and biopsy-guided therapy, dogs with CH can have a favorable long-term prognosis. However, if the cause remains untreated, CH is a progressive disease that can lead to death or euthanasia of the patient. In a combined analysis of 374 dogs from different studies, the median survival time was 561 days (Webster et al. 2019). Indicators of advanced disease are associated with a less favorable prognosis and include ascites, hyperbilirubinemia, prolonged bleeding times, and advanced fibrosis/cirrhosis (Raffan et al. 2009; Gomez Selgas et al. 2014; Sevelius 1995; Shih et al. 2007).

REFERENCES

Andersson, M. and Sevelius, E. (1992). Circulating autoantibodies in dogs with chronic liver disease. *Journal of Small Animal Practice* 33: 389–394.

Bayton, W., Watson, P.J., and Bexfield, N.H. (2020). Prednisolone therapy for chronic hepatitis in English springer spaniels: a prospective study of 12 cases. *Veterinary Record* 186: e21.

Bexfield, NH. (2014). Ascites and hepatic encephalopathy therapy for liver disease. In: *Kirk's Current Veterinary Therapy* (eds. I.D. Bonagura and D.C. Twedt), 15e, 591–594. St. Louis: Elsevier Saunders.

Bexfield, N.H., Watson, P.J., Aguirre-hernandez, J. et al. (2012). DLA class II alleles and haplotypes are associated with risk for and protection from chronic hepatitis in the English Springer spaniel. *PLoS One* 7: e42584.

Buob, S., Johnston, A.N., and Webster, C.R. (2011). Portal hypertension: pathophysiology, diagnosis, and treatment. *Journal of Veterinary Internal Medicine* 25: 169–86.

Center, S.A., Mcdonough, S.P., and Bogdanovic, L. (2013). Digital image analysis of rhodanine-stained liver biopsy specimens for calculation of hepatic copper concentrations in dogs. *American Journal of Veterinary Research* 74: 1474–1480.

Dyggve, H., Meri, S., Spillmann, T. et al. (2017). Antihistone autoantibodies in dobermans with hepatitis. *Journal of Veterinary Internal Medicine* 31: 1717–1723.

Favier, R.P., Poldervaart, J.H., Van Den Ingh, T.S. et al. (2013). A retrospective study of oral prednisolone treatment in canine chronic hepatitis. *Veterinary Quarterly* 33: 113–120.

Gaschen, L. (2009). Update on hepatobiliary imaging. *Veterinary Clinics: Small Animal Practice* 39: 439–467.

Gomez Selgas, A., Bexfield, N., Scase, T.J. et al. (2014). Total serum bilirubin as a negative prognostic factor in idiopathic canine chronic hepatitis. *Journal of Veterinary Diagnostic Investigation* 26: 246–251.

Hackett, E.S., Twedt, D.C., and Gustafson, D.L. (2013). Milk thistle and its derivative compounds: a review of opportunities for treatment of liver disease. *Journal of Veterinary Internal Medicine* 27: 10–16.

Hennes, E.M., Zeniya, M., Czaja, A.J. et al. (2008). Simplified criteria for the diagnosis of autoimmune hepatitis. *Hepatology* 48: 169–176.

Johnston, A.N., Center, S.A., Mcdonough, S.P. et al. (2009). Influence of biopsy specimen size, tissue fixation, and assay variation on copper, iron, and zinc concentrations in canine livers. *American Journal of Veterinary Research* 70: 1502–1511.

Mandigers PJ, van den Ingh TS, Spee B, et al. (2004). Chronic hepatitis in Doberman pinschers. A review. *Veterinary Quarterly* 26: 98–106.

Navarro, V.J. and Seeff, L.B. (2013). Liver injury induced by herbal complementary and alternative medicine. *Clinics in Liver Disease* 17: 715–735.

Pesavento, P.A., Jackson, K., Hampson, T. et al. (2019). A novel hepadnavirus is associated with chronic hepatitis and hepatocellular carcinoma in cats. *Viruses* 11 (10): 969.

Poldervaart, J.H., Favier, R.P., Penning, L.C., et al. (2009). Primary hepatitis in dogs: a retrospective review (2002–2006). *Journal of Veterinary Internal Medicine* 23: 72–80.

Prentice, K.D., Callahan-Clark, J.E., Parry, N.M. et al. (2024). Characterization of clinical presentation, histological features, ultrasonographic findings, and survival in 29 dogs with granulomatous hepatitis. *Journal of Veterinary Internal Medicine* 38: 167–175.

Proot, S., Biourge, V., Teske, E. et al. (2009). Soy protein isolate versus meat-based low-protein diet for dogs with congenital portosystemic shunts. *Journal of Veterinary Internal Medicine* 23: 794–800.

Raffan, E., Mccallum, A., Scase, T.J. et al. (2009). Ascites is a negative prognostic indicator in chronic hepatitis in dogs. *Journal of Veterinary Internal Medicine* 23: 63–66.

Respess, M., O'toole, T.E., Taeymans, O. et al. (2012). Portal vein thrombosis in 33 dogs: 1998–2011. *Journal of Veterinary Internal Medicine* 26: 230–237.

Serrano, G., Devriendt, N., De Rooster, H. et al. (2022). Comparison of diet, lactulose, and metronidazole combinations in the control of pre-surgical clinical signs in dogs with congenital extrahepatic portosystemic shunts. *Journal of Veterinary Internal Medicine* 36: 1258–1266.

Sevelius, E. (1995). Diagnosis and prognosis of chronic hepatitis and cirrhosis in dogs. *Journal of Small Animal Practice*, 36: 521–528.

Shih, J.L., Keating, J.H., Freeman, L.M. et al. (2007). Chronic hepatitis in Labrador Retrievers: clinical presentation and prognostic factors. *Journal of Veterinary Internal Medicine* 21: 33–39.

Strombeck, D.R., Miller, L.M., and Harrold, D. (1988). Effects of corticosteroid treatment on survival time in dogs with chronic hepatitis: 151 cases (1977–1985). *Journal of the American Veterinary Medical Association* 193: 1109–1113.

Tolbert, K., Bissett, S., King, A. et al. (2011). Efficacy of oral famotidine and 2 omeprazole formulations for the control of intragastric pH in dogs. *Journal of Veterinary Internal Medicine* 25: 47–54.

Ullal, T., Ambrosini, Y., Rao, S. et al. (2019). Retrospective evaluation of cyclosporine in the treatment of presumed idiopathic chronic hepatitis in dogs. *Journal of Veterinary Internal Medicine* 33: 2046–2056.

Van Den Ingh, T.S.G.A.M., Van Winkle, T.J., Cullen, J.M. et al. (2006). Morphological classification of parenchymal disorders of the canine and feline liver: hepatocellular death, hepatitis, and cirrhosis-2 (updated version) WSAVA Standards for Clinical and Histological Diagnosis of Canine and Feline Liver

Diseases. *Society of Comparative Hepatology*. https://comparativehepatology.org/wsava-liver-standards/

Wagner, K.A., Hartmann, F.A., and Trepanier, L.A. (2007). Bacterial culture results from liver, gallbladder, or bile in 248 dogs and cats evaluated for hepatobiliary disease: 1998–2003. *Journal of Veterinary Internal Medicine* 21: 417–424.

Wallisch, K. and Trepanier, L.A. (2015). Incidence, timing, and risk factors of azathioprine hepatotoxicosis in dogs. *Journal of Veterinary Internal Medicine* 29: 513–518.

Watson, P.J., Roulois, A.J., Scase, T.J. et al. (2010). Prevalence of hepatic lesions at post-mortem examination in dogs and association with pancreatitis. *Journal of Small Animal Practice* 51: 566–572.

Webster, C.R. (2017). Hemostatic disorders associated with hepatobiliary disease. *Veterinary Clinics: Small Animal Practice* 47: 601–615.

Webster, C.R. and Cooper, J. (2009). Therapeutic use of cytoprotective agents in canine and feline hepatobiliary disease. *Veterinary Clinics: Small Animal Practice* 39: 631–652.

Webster, C.R.L., Center, S.A., Cullen, J.M. et al. (2019). ACVIM consensus statement on the diagnosis and treatment of chronic hepatitis in dogs. *Journal of Veterinary Internal Medicine* 33: 1173–1200.

Copper-associated Hepatopathy

CHAPTER 13

Daniel K. Langlois

Department of Small Animal Clinical Sciences, College of Veterinary Medicine, Michigan State University, East Lansing, MI, USA

KEY POINTS

- High dietary copper intake likely has exacerbated underlying genetic susceptibilities in many dogs, but the exact etiology of copper-associated hepatopathy (CAH) remains a controversial topic.
- Genetic testing is not a reliable predictor of CAH phenotype in most breeds of dog.
- Copper chelation often is advised earlier in the course of CAH and with less severe hepatic copper burden as compared with traditional recommendations.
- Some dogs with CAH have persistent hepatitis despite appropriate hepatic decuprification; this phenomenon might represent concurrent or subsequent immune-mediated chronic hepatitis.

BACKGROUND

Pathologic hepatic copper accumulation is a common cause of progressive and potentially fatal liver disease in dogs (Dirksen and Fieten 2017; Webster et al. 2019). Copper is an essential micronutrient and cofactor for hundreds of enzymatic reactions throughout the body, but excessive tissue copper promotes free radical formation and oxidative injury (Pereira et al. 2016). The liver often is affected in states of copper overload because of its central role in copper storage and metabolism. Normal hepatic copper concentrations in dogs are poorly defined. As hepatic copper concentrations have increased over time, dogs tolerate a greater degree of hepatic copper than other species, and there is no clear cut-point that distinguishes between healthy and diseased dogs (Thornburg et al. 1990; Thornburg 2000; Twedt et al. 1979). Still, most laboratories consider a hepatic copper concentration of 400 μg/g (dry matter basis) to be the upper-end of normal, and this cut-point correlates with a copper burden that is often detectable with histochemical stains such as rhodanine or rubeanic acid (Webster et al. 2019). Hepatic injury is common when hepatic copper concentrations exceed 1000 μg/g (Dirksen and Fieten 2017; Webster et al. 2019; Thornburg et al. 1990). However, copper concentrations in the 600–800 μg/g range are associated with hepatitis in some dogs whereas other dogs can have copper concentrations > 1500 μg/g with no evidence of hepatitis (Webster et al. 2019; Thornburg et al. 1990; Thornburg 2000; Twedt et al. 1979). These caveats should be considered in the diagnosis and management of CAH in dogs. Regardless, copper-associated hepatopathy (CAH) was once thought to be a rare disease affecting only Bedlington terriers, but CAH now is recognized as a leading cause of chronic hepatitis in many breeds of dog (Dirksen and Fieten 2017; Webster et al. 2019).

ETIOLOGY

The precise etiology of CAH remains a source of debate, but mounting evidence suggests that both heritable factors and copper intake contribute to CAH development (Fieten et al. 2016; Johnston et al. 2013; Strickland et al. 2018; van De Sluis et al. 2002; Yuzbasiyan-Gurkan et al. 1997). Breeds considered to be at risk for CAH include Labrador retrievers, Doberman pinschers, Dalmatians, West Highland

Disorders of the Liver, Exocrine Pancreas, and Gastrointestinal Tract in Dogs and Cats, First Edition. Edited by Harry Cridge et al. Published 2026 by John Wiley & Sons, Inc. Companion Website: www.wiley.com/go/cridge/disorders

White terriers, Skye terriers, and Bedlington terriers, amongst others (Dirksen and Fieten 2017; Webster et al. 2019). Beyond breed predispositions, the potential for a genetic basis of disease is supported by several studies. Copper toxicosis in Bedlington terriers is a well-characterized autosomal recessive disorder, and most cases result from an exon 2 deletion of the *COMMD1* gene (van De Sluis et al. 2002; Yuzbasiyan-Gurkan et al. 1997). Selective breeding strategies have dramatically decreased the prevalence of CAH in Bedlington terriers, but CAH has been increasingly recognized in many other breeds in recent decades. Variants in the *ATP7B* gene might predispose some Labrador retrievers and Doberman pinschers to CAH, whereas variants in the *ATP7A* gene might have a slight protective effect against CAH in Labrador retrievers, but these variants only account for a small proportion of the variation in hepatic copper concentrations (Fieten et al. 2016; Wu et al. 2019; Langlois et al. 2022). Indeed, approximately 50% of Labrador retrievers with CAH lack an *ATP7B* variant allele and 25% of healthy Labrador retrievers possess an *ATP7B* variant allele (Langlois et al. 2022). Other genetic variants might influence susceptibility to disease, but no overt causative mutations have been identified in non-Bedlington terrier breeds despite several investigations (Wu et al. 2020).

The lack of a clear hereditary pattern, failure to identify causative mutations, and increased recognition of CAH in breeds of dog that are not historically considered to be at risk of CAH have spurred concerns that environmental copper exposures are involved in CAH pathogenesis (Webster et al. 2019; Center et al. 2021). In support of this premise, the copper content of many commercial dog foods far exceeds minimum regulatory requirements even though clinically relevant copper deficiency has never been problematic in dogs that eat a commercial diet (Webster et al. 2019). Regulatory changes in dietary copper supplementation practices in the mid-1990s also led to higher amounts of bioavailable copper in commercial dog food, which coincided with observed increases in hepatic copper concentrations in dogs (Johnston et al. 2013; Strickland et al. 2018). In one study, <5% of specimens from Labrador retrievers that were obtained prior to 1997 had copper concentrations > 1000 μg/g, whereas nearly 25% of specimens from Labrador retrievers that were obtained in 1997 and onward had copper concentrations > 1000 μg/g (Strickland et al. 2018). Even breeds not considered to be at risk for CAH had a median increase in hepatic copper concentrations of 100 μg/g after this time point. These observations provide support that dietary copper supplementation practices are contributing to CAH, but the exact etiology likely is multifactorial and involves a complex interplay of dietary copper intake and genetic susceptibilities.

CLINICAL FEATURES

Pathologic copper accumulation is a gradual process, and a subclinical phase of months to years precedes the development of biochemical abnormalities and overt clinical signs. Further confounding matters is the fact that some dogs can have severe hepatic copper accumulation with virtually no histologic abnormalities, and even if low-level inflammation is present, increased liver enzyme activities are not always observed (Dirksen et al. 2017; Vincent et al. 2021). As such, most dogs are middle-aged (i.e., 4–9 years) at the time of CAH diagnosis and have substantial copper accumulation (Dirksen and Fieten 2017; Webster et al. 2019). However, dogs ranging in age from 1 to over 13 years have been reported. A female predisposition and earlier onset of disease have been described in Doberman pinschers, and a slight female predisposition might exist in Labrador retrievers and Dalmatians, but study results are conflicting (Dirksen and Fieten 2017; Webster et al. 2019; Vincent et al. 2021; Hoffmann et al. 2006; Langlois et al. 2013b; Webb et al. 2002).

Clinical signs are not uniformly present as many seemingly healthy dogs are diagnosed with CAH after increased liver enzyme activities are discovered during routine wellness or preanesthetic evaluations. Clinical features of CAH, when present, are nonspecific and similar to those of any progressive liver disease (Webster et al. 2019; Hoffmann et al. 2006). Dogs with moderate-to-severe disease often experience varying combinations of hyporexia, lethargy, weight loss, and nausea/vomiting. Clinical signs such as gastrointestinal bleeding, jaundice, hepatic encephalopathy, ascites, polyuria, and polydipsia are less common and more likely in advanced disease.

Clinical biochemistry results are nonspecific and suggestive of liver injury and potentially liver dysfunction. A mild to moderately increased ALT activity is the hallmark biochemical feature, and this might be the only abnormality early in the course of disease (Webster et al. 2019). Increased ALP activity also is observed in most affected dogs, but the magnitude of increase is typically much less than that of ALT activity (Dirksen and Fieten 2017; Webster et al. 2019; Hoffmann et al. 2006). However, the hepatic enzymopathy can shift in more advanced disease such as cirrhosis, with ALP activity sometimes exceeding ALT activity. Biomarkers of liver function (e.g., albumin, cholesterol, urea, bilirubin, etc.) are variably affected in 20–70% of cases dependent upon the stage and severity of disease. Some dogs experience an acute onset of clinical signs in association with severely increased liver enzyme activities (i.e., ALT > 1000–2000 U/L) and hyperbilirubinemia that can mimic an acute liver injury or acute liver failure (Hoffmann et al. 2006; Webb et al. 2002). These cases often are not recognized as potential CAH until after initial supportive measures improve clinical signs but fail to completely resolve liver enzyme abnormalities.

Other less common biochemical features of CAH include renal glucosuria or Fanconi syndrome, often in conjunction with a normal anion gap metabolic acidosis (Langlois et al. 2013b). Renal tubular dysfunction in these dogs is associated with renal tubular copper accumulation. Release of excess hepatic copper is speculated to be involved in this process because most affected dogs have severe hepatic copper burdens and moderate-to-severe centrilobular hepatocyte necrosis (Langlois et al. 2013b). Given the rarity of renal tubular disorders, the combination of hepatic disease and renal tubular dysfunction should prompt consideration of CAH. Finally, acute hemolytic crises associated with massive release of copper into the bloodstream are possible, but exceedingly rare (Dirksen and Fieten 2017).

Abdominal ultrasound is the preferred imaging modality in the assessment of dogs with suspected CAH, but its primary value is exclusion of other causes of liver disease (e.g., hepatocellular carcinoma) and identification of clinically relevant comorbidities (e.g., gallbladder mucocele). Ultrasound changes in dogs with CAH are diffuse but not necessarily uniform. Heterogenous or hyperechoic hepatic echotexture are common, and small irregular hypoechoic nodules and microhepatica can occur with more advanced CAH (Webster et al. 2019). Conversely, minimal to no sonographic abnormalities are present in dogs with early CAH. These changes are not unique and can occur with any form of chronic hepatitis. Ultrasound examination can also be used to facilitate tissue acquisition.

DIAGNOSIS

Various noninvasive biomarkers including serum microRNAs, measures of plasma oxidant status, and serum and urinary copper levels have been investigated as diagnostic tools for CAH, but these tests are limited by overlap between affected and unaffected dogs, complicated sample handling and processing, or complex analytical methods (Vincent et al. 2021; Dirksen et al. 2016; Fieten et al. 2013b). Cytologic assessments of liver aspirates might reveal intracytoplasmic copper, but cytology cannot be used to definitively diagnose CAH because inflammatory infiltrates often are missed, the degree of copper accumulation cannot be determined, and the degree of remodeling/fibrosis cannot be assessed (Webster et al. 2019). Genetic testing is available for the exon 2 deletion of the *COMMD1* gene as well as for variants in the *ATP7B* and *ATP7A* genes. However, *COMMD1*-associated CAH is limited to Bedlington terriers, some Bedlington terriers develop CAH for other reasons, and most *ATP7A* and *ATP7B* genotypes are poor predictors of CAH phenotype in other dog breeds (van De Sluis et al. 2002; Langlois et al. 2022). Labrador retrievers that are homozygous for the *ATP7B* variant do seem likely to develop CAH, but this genotype is extremely uncommon in the general dog population and also uncommon in Labrador retrievers with CAH (Fieten et al. 2016; Langlois et al. 2022; Pindar and Ramirez 2019).

As such, hepatic biopsy is required to definitively diagnose CAH (Webster et al. 2019). Hepatic biopsy should be considered in (i) clinically normal dogs with persistently increased ALT activity in which other causes are not apparent, (ii) dogs with acute hepatocellular hepatopathies in which clinical signs resolve with supportive treatment but ALT activity fails to normalize, and (iii) unwell dogs with biochemical and imaging evidence of chronic liver disease. More detailed descriptions of techniques and considerations for hepatic biopsy can be found elsewhere (see Chapters 4 and 12.

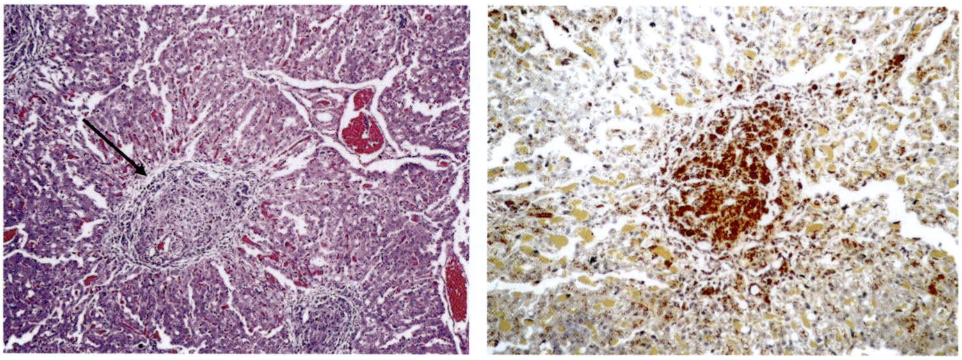

FIGURE 13.1 Photomicrographs (40×) of H&E (left) and rhodanine (right) stained sections of liver from a Labrador retriever with CAH. The left panel demonstrates a centrilobular-focused chronic hepatitis (the arrow), whereas the right panel demonstrates severe centrilobular copper accumulation (orange–red granules) within hepatocytes and macrophages, which corresponds to a rhodanine grade of 4. Images were courtesy of Rebecca Smedley

Regardless of biopsy method, more than one lobe should be sampled and a total of at least four and ideally five specimens should be obtained. One piece should be used for determination of quantitative copper concentrations, one piece should be used for bacterial cultures, and the remaining specimens should be placed in formalin for histologic assessments. Rhodanine or rubeanic acid staining should be performed as part of the histologic assessments and scored (i.e., scores of 0–5, normal ≤1) according to published guidelines to semiquantitatively assess copper accumulation and lobular localization (Webster et al. 2019; Center et al. 2013).

Classically, dogs with CAH have histologic evidence of chronic hepatitis in association with centrilobular copper accumulation, rhodanine scores ≥3, and quantitative copper concentrations > 1000 μg/g (Figure 13.1) (Dirksen and Fieten 2017; Webster et al. 2019). Panlobular copper accumulation and associated hepatitis also can be observed in severe cases. However, CAH diagnosis is not always straightforward because fibrosis and regenerative nodule formation can preclude accurate determination of the lobular distribution of copper. Fibrous tissue and regenerative nodules also have minimal copper as compared to adjacent parenchyma and can thereby decrease measured copper concentrations (Webster et al. 2019). Some dogs develop chronic hepatitis in association with hepatic copper concentrations between 600 and 1000 μg/g, a range which is often considered a "gray zone". Finally, some dogs can have moderate-to-severe hepatic copper accumulation that is not located in centrilobular regions. These challenging scenarios must be assessed on a case-by-case basis while integrating clinical and histologic features. Collaboration with a pathologist with expertise in hepatopathology is critical in these cases.

MANAGEMENT

Therapy for CAH should be tailored to individuals with consideration given to clinical severity and hepatic histopathologic features. The principals of treatment are to reduce the hepatic copper burden and mitigate the consequences of excess copper. Dietary copper restriction, copper chelation, or zinc salt administration can be used to lower hepatic copper concentrations. Dietary copper restriction (i.e., <0.18 mg copper per 100 kcal) is indicated for all dogs with CAH, and life-long restriction is appropriate in most cases (Webster et al. 2019). Therapeutic hepatic diets with <0.12 mg copper per 100 kcal (Hills® Prescription Diet l/d and Royal Canin Veterinary Diet® Hepatic) are often used, but the degree of protein restriction in these diets might warrant additional protein supplementation. Home-prepared low-copper diets, formulated by a board-certified veterinary nutritionist to ensure they are balanced for long-term feeding, can also be considered. Other therapeutic diets as well as commercially available diets that have copper contents closer to the AAFCO minimum of 0.18 mg copper per 100 kcal are also likely suitable diets. Some dogs with CAH achieve normalization of hepatic copper with dietary therapy alone, but this is a very slow process (Hoffmann et al. 2009; Fieten et al. 2015). Dietary copper restriction might be reasonable as sole treatment in dogs with low-level copper accumulation (i.e., < 600–800 μg/g or rhodanine scores ≤2) and minimal to absent chronic hepatitis, but otherwise should be considered as a component of a broader treatment strategy. Furthermore, normalization of hepatic copper does not occur in some dogs being fed a therapeutic hepatic diet, and a smaller subset of dogs will continue to accumulate copper (Fieten et al. 2015).

Copper chelation with d-penicillamine (10–15 mg/kg PO twice daily) is the treatment of choice for CAH and is most effective when combined with dietary copper restriction (Webster et al. 2019; Fieten et al. 2013a). Compounded d-penicillamine preparations often are used because of cost concerns with commercially available products. The drug should be given on an empty stomach, as coadministration with food reduces bioavailability by approximately 70% (Langlois et al. 2013a). Gastrointestinal side effects occur in approximately 20% of d-penicillamine-treated dogs, but these effects usually can be minimized with dose-escalation strategies, anti-nausea medications, or administration of d-penicillamine with a very small piece of food. If gastrointestinal adverse effects persist, the author recommends a lower dose (e.g., 4–6 mg/kg) on an empty stomach rather than a standard dose coadministered with a meal. Other adverse effects of d-penicillamine such as blood dyscrasias, proteinuria, and dermatologic reactions are uncommon but warrant routine clinical and biochemical monitoring. Other copper chelators such as ammonium tetrathiomolybdate or trientine are not well-studied in dogs but can be considered in cases of d-penicillamine intolerance.

Historically, copper chelation was initiated if hepatic copper concentrations exceeded 1500 μg/g, but chelation is now recommended for any CAH case in which copper concentrations exceed 1000 μg/g. Many veterinary hepatologists will initiate copper chelation when copper concentrations exceed 800 μg/g or rhodanine scores are ≥3, and some veterinary hepatologists even treat when copper concentrations exceed 600 μg/g or rhodanine scores are ≥2. Treatment should be considered in this lower range if chronic hepatitis is present and associated with copper deposits or if advanced parenchymal disease might be artifactually skewing copper concentrations downward. The duration of treatment is variable and loosely correlated with the severity of copper accumulation. The author typically advises 3–4 months, 4–6 months, or 6–12 months of chelation for copper concentrations < 1200 μg/g, 1200–2000 μg/g, or > 2000 μg/g, respectively. Repeat hepatic biopsies should be performed to guide treatment duration. However, continuing chelation therapy for several weeks beyond resolution of abnormal ALT activity is advised if repeat biopsy is not possible.

Zinc salt administration (5 mg/kg elemental zinc PO twice daily; ideally administered on an empty stomach to avoid binding with dietary phytates) induces intestinal metallothionein expression and blocks intestinal copper absorption (Webster et al. 2019). This treatment can effectively lower hepatic copper in dogs with high copper burdens, but similar to diet, decuprification is slow (Brewer et al. 1992). Zinc salts are inexpensive but can cause treatment-limiting gastrointestinal upset in some dogs. This might be offset by using zinc gluconate as opposed to other zinc salts and coadministering zinc with a small amount of canned tuna or other food that lacks phytates. Zinc salts also should not be administered during d-penicillamine chelation therapy. The author occasionally uses zinc as maintenance treatment after successful copper chelation, but gastrointestinal adverse effects are frequently encountered.

Treatments targeting oxidative stress and inflammation are used frequently for CAH because months of decuprification is needed before clinically relevant reductions in hepatic copper occur. CAH is a disease of oxidative injury, and antioxidants are generally recommended despite limited evidence of efficacy (Webster et al. 2019). Vitamin E or S-adenosyl-methionine (SAMe) is recommended for this purpose. The role of glucocorticoids is poorly studied in CAH, although glucocorticoid administration increased survival in several retrospective studies of chronic hepatitis that probably included dogs with CAH (Webster et al. 2019; Strombeck et al. 1988; Favier et al. 2013). Short to intermediate courses of anti-inflammatory glucocorticoids (e.g., 0.5 mg/kg/day prednisolone for 3–4 weeks and then tapered over an additional two weeks) can be used in dogs that are clinically unwell and have advanced chronic hepatitis with substantial parenchymal remodeling. Anecdotally, glucocorticoids help many dogs feel better quickly, improve d-penicillamine tolerance, and improve hepatitis prior to reductions in copper. Glucocorticoids are not recommended in dogs that are clinically well or have only mild-to-moderate CAH.

The prognosis for CAH is fair to good with dogs diagnosed early in the disease process typically experiencing years of survival. Long-term outcomes are highly variable for dogs with more advanced parenchymal disease or cirrhosis. In addition to life-long dietary copper restriction, some dogs require low-dose intermittent d-penicillamine (5 mg/kg PO every other day) or zinc salt administration to maintain normal hepatic copper concentrations. Some CAH-affected dogs have persistent chronic hepatitis despite normalization of hepatic copper. Whether this represents concurrent or subsequent immune-mediated hepatitis is unknown, but immune modulation is required.

COPPER ASSOCIATED HEPATOPATHY IN CATS

CAH is an uncommon to rare cause of liver disease in cats, although cases might be overlooked because CAH is seldom considered a differential for feline liver disease (Hurwitz et al. 2014; Yamkate et al. 2021). Variants in the *ATP7B* gene might be involved in pathogenesis in some cases, whereas environmental copper exposure was hypothesized to be involved in another case, but overall evidence to support these speculations is limited (Asada et al. 2020). Copper accumulation secondary to cholestasis might occur in some cats. Cats with CAH share many similarities with dogs in terms of clinical signs and biochemical abnormalities. Vomiting, lethargy, and hyporexia are common, and CAH-affected cats generally have increased ALT activity and predominantly centrilobular copper accumulation (Hurwitz et al. 2014). However, cats with CAH are often diagnosed at a younger age (median age of two years) than dogs, and no sex predisposition has been identified in cats. Treatment is poorly described, but several reports suggest similar treatment approaches to those used in dogs such as d-penicillamine chelation (10–15 mg/kg PO twice daily), dietary modification, and hepatoprotective medications. Long-term prognosis is largely unknown though because of limited data, but variable survival times of weeks to years have been observed. Interestingly, the pathologic copper accumulation might predispose some CAH-affected cats to subsequent development of hepatocellular carcinoma (Hurwitz et al. 2014).

REFERENCES

Asada, H., Kojima, M., Nagahara, T. et al. (2020). Variations in ATP7B in cats with primary copper-associated hepatopathy. *Journal of Feline Medicine and Surgery* 33 (2): 874–878.

Brewer, G.J., Dick, R.D., Schall, W. et al. (1992). Use of zinc acetate to treat copper toxicosis in dogs. *Journal of the American Veterinary Medical Association* 201: 564–568.

Center, S.A., McDonough, S.P., and Bogdanovic, L. (2013). Digital image analysis of rhodanine-stained liver biopsy specimens for calculation of hepatic copper concentrations in dogs. *American Journal of Veterinary Research* 74 (12): 1474–1480.

Center, S.A., Wakshlag, J.J., Cullen, J.M. et al. (2021). Possible diet-related increase in copper-associated liver disease in dogs. *Veterinary Record* 189: 117.

Dirksen, K. and Fieten, H. (2017). Canine copper-associated hepatitis. *Veterinary Clinics: Small Animal Practice* 47 (3): 631–644.

Dirksen, K., Burgener, I.A., Rothuizen, J. et al. (2017). Sensitivity and specificity of plasma ALT, ALP, and bile acid for hepatitis in labrador retrievers. *Journal of Veterinary Internal Medicine* 31: 1017–1027.

Dirksen, K., Verzijl, T., van den Ingh, T.S.G.A.M. et al. (2016). Hepatocyte-derived microRNAs as sensitive serum biomarkers of hepatocellular injury in labrador retrievers. *The Veterinary Journal* 211: 75–81.

Favier, R.P., Poldervaart, J.H., van den Ingh, T.S. et al. (2013). A retrospective study of oral prednisolone treatment in canine chronic hepatitis. *Veterinary Quarterly* 33: 113–120.

Fieten, H., Biourge, V.C., Watson, A.L. et al. (2015). Rothuizen J. Dietary management of Labrador retrievers with subclinical hepatic copper accumulation. *Journal of Veterinary Internal Medicine* 29: 822–827.

Fieten, H., Dirksen, K., van den Ingh, T.S. et al. (2013a). D-penicillamine treatment of copper-associated hepatitis in Labrador retrievers. *The Veterinary Journal* 196: 522–527.

Fieten, H., Gill, Y., Martin, A.J. et al. (2016). The Menkes and Wilson disease genes counteract in copper toxicosis in labrador retrievers: a new canine model for copper-metabolism disorders. *Disease Models & Mechanisms* 9 (1): 25–38.

Fieten, H., Hugen, S., van den Ingh, T.S.G.A.M. et al. (2013b). Urinary excretion of copper, zinc and iron with and without D-penicillamine administration in relation to hepatic copper concentration in dogs. *The Veterinary Journal* 197: 468–473.

Hoffmann, G., Jones, P.G., Biourge, V. et al. (2009). Dietary management of hepatic copper accumulation in Labrador Retrievers. *Journal of Veterinary Internal Medicine* 23: 957–963.

Hoffmann, G., van den Ingh, T.S.G.A.M., Bode, P. et al. (2006). Copper-associated chronic hepatitis in labrador retrievers. *Journal of Veterinary Internal Medicine* 20 (4): 856–861.

Hurwitz, B.M., Center, S.A., Randolph, J.F. et al. (2014). Presumed primary and secondary hepatic copper accumulation in cats. *Journal of the American Veterinary Medical Association* 244 (1): 68–77.

Johnston, A.N., Center, S.A., McDonough, S.P. et al. (2013). Hepatic copper concentrations in Labrador Retrievers with and without chronic hepatitis: 72 cases (1980–2010). *Journal of the American Veterinary Medical Association* 242 (3): 372–380.

Langlois, D.K., Lehner, A.F., Buchweitz, J.P. et al. (2013a). Pharmacokinetics and relative bioavailability of D-penicillamine in fasted and nonfasted dogs. *Journal of Veterinary Internal Medicine* 27: 1071–1076.

Langlois, D.K., Nagler, B.S.M., Smedley, R.C. et al. (2022). ATP7A, ATP7B, and RETN genotypes in Labrador Retrievers with and without copper-associated hepatitis. *Journal of the American Veterinary Medical Association* 260: 1–8.

Langlois, D.K., Smedley, R.C., Schall, W.D. et al. (2013b). Acquired proximal renal tubular dysfunction in 9 Labrador Retrievers with copper-associated hepatitis (2006–2012). *Journal of Veterinary Internal Medicine* 27 (3): 491–499.

Pereira, T.C., Campos, M.M., and Bogo, M.R. (2016). Copper toxicology, oxidative stress, and inflammation using zebrafish as experimental model. *Journal of Applied Toxicology* 36: 876–885.

Pindar, S. and Ramirez, C. (2019). Predicting copper toxicosis: relationship between the ATP7A and ATP7B gene mutations and hepatic copper quantification in dogs. *Human Genetics* 138: 541–546.

Strickland, J.M., Buchweitz, J.P., Smedley, R.C. et al. (2018). Hepatic copper concentrations in 546 dogs (1982–2015). *Journal of Veterinary Internal Medicine* 32: 1943–1950.

Strombeck, D.R., Miller, L.M., and Harrold, D. (1988). Effects of corticosteroid treatment on survival time in dogs with chronic hepatitis: 151 cases (1977–1985). *Journal of the American Veterinary Medical Association* 193: 1109–1113.

Thornburg, L.P. (2000). A perspective on copper and liver disease in the dog. *Journal of Veterinary Diagnostic Investigation* 12: 101–110.

Thornburg, L.P., Rottinghaus, G., McGowan, M. et al. (1990). Hepatic copper concentrations in purebred and mixed-breed dogs. *Veterinary Pathology* 27: 81–88.

Twedt, D.C., Sterlieb, I., and Gilbertson, S.R. (1979). Clinical, morphologic, and chemical studies on copper toxicosis of Bedlington Terriers. *Journal of the American Veterinary Medical Association* 175: 269–275.

van De Sluis, B., Rothuizen, J., Pearson, P. et al. (2002). Identification of a new copper metabolism gene by positional cloning in a purebred dog population. *Human Molecular Genetics* 11 (2): 165–173.

Vincent, A.M., Sordillo, L.M., Smedley, R.C. et al. (2021). Peripheral markers of oxidative stress in Labrador Retrievers with copper-associated hepatitis. *Journal of Small Animal Practice* 62 (10): 866–873.

Webb, C.B., Twedt, D.C., and Meyer, D.J. (2002). Copper-associated liver disease in Dalmatians: a review of 10 dogs (1998–2001). *Journal of Veterinary Internal Medicine* 16: 665–668.

Webster, C.R.L., Center, S.A., Cullen, J.M., et al. (2019). ACVIM consensus statement on the diagnosis and treatment of chronic hepatitis in dogs. *Journal of Veterinary Internal Medicine* 33 (3): 1173–1200.

Wu, X., Mandigers, P.J.J., Fieten, H. et al. (2020). Evaluation of COMMD1 in copper toxicosis in Labradors retrievers and Dobermans. *The Veterinary Journal* 265: 105561.

Wu, X., Mandigers, P.J.J., Watson, A. et al. (2019). Association of canine ATP7A and ATP7B with hepatic copper accumulation in Dobermann dogs. *Journal of Veterinary Internal Medicine* 33 (4): 1646–1652.

Yamkate, P., Gold, R.M., Xenoulis, P.G. et al. (2021). Assessment of copper accumulation in archived liver specimens from cats. *Journal of Feline Medicine and Surgery* 23 (6): 526–533.

Yuzbasiyan-Gurkan, V., Blanton, S.H., Cao, Y. et al. (1997). Linkage of a microsatellite marker to the canine copper toxicosis locus in Bedlington Terriers. *American Journal of Veterinary Research* 58 (1): 23–27.

CHAPTER 14 Hepatocutaneous Syndrome

Rommaneeya Leela-arporn[1] *and Cynthia R. L. Webster*[2]

[1] *Department of Clinical Sciences, College of Veterinary Medicine and Biomedical Sciences, Colorado State University, Fort Collins, CO, USA*
[2] *Department of Clinical Sciences, Cummings School of Veterinary Medicine at Tufts University, North Grafton, MA, USA*

KEY POINTS

- Hepatocutaneous syndrome (HCS) is an uncommon metabolic disorder with a predilection for affecting middle-aged to older male dogs.
- The pathogenesis of HCS remains unclear but likely involves impaired protein metabolism leading to profound plasma hypoaminoacidemia, which in turn results in the development of characteristic skin lesions (superficial necrolytic erythema) and hepatic pathology (degenerative vacuolar hepatopathy) with long-term sequelae that include diabetes mellitus and hepatocellular carcinoma.
- The diagnosis of the HCS is made by the detection of plasma hypoaminoacidemia in a dog with typical hyperkeratotic, crusting and erosive skin lesions, and the characteristic honeycomb appearance of the liver on ultrasound.
- Treatment is multimodal and includes parenteral amino acid infusions, enteral supplementation of oral amino acids, antioxidants, +/– zinc, +/– omega-3 fatty acids, a high-protein diets, and treatment of secondary sequelae.

INTRODUCTION

Hepatocutaneous syndrome (HCS), also referred to as aminoaciduria canine hypoaminoacidemic hepatopathy syndrome (ACHES), is a rare metabolic disorder. HCS is characterized by distinctive skin lesions known as superficial necrolytic dermatitis (SND) and hepatic pathology, both of which are the result of profound amino acid depletion (DeMarle et al. 2021; Outerbridge et al. 2002; Loftus et al. 2017; Loftus et al. 2022a; Byrne 1999; Hall-Fonte et al. 2016; Leela-arporn et al. 2025; Loftus et al. 2022b). HCS predominantly affects dogs (DeMarle et al. 2021; Outerbridge et al. 2002; Loftus et al. 2017; Loftus et al. 2022a; Byrne 1999; Hall-Fonte et al. 2016; Leela-arporn et al. 2025), but rare occurrences have been reported in cats (Kimmel et al. 2003; Asakawa et al. 2013). HCS can present a diagnostic and therapeutic challenge; however, advances in understanding of the disease have improved recognition and facilitated the development of treatment interventions which have improved prognosis (DeMarle et al. 2021; Outerbridge et al. 2002; Loftus et al. 2022b). This chapter provides a broad overview of HCS, emphasizing how to make a prompt diagnosis and discussing a therapeutic approach that can be successful in many dogs. For a more detailed discussion of the syndrome readers are referred to recent reviews (DeMarle et al. 2021; Loftus et al. 2022a; Byrne 1999; Loftus et al. 2022b).

ETIOLOGY AND PATHOPHYSIOLOGY

The etiopathogenesis of HCS is not fully understood but is believed to reflect a metabolic disorder that results in severe plasma hypoaminoacidemia, which sequentially triggers characteristic hepatic and skin pathology. Quantification of plasma amino acids in HCS patients demonstrates a 50–85%

Disorders of the Liver, Exocrine Pancreas, and Gastrointestinal Tract in Dogs and Cats, First Edition. Edited by Harry Cridge et al. Published 2026 by John Wiley & Sons, Inc. Companion Website: www.wiley.com/go/cridge/disorders

decrease in characteristic amino acids (Table 14.1) (DeMarle et al. 2021; Outerbridge et al. 2002; Loftus et al. 2022a; Byrne 1999; Leela-arporn et al. 2025; Loftus et al. 2022b).

The genesis of the profound hypoaminoacidemia in HCS has not been determined. A similar plasma hypoaminoacidemia leading to SND occurs in dogs with glucagonomas (DeMarle et al. 2021; Byrne 1999). In this case, excessive glucagon secretion from the tumor accelerates hepatic breakdown of gluconeogenic amino acids that are then consumed in gluconeogenesis (DeMarle et al. 2021; Loftus et al. 2022a; Byrne 1999). However, dogs with HCS typically have glucagon levels that are within normal limits or mildly increased (DeMarle et al. 2021; Byrne 1999). There is some evidence to suggest the plasma hypoaminoacidemia in HCS associated with urinary loss of amino acids; however, the aminoacidurias reported in dogs with HCS have been limited to only three amino acids, lysine, l-methyl histidine, and proline (Loftus et al. 2017). Zinc deficiency, mycotoxin ingestion, and the administration of anticonvulsants, such as phenobarbital and primidone, have been proposed as risk factors for the development of HCS, although a pathological basis for these relationships has not been determined (Byrne 1999; March et al. 2004). A recent metabolomic study of dogs with HCS revealed altered metabolic pathways related to cellular energetics, amino acid, and lipid metabolism, providing some insight into possible pathogenic mechanisms (Loftus et al. 2023).

CLINICAL PRESENTATION

HCS is most commonly reported in middle-aged to older, small-breed dogs, and affects male dogs at 2:1 male-to-female ratio (DeMarle et al. 2021; Outerbridge et al. 2002; Loftus et al. 2017; Loftus et al. 2022a; Byrne 1999; Hall-Fonte et al. 2016; Leela-arporn et al. 2025). Shi Tzus are overrepresented (Hall-Fonte et al. 2016).

Dermatological manifestations include hyperkeratotic, erythematous plaques, ulcers, crusts, and erosions, most often affecting the footpads, periorbital areas, perineum, and muzzle (Figure 14.1) (DeMarle et al. 2021; Outerbridge et al. 2002; Byrne 1999). The initial lesion is most often hyperkeratosis of the footpads, which subsequently progresses to thickened crusts and fissures that can lead to secondary infections (DeMarle et al. 2021; Outerbridge et al. 2002; Byrne 1999). These lesions can become pruritic and be a source of considerable pain. The appearance of these SND skin lesions can mimic other more common dermatologic disorders in dogs including bacterial, allergic, immune, and fungal diseases, which may lead to a delay in diagnosis.

Systemic signs of HCS include lethargy, vomiting, diarrhea, weight loss, anorexia, and, in more severe cases, polyuria and polydipsia (DeMarle et al. 2021; Outerbridge et al. 2002; Loftus et al. 2017; Loftus et al. 2022a; Byrne 1999; Hall-Fonte et al. 2016; Leela-arporn et al. 2025). On abdominal palpation, hepatomegaly may be noted. Laboratory findings include elevations in serum liver enzyme activity with serum alkaline phosphatase typically higher than the serum transaminases.

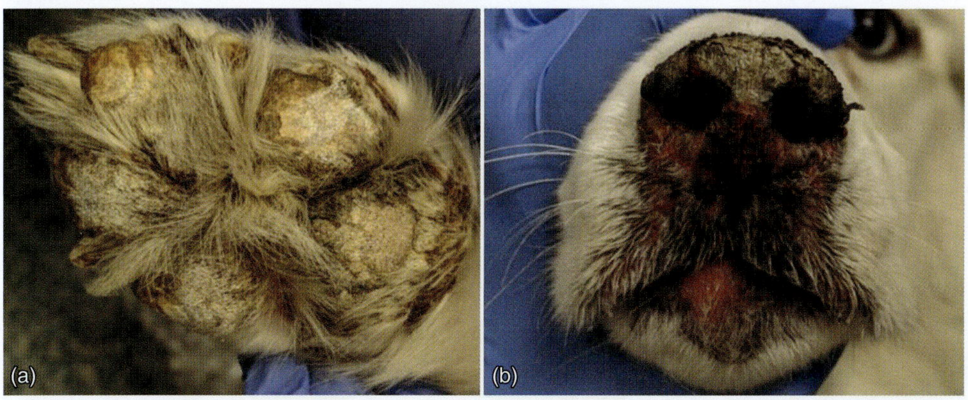

FIGURE 14.1 Photographs of skin lesions in a dog with hepatocutaneous syndrome demonstrate marked footpad hyperkeratosis (a), as well as alopecia with erosive, ulcerative, and crusted lesions on the muzzle (b)

A mild anemia with a microcytosis is often reported (DeMarle et al. 2021; Outerbridge et al. 2002; Loftus et al. 2017; Loftus et al. 2022a; Byrne 1999; Hall-Fonte et al. 2016; Leela-arporn et al. 2025; Loftus et al. 2022b; Kimmel et al. 2003; Asakawa et al. 2013; March et al. 2004). Some dogs may have diabetes mellitus at diagnosis or hyperglycemia either associated with glucose intolerance or accelerated gluconeogenesis.

DIAGNOSTIC IMAGING

Abdominal ultrasound of the liver is helpful in making a diagnosis of HCS. A hallmark finding on hepatic ultrasound is the presence of disseminated hypoechoic nodules surrounded by hyperechoic bands, often described as a "honeycomb" or "Swiss cheese" pattern (Figure 14.2) (DeMarle et al. 2021; Loftus et al. 2022a; Byrne 1999; Hall-Fonte et al. 2016; Nyland et al. 1996; Jacobson et al. 1995). This lesion is unique to dogs with HCS and is not seen in dogs with SND associated with glucagonomas (DeMarle et al. 2021).

HISTOPATHOLOGY

Skin biopsies from affected areas typically reveal characteristic histologic features, including diffuse parakeratotic hyperkeratosis, inter- and intracellular edema, and basal cell hyperplasia, resulting in a distinctive "red, white, and blue" appearance on hematoxylin and eosin-stained skin sections. These findings are considered pathognomonic for SND (also known as necrolytic migratory erythema) a hallmark of the disease (DeMarle et al. 2021; Outerbridge et al. 2002).

Histological examination of the liver reveals a vacuolar hepatopathy (glycogen and lipid) characterized by multifocal to coalescing foci of hepatocytes with severe ballooning degeneration, intermixed with hepatocyte proliferation, and areas of parenchymal collapse (DeMarle et al. 2021).

There are three reports of HCS occurring in dogs without the characteristic liver lesions, and in each case the dog had underlying inflammatory/fibrotic disease including two dogs with copper associated hepatitis (DeMarle et al. 2021; Talbot et al. 2023).

DIAGNOSIS

The diagnosis of HCS should be accomplished efficiently, so that treatment can be initiated promptly. A diagnostic algorithm that does not require an invasive skin or hepatic biopsy is shown in Figure 14.3. In dogs with the gross appearance of skin lesions typical of HCS, a plasma amino acid panel should be done early on. Plasma hypoaminoacidemia is an accurate biomarker of SND. Since SND can occur

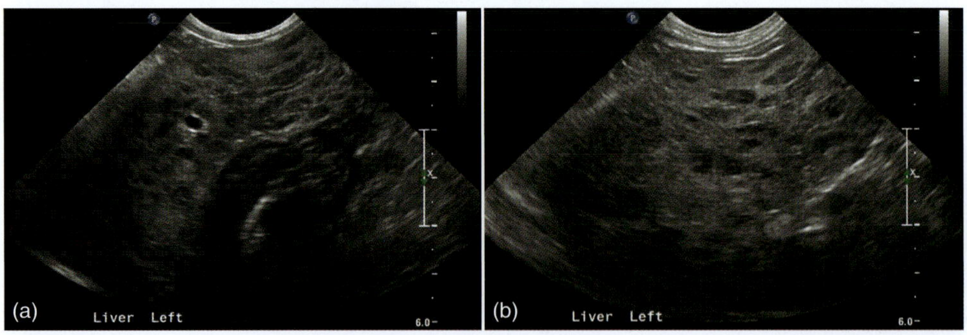

FIGURE 14.2 Liver ultrasound images of a dog with hepatocutaneous syndrome (HCS) show disseminated hypoechoic nodules surrounded by hyperechoic bands, creating a "honeycomb" or "Swiss cheese" appearance, a characteristic of HCS

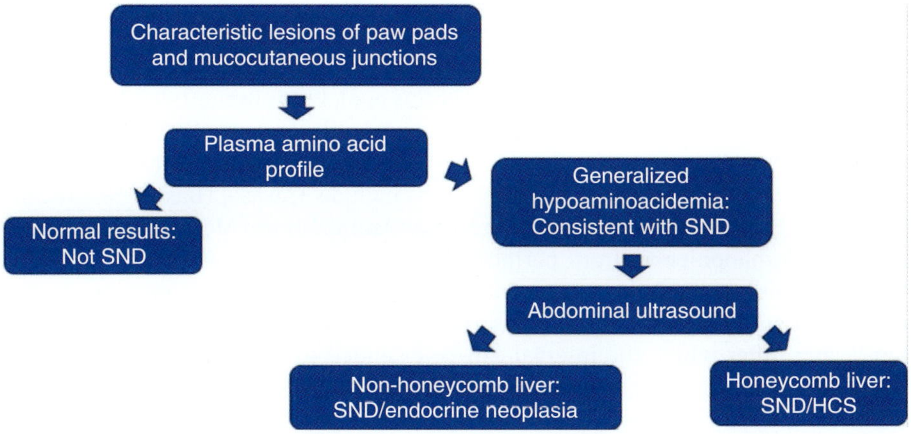

FIGURE 14.3 Algorithm for the diagnosis of the hepatocutaneous syndrome (HCS). SND, superficial necrolytic dermatitis

in dogs as a paraneoplastic syndrome or be associated with the HCS, the next step in the diagnostic algorithm is to demonstrate hepatic involvement. An abdominal ultrasound showing the characteristic honeycomb-like pattern of the liver parenchyma accomplishes this. Although the detection of serum liver enzyme elevations can also provide evidence of hepatic involvement, dogs with glucagonomas can have elevations in serum liver enzymes due to the presence of hepatic metastasis (DeMarle et al. 2021).

The value of the proposed algorithm is supported by a retrospective review of the literature which showed that all dogs with confirmed HCS have profound hypoaminoacidemia (DeMarle et al. 2021).

Hypoaminoacidemia is 100% sensitive for the detection of this disorder (DeMarle et al. 2021). Several studies have confirmed this profound deficiency of amino acids does not accompany other hepatocellular disorders including hepatocellular cancer, gallbladder mucoceles, chronic hepatitis, acute liver failure, portosystemic shunts, ductal plate abnormalities, and vacuolar hepatopathies (DeMarle et al. 2021; Leela-arporn et al. 2025). Amino acid analysis thus plays a key role in confirming the diagnosis of HCS and differentiating it from other conditions with similar dermatologic signs. Although typically plasma amino acid panels in dogs with HCS show decreases in 13–15 amino acids, a recent study has simplified evaluation of the 27 amino acid panel by showing that detection of decreases of greater than 70% in the plasma level of just 5 amino acids (glycine, glutamine, citrulline, arginine, and proline) has a 100% sensitivity and specificity for the diagnosis of SND in the dog (Leela-arporn et al. 2025).

Recent studies have demonstrated that the hypoaminoacidemic hepatopathy of HCS can be present in the absence of skin lesions, presumably representing an earlier stage of disease (Loftus et al. 2017; Loftus et al. 2022a; Hall-Fonte et al. 2016). Longitudinal evaluation shows that some of these dogs go on to develop the skin lesions of SND (Loftus et al. 2017; Hall-Fonte et al. 2016). These so-called ACHES cases are most often discovered when the characteristic honeycomb liver is detected on abdominal ultrasound in a dog being evaluated for asymptomatic increases in serum liver enzyme activity. The presence of HCS is confirmed by detecting plasma hypoaminoacidemia. Whether treatment for the hypoaminoacidemia forestalls the development of future skin lesions has not been demonstrated.

TREATMENT

There is still much to be learned about the optimal management of dogs with HCS, and this will ultimately depend on the discovery of the metabolic basis for the disorder. Currently, a multimodal treatment strategy, which includes parenteral infusions of amino acids, enteral supplements, and nutritional management, is recommended (DeMarle et al. 2021; Outerbridge et al. 2002; Byrne 1999; Loftus et al. 2022b).

PARENTERAL INFUSIONS

Intravenous administration of amino acid solutions is considered the gold standard for treating dogs with HCS (DeMarle et al. 2021; Outerbridge et al. 2002; Loftus et al. 2017; Byrne 1999; Loftus et al. 2022b). Multiple intravenous amino acid infusion protocols are available, typically recommending the administration of 25–50 ml/kg of 8.5–10% intravenous amino acid solutions over 6–8 hours via a peripheral or central catheter. Examples of these solutions include Travasol (Baxter Healthcare, Deerfield, Ill), Aminosyn (Hospira, Lake Forest, Ill), and TrophAmine (Braun Medical Inc, Prospect, Ill). While the risk of thrombophlebitis from peripheral catheter use exists when administering these high-osmolality amino acid solutions, a recent study show that this is uncommon (Loftus et al. 2022b; Arsenault et al. 2024). Repeat infusions every 7–10 days are recommended until the resolution of skin lesions, after which the interval can be extended to every 3–6 weeks based on individual response and recurrence of skin lesions. Although these infusions seldom correct the plasma hypoaminoacidemia, they have been shown to improve skin pathology. The time to response is highly variable and not necessarily predictive of long-term prognosis.

While fatty acid deficiencies have not been documented in dogs with HCS, they accompany some humans with SND (Alexander et al. 2002). A single case report describes successful management of HCS with a protocol that involved lipid infusion (Bach and Glasser 2013). Therefore, lipid emulsions (typically 20% solutions at 7 ml/kg), particularly in refractory cases, may be considered unless contraindicated such as in hyperlipidemic patients.

ENTERAL SUPPLEMENTS

Oral amino acid supplementation targeting the abnormally low plasma amino acid concentrations is also advocated. Whey protein sources such as Beneprotein (Nestle Health Science, Bridgewater, NJ) or supplementation of individual amino acids such as arginine, ornithine and proline (500–750 mg) have been advocated. It is particularly important to supplement amino acids that are known to be deficient in dogs with HCS but may not be contained in the IV infusion selected for treatment (Table 14.1).

In addition to amino acid supplementation, other oral supplements used to treat HCS include antioxidants such as S-adenosylmethionine tosylate salt (20 mg/kg PO) (Denosyl or Denamarin, Nutramax Laboratories, Lancaster, PA) to increase glutathione levels, zinc (2.2 mg elemental zinc/kg), and omega 3 fatty acids (combined eicosapentaenoic acid and docosahexaenoic acid dose of 125–140 mg/kg$^{0.75}$) (Leela-arporn et al. 2025; Loftus et al. 2022b; Jaffey et al. 2020).

Table 14.1 Typical Plasma Amino Acid Patterns in Dogs with Hepatocutaneous Syndrome

Decreased	Increased
Glutamine[a]	Phenylalanine
Glycine[a]	Glutamic acid
Citrulline[a]	Tryptophan
Arginine[a]	α-aminobutyric acid
Proline[a]	—
Threonine	—
Ornithine	—
Hydroxyproline	—
Asparagine	—
Alanine	—
Serine	—
Aspartate	—
Lysine	—
Methionine	—

[a]30% or greater decreases in these amino acids is typical in dogs with superficial necrolytic dermatitis.

Thus far, no studies have determined the efficacy of individual supplements in a way that would establish one as superior to the others or demonstrate a direct impact on survival time. However, a single study suggests that the most effective treatment, which results in the longest survival time, involves the use of at least three enteral supplements in addition to intravenous amino acid infusions (Loftus et al. 2022b).

NUTRITIONAL MANAGEMENT

A high-quality, easily digestible, high-protein diet with protein levels targeted at greater than 35% of metabolizable energy are recommended. These can either be commercial diets or home-cooked diets formulated by a veterinary nutritionist (Outerbridge et al. 2002; Loftus et al. 2022b; Bach and Glasser 2013). There is some evidence to suggest that formulated homemade diets may promote better long-term survival (Loftus et al. 2022b).

Although multimodal treatment is optimal, less intensive treatment approaches may be considered when multimodal treatment is not feasible due to financial or logistic constraints. These treatment options should ideally always include a strategy to increase amino acid and protein intake.

In addition to specific treatment for HCS, supportive care for secondary bacterial or yeast infections on the skin is important, which includes the use of appropriate topical or systemic antibiotics or antifungal medications. Pain management is critical in dogs with severe skin ulcerations or fissures. Glucocorticoids should be avoided due to the risk of potentiating the development of diabetes mellitus and inhibiting wound healing.

MONITORING

Patients with HCS require regular monitoring. Clinical signs, particularly the nature of skin lesions, evaluation of biochemical parameters, including serum liver enzyme activity, albumin, glucose, and evaluation of nutritional status (body weight and body and muscle condition scores), are used to assess response to therapy and to detect any signs of recurrence. Repeat plasma amino acid profiles may be indicated to assess persistent amino acid deficiencies, but the limited studies in which patients have been serially monitored have shown that amino acid deficiencies are typically not fully corrected even in animals that are clinically responsive to therapy. Thus, the utility of repeat profiles is questionable, but may be useful to adjust therapy in poorly responsive dogs. Since diabetes mellitus develops during treatment in many dogs, close attention to the detection of clinical signs of diabetes and serial blood glucose monitoring is warranted. Periodic abdominal ultrasound is suggested to monitor for the development of hepatocellular carcinoma.

PROGNOSIS

The prognosis for HCS has improved as treatment protocols have become more standardized, and veterinarian's awareness of the disease facilitates prompt recognition and more timely intervention. The most common reason for euthanasia in dogs with HCS is a perceived decline in quality of life due to uncontrolled symptoms, especially those affecting the foot pads, which can cause severe pain and impair mobility (DeMarle et al. 2021; Byrne 1999). Early recognition of the disease, prior to the development of skin lesions, may enhance survival time (Loftus et al. 2017; Loftus et al. 2022a; Hall-Fonte et al. 2016; Loftus et al. 2022b). Nonetheless, with proper management and monitoring, some animals can experience prolonged periods of remission and achieve optimal outcomes.

The two largest retrospective studies looking at survival in dogs treated with a variety of protocols but all receiving some form of amino acid support show median survival times of 180 days (range 2–960, n = 30) (Outerbridge et al. 2002) and 90 days (range 2–1920, n = 24) (DeMarle et al., 2021). However, these studies as well as single case reports show that there is a population of dogs that can have long-term survival up to 3–5 years (DeMarle et al. 2021; Byrne 1999; Loftus et al. 2022b).

Age, sex, or the severity of skin lesions do not effect survival, but feeding a veterinary nutritionist-formulated homemade diet and the presence of diabetes mellitus are associated with decreased risk. The latter may be associated with the positive effect of insulin therapy on wound healing (Bach and Glasser 2013).

REFERENCES

Alexander, E.K., Robinson, M., Staniec, M. et al. (2002). Peripheral amino acid and fatty acid infusion for the treatment of necrolytic migratory erythema in the glucagonoma syndrome. *Clinical Endocrinology* 57: 827–831.

Arsenault, A.C., Loftus, J.P., and Rishniw, M. (2024). Short-term parenteral infusions with high-osmolality amino acid solutions can be safely administered through peripheral catheters in dogs treated for hypoaminoacidemia-related conditions. *Journal of the American Veterinary Medical Association* 262: 1–6.

Asakawa, M.G., Cullen, J.M., and Linder, K.E. (2013). Necrolytic migratory erythema associated with a glucagon-producing primary hepatic neuroendocrine carcinoma in a cat. *Veterinary Dermatology* 24: 466–469.

Bach, J.F. and Glasser, S.A. (2013). A case of necrolytic migratory erythema managed for 24 months with intravenous amino acid and lipid infusions. *The Canadian Veterinary Journal* 54: 873–875.

Byrne, K.P. (1999). Metabolic epidermal necrosis-hepatocutaneous syndrome. *Veterinary Clinics of North America: Small Animal Practice* 29: 1337–1355.

DeMarle, K.B., Webster, C.R.L., Penninck, D. et al. (2021). Approach to the diagnosis of hepatocutaneous syndrome in dogs: a retrospective study and literature review. *Journal of the American Animal Hospital Association* 57: 15–25.

Hall-Fonte, D.L., Center, S.A., McDonough, S.P. et al. (2016). Hepatocutaneous syndrome in Shih Tzus: 31 cases (1996–2014). *Journal of the American Veterinary Medical Association* 248: 802–813.

Jacobson, L.S., Kirberger, R.M., and Nesbit, J.W. (1995). Hepatic ultrasonography and pathological findings in dogs with hepatocutaneous syndrome: new concepts. *Journal of Veterinary Internal Medicine* 9: 399–404.

Jaffey, J.A., Backus, R.C., Sprinkle, M. et al. (2020). Successful long-term management of canine superficial necrolytic dermatitis with amino acid infusions and nutritionally balanced home-made diet modification. *Frontiers in Veterinary Science* 7: 28.

Kimmel, S.E., Christiansen, W., and Byrne, K.P. (2003). Clinicopathological, ultrasonographic, and histopathological findings of superficial necrolytic dermatitis with hepatopathy in a cat. *Journal of the American Animal Hospital Association* 39: 23–27.

Leela-arporn, R., DeMarle, K.B., Heinze, C.R. et al. (2025). Comparison of plasma amino acid profiles between dogs with the hepatocutaneous syndrome and dogs with other chronic liver diseases. *Journal of Veterinary Internal Medicine* 39: e17285.

Loftus, J.P., Center, S.A., Lucy, J.M. et al. (2017). Characterization of aminoaciduria and hypoaminoacidemia in dogs with hepatocutaneous syndrome. *American Journal of Veterinary Research* 78: 735–744.

Loftus, J.P., Center, S.A., Astor, M. et al. (2022a). Clinical features and amino acid profiles of dogs with hepatocutaneous syndrome or hepatocutaneous-associated hepatopathy. *Journal of Veterinary Internal Medicine* 36: 97–105.

Loftus, J.P., Miller, A.J., Center, S.A. et al. (2022b). Treatment and outcomes of dogs with hepatocutaneous syndrome or hepatocutaneous-associated hepatopathy. *Journal of Veterinary Internal Medicine* 36: 106–115.

Loftus, J.P., Rubio, M.E.D., Yant, J. et al. (2023). Untargeted metabolomic profiles reveal widespread metabolic perturbations and identify candidate biomarkers in aminoaciduric canine hypoaminoacidemic hepatopathy syndrome. *American Journal of Veterinary Research* 84: ajvr.23.08.0186.

March, P.A., Hillier, A., Weisbrode, S.E. et al. (2004). Superficial necrolytic dermatitis in 11 dogs with a history of phenobarbital administration (1995–2002). *Journal of Veterinary Internal Medicine* 18: 65–74.

Nyland, T.G., Barthez, P.Y., Ortega, T.M. et al. (1996). Hepatic ultrasonographic and pathologic findings in dogs with canine superficial necrolytic dermatitis. *Veterinary Radiology & Ultrasound* 37: 200–205.

Outerbridge, C.A., Marks, S.L., and Rogers, Q.R. (2002). Plasma amino acid concentrations in 36 dogs with histologically confirmed superficial necrolytic dermatitis. *Veterinary Dermatology* 13: 177–186.

Talbot, C., Kearns, S., and Mouser, P.J. (2023). Treatment of superficial necrolytic dermatitis with copper chelation in a dog with copper-associated hepatitis. *Journal of the American Animal Hospital Association* 59: 1–8.

Vacuolar Hepatopathy

CHAPTER 15

Sharon A. Center[1] *and Andrea N. Johnston*[2]

[1] *Department of Clinical Sciences and Biomedical Sciences, College of Veterinary Medicine, Cornell University, Ithaca, NY, USA*
[2] *Departments of Pathobiology and Diagnostic Investigation/Small Animal Clinical Sciences, College of Veterinary Medicine, Michigan State University, East Lansing, MI, USA*

KEY POINTS

- Risk factors for Glycogen-type Vacuolar Hepatopathy (G-VH) include exogenous glucocorticoid administration, endogenous hypercortisolemia, or high endogenous steroidogenic hormones associated with hyperadrenal function (or adrenal neoplasia), hepatocyte response to inflammation, acute phase response, systemic stress derived from numerous systemic disorders, and several unique metabolic syndromes (dyslipidemia, HCS, and Scottish Terrier Hepatopathy).
- If endogenous and exogenous hypercortisolemia and sex hormone excess are ruled out, a diagnostic search is undertaken to detect a provocative cause that might be directly treated.
- Degenerative G-VH predisposes dogs with adrenal hormone excess (especially sex hormones) to hepatocellular dysplasia, adenoma, and carcinoma. Annual or biannual abdominal imaging should be performed in these patients if surgical excision is considered a viable option by owners.

INTRODUCTION

Hepatocyte vacuolation signifies altered *in vivo* biometabolism, reactive glycogen accumulation, or artifacts induced by tissue processing. Histologically, hepatocyte vacuolation can reflect membrane-delimited (lipid, metabolic storage products) or non-membrane confined product accumulation. Vacuolation reflects extraction of cytosolic materials during tissue processing. Domestic dogs have a unique propensity for hepatocyte glycogen accumulation and development of Glycogen-type Vacuolar Hepatopathy (G-VH). As a dynamic glucose polymer, glycogen functions as an energy storage depot with glycogenolysis able to replete low systemic glucose concentrations. Non-membrane confined cytosolic glycogen imparts a rarified or diaphanous appearance to hepatocytes (Figures 15.1 and 15.2).

Although G-VH is the preferred nomenclature, inconsistent terminology confuses this diagnosis: e.g., Vacuolar Hepatopathy, Steroid Hepatopathy, Glucocorticoid Hepatopathy, Vacuolar Degeneration, Hepatocellular Degeneration, Hepatocyte "Granulation", and Glycogen Storage Hepatopathy. Mild-to-moderate non-degenerative G-VH is benign. However, confluently affected hepatocytes with a 3–7-fold dimensional expansion restrict sinusoidal perfusion and are associated with hepatocyte ballooning degeneration and parenchymal collapse. This process leads to parenchymal nodularity/remodeling without regenerative nodule formation or inflammation, reflecting progressive decline in cell membrane viability and the impact of impaired sinusoidal perfusion (Sepesy et al. 2006). When severe, this process may impact continuity of canalicular bile flow (Sepesy et al. 2006). In a subset of dogs, chronic severe VH seemingly provokes development of primary hepatic neoplasia (carcinomas and adenomas) (Cortright et al. 2014; Zimmerman et al. 2010). Unfortunately, diagnosis of G-VH is subjective, with reported severity widely variable among examining pathologists. Indeed, G-VH may be too liberally declared by some pathologists

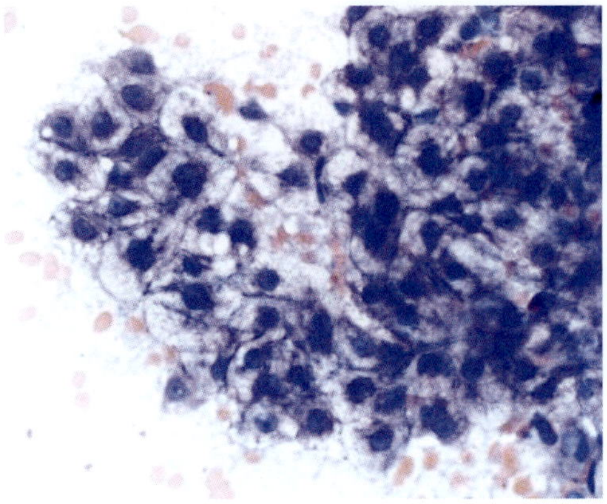

FIGURE 15.1 Photomicrograph of cytologic appearance of hepatocytes from a dog with Glycogen-type Vacuolar Hepatopathy stained with Wright Giemsa. Hepatocytes are distended with glycogen. The cytosol contains multiple, small, indistinct vacuoles. Image was provided by Dr. Shannon Dehghanpir, LSU School of Veterinary Medicine

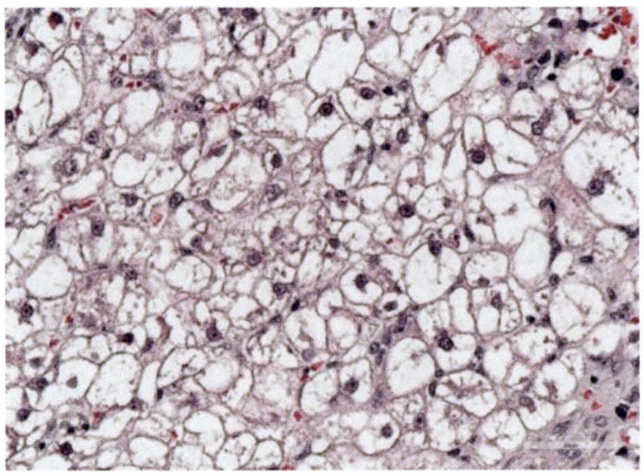

FIGURE 15.2 Liver biopsy stained with H&E, 400×: hepatocytes are diffusely distended with glycogen washed out during tissue processing. This imparts a "rarefied or diaphanous" appearance to the cytologic compartment. Irregular cell expansion increases resistance to transhepatic perfusion. Note: bright red RBCs with limited sinusoidal space. Hepatic cords are distorted due to diversity of hepatocyte glycogen expansion and parenchymal collapse. Image: SA Center, Cornell College of Veterinary Medicine, Cornell University, Ithaca, NY

considering that non-distending cytosolic glycogen is a normal hepatocyte characteristic in clinically healthy well-fed dogs. Look for qualifying morphologic features: diffuse, severe, ballooning degeneration, stromal collapse, and nodularity to appreciate G-VH severity. Mild-to-moderate focal G-VH is common.

ETIOLOGY AND RISK FACTORS

As the most common histopathologic feature reported in canine liver biopsies, G-VH represents a syndromic phenomenon (Table 15.1). Common associations exist with glucocorticoid exposure (idiopathic adrenal disease, iatrogenic [any exposure route]), systemic stress, and acute phase response. A G-VH also may derive from non-glucocorticoid drugs, as a defensive/reparative hepatocyte response to various hepatotoxins (e.g., herbal, Chinese medicinal extracts, holistic compounds, environmental and chemical toxins) or secondary to food-borne endocrine hormone ingestion (raw foods). Thus, meticulous review of environmental exposures, supplements, and novel foods should be undertaken. Potential for the histologic diagnosis of G-VH should be anticipated in non-jaundiced dogs with markedly increased ALP before liver biopsy. This should be thoughtfully discussed with owners, as a G-VH diagnosis will initiate concern for an overlooked causal illness.

Table 15.1 Factors Associated with Canine Glycogen-type Vacuolar Hepatopathy (Sepesy et al. 2006)

Category	Potential risk factor
Drugs/Toxins	Glucocorticoids, Progestogens: idiopathic, medications, food ingestion
	Holistic or herbal remedies, numerous hepatotoxins (induced response)
Endocrinopathies	Cushing's syndrome, Dysregulated adrenal steroidogenesis
	Diabetes mellitus, Hypothyroidism
Dyslipidemia	Hypertriglyceridemia (primary or secondary)
	Hypercholesterolemia
Acute Phase Response Hepatocyte:	Atopic dermatitis (severe)
Adaptive Injury Response	Cardiovascular disease
Systemic Inflammation	Severe dental disease
Systemic Stress	Gastrointestinal / Pancreatic inflammation
	Immune-mediated disorders
	Infectious disorders
	Necroinflammatory and Neoplastic Hepatobiliary Disorders
	e.g., Copper-associated hepatitis, d-penicillamine induction, idiopathic chronic hepatitis, gallbladder mucocele, cholangitis, bacterial cholecystitis, hepatocellular carcinoma.
	Neoplasia: primary hepatic, lymphoma, splenic hemangiosarcoma, others
	Neurologic maladies: with and without glucocorticoid intervention
	Renal disease: pyelonephritis, chronic cystitis
Syndromes	Scottish Terrier Hepatopathy: risk for hepatocellular carcinoma
	Hepatocutaneous Syndrome
	Inherited or Congenital Glycogen Storage Disease (genetic mutation)

CLINICAL DIAGNOSIS OF GLYCOGEN-TYPE VACUOLAR HEPATOPATHY

SIGNALMENT

Most dogs are mature or geriatric adults; a large retrospective study found a predisposition for neutered females (Sepesy et al. 2006). G-VH can affect any dog breed (rare diagnosis in cats). A progressive G-VH syndrome is common in middle-to-mature-aged Scottish Terriers, where it is associated with increased progestins and androgens, and 34% risk for hepatocellular carcinoma (Cortright et al. 2014; Zimmerman et al. 2018). Genomic analysis of Scottish Terriers implicated suppressed hydroxysteroid 17-beta dehydrogenase-2 (HSD17B2) function, speculated to provoke chronic high androstenedione concentrations in hepatocytes. Treatment of affected Scottish Terriers with trilostane or lysodren has not halted G-VH progression and may be hazardous (Cortright et al. 2014). A unique G-VH lesion is associated with hepatocutaneous syndrome (HCS), also known as aminoaciduric canine hypoaminoacidemic hepatopathy syndrome (ACHES). This can affect numerous breeds but is more common in West Highland White Terriers, Cocker Spaniels, Shetland Sheepdogs, and a large Shih Tzu kindred (Hall-Fonte et al. 2016; Loftus 2025).

CLINICAL SIGNS AND PHYSICAL EXAMINATION FINDINGS

Dogs with glucocorticoid-induced G-VH often are polyphagic, polydipsic, and polyuric, and display hepatomegaly, endocrine truncal alopecia, and typical glucocorticoid dermatopathy. Acute or chronic illness can provoke G-VH (i.e., physiologic stress) with clinical features reflecting causal conditions (organ-specific disorders). Benign G-VH with mild-to-moderate non-degenerative features may be asymptomatic sans trivial to moderate induction of ALP activity with no other behavioral, physical, or clinicopathologic features. Unique painful cutaneous lesions in dogs with ACHES/HCS typically manifest late, after recognition of hepatic ultrasound lesions, hypoaminoacidemia, and liver biopsy (Loftus 2025).

CLINICOPATHOLOGIC ABNORMALITIES

Most dogs with G-VH display increased serum ALP activity. Testing for glucocorticoid-ALP isoenzyme induction does not help distinguish causal factors (Syakalima et al. 1998). Many dogs with or without glucocorticoid-induced G-VH may display increased GGT activity and increased total cholesterol. Increased transaminase activity accompanies moderate-to-severe progressive G-VH, reflecting glycogen-associated cellular injury (restricted sinusoidal perfusion, membrane injury, dysplastic or neoplastic hepatocyte proliferation). Because increased transaminase, ALP, and GGT activities also accompany G-VH and other primary hepatobiliary disorders, biochemical features alone cannot distinguish G-VH. However, G-VH induced by excessive glucocorticoid exposure is usually associated with erythrocytosis, thrombocytosis, and canine glucocorticoid leukocytic stress response (mature neutrophilic leukocytosis, monocytosis, lymphopenia, and eosinopenia), isosthenuria (reflecting polyuria and polydipsia), and modest proteinuria (glomerular). Adrenal functional assessment may be indicated if hyperadrenocorticism is suspected. Rarely, dogs with severe G-VH develop increased total serum bile acid concentrations reflecting compromised canalicular bile flow (compression from hepatocyte distention, membrane injury, or hepatic remodeling) (Sepesy et al. 2006; Tinted et al. 2023; Solter et al. 1994). Hyperbilirubinemia is rare. Dogs with VH associated with ACHES/HCS have predisposition to diabetes mellitus (~50%). Typical clinicopathologic features include microcytic anemia and markedly increased ALP activity. Definitive diagnosis requires documentation of hypoaminoacidemia, unique ultrasonography features, and hepatic histopathology.

DIAGNOSTIC IMAGING

Dogs with moderate-to-severe G-VH usually display palpable and radiographic hepatomegaly. Otherwise, radiography may disclose features implicating a causal disorder. Abdominal ultrasonography (US) enables assessment of hepatic parenchymal echogenicity and homogeneity, mass lesion detection, critical assessment of other abdominal organs (including adrenal size and nodularity), and discovery of asymptomatic compartmentalized effusions implicating a causal disorder. Hyperechoic echogenicity typifies G-VH with the development of scattered hypoechoic nodules with progressive G-VH degeneration. Definite assessment of a nodular ultrasonography pattern requires liver biopsy to differentiate nodular regeneration (advanced-stage liver disease/post-necrotic scarring), benign nodular hyperplasia (usually few small nodules), and primary or infiltrative hepatic neoplasia (color-flow doppler interrogation). A unique honeycomb or Swiss cheese nodular hepatopathy is a common initial feature of ACHES (HCS). Because Scottish Terriers with progressive G-VH have a risk for hepatocellular carcinoma, six month or yearly ultrasonography surveillance is advised but indicated only if surgical mass resection is a considered intervention.

For a more comprehensive overview of diagnostic imaging for dogs with VH, please see Chapter 2: Diagnostic Imaging of the Hepatobiliary System.

HEPATIC CYTOPATHOLOGY AND HISTOPATHOLOGY

Cytologic features of G-VH include cytosolic rarefaction (indistinct feathery-wispy cytoplasmic protrusions intersecting empty space; Figure 15.1), foci of extramedullary hematopoiesis, and occasional canalicular bile casts. Although cytologic features are easily recognized, similar findings accompany primary necroinflammatory and neoplastic hepatic disorders that require liver biopsy for diagnosis. The small size of cytologic samples deprives estimation of lesion distribution, degenerative severity, parenchymal collapse, hepatic cord disorganization, and the all-too-common pathologic accumulation of copper. Thus, important primary necroinflammatory, copper-associated hepatopathy, and neoplastic conditions are overlooked if sampling is limited to cytology.

Histopathology of early G-VH may display an initial periacinar zonal distribution (suspected zone 3 upregulated glycogen synthase activity) (Sepesy et al. 2006). Severity of G-VH is semiquantitatively categorized as mild, moderate, or severe. Diffuse vacuolation with parenchymal collapse (hepatocyte degeneration causing stromal collapse) is classified as severe; see Figures 15.2 and 15.3. Injury does not associate with inflammation or overt necrosis. Hepatocellular nodules (dysplastic or neoplastic) evolve in G-VH associated with increased adrenal sex hormones (androgens, progestogens) and fewer dogs with ACHES/HCS. Other variable histologic features include multifocal extramedullary hematopoiesis and centrilobular copper accumulation (reflecting supraphysiologic dietary copper in commercial dog foods derived from over-formulated pre-mix supplements). Unique histologic features characterizing ACHES/HCS include diffuse degenerative G-VH and lipid-VH with a moth-eaten irregular intersection between VH affected and non-vacuolated proliferative hepatocytes; Figure 15.4.

For a more comprehensive overview of liver cytopathology please see Chapter 3.

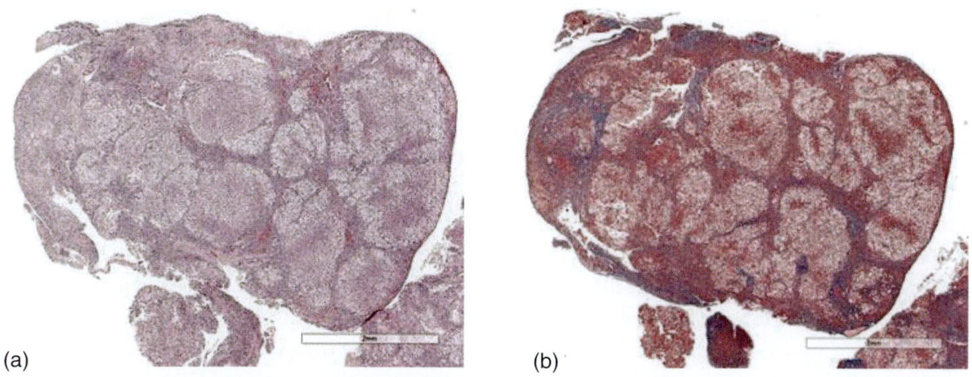

FIGURE 15.3 Overview of liver section stained with H&E, 40×(a) and with Masson's trichrome, 40× for fibrosis(b). This nodular G-VH evolved from chronic hepatocyte degeneration. Nodules are marginated by collapsed parenchyma and trivial extracellular matrix and collagen without inflammatory infiltrates. (b) A paucity of fibrosis and extracellular matrix (blue staining material) marginating nodules. Image: SA Center, Cornell College of Veterinary Medicine, Cornell University, Ithaca, NY

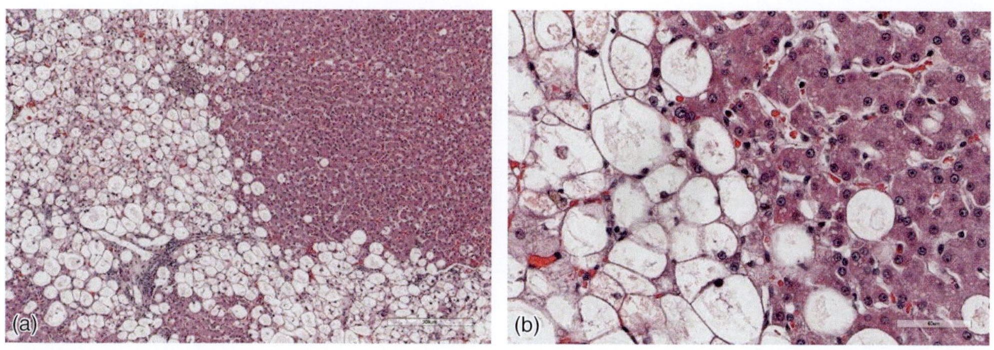

FIGURE 15.4 Photomicrographs of liver sections stained with H&E from a dog with ACHES/HCAS. (a): overview of irregular "moth-eaten" interface between severely vacuolated and non-vacuolated proliferative hepatocytes. Proliferative parenchyma corresponds to hypoechoic nodules in the Swiss cheese ultrasound pattern contrasted against the hyperechogenic G-VH. (b): higher magnification displays degenerative G-VH hepatocytes and proliferative parenchyma with disorganized hepatic cords and hepatocyte nuclei displaced to sinusoidal margins (common with proliferative response). Images: SA Center, College of Veterinary Medicine, Cornell University, Ithaca, NY

TREATMENT AND MONITORING

Diet

Nutrition should be individualized for each patient. Generally, dogs with G-VH do not require protein restriction. In progressive degenerative G-VH of ACHES/HCS, protein restriction compromises metabolic stabilization and resolution of severe VH (Loftus 2025; Loftus et al. 2022). Dietary fat restriction and hypolipidemic medications (e.g., fibrates) may benefit G-VH associated with serious hypertriglyceridemia (De Marco et al. 2017; Miceli et al. 2021).

For a more comprehensive overview of diagnosis and treatment of HCS please see Chapter 14.

Medical Therapy

Antioxidant supplements are recommended to help attenuate lipid peroxidation of hepatocellular membranes due to impaired sinusoidal perfusion and adverse effects of cytosolic glycogen distention on cell/organelle membranes. Water-soluble vitamin E ± phosphatidylcholine is recommended for dogs with fibrosis (uncommon in G-VH). Ursodeoxycholic acid is recommended for dogs with increased total serum bile acid concentrations or with conspicuous canalicular bile stasis on cytologic or histologic assessment. None of the above interventions will reverse G-VH without resolution of the underlying cause.

Monitoring

In dogs with moderate-to-severe VH, especially those with abnormal sex hormone accumulation with risk for dysplastic/neoplastic hepatocellular foci (i.e., Scottish terriers, dogs with adrenal hyperplasia/neoplasia syndromes, ACHES/HCS), serial biochemical analyses and hepatic US are recommended for early mass detection. A marked increase in cholestatic or hepatocellular leakage enzymes should prompt urgent US surveillance for causal disorders. Fine needle aspirate cytology can only define poorly differentiated/anaplastic hepatocellular neoplasms, with low sensitivity detection of well-differentiated hepatocellular carcinoma. Biopsy or tumor resection is indicated for large (>5 cm), rapidly growing, or well-vascularized neoplasms in dogs with G-VH.

REFERENCES

Cortright, C.C., Center, S.A., Randolph, J.F. et al. (2014). Clinical features of progressive vacuolar hepatopathy in Scottish Terriers with and without hepatocellular carcinoma: 114 cases (1980–2013). *Journal of the American Veterinary Medical Association* 245: 797–808.

De Marco, V., Noronha, K.S.M., Casado, T.C. et al. (2017). Therapy of canine hyperlipidemia with bezafibrate. *Journal of Veterinary Internal Medicine* 31 (3): 717–722. https://doi.org/10.1111/jvim.14701.

Hall-Fonte, D.L., Center, S.A., McDonough, S.P. et al. (2016). Hepatocutaneous syndrome in Shih Tzus: 31 cases (1996–2014). *Journal of the American Veterinary Medical Association* 248: 802–813.

Loftus, J.P. (2025). Aminoaciduric canine hypoaminoacidemic hepatopathy syndrome. *Veterinary Clinics of North America: Small Animal Practice* 55 (4): 595–613. https://doi.org/10.1016/j.cvsm.2025.03.009.

Loftus, J.P., Miller, A.J., Center, S.A. et al. (2022). Treatment and outcomes of dogs with hepatocutaneous syndrome or hepatocutaneous-associated hepatopathy. *Journal of Veterinary Internal Medicine* 36 (1): 106–115. https://doi.org/10.1111/jvim.16323.

Miceli, D.D., Vidal, V.P., Blatter, M.F.C. et al. (2021). Fenofibrate treatment for severe hypertriglyceridemia in dogs. *Domestic Animal Endocrinology* 74: 106578. https://doi.org/10.1016/j.domaniend.2020.106578.

Sepesy, L.M., Center, S.A., Randolph, J.F. et al. (2006). Vacuolar hepatopathy in dogs: 336 cases (1993–2005). *Journal of the American Veterinary Medical Association* 229: 246–252.

Solter, P.F., Hoffmann, W.E., Chambers, M.D. et al. (1994). Hepatic total 3 alpha-hydroxy bile acids concentration and enzyme activities in prednisone-treated dogs. *American Journal of Veterinary Research* 55: 1086–1092.

Syakalima, M., Takiguchi, M., Yasuda, J. et al. (1998). The canine alkaline phosphatases: a review of the isoenzymes in serum, analytical methods and their diagnostic application. *Japanese Journal of Veterinary Research* 46: 3–11.

Tinted, N., Pongcharoenwanit, S., Ongvisespaibool, T. et al. (2023). Serum bile acids concentrations and liver enzyme activities after low-dose trilostane in dogs with hyperadrenocorticism. *Animals (Basel)* 13: 3244.

Zimmerman, K.L., Panciera, D.L., Hoeschele, I. et al. (2018). Adrenocortical challenge response and genomic analyses in Scottish Terriers with increased alkaline phosphate activity. *Frontiers in Veterinary Science* 5: 231.

Zimmerman, K.L., Panciera, D.L., Panciera, R.J. et al. (2010). Hyperphosphatasemia and concurrent adrenal gland dysfunction in apparently healthy Scottish Terriers. *Journal of the American Veterinary Medical Association* 237: 178–186.

CHAPTER 16

Infectious Biliary Tract and Gallbladder Disease

Emma J. O'Neill

School of Veterinary Medicine, University College Dublin, Belfield, Dublin, Ireland

KEY POINTS

- Lethargy, vomiting, hyporexia, and jaundice are the most common clinical signs of biliary tract infections in dogs and cats. While jaundice, abdominal discomfort, and pyrexia elevate the index of suspicion, they are not recognized in all cases. Jaundice is reported in approximately 40–50% of feline and canine cholangitis cases, and abdominal discomfort and pyrexia are noted in approximately 25–33% of cholangitis and cholecystitis cases.
- Elevated liver enzyme activities, hyperbilirubinemia, and an inflammatory leukogram are frequently observed clinicopathologic abnormalities although leukogram changes are only reported in approximately 33% of cholangitis cases.
- Hepatobiliary ultrasound is a critical component of clinical decision-making, helping to identify patients that require surgical management.
- Bile sampling should be performed for cytology and aerobic/anaerobic bacterial culture. Rational clinical decision-making and appropriate antimicrobial stewardship should guide therapy.

INTRODUCTION

Biliary tract diseases target the intra- or extra-hepatic bile ducts or the gallbladder and can progress to involve the liver parenchyma in more severe cases. Biliary disorders were classified by the World Small Animal Veterinary Association (WSAVA) Liver Standardization Group (LSG) into four main groups, with subclassification of cholangitis and gallbladder diseases (Cullen et al. 2006). This classification scheme is shown along with the reported prevalence of different conditions in cats and dogs (where available), expressed as the percentage of total liver pathology submissions. Overall biliary disease are reported to account for 35–36% of feline liver submissions (Bayton et al. 2018; Fluen et al. 2019) and 11% of canine submissions (Bandara et al. 2021).

WSAVA LSG Classification of Biliary Disorders (Cullen et al. 2006) (cats/dogs) is as follows:

1. Biliary cystic diseases (2.6–5.7% [Bayton et al. 2018; Fluen et al. 2019]/0.4 % [Bandara et al. 2021]) and biliary atresia
2. Cholestasis (2.7% [Bayton et al. 2018]/1.3% [Bandara et al. 2021])
3. Cholangitis:
    - Neutrophilic cholangitis (9.7–24% [Hirose et al. 2014; Bayton et al. 2018; Fluen et al. 2019]/3.0–14.7% [Hirose et al. 2014; Tamborini et al. 2016; Bandara et al. 2021])
    - Lymphocytic cholangitis (6.8–20% [Hirose et al. 2014; Bayton et al. 2018; Fluen et al. 2019]/0.3% [Bandara et al. 2021])
    - Destructive cholangitis
    - Chronic cholangitis associated with liver fluke (cats >> dogs)

4. Diseases of the gallbladder (figure not reported/6.4% [Bandara et al. 2021]):
   - Agenesis or duplication (cats > dogs)
   - Cystic mucinous hyperplasia and gallbladder mucocele (dog 3.6% [Bandara et al. 2021])
   - Cholecystitis (cat 0.4% [Bayton et al. 2018])
   - Infarction
   - Lithiasis

Neutrophilic cholangitis (NC) and cholecystitis are the biliary disorders most frequently associated with an infectious etiology in cats and dogs. However, many biliary diseases have the potential to promote or be exacerbated by infection (Center 2009), as is discussed further in the section exploring biliary defense mechanisms. Bacterial infections are the most frequent infectious etiology and the focus of this book chapter. Other infectious causes include liver flukes, protozoa, or fungi.

The liver is the largest solid organ in the body and plays a central role in a broad range of metabolic pathways. The functions that are of most relevance to biliary diseases include excretory and digestive roles, the removal of endogenous and exogenous toxins, and immune surveillance. Key to these roles is its unique blood supply, receiving blood from both the hepatic portal vein (80%) and hepatic artery (20%), effectively positioning the liver between the splanchnic and systemic circulations (Center 2009). While this supports the liver in its core functions, it leaves the liver at risk of injury resulting from drugs, toxins, or infectious organisms.

The main function of the biliary tract is transportation, modification, and storage of bile before its ultimate delivery to the duodenum to perform its roles in digestion, absorption, excretion, and immune function. The final part of the biliary tree, the common bile duct (CBD), courses through the pancreas and then intramurally within the duodenum before entering its lumen several centimeters distal to the pylorus. Important differences in canine and feline biliary anatomy have been proposed as an explanation for the differing incidence of biliary disease in the two species (Center 2009). In dogs, the CBD enters the duodenum at the major duodenal papilla via the sphincter of Oddi, along with the smaller of two pancreatic ducts (minor pancreatic duct). The second, accessory pancreatic duct, is the primary channel for secretions from the pancreas in this species and enters the duodenum at the minor duodenal papilla approximately 2 cm distally to this. In cats, the CBD is far longer and more tortuous than in dogs and, in most cats, fuses with the pancreatic duct in an ampulla before entering the duodenum through a common orifice at the sphincter of Oddi. It is widely accepted that only about 20% of cats have an accessory pancreatic duct (Center 2009), although there is limited data on this and huge interindividual variation in biliary anatomy in this species.

BILIARY DEFENSE MECHANISMS

Overall, the liver plays a crucial role in the immune system, providing an important defense against pathogen and toxin exposure, and actively involved in the maintenance of immune tolerance. Biliary defense mechanisms comprise both immunological and mechanical components, which together help to prevent microbial invasion, adhesion, and colonization, as shown in Figure 16.1. Collectively, these mechanisms protect against bacteria or toxin exposure that can occur by transfer from the portal bloodstream, hematogenous dissemination, or by direct ascension from the gastrointestinal tract (GIT) (Sykes et al. 2021).

IS THERE A NORMAL GALLBLADDER FLORA?

Culture-independent methods have allowed identification of a complex microbiota in the normal, healthy human gallbladder, and recognition that, much like the situation in the gut, homeostatic mechanisms balance protection of the host from both pathogen invasion and unnecessary immune responses to commensal organisms. The hepatic immune system's default setting is tolerance, with any disruption to the normal balance predisposing to biliary colonization and/or inflammation. In humans, a variety of conditions predispose to biliary infection, including increased biliary pressure,

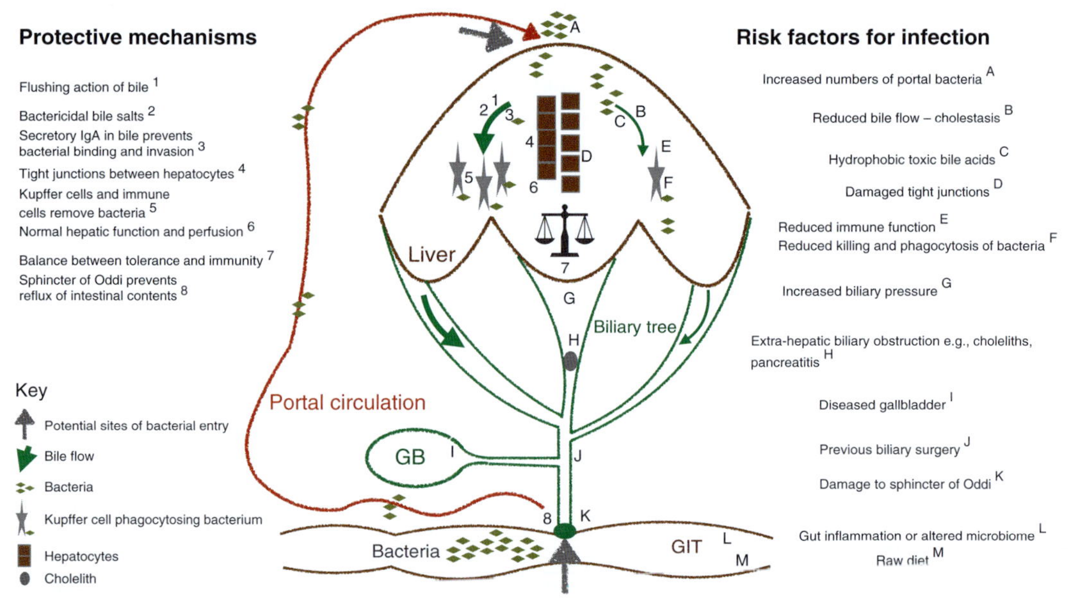

FIGURE 16.1 Biliary protective mechanisms and risk factors for infection. This diagram provides a schematic representation of the liver, bile flow, and the portal circulation. It indicates the enterohepatic circulation of bacteria from the GIT via the portal circulation to the liver. Protective mechanisms normally operating in the liver to protect against hepatobiliary infections are shown on the left side of the diagram. Factors that can disrupt these normal defense mechanisms and increase the risk of hepatobiliary infection are shown on the right. The two gray arrows indicate the potential sites of bacterial entry; portal translocation (or hematogenous dissemination) or ascension from the GIT. *Source*: O'Neill (2025) with permission of Elsevier

biliary stasis, biliary tract obstruction, and gastrointestinal (GI) dysbiosis. In addition, an exaggerated, inappropriate immune response to bacteria or their components can also result in biliary inflammation.

Bactibilia is uncommonly identified in cats and dogs without biliary pathology, although transient bactibilia has been reported in kenneled dogs. While the situation is likely to be similar to that in humans, there is currently limited information available about the canine biliary microbiome (Gookin et al. 2023), with a single study failing to identify a core biliary microbiome in cats (Slead et al. 2023). There is far more information available about the organisms most frequently isolated in canine and feline biliary infections, with *Bacteroides* spp., *Clostridium* spp., *Escherichia coli (E. coli), Enterococcus* spp., and *Streptococcus* spp. being the most commonly identified bacteria in both species, irrespective of the underlying biliary pathology (Wagner et al. 2007; Church and Matthiesen 1988; Tamborini et al. 2016; Harrison et al. 2018; Kirpensteijn et al. 1993; Center et al. 2022b).

OVERVIEW OF NEUTROPHILIC CHOLANGITIS AND CHOLECYSTITIS

HISTOPATHOLOGICAL DESCRIPTIONS

Neutrophilic Cholangitis

NC is the most commonly occurring type of cholangitis in dogs and, in many studies, also in cats, with both acute and chronic stages recognized histopathologically by the WSAVA LSG (Cullen et al. 2006). Acute NC is characterized by neutrophilic inflammation, whereas in chronic cases, the inflammatory cell population is mixed, consisting of neutrophils, plasma cells, and lymphocytes. The inflammatory infiltrate occurs periportally and within intrahepatic bile ducts. The severity and distribution varies considerably between cases, with inflammatory infiltrates breaching the limiting plate in some cases (cholangiohepatitis). With chronicity, ductular reaction and varying degrees of fibrosis can occur, depending on the duration and severity of disease (Cullen et al. 2006). Lesion severity can also be very variable and irregular in distribution within a given animal, which is important to remember when interpreting biopsy findings.

Cholecystitis

The WSAVA LSG characterized neutrophilic cholecystitis as "frequently" observed in the cat but "rarely" observed in the dog (Cullen et al. 2006). Lymphoplasmacellular and follicular cholecystitis were mentioned but not described further. Acute neutrophilic cholecystitis is described as an intramural, epithelial, and luminal neutrophilic infiltrate, which with chronicity progresses to involve a more mixed inflammatory infiltrate (Cullen et al. 2006). Mucosal erosion or ulceration may occur in acute cases and, with increased severity under certain conditions, necrosis of the gallbladder wall can occur (Cullen et al. 2006). The latter is also recognized to occur as a sequel to infarction (Holt et al. 2004). Gallbladder rupture and bile peritonitis is associated with gallbladder wall necrosis in dogs (Crews et al. 2009). Occasionally, emphysematous cholecystitis results in gas identifiable within the gallbladder wall and lumen, a condition mainly described in dogs (Center 2009) and only more recently in cats (Hernandez Perello et al. 2025).

DESCRIPTIONS IN THE LITERATURE

Neutrophilic Cholangitis

Reports of NC are limited for both dogs and cats, despite being clinically recognized far more commonly in the latter (Table 16.1).

Cholecystitis

The key reported features of feline and canine cholecystitis are summarized in Table 16.2, with two important points of note. Firstly, the very limited published studies, particularly for cats, which significantly impacts the objective information available on this topic. Secondly, the literature is heavily biased toward more severely affected cases by virtue of study selection criteria. In dogs, much of the clinical information comes from surgical case series (Church and Matthiesen 1988) or those reporting biliary tract obstruction (Kirpensteijn et al. 1993) or rupture with bile peritonitis (Parchman and Flanders 1990; Crews et al. 2009). Other case series of dogs have identified cholecystitis concurrently with NC (Tamborini et al. 2016; Harrison et al. 2018), symptomatic cholelithiasis (Kirpensteijn et al. 1993), or other gallbladder diseases (Worley et al. 2004; Crews et al. 2009). Despite being recognized to occur more frequently from a clinical perspective, there are only two very small feline case series, one detailing cholecystitis and NC (Brain et al. 2006), the other emphysematous cholecystitis (Hernandez Perello et al. 2025).

Within the canine case series, where histopathological descriptions of the cholecystitis are available, they identify lymphoplasmacytic inflammation of the gallbladder as a common feature of canine cholecystitis (Azuma et al. 2024; Kirpensteijn et al. 1993; Mitsui et al. 2021). Overall, very few dogs had neutrophilic inflammation and when present, it was typically associated with acute-on-chronic inflammation, although in a small number of cases with necrotic cholecystitis, macrophages and neutrophils were predominant. Whilst far less information is available about cats, neutrophilic inflammation does appear to be more common in this species (Simpson et al. 2022).

ETIOPATHOGENESIS

Bacterial infection is accepted to relate to NC (Cullen et al. 2006; Center 2009); however, bacteria have only been cultured in approximately 70% of feline (Center et al. 2022b) and 50% of canine cases (Harrison et al. 2018). Enteric bacteria predominate, which supports the theory that bacteria arise from ascending infection from the GIT or bacterial translocation from the portal circulation (Center 2009). False negative bacterial cultures may result from antimicrobial therapy. A study using immunohistochemical detection of bacteria and endotoxin provided evidence of a bacterial etiology in a far greater proportion of feline cases than was identified purely replying on bacterial culture (Center et al. 2022b). Cholecystitis can also have a bacterial etiology, although limited frequency data are available in

Table 16.1 Summary of the Key Findings Reported in Case Series of Feline and Canine Cholangitis

	Cats	Dogs
Signalment		
Age	**Median 7–9.2 years** based on 3 largest reports (Bayton et al. 2018; Fluen et al. 2019; Center et al. 2022a)	**Mean 8.9–9.7 years** based on 2 reports (Harrison et al. 2018; Tamborini et al. 2016)
Breed	No breed predispositions noted in cholangitis studies (Hirsch and Doige 1983; Gagne et al. 1999; Clark et al. 2011; Center et al. 2022a), however, 5/6 were purebred in 1 report (Brain et al. 2006) and BSH, Burmese, DLH, Persian, and Siamese were identified in a larger pathology study (Bayton et al. 2018)	No breed predispositions noted in cholangitis studies (Harrison et al. 2018; Tamborini et al. 2016) Median body weight 11–15 kg (Harrison et al. 2018; Tamborini et al. 2016) Border terrier and bull terrier reported increased incidence – pathology study (Bandara et al. 2021)
Clinical signs		
Duration	Only recorded in 2 reports. All acute (<3 weeks) in small report (Brain et al. 2006) Median of 30 days (very wide range) for time to diagnosis in large report (Center et al. 2022a)	Median of 3 days (range 0–56 days) (Harrison et al. 2018) 22/31 < 3-week history 9/31 chronic waxing and waning signs (O'Neill et al. 2006; Tamborini et al. 2016)
Main recorded clinical signs	Lethargy (73%), vomiting (72%), anorexia/hyporexia (70%), jaundice (56%), weight loss (54%), pyrexia (40%), hepatomegaly* (31%), abdominal discomfort** (25%), diarrhea** (19%) Percentage of reported signs in 239 cats (Hirsch and Doige 1983; Brain et al. 2006; Gagne et al. 1999; Clark et al. 2011; Center et al. 2022a), where * indicates 208 cats (Clark et al. 2011; Center et al. 2022a) and ** 174 cats (Brain et al. 2006; Center et al. 2022a) Ptyalism 3/11 in the 2 reports this was documented.	Vomiting (79%), lethargy* (69%), hyporexia* (67%), jaundice (39%), diarrhea (35%), abdominal discomfort* (33%), pyrexia (32%) Percentage of reported signs in 85 dogs (O'Neill et al. 2006; Tamborini et al. 2016; Harrison et al. 2018), where * indicates out of 81 dogs (Harrison et al. 2018; Tamborini et al. 2016) Jaundice was present in 61% of the 31 dogs with confirmed bactibilia (O'Neill et al. 2006; Tamborini et al. 2016)
Clinical pathology		
Neutrophilia	**36%** (65/179) (Hirsch and Doige 1983; Brain et al. 2006; Gagne et al. 1999; Center et al. 2022a) 9/27 "leukocytosis" (Clark et al. 2011)	Overall, **approximately 50%** of all cases **33%** (16/48) "leukocytosis" (Harrison et al. 2018) **89%** (25/28) an inflammatory leukogram, **79%** neutrophilia of + bactibilia cases
Band shift	**15%** (31/211) All 5 studies 35% (18/51) (Hirsch and Doige 1983; Brain et al. 2006; Gagne et al. 1999, Clark et al. 2011) Lower figure 8% was recorded in the large study (Center et al. 2022a)	**30%** (23/76) Toxic changes reported in 5/24 (Tamborini et al. 2016)
Hyperbilirubinemia	**73%** (38/53) Hirsch and Doige (1983); Gaigne et al. (1999); Brain et al. (2006); CLark et al. (2011) **80%** (134/168) "more than twofold increase" (Center et al. 2022a)	**70%** (56/80) (O'Neill et al. 2006; Tamborini et al. 2016; Harrison et al. 2018) **80%** (24/30) + bactibilia (O'Neill et al. 2006; Tamborini et al. 2016)
Increased ALT activity	**67%** (179/216)	**91%** (72/79) (O'Neill et al. 2006; Tamborini et al. 2016; Harrison et al. 2018) 97% (29/30) + bactibilia (O'Neill et al. 2006; Tamborini et al. 2016)

Increased AST activity	**82%** (121/147)	**80%** (33/41) (O'Neill et al. 2006; Harrison et al. 2018)
Increased ALP activity	**58%** (126/217)	**97%** (76/78)
Increased GGT activity	**67%** (100/150) (Clark et al. 2011; Center et al. 2022a)	**52%** (15/29) (Harrison et al. 2018)
Hypercholesterolemia	**24%** (36/140) (Center et al. 2022a) Reported in only 5% of cats with EHBO (Mayhew et al. 2002)	**58%** (40/69) (O'Neill et al. 2006; Tamborini et al. 2016; Harrison et al. 2018)
Hyperglobulinemia	**27%** (45/166) (Gagne et al. 1999; Center et al. 2022a)	**23%** (7/30) (O'Neill et al. 2006; Tamborini et al. 2016)
Hepatic ultrasound		
Enlarged liver	**42%** (14/33) (Clark et al. 2011; Marolf et al. 2012)	**35%** (17/49) (Tamborini et al. 2016; Harrison et al. 2018)
Hepatic echogenicity	Hyperechoic **42%** (14/33) (Clark et al. 2011; Marolf et al. 2012) Hypoechoic **0%** (0/35) (Clark et al. 2011; Marolf et al. 2012) Normal **62%** (16/26) (Gagne et al. 1999; Marolf et al. 2012)	Hyperechoic **31%** (23/75) Mixed echogenicity **31%** (23/75) (O'Neill et al. 2006; Tamborini et al. 2016; Harrison et al. 2018)
Thickened gallbladder wall	5/5 + bactibilia (Brain et al. 2006) 4/26 cats with cholangitis (lymphocytic or neutrophilic) (Marolf et al. 2012)	**30%** (9/30) >3 mm (O'Neill et al. 2006; Tamborini et al. 2016) 3/4 > 1.3 mm (O'Neill et al. 2006)
Enlarged common bile duct	**4/4** + bactibilia (Brain et al. 2006) Dilated bile ducts 45% (18/40) (Brain et al. 2006; Clark et al. 2011; Marolf et al. 2012)	**33%** (10/30) (O'Neill et al. 2006; Tamborini et al. 2016) Dilated bile ducts 53% (24/45) (Harrison et al. 2018)
Gallbladder sediment	**38%** (15/39) (Brain et al. 2006; Clark et al. 2011; Marolf et al 2012)	**51%** (38/75) (O'Neill et al. 2006; Tamborini et al. 2016; Harrison et al. 2018)
Biliary/hepatic abnormalities	Noted general biliary abnormalities in results **71%** (20/28) (Brain et al. 2006; Clark et al. 2011)	"Liver and GB abnormalities" 84% (38/45) cases but includes GB sediment (Harrison et al. 2018) 4/4 GB abnormalities (O'Neill et al. 2006) 19/27 US indicated potential need for Sx (e.g., gas in GB, CL, etc.), 4 additional cases showing GB wall changes. Only 1/27 US "not directly instrumental in Mx decision" (Tamborini et al. 2016)

(*continued*)

Table 16.1 *(continued)*

	Cats	Dogs
Intercurrent disease		
Intercurrent diseases described in these case series	78% (67/86) pancreatitis (histopathology) (Hirsch and Doige 1983; Brain et al. 2006; Clark et al. 2011; Center et al. 2022a) 74% (78/106) GI inflammation or neoplasia (histopathology) (Brain et al. 2006; Clark et al. 2011; Center et al. 2022a) 40% (69/173) CC, 41% (73/179) CL (Hirsch and Doige 1983; Brain et al. 2006; Center et al. 2022a) 5/5 GB US wall thickness suggested cholecystitis (Brain et al. 2006) Biliary/GB developmental abnormalities 42% (76/179) (Hirsch and Doige 1983; Brain et al. 2006; Center et al. 2022a) 14 cases of NC in an EHBO series; 8 of 9 that GB histopathology had confirmed concurrent CC, 4 had CL, 6 pancreatitis, 2 pancreatic adenocarcinoma. Only 2 cases had no identified concurrent disease (Mayhew et al. 2002)	2/4 CC + one suspected based on US, 1/4 cholelithiasis (O'Neill et al. 2006) 14/20 cases cholecystitis overall 20/27 GB disease (GBM 8, cholelithiasis 5) All had underlying cause; GB/GI disease/suspected pancreatitis or immunosuppressants (Tamborini et al. 2016) 30/31 GB or GIT disease confirmed histopathologically; 7 had GI disease, 25 GB disease (CC 11, infarcts, GBM) (Harrison et al. 2018)

ALP: alkaline phosphatase ALT: alanine aminotransferase; AST: aspartate aminotransferase; BSH: British short hair; CC: cholecystitis; CL: cholelithiasis; DLH: Domestic long hair; EHBO: Extra-hepatic biliary obstruction; GB: gallbladder; GBM: gallbladder mucocele; GGT: gamma-glutamyltransferase; GI: gastrointestinal; GIT: gastrointestinal tract; Mx: Management; Sx: Surgery; US: ultrasound; + bactibilia identification of bacteria in bile (positive culture or cytology).

Table 16.2 Summary of the Key Findings Reported in Case Series of Feline and Canine Cholecystitis

	Feline	Canine
Signalment		
Age	Median age 8.0 years (range 4–13 years)	Mean age 6.9–9.5 years
Breed	No breed predispositions	No breed predispositions
Clinical signs		
Duration	**Typically acute presentation**	**90%** (35/39) acute (<3 weeks)
	Median duration 11 days (range 0–365 days) (Hernandez Perello et al. 2025)	
	6/6 acute history (<7 days), although at least one acute on chronic (Brain et al. 2006)	
Main recorded clinical signs	Anorexia/hyporexia (100%), pyrexia* (83%), lethargy (82%), vomiting (64%), jaundice (64%), abdominal discomfort (45%), diarrhea* 33%), ptyalism* (33%), weight loss (27%), PU/PD (18%)	Anorexia/hyporexia (70%), vomiting (53%), abdominal discomfort (36%), jaundice (30%), pyrexia (27%), lethargy (16%), diarrhea (9%), no signs (4%)
	Percentages of 11 cats (Brain et al. 2006; Hernandez Perello et al. 2025) or * indicates 6 cats	Percentages of the 79 dogs from the larger studies listed and 10 case reports/small case series
Clinical pathology	Unless stated otherwise includes the 2 CC case series	Unless stated otherwise includes all the studies
		+/− occasional case studies where information is not provided
Neutrophilia	**45%** (5/11)	**61%** (45/74)
Band shift	**33%** (2/6) (Brain et al. 2006)	**35%** (26/74)
Monocytosis	**27%** (3/11)	**60%** (24/40) (Kirpensteijn, 1993; Oswald 1994; Lawrence 2015)
Hyperbilirubinemia	**73%** (8/11)	**54%** (43/79)
Elevation of ALT	**91%** (10/11)	**81%** (59/78)
		Lower proportion reported in dogs presenting with necrotizing cholecystitis/symptomatic cholelithiasis (Church and Matthiesen, 1988; Kirpensteijn et al. 1993)
Elevation of ALP	**64%** (7/11)	**82%** (64/78)
		Lower proportion reported in dogs presenting with necrotizing cholecystitis/symptomatic cholelithiasis (Church and Matthiesen 1988; Kirpensteijn et al. 1993)

(*continued*)

Table 16.2 (*continued*)

	Feline	Canine
Hepatic ultrasound		
Size/echogenicity	4/4 cases normal size with heterogeneous echotexture 2/4 (Hernandez Perello et al. 2025) Inconsistently described in second series (Brain et al. 2006)	Unavailable, infrequently recorded
Thickened gallbladder wall	3/4 thickened (noted on US) (Hernandez Perello et al. 2025) 5/5 cases where it was measured (Brain et al. 2006) 4/4 cases luminal and /or intra-luminal hyperechoic non-shadowing foci with reverberation artifact at US – inclusion criteria for emphysematous cholecystitis 2/2 had gas-attenuating foci at CT (Hernandez Perello et al. 2025)	10/12 where it was reported, often the reference value used was not indicated
Enlarged common bile duct	At least one of the biliary ducts described as "mildly–severely dilated" but not quantified in 4/4 cases at US and 2/2 cases at CT (Hernandez Perello et al. 2025) 4/4 cases where it was measured, no comment on appearance in the other 2 cases (Brain et al. 2006)	Very infrequently commented on 3/14 "distended" (Kirpensteijn et al. 1993). 1/1 "tortuous" but not measured, 2/2 "not visualized"
Gallbladder sediment	2/6 (Brain et al. 2006) Not commented on (Hernandez Perello et al. 2025)	Inconsistently reported
Additional information		
Bacterial growth	**68%** (2/5) growth of aerobes **0%** (0/5) growth of anaerobes Positive culture was an inclusion criterion for second study. 1/6 cases included an anaerobe, 6/6 aerobes. Two of these 6 cases grew 2 organisms 65% (15/23) positive culture but not all CC (Simpson et al. 2022), not stated if aerobic or anaerobic. 5/23 culturing multiple species. Multidrug-resistant bacteria identified 10 cats; only 4 resistant to penicillin antibiotics 5/5 of the CC cases cultured with EHBO had positive results (Mayhew et al. 2002)	**72%** (43/60) growth of aerobes **29%** (17/58) growth of anaerobes Where it was noted 33% (8/24) >1 organism Including data from all reports where it was available (In addition, at least 6 of 31 also >1 organism but difficult to discern exact numbers in two larger reports) (Church and Matthiesen 1988; Kirpensteijn et al. 1993)

Concurrent disease	3/6 cases had histologically confirmed pancreatitis (2 cases) or low-grade intestinal lymphoma (1 case). The other 3 cases had no pancreatic/GI sampling (Brain et al. 2006).	6/6 hepatic disease and lymphoplasmacytic/lymphohistiocytic cholecystitis and 3/4 inflammatory GI disease on biopsy (Lawrence et al. 2015)
	Limited information provided in emphysematous cholecystitis series – none of the cases were diabetic (Hernandez Perello et al. 2025)	6/23 cholelithiasis, 5/23 emphysema in biliary tract (Church and Matthiesen 1988)
	4/8 cases with CC in case series with EHBO had CL (Mayhew et al. 2002)	3/3 inflammatory liver disease, 3/3 underlying causes (immunosuppression/biliary surgery) (Rivers et al. 1997).
		17/17 cholecystitis, 16/21 cholangitis, 1/21 acute hepatitis (Kirpensteijn et al. 1993).
Survival information	Limited information available	Very difficult to gain a clear information
	3/5 cats with emphysematous cholecystitis survived hospital discharge. (Hernandez Perello et al. 2025). 5/6 survived at least 1 year (Brain et al. 2006)	Dogs requiring surgery for acute presentation have lower survival rates (Church and Matthiesen, 1988)
	Perioperative mortality for cholecystectomy was 22% in case series comprising >=70% CC. Long-term outcome was available for 16/22 cats; 15 survived >6 months and 8 (44.4%) surviving >3 years	

CC: cholecystitis; CL: cholelithiasis; CT: computed tomography; EHBO: Extra-hepatic biliary obstruction; GB: gallbladder; GBM: gallbladder mucocele; Mx: Management; Sx: Surgery; US: ultrasound; + bactibilia identification of bacteria in bile (positive culture or cytology).

either species. In a canine surgical case series, 80% were reported to be culture positive (Church and Matthiesen 1988) and 5/5 cats with CC that had culture performed in an EHBO case series had positive results (Mayhew et al. 2002). However, a wide variety of insults have been found either experimentally or clinically to result in cholecystitis (Otte et al. 2017; Center 2009). These include lipopolysaccharide administration, cystic duct obstruction and cholestasis, a local inflammatory process, and cystic arterial occlusion; overall surface mucosal irritation and impaired cystic duct flow are believed to be important underlying features. In view of this, cholecystitis often occurs concurrently with cholelithiasis (Kirpensteijn et al. 1993) or other gallbladder diseases (Crews et al. 2009), for example, in dogs, gallbladder mucocele.

The possible interrelationship between NC and cholecystitis in dogs has been suggested by many authors (O'Neill et al. 2006; Tamborini et al. 2016; Harrison et al. 2018). This has also been suggested in cats (Otte et al. 2017), although many historical reports of feline cholangitis cases have not provided information about the gallbladder. Overall, it is unclear if the co-presentation of NC and cholecystitis simply reflects shared predisposing factors (Center 2009) or an interconnected etiology. Inflammatory liver disease occurs in a proportion of dogs with cholecystitis (Church and Matthiesen 1988; Kirpensteijn et al. 1993; Mitsui et al. 2021); the proportion of cases with gallbladder disease is still higher in dogs with cholangitis (O'Neill et al. 2006; Tamborini et al. 2016; Harrison et al. 2018). About 40% of cats had cholecystitis in a series of 168 cats with NC (Center et al. 2022a). A smaller study identified cholecystitis in 8 of the 9 cases of extrahepatic bile duct obstruction (EBDO) that had gallbladder histopathology; 7 had concurrent NC (Mayhew et al. 2002). It would seem plausible that gallbladder disease could drive inflammation and bacterial infection involving the biliary tree and liver.

APPROACH TO A CASE

The overall approach to cats and dogs with clinical signs compatible with a biliary tract infection is very similar and is outlined in Figure 16.2. Tables 16.1 and 16.2 provide more detailed information.

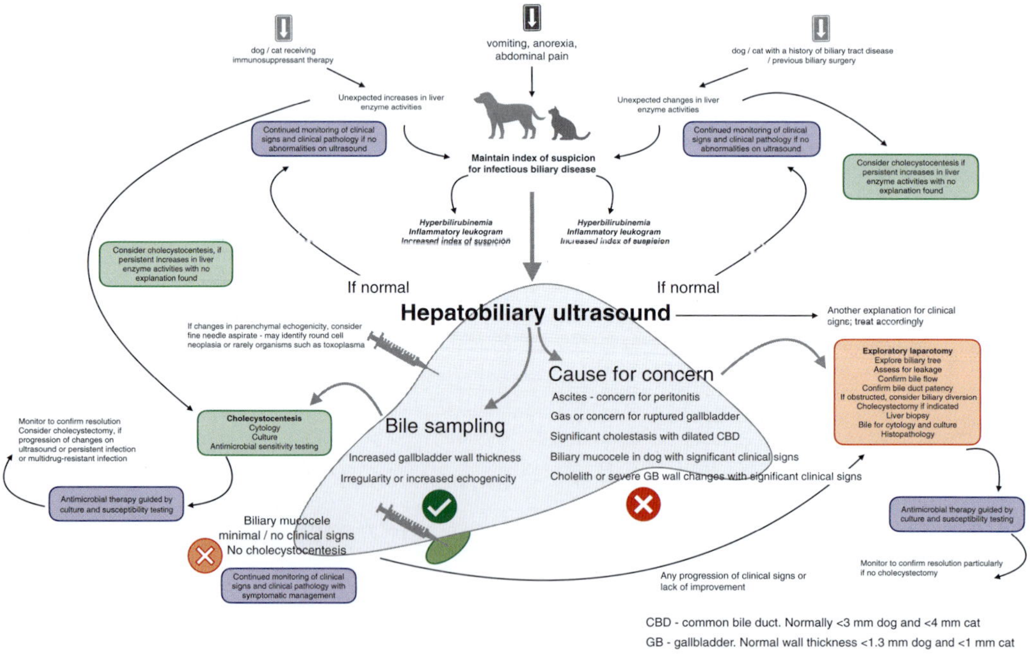

FIGURE 16.2 Flowchart showing the approach to a case. Dogs or cats typically present with one of the three main scenarios shown by the boxed arrows at the top of the diagram. The flowchart depicts a step-by-step approach to case diagnosis and management. *Source*: Adapted from O'Neill (2025).

SIGNALMENT AND HISTORY

Clinical signs of biliary tract infections vary and overlap considerably with those that occur with a wide variety of other conditions. Infections can complicate preexisting hepatobiliary disease, or other conditions that disrupt normal biliary-immune homeostasis, such as previous biliary tract surgery/trauma, endocrinopathies, or immunomodulatory therapies (Center 2009).

The majority of cats and dogs presenting with cholecystitis or NC are middle aged to older (Church and Matthiesen 1988; Brain et al. 2006; Center et al. 2022a; Tamborini et al. 2016; Harrison et al. 2018). Younger cases may have underlying conditions such as congenital biliary abnormalities (Center et al. 2022a; Church and Matthiesen 1988), previous biliary trauma (Rivers et al. 1997), or altered immune function (Rivers et al. 1997; Timofte et al. 2011). Most reported studies are retrospective and use histopathological diagnosis as an inclusion criteria, impacting their interpretation. Firstly, while histopathological confirmation allows the accurate identification of cases, it immediately biases toward more severely affected cases, particularly for cholecystitis as tissue samples typically require cholecystectomy. Secondly, calculations of the prevalence of presenting signs/features are likely to be far less accurate when using information gleaned from retrospective studies.

Although the majority of cats and dogs present acutely with cholecystitis and NC, some have waxing and waning signs, or an acute-on-chronic presentation (Center et al. 2022a; Tamborini et al. 2016); histopathologic evidence indicates that this acute-on-chronic presentation actually occurs commonly in both dogs (Tamborini et al. 2016; Harrison et al. 2018) and cats (Center et al. 2022a). In people, Charcot's triad (upper right quadrant pain, fever and jaundice) is reported in approximately one-third of patients. In dogs with NC, approximately one-third of cases have abdominal pain and pyrexia, and approximately 40% are jaundiced (O'Neill et al. 2006; Tamborini et al. 2016; Harrison et al. 2018). In cats, the figures are slightly higher for pyrexia (40%) and jaundice (56%), with approximately 25% recognized to present with abdominal discomfort (Bayton et al. 2018; Fluen et al. 2019; Center et al. 2022a).

CLINICAL PATHOLOGY

The first clue that biliary infection might be occurring is often provided by clinicopathological abnormalities. Hyperbilirubinemia is reported in just over half of the canine and 70% of the feline (very small numbers) cholecystitis cases, and 70–80% of NC cases in both species. Significant increases in liver enzyme activities are also an important feature of both conditions, with the proportion of cholangitis cases showing elevations higher in dogs than cats, as would be expected in view of the shorter enzyme half-lives in cats (91% and ~80% of canine cholangitis and cholecystitis cases respectively had increased alanine aminotransferase (ALT) activity, with figures of 67% and 91% for cats). The figure for cholecystitis cats should be interpreted with caution in view of the very small case numbers. Unexpected liver enzyme elevation in cases receiving immunosuppressive therapy or naturally immunosuppressed (e.g., hyperadrenocorticism) can be an important indicator of the potential for biliary infection.

The presence of an inflammatory leukogram in a cat or dog with biochemical evidence of a cholestatic hepatopathy raises the index of suspicion for inflammatory, and potentially infectious, biliary disease. In the literature, 60% of canine and 45% of feline cholecystitis cases had a neutrophilia, and approximately one-third had a left shift. In the canine NC cases, just over 50% had an inflammatory leukogram (O'Neill et al. 2006; Tamborini et al. 2016; Harrison et al. 2018). This figure increases to just under 90% when only confirmed bactibilic cases are considered (O'Neill et al. 2006; Tamborini et al. 2016). About one-third of the canine cases had a left shift identified (O'Neill et al. 2006; Tamborini et al. 2016; Harrison et al. 2018), a finding only identified in 15% of feline NC cases (Hirsch and Doige 1983; Brain et al. 2006; Gagne et al. 1999; Center et al. 2022a).

DIAGNOSTIC IMAGING

Abdominal Radiography

While abdominal radiography is an insensitive method for the diagnosis of biliary diseases in dogs and cats, it allows a holistic overview evaluation of the abdomen prior to abdominal ultrasound. It enables visualization of mineral opacification of bile ducts or luminal choleliths. It also enables identification of emphysematous cholecystitis.

ABDOMINAL ULTRASOUND

Abdominal ultrasound is a critical to the diagnosis of biliary disease and is indicated in any patient presenting with hyperbilirubinemia or unexplained increases in their liver enzyme activities (Center 2009). Readers are referred to Chapter 2, "Hepatobiliary Diagnostic Imaging" for more detailed information.

In any icteric patient, an important priority is to evaluate for bile duct obstruction. In addition, evaluation for features that might raise the index of suspicion of biliary tract rupture, such as peritoneal effusion, is also important, although bile peritonitis is extremely uncommon in cats and more typically traumatic in origin. While there are ultrasonographic features that might raise concern for gallbladder rupture (Crews et al. 2009), it is important to remain vigilant and aware of the limitations of this modality (low sensitivity for the detection of rupture), considering computed tomography (CT) if there is concern. Sonographic changes within the biliary tree and gallbladder are more frequently recognized in animals with cholecystitis or NC than hepatic parenchymal abnormalities (Tables 16.1 and 16.2) (Rivers et al. 1997; O'Neill et al. 2006; Crews et al. 2009; Tamborini et al. 2016). Historically, normal gallbladder wall thickness in dogs was taken as 2–3 mm, based on a reference without supporting data (Spaulding 1993). A considerably lower upper limit of 1.3 mm has been proposed in a recent study (Martinez et al. 2023), a finding corroborated by data included in other reports (Schiborra et al. 2017). In cats, the recognized upper limit for gallbladder wall thickness is 1 mm (Hittmair et al. 2001) Figure 16.3, and cats with gallbladder wall thickness above >1 mm were shown to have histopathological evidence of cholecystitis, although some cats with cholecystitis had values below this cutoff. The identification of sonographic gallbladder abnormalities has a high sensitivity (96%) but low specificity (49%) for bactibilia in cats (Policelli Smith et al. 2017). These figures were considerably lower in dogs (81% and 31%, respectively), based on a gallbladder wall thickness of 2 mm (Policelli Smith et al. 2017). However, it is important to note that cholecystitis is not synonymous with bactibilia and may occur in its absence reflecting multiple likely etiologies for cholecystitis.

The interpretation of gallbladder content raises some areas of controversy. In dogs, a small-to-moderate amount of biliary sludge (hyperechoic, gravity-dependent material) is commonly observed and, in view of this, is generally considered normal, although there is some debate on this.

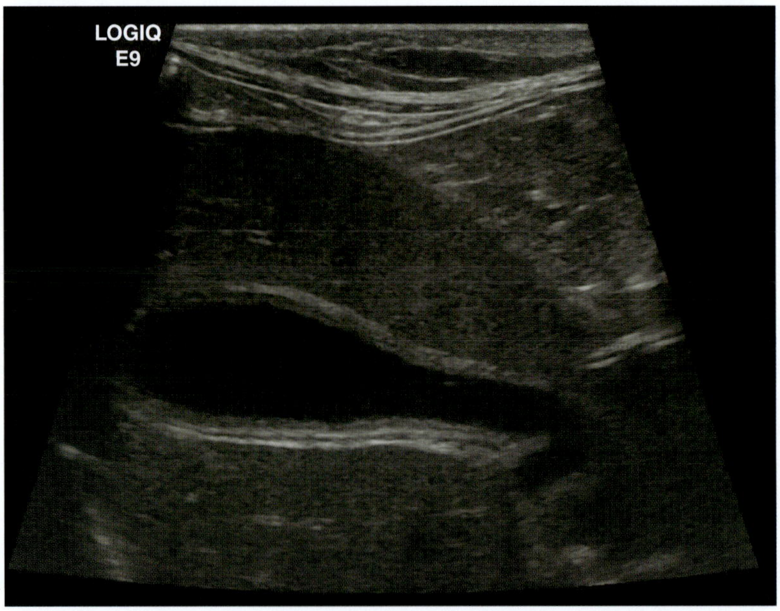

FIGURE 16.3 Ultrasound image from a 2-year-old neutered female domestic shorthair cat with cholecystitis. The gallbladder is poorly distended with a uniformly mildly thickened hyperechoic wall measuring 1.3 mm. There is a small amount of hyperechoic mobile gallbladder sludge. Bile culture yielded a pure growth of *Salmonella typhimurium* and liver biopsies yielded a diagnosis of neutrophilic cholangitis. The cat also had ultrasonographic findings suggestive of acute pancreatitis

Uncertainty increases when there is more marked sludge accumulation, especially if it is adherent. In cats, any biliary sludge is generally considered abnormal (Marolf et al. 2012). There are two things of particular relevance to potential biliary infections; firstly, cholecystocentesis should not be performed if there is a suspected gallbladder mucocele, and secondly, in the author's view, progressive changes in biliary sludge over time in dogs should be investigated, particularly if there are concurrent progressive increases in liver enzyme activities. Biliary stones can be recognized within the biliary tract as single or multiple hyperechoic foci with or without accompanying acoustic shadows, dependent on their size and composition. They are reported most commonly within the gallbladder (~90% of cases) but also occur within the CBD (choledocholith) or other intra- or extrahepatic bile ducts. They are considered to be incidental findings in a large proportion of cases (Ward et al. 2020); however, they can cause biliary obstruction, rupture, and be associated with chronic cholecystitis, biliary infections, and abdominal pain (Kirpensteijn et al. 1993). In view of this, it is always important to consider the clinical context. From a hepatobiliary infection perspective, they have been shown experimentally and clinically to have the potential to act as a nidus for infection.

DIAGNOSTIC SAMPLING

When managing animals suspected of having infectious biliary disease, the overall aims of diagnostic sampling are essentially to confirm a diagnosis and gain samples for bacteriological culture. While the definitive diagnosis of NC or cholecystitis requires histopathological evaluation of a liver biopsy or gallbladder tissue, respectively, and confirmation of an infectious etiology requires the culture of organisms, or their identification on cytology, in combination with a compatible clinicopathological presentation, from a practical perspective this is not always pursued. A tissue diagnosis is not necessarily required, particularly where the clinical suspicion is one of cholecystitis or NC in an acutely presenting patient. In these cases, identification of bactibilia in an animal with appropriate clinical signs and imaging findings is often sufficient to guide clinical management, working with a presumptive diagnosis of a bacterial biliary tract infection. The potential risk versus the overall benefit of biopsy needs to be carefully considered. In acute cases, the initial approach of managing the animal with a presumptive diagnosis guided by the bacteriology findings is entirely appropriate. However, a suboptimal or failed response to therapy should prompt reevaluation and consideration of biopsy.

Bile Sampling

Bile sampling is recommended as it serves several important purposes in animals suspected to have biliary infections:

- Significant bactibilia (cytologically or culture) in an animal with compatible clinical signs provides a working diagnosis and helps to guide appropriate antimicrobial management.
- Alternate organisms may also be detected, including protozoa, for example, *Toxoplasma gondii* in cats and *Hammondia heydorni* in dogs, fungi, or flukes, guiding therapy accordingly.
- Aerobic and anaerobic bacterial cultures are important for the following reasons:
  - Polymicrobial infections are identified in a proportion of patients, most commonly dogs (Wagner et al. 2007; Tamborini et al. 2016), and the organisms identified can change over time (O'Neill et al. 2006).
  - Several reports have highlighted growth of obligate or facultative anaerobes in cats and dogs (Wagner et al. 2007; Tamborini et al. 2016).
  - Occasionally, organisms with public health relevance are identified.
- Antimicrobial susceptibility guides appropriate treatment options:
  - Antimicrobial resistance is a recognized problem in bacteria isolated from cats and dogs with hepatobiliary disease (Wagner et al. 2007; Tamborini et al. 2016).
  - Reports that have documented changes in the antimicrobial resistance patterns of organisms over time (O'Neill et al. 2006; Timofte et al. 2011).

- An observed clinical response, even with an improvement in clinical pathology results, does not always correlate with resolution of the bactibilia (Lawrence et al. 2015); repeat sampling confirms resolution.
- Good antimicrobial stewardship and prudent use principles should guide decision-making. (Caneschi et al. 2023).

Percutaneous ultrasound-guided cholecystocentesis (PUC), used in both cats and dogs, offers a minimally invasive method for gaining bile samples for cytology and culture. An overall risk of bile peritonitis as a complication was identified in 0.7–2% of procedures in two large studies, with cats appearing to be at lower risk of complications than dogs (Peters et al. 2016; Schiborra et al. 2017). Bile cytology provides evidence of inflammation and microorganisms, which commonly occur together in bactibilic cats. In contrast, dogs often have few or no inflammatory cells present, even when significant bactibilia is evident. Overall, cytological evaluation of bile is valuable, allowing the early confirmation and characterization of organisms, and identification of mixed bacterial infections or occasionally parasites (Peters et al. 2016). There is not always agreement between cytology and culture results; combining cytology with culture increases the sensitivity for detecting bactibilia (Peters et al. 2016; Schiborra et al. 2017). Culturing gallbladder wall or choleliths, where material is available, can increase the proportion of positive results (Center et al. 2022a). In contrast, liver tissue culture typically yields fewer positive results than bile (Wagner et al. 2007).

Histopathology

A definitive diagnoses of NC or cholecystitis requires tissue histopathology of liver or gallbladder tissue respectively. While this information may not substantially influence the management plan in acutely presenting cases, the information gleaned can aid planning in more chronic cases, providing additional prognostic information. For more detailed information about liver biopsy interested readers are referred to Chapter 4.

MANAGEMENT

The severity of clinical signs observed in dogs and cats presenting with infectious biliary disease varies markedly, ranging from vague waxing and waning signs through to septic shock or septic peritonitis. In view of this, the requirements for intravenous fluids, antiemetics, and supplemental feeding, along with decisions about the requirement for surgical management or intensive care, will vary considerably. Broad spectrum antimicrobial therapy is the mainstay of treatment for cholecystitis and NC, particularly with culture or cytology confirmed bactibilia (Center 2009). The aim being to select a drug excreted in bile in an active form with good activity against enteric bacteria. Amoxicillin clavulanate is a reasonable empirical first choice, particularly when taking account of antimicrobial stewardship (Caneschi et al. 2023). However, it is important to make adjustments based on antimicrobial sensitivity testing (Wagner et al. 2007). A canine cholangitis study of cases from four referral hospitals reported *E. coli* isolates in 62% (16/26) cases (roughly 40% of the overall isolates) with resistance to amoxicillin clavulanate in about two-third of these cases (Tamborini et al. 2016). Similar results were gained in the six isolates evaluated in another study (Wagner et al. 2007). However, the rate of resistance was far lower in different study (25% [4/16] isolates – two from one dog) (Harrison et al. 2018) and is likely to be lower still in acutely presenting first opinion cases. The clinical bottom line is that antimicrobial therapy requires individualized care dictated by the clinical presentation, along with careful monitoring (Lawrence et al. 2015).

Generally, treatment for 6–8 weeks has been the recommendation for cats and dogs (Center 2009). However, in human medicine, initial management strategies now utilize much shorter treatment times, and then if an initial short course of therapy proves suboptimal, establishing bile flow is prioritized. The primary antimicrobial course in the author's institution is given, based on culture results, for approximately three weeks before resampling. However, overall clinical decision-making should be informed by the combination of response to treatment, monitoring biochemical and sonographic markers (O'Neill et al. 2006), and repeat sampling (Lawrence et al. 2015). If appropriate medical therapy fails, cholecystectomy should be considered, as retrospective studies in both species have linked cholecystectomy to improved outcomes (Harrison et al. 2018; Center et al. 2022a).

A strong theoretical case can be made for the use of ursodeoxycholic acid (UDCA) for choleresis (Center 2009), and additionally for the use of antioxidant agents, but there are no supporting clinical trial data. Symptomatic cholelithiasis should be treated with cholecystectomy (Kirpensteijn et al. 1993). There is also evidence to suggest cholecystectomy should be considered where there are severe or progressive gallbladder wall changes noted ultrasonographically, or when there is a lack of response to medical therapy (Harrison et al. 2018; Center et al. 2022a). The recognition and management of any potential underlying or exacerbating conditions (Figure 16.1) is also likely to be important. Cats with NC are frequently noted to have concurrent pancreatitis (50–70%), chronic inflammatory enteropathy (CIE) (40–80%), or both (30–50%); the reason for this remains unknown but is thought to reflect either a bacterial and/or immune-mediated etiopathogenesis. There is limited data available about the rate of occurrence of pancreatitis and CIE in dogs with biliary disease, but GI disease was noted in a considerable proportion of NC cases in one study (Harrison et al. 2018). A large feline NC study commonly identified comorbidities including extrahepatic bile duct obstruction, cholelithiasis, cholecystitis, congenital biliary disease, pancreatitis, and CIE (Center et al. 2022a).

Management of cases where culture is negative, is less clear, particularly those with chronic NC and mixed inflammatory infiltrates on histopathology. It is prudent to initially trial antimicrobials and standard supportive therapy, carefully evaluating the patient for their response to therapy as detailed above. Corticosteroids may be considered in refractory cases to blunt the inflammation, considered likely to be an aberrant ongoing, dysregulated immune response.

Overall, NC and uncomplicated cholecystitis have a good prognosis, with cats and dogs that survive initial management and are discharged from hospital being reported to survive for several years (Tamborini et al. 2016; Harrison et al. 2018; Center et al. 2022a). In dogs, biliary tract rupture and bile peritonitis are poor prognostic indicators (Church and Matthiesen 1988) that occur secondary to gallbladder necrosis, severe cholecystitis, mucoceles, or cholelithiasis (Crews et al. 2009). Bile peritonitis associated with biliary disease is far less commonly recognized in the cat (Otte et al. 2017).

SUMMARY

Bacterial biliary diseases, such as NC or cholecystitis, are an important differential in any animal presenting with hyperbilirubinemia, abdominal pain, and pyrexia. While both conditions occur more commonly in cats than dogs, there is relatively limited literature in this species, particularly for cholecystitis. The prognosis is generally thought to be good for NC and cholecystitis, particularly if patient care is individualized and carefully adjusted based on clear identification of the organisms involved and their antimicrobial susceptibility, ongoing patient monitoring, and consideration of any potential underlying causes. Cholecystectomy should be considered promptly in patients showing signs of being refractory to medical management.

DISCLOSURES

The author has no commercial or financial conflicts of interest to disclose.

The author holds a grant from the ECVIM Clinical Studies Fund to explore the role of bacteria in canine neutrophilic cholangitis.

REFERENCES

Azuma, K., Mason, G., and Monnet, E. (2024). Examination of the thickness of the different components of gallbladder wall in cases with mucocele and/or cholecystitis. *American Journal of Veterinary Research* 85: ajvr.24.03.0058.

Bandara, Y., Bayton, W.A., Williams, T.L. et al. (2021). Histopathological frequency of canine hepatobiliary disease in the United Kingdom. *Journal of Small Animal Practice* 62: 730–736.

Bayton, W.A., Westgarth, C., Scase, T. et al. (2018). Histopathological frequency of feline hepatobiliary disease in the UK. *Journal of Small Animal Practice* 59: 404–410.

Brain, P.H., Barrs, V.R., Martin, P. et al. (2006). Feline cholecystitis and acute neutrophilic cholangitis: clinical findings, bacterial isolates and response to treatment in six cases. *Journal of Feline Medicine and Surgery* 8: 91–103.

Caneschi, A., Bardhi, A., Barbarossa, A. et al. (2023). The use of antibiotics and antimicrobial resistance in veterinary medicine, a complex phenomenon: a narrative review. *Antibiotics (Basel)* 12: 487.

Center, S.A. (2009). Diseases of the gallbladder and biliary tree. *Veterinary Clinics of North America, Small Animal Practice* 39: 543–598.

Center, S.A., Randolph, J.F., Warner, K.L. et al. (2022a). Clinical features, concurrent disorders, and survival time in cats with suppurative cholangitis-cholangiohepatitis syndrome. *Journal of the American Veterinary Medical Association* 260: 212–227.

Center, S.A., Randolph, J.F., Warner, K.L. et al. (2022b). Bacterial culture and immunohistochemical detection of bacteria and endotoxin in cats with suppurative cholangitis-cholangiohepatitis syndrome. *Journal of the American Veterinary Medical Association* 260: 194–211.

Church, E.M. and Matthiesen, D.T. (1988). Surgical treatment of 23 dogs with necrotizing cholecystitis. *Journal of the American Animal Hospital Association* 24: 305–310.

Clark, J.E.C., Haddad, J.L., Brown, D.C. et al. (2011). Feline cholangitis: a necropsy study of 44 cats (1986-2008). *Journal of Feline Medicine and Surgery* 13: 570–576.

Crews, L.J., Feeney, D.A., Jessen, C.R. et al. (2009). Clinical, ultrasonographic, and laboratory findings associated with gallbladder disease and rupture in dogs: 45 cases (1997–2007). *Journal of the American Veterinary Medical Association* 234: 359–366.

Cullen, J., Van Den Ingh, T., Bunch, S. et al. (2006). *WSAVA Standards for Clinical and Histological Diagnosis of Canine and Feline Liver Disease*. Philadelphia: Elsevier Saunders.

Fluen, T., Hardcastle, M., Smith, H.L. et al. (2019). Retrospective study of the relative frequency of feline hepatobiliary disease in New Zealand based on 10 years of hepatic biopsy samples. *Veterinary Record Open* 6: e000367.

Gagne, J.M., Armstrong, P.J., Weiss, D.J. et al. (1999). Clinical features of inflammatory liver disease in cats: 41 cases (1983–1993). *Journal of the American Veterinary Medical Association* 214: 513–516.

Gookin, J.L., Hartley, A.N., Aicher, K.M. et al. (2023). Gallbladder microbiota in healthy dogs and dogs with mucocele formation. *PLoS One* 18: e0281432.

Harrison, J.L., Turek, B.J., Brown, D.C. et al. (2018). Cholangitis and cholangiohepatitis in dogs: a descriptive study of 54 cases based on histopathologic diagnosis (2004–2014). *Journal of Veterinary Internal Medicine* 32: 172–180.

Hernandez Perello, M., Prior, C., Moloney, M. et al. (2025). Clinicopathological features of feline emphysematous cholecystitis: five cases (2017–2022). *Journal of Small Animal Practice* 66: 816–823.

Hirose, N., Uchida, K., Kanemoto, H. et al. (2014). A retrospective histopathological survey on canine and feline liver diseases at the University of Tokyo between 2006 and 2012. *Journal of Veterinary Medical Science* 76: 1015–1020.

Hirsch, V.M. and Doige, C.E. (1983). Suppurative cholangitis in cats. *Journal of the American Veterinary Medical Association* 182: 1223–1226.

Hittmair, K.M., Vielgrader, H.D., and Loupal, G. (2001). Ultrasonographic evaluation of gallbladder wall thickness in cats. *Veterinary Radiology & Ultrasound* 42: 149–155.

Holt, D.E., Mehler, S., Mayhew, P.D. et al. (2004). Canine gallbladder infarction: 12 cases (1993-2003). *Veterinary Pathology* 41: 416–418.

Kirpensteijn, J., Fingland, R.B., Ulrich, T. et al. (1993). Cholelithiasis in dogs: 29 cases (1980-1990). *Journal of the American Veterinary Medical Association* 202: 1137–1142.

Lawrence, Y.A., Ruaux, C.G., Nemanic, S. et al. (2015). Characterization, treatment, and outcome of bacterial cholecystitis and bactibilia in dogs. *Journal of the American Veterinary Medical Association* 246: 982–989.

Marolf, A.J., Leach, L., Gibbons, D.S. et al. (2012). Ultrasonographic findings of feline cholangitis. *Journal of the American Animal Hospital Association* 48: 36–42.

Martinez, C., Davies, D., Hoey, S. et al. (2023). Ultrasonographic measurement of gallbladder wall thickness in fasted dogs without signs of hepatobiliary disease. *Journal of Veterinary Internal Medicine* 37: 1766–1771.

Mayhew, P.D., Holt, D.E., McLear, R.C. et al. (2002). Pathogenesis and outcome of extrahepatic biliary obstruction in cats. *Journal of Small Animal Practice* 43: 247–253.

Mitsui, I., Ohtsuki, S., and Uchida, K. (2021). Chronic cholecystitis of dogs: clinicopathologic features and relationship with liver. *Animals (Basel)* 11: 3324.

O'neill, E.J. (2025). Biliary tract infections in dogs. *Veterinary Clinics: Small Animal Practice* 55: 647–664.

O'neill, E.J., Day, M.J., Hall, E.J. et al. (2006). Bacterial cholangitis/cholangiohepatitis with or without concurrent cholecystitis in four dogs. *Journal of Small Animal Practice* 47: 325–335.

Oswald, G., Twedt, D.C., and Steyn, P.F. (1994). *Campylobacter jejuni* bacteremia and acute cholecystitis in two dogs. *Journal of the American Animal Hospital Association* 30: 165–169.

Otte, C.M., Penning, L.C., and Rothuizen, J. (2017). Feline biliary tree and gallbladder disease: aetiology, diagnosis and treatment. *Journal of Feline Medicine and Surgery* 19: 514–528.

Parchman, M. and Flanders, J. (1990). Extrahepatic biliary tract rupture: evaluation of the relationship between the site of rupture and the cause of rupture in 15 dogs. *Cornell Veterinarian* 80: 267–272.

Peters, L.M., Glanemann, B., Garden, O.A. et al. (2016). Cytological findings of 140 bile samples from dogs and cats and associated clinical pathological data. *Journal of Veterinary Internal Medicine* 30: 123–131.

Policelli Smith, R., Gookin, J.L., Smolski, W. et al. (2017). Association between gallbladder ultrasound findings and bacterial culture of bile in 70 cats and 202 dogs. *Journal of Veterinary Internal Medicine* 31: 1451–1458.

Rivers, B.J., Walter, P.A., Johnston, G.R. et al. (1997). Acalculous cholecystitis in four canine cases: ultrasonographic findings and use of ultrasonographic-guided, percutaneous cholecystocentesis in diagnosis. *Journal of the American Animal Hospital Association* 33: 207–214.

Schiborra, F., McConnell, J.F., and Maddox, T.W. (2017). Percutaneous ultrasound-guided cholecystocentesis: complications and association of ultrasonographic findings with bile culture results. *Journal of Small Animal Practice* 58: 389–394.

Simpson, M., Neville-Towle, J., Lee, K. et al. (2022). Cholecystectomy in 23 cats (2005–2021). *Veterinary Surgery* 51: 109–116.

Slead, T.S., Callahan, B.J., Schreeg, M.E. et al. (2023). Microbiome analysis of bile from apparently healthy cats and cats with suspected hepatobiliary disease. *Journal of Veterinary Internal Medicine* 37: 2178–2187.

Spaulding, K.A. (1993). Ultrasound corner gallbladder wall thickness. *Veterinary Radiology & Ultrasound* 34: 270–272.

Sykes, J.E., Marsilio, S., and Marks, S.L. (2021). 126 - hepatobiliary infections. In: *Greene's Infectious Diseases of the Dog and Cat*, 5e (ed. J.E. Sykes). Philadelphia: W.B. Saunders.

Tamborini, A., Jahns, H., McAllister, H. et al. (2016). Bacterial cholangitis, cholecystitis, or both in dogs. *Journal of Veterinary Internal Medicine* 30: 1046–1055.

Timofte, D., Dandrieux, J., Wattret, A. et al. (2011). Detection of extended-spectrum-beta-lactamase-positive Escherichia coli in bile isolates from two dogs with bacterial cholangiohepatitis. *Journal of Clinical Microbiology* 49: 3411–3414.

Wagner, K.A., Hartmann, F.A., and Trepanier, L.A. (2007). Bacterial culture results from liver, gallbladder, or bile in 248 dogs and cats evaluated for hepatobiliary disease: 1998-2003. *Journal of Veterinary Internal Medicine* 21: 417–424.

Ward, P.M., Brown, K., Hammond, G. et al. (2020). Cholelithiasis in the dog: prevalence, clinical presentation, and outcome. *Journal of the American Animal Hospital Association* 56: 152–152.

Worley, D.R., Hottinger, H.A. and Lawrence, H.J. (2004). Surgical management of gallbladder mucoceles in dogs: 22 cases (1999–2003). *Journal of the American Veterinary Medical Association* 225: 1418–1422.

CHAPTER 17 Gallbladder Mucoceles

Jared A. Jaffey

Chief of Small Animal Internal Medicine, Midwestern University College of Veterinary Medicine, Glendale, AZ, USA

KEY POINTS

- Gallbladder mucoceles (GBMs) have a broad spectrum of disease severity ranging from subclinical-to-severe and even death.
- Abdominal ultrasonography can be used to diagnose GBMs and categorize them into six different types based upon their unique sonographic appearance, which may provide added value for risk of developing clinical disease and surviving surgery.
- Ultrasonography has a poor sensitivity but moderate-to-good specificity for detection of gallbladder rupture in dogs with acute illness from GBM.
- Cholecystectomy is recommended for dogs with GBM and acute illness regardless of severity, but medical treatment can be pursued in mild cases that do not have biliary rupture or obstruction.
- Prophylactic cholecystectomy in subclinical dogs with GBM conveys a lower mortality rate (<5%) than emergent surgery is pursued with acute illness (~20%).

INTRODUCTION

Gallbladder mucocele (GBM) is a common extrahepatic biliary disorder in dogs that has been diagnosed with increased frequency over the last 25 years but is extremely rare in cats. GBMs are characterized by an accumulation of inspissated, rubber-like, immobile mucus and bile within the gallbladder on gross examination (Figure 17.1a). Histologically, gallbladders display proliferated mucosa with long, thin and branching fronds of well-differentiated gallbladder epithelial cells that contain mucus-filled cysts (Figure 17.1b) (Cullen et al. 2016; Kesimer et al. 2015). The mucosa and luminal surface are typically saturated with abundant eosinophilic homogeneous material (mucus).

This biliary disorder is found more frequently in older aged dogs (median, 10 years) but can be identified in a wide range of ages (2–17 years), and there is no sex predisposition (Jaffey et al. 2019). Small-to-medium-sized breed dogs tend to be overrepresented with common breeds, including Shetland sheepdog, Cocker spaniel, Miniature schnauzer, Bichon frise, Beagle, Pomeranian, Border terrier, Chihuahua, Yorkshire terrier, and Shih tzu (Jaffey et al. 2019).

ETIOLOGY AND RISK FACTORS

The etiology for GBM formation is unclear, but recent research has outlined several important acquired phenotypic derangements that provide insight into their development. One such study utilized immunohistochemical, ultrastructural, biochemical/biophysical, and proteomic analyses to provide a comprehensive assessment of gallbladder mucosal and mucin abnormalities in dogs with GBM (Kesimer et al. 2015). First, the study observed that the gallbladder epithelium develops a mucin hypersecretory phenotype more befitting of a histologic classification of cystic mucosal hypertrophy rather than "glandular hyperplasia," the term commonly used to describe the gallbladder mucosa

Disorders of the Liver, Exocrine Pancreas, and Gastrointestinal Tract in Dogs and Cats, First Edition. Edited by Harry Cridge et al. Published 2026 by John Wiley & Sons, Inc. Companion Website: www.wiley.com/go/cridge/disorders

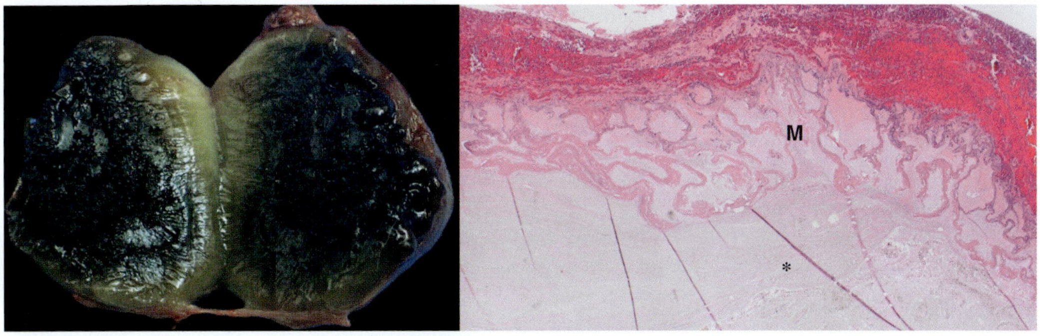

(a) (b)

FIGURE 17.1 (a) Gross appearance of a transected gallbladder with mucocele formation. The gallbladder is distended and turgid because of distension from solidified mucus and remains adhered to the mucosal surface. The central mucus is darkly stained because of exposure to bile pigments. (b) Histopathologic appearance of gallbladder with mucocele formation. The mucosal epithelium (M) is hypertrophied into long thin folds and glands are variably dilated and cystic. Pale eosinophilic mucinous material (*) fills glands and gallbladder lumen. The muscularis and adventitia are expanded by large amounts of hemorrhage. Courtesy of Tamara Chamberlin DVM, PhD, DACVP (Midwestern University College of Veterinary Medicine)

in cases with GBM (Kesimer et al. 2015). Next, there were several abnormalities related to the compositional properties of mucin that were speculated to alter the physical and functional properties of mucus making it thick and inspissated. Specifically, there was a disproportionate increase in MUC5AC relative to MUC5B along with defective mucin un-packaging and a unique composition of proteins that interact with mucus (Kesimer et al. 2015).

Hydration of the mucosal surface and luminal mucus is essential for normal gallbladder homeostasis. Disruptions in mucus composition combined with defective fluid secretion and unabated absorption can lead to adhesion of the mucus layer to the epithelial surface with continued desiccation of luminal contents. Results from a recent study provide support for this hypothesis, as dogs with GBM were found to have decreased function and membrane presence of cystic fibrosis transmembrane conductance regulatory protein (CFTR) (Gookin et al. 2024). Normal function of CFTR enables transmembrane anion secretion that is essential for mucosal hydration.

The aforementioned studies provide key insight into the mechanistic underpinnings for GBM formation but were unable to identify causes for the described acquired phenotype. Gallbladder hypomotility, alterations to bile fraction composition, or an interplay between the two have been proposed by experts to be important contributors, but definitive evidence for causation is lacking. Hydrophobic bile acids stimulate mucin secretion, inhibit smooth muscle contraction, and induce cytotoxicity of dog gallbladder epithelium in vitro (Klinkspoor et al. 1998). Gallbladder hypomotility causes supersaturation of bile constituents, which may incite a cycle of mucosal injury, mucus hypersecretion, and continued impairment of gallbladder emptying. Several potential risk factors have been identified for GBM formation, including hyperlipidemia, endocrinopathies, hyperleptinemia, decreased serum vitamin D concentrations, gluten sensitivity in Border terriers, and imidacloprid administration in Shetland sheepdogs (Jaffey et al. 2020; Lee et al. 2017; Gookin et al. 2015; Mesich et al. 2009; Barker et al. 2020). Interestingly, most of the previously mentioned variables also directly or indirectly affect gallbladder motility, bile acid composition, or both. To date, there have been no genetic variants linked with GBM formation.

CLINICAL DIAGNOSIS OF GALLBLADDER MUCOCELE

The clinical presentation of GBM is broad (Jaffey et al. 2019). Most dogs that develop clinical disease have an acute onset of clinical signs (median, four days) (Jaffey et al. 2019). Anecdotally, there is an increasing recognition of a subpopulation of dogs with GBM that have a chronic form of disease with mild intermittent clinical signs and a substantial number of dogs that are subclinical. Taken together, the clinical spectrum can vary from subclinical-to-severe disease and death. Dogs with clinically severe disease present with some combination of vomiting, diarrhea, decreased appetite, lethargy, dehydration, jaundice, and abdominal pain (Jaffey et al. 2019). Dogs with mild-to-moderate clinical disease can demonstrate similar, albeit milder clinical signs. Given the broad clinical spectrum of GBM, it is important to maintain this biliary disorder on the initial list of differential diagnoses in any dog with biochemical evidence of liver enzymopathy, nonspecific lethargy, jaundice, or that demonstrates gastrointestinal tract signs.

There are no specific findings on CBC or biochemical panels for GBM. Most dogs have some degree of a liver enzymopathy identified with a cholestatic pattern being most frequent. Many dogs will have hypercholesterolemia, hypertriglyceridemia, or both. Other abnormalities are heavily impacted by comorbid conditions and GBM-associated complications (e.g., extrahepatic bile duct obstruction [EHBDO], gallbladder rupture, infection). Hyperbilirubinemia is a common abnormality in dogs with acute illness and can range in severity from mild to severe (Jaffey et al. 2019; Jaffey et al. 2022). Most of these cases tend to be mild-to-moderate unless another issue is present, such as EHBDO, severe pancreatitis, cholestasis of sepsis, severe functional hepatobiliary disease, biliary rupture, or infection. Importantly, gallbladder rupture has the potential to either increase or decrease the total blood bilirubin concentration relative to baseline results. Moreover, it is possible for dogs with GBM and rupture to be normobilirubinemic (Wilson et al. 2020).

GBMs are readily diagnosed with abdominal ultrasonography. The ultrasonographic criteria used for diagnosis have evolved since they were first described more than 20 years ago (Besso et al. 2000). Historically, they were described as immobile contents with a hypoechoic rim and patterns consistent with echogenic striations, stellates, or both (Besso et al. 2000). Visualization of the gallbladder with this specific description in a transverse plane has an uncanny resemblance to a "kiwi-fruit". GBMs are now categorized into six different types based upon their ultrasonographic appearance (Figure 17.2) (Jaffey et al. 2022). GBM types 1, 2, and 4 have been reported in 2 studies to be the most common, whereas a type 6 (classic kiwi-fruit appearance) was the least identified form (Jaffey et al. 2022). Utilization of this classification scheme has improved detection of GBM because it accounts for the wide spectrum of appearances and captures cases that had previously been referred to as "early or developing GBM". There is a lack of prospective longitudinal studies to determine whether there is a sequential progression in GBM types wherein lower GBM types evolve to higher types. Anecdotally, this author views GBM types 1–3 as being immature and types 4–6 as mature. Utilization of the GBM ultrasonographic classification system not only improves case capture, but it also may convey clinically important patient information. One study identified that the risk for death increased along with GBM type in dogs that had surgery (Parkanzky et al. 2019). Another study found that dogs with higher GBM types were more likely to demonstrate clinical signs related to biliary tract disease (e.g., vomiting, diarrhea, decreased appetite, lethargy, dehydration, jaundice, and abdominal pain) than lower types (Jaffey et al. 2022).

Gallbladder rupture occurs in approximately 20% of dogs with GBM with acute illness and is a risk factor for death; therefore, ideally it should be identified as early as possible so that surgery can be pursued (Parkanzky et al. 2019; Malek et al. 2013; Jaffey et al. 2018; Choi et al. 2014). Commonly used

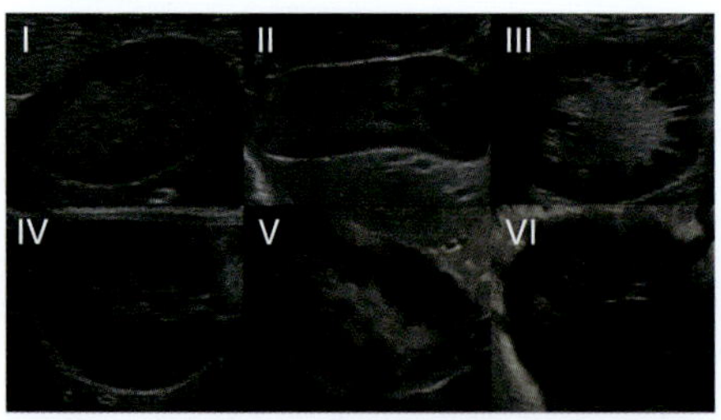

FIGURE 17.2 Representative ultrasonogram images of six gallbladder mucocele types: (I) organized echogenic debris occupying >30% of lumen, (II) combination of organized echogenic debris with partial stellate strands adhered to the gallbladder wall, (III) stellate pattern, (IV) combination of stellate and kiwi pattern, (V) kiwi pattern with echogenic debris, and (VI) kiwi pattern. Courtesy of Eric T. Hostnik DVM, MS, DACVR-DI, DACVR-EDI (Ohio State University, College of Veterinary Medicine)

ultrasonographic features to diagnose gallbladder rupture include detection of a discontinuous gallbladder wall or pericholecystic free fluid or steatitis (Jaffey et al. 2018). Extruded GBM is an uncommon phenomenon that is highly specific for gallbladder rupture. Conventional ultrasonography has a poor sensitivity and moderate-to-good specificity to identify gallbladder rupture in dogs with GBM. This means that gallbladder rupture cannot be ruled out with ultrasonography, but its detection can typically be trusted. Computed tomography is superior to ultrasonography for the identification of gallbladder rupture in people, and a study is currently ongoing in dogs with GBM. When imaging results for gallbladder rupture are inconclusive, measurement of bilirubin or bile acid concentrations as well as cytological examination of peritoneal fluid are useful for diagnosing biliary rupture.

GALLBLADDER MUCOCELE TREATMENT AND PROGNOSIS

Dogs can be treated medically or with surgery. Cholecystectomy is recommended in dogs that demonstrate biliary tract signs or have moderate-to-severe clinicopathologic abnormalities. Surgery or euthanasia must be considered in cases with a high level of suspicion or confirmation of biliary rupture or EHBDO. Delaying surgery in dogs with acute illness can result in potentially life-threatening complications such as biliary rupture, bile peritonitis, sepsis, systemic inflammatory response syndrome, multiple organ dysfunction syndrome, and death. Two recent studies highlighted that dogs with mild acute clinical disease and no evidence of biliary rupture or EHBDO can have good outcomes without surgery (Jaffey et al. 2022; Allerton et al. 2018). The decision to pursue cholecystectomy should be reexamined if the dog fails to improve or worsens within 7–10 days of initiating medical therapy.

Most dogs with acute illness related to GBM require hospitalization regardless of whether cholecystectomy is pursued. Medical therapy includes intravenous fluids with electrolyte support, ursodeoxycholic acid, S-adenosylmethionine (or N-acetylcysteine IV), broad-spectrum antimicrobials (potentiated penicillin and fluoroquinolone), supplemental nutrition, and other treatments that will vary on a case-by-case basis, such as analgesia, antiemetics, prokinetics, and proton pump inhibitors. Complete EHBDO and biliary rupture are the only two clinical scenarios in which ursodeoxycholic acid administration is contraindicated. Generally, routine antibiotic administration is not indicated without a confirmed or high level of suspicion for infection, but this is difficult to achieve in GBM cases. Therefore, out of an abundance of caution, early empiric broad-spectrum antimicrobials are recommended with the intention of deescalating with guidance from the antimicrobial susceptibility panel after surgery.

There is an increasing recognition of a subpopulation of dogs with GBM that demonstrate mild episodic clinical signs that include vomiting, lethargy, diarrhea, decreased appetite, abdominal discomfort, and exercise avoidance. The specific cause for clinical signs is unknown but may be the result of chronic cholecystitis, biliary colic, or both. Biliary colic is a common phenomenon in people with cholecystolithiasis, or gallbladder sludge characterized by increases in intraluminal gallbladder pressure following contraction against a transient cystic duct obstruction. While not yet formally described in veterinary medicine, it is reasonable to suspect a similar syndrome may occur in dogs with GBM. It is important to thoroughly investigate other more common disorders such as primary gastrointestinal tract disease, pancreatitis, hypoadrenocorticism, other hepatobiliary disorders, and musculoskeletal disease before designating GBM as the likely culprit for clinical signs. Anecdotally, medical treatment and even surgery in some cases with chronic signs related to GBM are beneficial.

Treatment recommendations for subclinical dogs are controversial and are predominately based on expert opinion. There is no evidence that demonstrates medical therapy significantly alters disease progression. General recommendations for subclinical dogs consist of ursodeoxycholic acid, S-adenosylmethionine, switching to a fat-restricted diet, as well as screening for and managing any potential contributing variables (e.g., naturally occurring Cushing's syndrome, corticosteroid administration, hypothyroidism, diabetes mellitus, hyperlipidemia). Serial ultrasound examinations are recommended once every 3–6 months to assess changes after institution of therapy. Typically, mature GBM (i.e., types 4–6) are examined once every three months because of the higher risk for clinical disease. Prophylactic cholecystectomy is recommended if there is failure of the GBM to resolve within 2–4 months of medical therapy and adequate control of any potentially contributing comorbid disorders.

Generally, dogs with GBM that have a cholecystectomy have a good prognosis if they survive the immediate postoperative period. The in-hospital mortality rate in dogs that are clinical or subclinical at the time of cholecystectomy is approximately 20% and < 5%, respectively (Jaffey et al. 2019; Jaffey et al. 2020; Malek et al. 2013; Jaffey et al. 2018). Negative prognostic indicators for survival in dogs with GBM that have cholecystectomy performed include higher GBM type, increased ALP activity, intraoperative and postoperative hypotension, increasing postoperative serum lactate concentrations, owner recognition of jaundice, concurrent hyperadrenocorticism, Pomeranian breed, increasing age or blood bilirubin concentrations, and the presence of clinical signs or gallbladder rupture (Jaffey et al. 2019; Parkanzky et al. 2019; Malek et al. 2013; Jaffey et al. 2018). One study investigated long-term outcome of dogs with GBM that survived at least 14 days after diagnosis and reported median survival times of 1,802 days, 1,340 days, and 203 days for the surgical, medical, and medical-then-surgical treatment groups, respectively (Parkanzky et al. 2019). Survival analyses in that study revealed dogs treated with surgery lived significantly longer than dogs treated with medical management (Parkanzky et al. 2019).

REFERENCES

Allerton, F., Swinbourne, F., Barker, L. et al. (2018). Gall bladder mucoceles in Border terriers. *Journal of Veterinary Internal Medicine* 32: 1618–1628.

Barker, L., Tivers, M.S., Kathrani, A. et al. (2020). Serological markers of gluten sensitivity in Border terriers with gall bladder mucocoeles. *Journal of Small Animal Practice* 61: 630–636.

Besso, J.G., Wrigley, R.H., Gliatto, J.M. et al. (2000). Ultrasonographic appearance and clinical findings in 14 dogs with gallbladder mucocele. *Veterinary Radiology & Ultrasound* 41: 261–271.

Choi, J., Kim, A., Keh, S. et al. (2014). Comparison between ultrasonographic and clinical findings in 43 dogs with gallbladder mucoceles. *Veterinary Radiology & Ultrasound* 55: 202–207.

Cullen, J.M. and Stalker, M.J. (2016). Liver and biliary system. In: *Jubb, Kennedy, and Palmer's Pathology of Domestic Animals* (ed. G.M. Maxie), 259–334. St. Louis, Missouri: Elsevier.

Gookin, J.L., Correa, M.T., Peters, A. et al. (2015). Association of gallbladder mucocele histologic diagnosis with selected drug use in dogs: a matched case-control study. *Journal of Veterinary Internal Medicine* 29: 1464–1472.

Gookin, J.L., Holmes, J., Clarke, L.L. et al. (2024). Acquired dysfunction of CFTR underlies cystic fibrosis-like disease of the canine gallbladder. *American Journal of Physiology-Gastrointestinal and Liver Physiology* 327: G513–G530.

Jaffey, J.A., Graham, A., Van Eerde, E. et al. (2018). Gallbladder mucocele: variables associated with outcome and the utility of ultrasonography to identify gallbladder rupture in 219 dogs (2007–2016). *Journal of Veterinary Internal Medicine* 32: 195–200.

Jaffey, J.A., Kreisler, R., Shumway, K. et al. (2022). Ultrasonographic patterns, clinical findings, and prognostic variables in dogs from Asia with gallbladder mucocele. *Journal of Veterinary Internal Medicine* 36: 565–575.

Jaffey, J.A, Matheson, J., Shumway, K. et al. (2020). Serum 25-hydroxyvitamin D concentrations in dogs with gallbladder mucocele. *PLoS One* 15: e0244102.

Jaffey, J.A., Pavlick, M., Webster, C.R. et al. (2019). Effect of clinical signs, endocrinopathies, timing of surgery, hyperlipidemia, and hyperbilirubinemia on outcome in dogs with gallbladder mucocele. *Veterinary Journal* 251: 105350.

Kesimer, M., Cullen, J., Cao, R. et al. (2015). Excess secretion of gel-forming mucins and associated innate defense proteins with defective mucin un-packaging underpin gallbladder mucocele formation in dogs. *PLoS One* 10: e0138988.

Klinkspoor, J.H., Yoshida, T., and Lee, S.P. (1998). Bile salts stimulate mucin secretion by cultured dog gallbladder epithelial cells independent of their detergent effect. *Biochemical Journal* 332: 257–262.

Lee, S., Kweon, O.K., and Kim, W.H. (2017). Increased leptin and leptin receptor expression in dogs with gallbladder mucocele. *Journal of Veterinary Internal Medicine* 31: 36–42.

Malek, S., Sinclair, E., Hosgood, G. et al. (2013). Clinical findings and prognostic factors for dogs undergoing cholecystectomy for gall bladder mucocele. *Veterinary Surgery* 42: 418–426.

Mesich, M.L., Mayhew, P.D., Paek, M. et al. (2009). Gall bladder mucoceles and their association with endocrinopathies in dogs: a retrospective case-control study. *Journal of Small Animal Practice* 50: 630–635.

Parkanzky, M., Grimes, J., Schmiedt, C. et al. (2019). Long-term survival of dogs treated for gallbladder mucocele by cholecystectomy, medical management, or both. *Journal of Veterinary Internal Medicine* 33: 2057–2066.

Wilson, K., Powers, D., Grasperge, B. et al. (2020). Dogs with biliary rupture based on ultrasound findings may have normal total serum bilirubin values. *Veterinary Radiology & Ultrasound* 62 (2): 236–245.

Other Non-infectious Biliary Tract and Gallbladder Diseases

CHAPTER 18

Frederik William Scott Allan

North Downs Specialist Referrals, Bletchingley, United Kingdom

KEY POINTS

- Cholelithiasis is frequently asymptomatic, and when identified in the symptomatic patient, it should prompt investigations for concurrent hepatobiliary disease and/or biliary tract obstruction.
- Hemocholecysts, cholecystitis, and sludge can mimic the sonographic appearance of gallbladder mucocele (GBM).
- The sensitivity of ultrasonography for detection of gallbladder rupture varies from 56 to 75%.
- The clinical relevance of gallbladder sludge is unclear. Routine monitoring is recommended in breeds at high risk of GBM and dogs with non-gravity-dependent sludge.

CHOLELITHIASIS

INTRODUCTION

While choleliths in humans are usually cholesterol-based, most choleliths in dogs and cats are pigment stones containing calcium carbonate and bilirubin pigments (Brunet et al. 2023). Patients with cholelithiasis are commonly encountered in clinical practice, with the prevalence of cholelithiasis estimated to be between 0.03 and 13% in dogs and 0.99% in cats (Brunet et al. 2023).

ETIOLOGY AND RISK FACTORS

Pathogenic factors promoting lithogenesis include bile stasis, mucin production, bacterial deconjugation of bilirubin, and biliary cholesterol supersaturation. Mechanisms of cholelith formation are multifactorial and vary between stone types. Bacterial infection and bile stasis are implicated in the formation of "brown" pigment stones (which are mostly composed of calcium bilirubinate), prolonged hyperbilirubinemia can lead to "black" pigment stone formation, and cholesterol-supersaturation of bile is an important factor in the formation of cholesterol-based stones. Risk factors for the development of cholelithiasis include hypercholesterolemia, hypertriglyceridemia, and bile stasis; small-breed dogs appear to be overrepresented (Allan et al. 2021). Hyperadrenocorticism is associated with gallbladder dysfunction and increases risk for GBM, and endocrinopathies associated with hyperlipidemia, such as hyperadrenocorticism and diabetes mellitus, could predispose patients to developing cholelithiasis. Humans with cholelithiasis have an increased incidence of hypercalcemia, and hyperparathyroidism has been documented in both humans and dogs with cholelithiasis (Allan et al. 2021).

DIAGNOSIS

Patients with cholelithiasis are often middle-aged to older at the time of diagnosis but can present at any age. The diagnosis of cholelithiasis is straightforward, with choleliths appearing as hyperechoic, curvilinear structures with acoustic shadowing on abdominal ultrasound (Figure 18.1a), although

Disorders of the Liver, Exocrine Pancreas, and Gastrointestinal Tract in Dogs and Cats, First Edition. Edited by Harry Cridge et al. Published 2026 by John Wiley & Sons, Inc. Companion Website: www.wiley.com/go/cridge/disorders

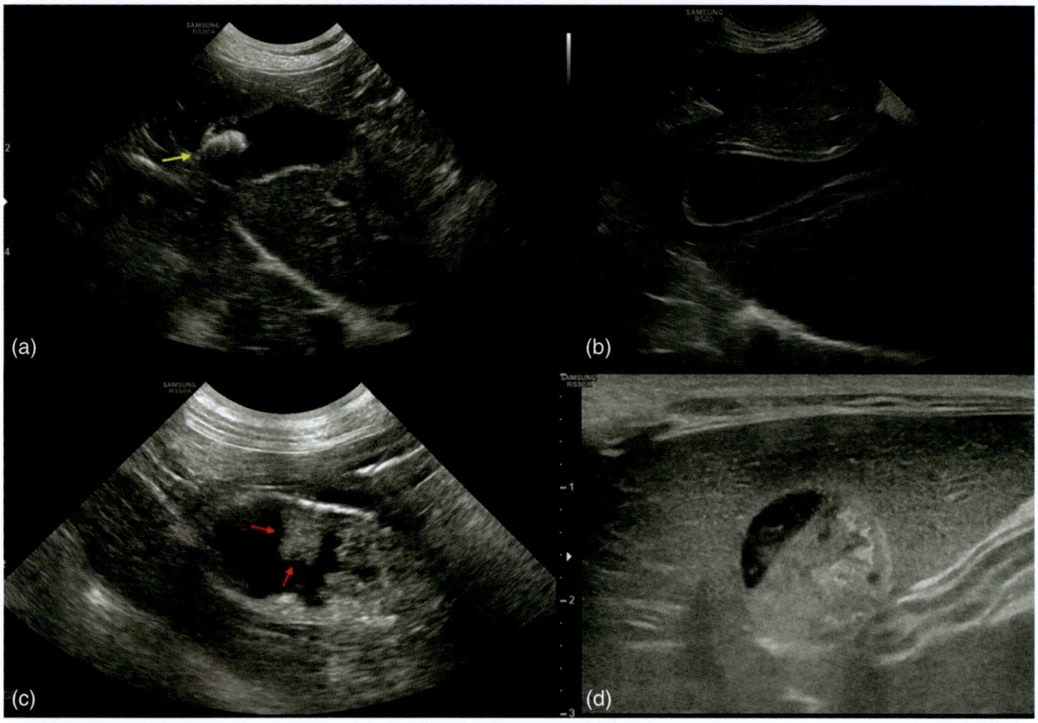

FIGURE 18.1 Ultrasonographic images of non-infectious gallbladder pathologies. (a) single cholelith appearing as an intraluminal curvilinear hyperechoic structure with acoustic shadowing, indicated by yellow arrow; (b) gallbladder wall edema, appearing as a striated, triple-layered, "hyperechoic-hypoechoic-hyperechoic" gallbladder wall; (c) multiple polypoid gallbladder lesions, with the largest lesion indicated by two red arrows; (d) hemocholecyst appearing as heterogenous echogenic content occupying the gallbladder lumen

stones in the common bile duct and cystic duct can be more difficult to identify. Radiopaque choleliths can be seen on abdominal radiography, but small or radiolucent stones may go undetected, and radiography is not useful for imaging the gallbladder or biliary tract. CT imaging can provide useful information regarding size, number, and location of choleliths in cases where ultrasound is not feasible, such as in large or deep-chested dogs. Ultrasonography allows for the assessment of biliary tract obstruction. Retrograde biliary dilatation from the point of blockage suggests obstruction, but the sensitivity of routine ultrasonography for detection of gallbladder rupture is variable, with recent studies reporting sensitivities from 56 to 75%. Contrast-enhanced gallbladder ultrasound has superior sensitivity and specificity to detect gallbladder rupture but is not widely available. The presence of free fluid in symptomatic patients should prompt investigation for biliary rupture, with sampling recommended to rule out bile peritonitis or septic effusion.

CLINICAL MANIFESTATIONS

Clinical signs are variable, and patients may be asymptomatic or present with abdominal pain, vomiting, hyporexia, lethargy, and jaundice. The presence of jaundice generally suggests bile duct obstruction, rupture, and/or concurrent hepatobiliary disease; however, some patients with biliary rupture can present without hyperbilirubinemia. The onset of hyperbilirubinemia with biliary obstruction can be delayed by several days. Decision-making regarding specific treatment for cholelithiasis should be based on the clinical presentation.

INCIDENTALLY DETECTED CHOLELITHIASIS

A notable proportion of cats and dogs are asymptomatic at presentation, with cholelithiasis representing an incidental finding in 52.6–86.9% of dogs and just under half of cats (Brunet et al. 2023).

Some asymptomatic patients may never progress to develop clinical signs; however, monitoring for development of complications is sensible. Close attention should be paid to patients with choledocholiths, younger dogs, and cats with multiple choleliths or choleliths in multiple locations, as these patients are more commonly symptomatic. Investigations for predisposing factors to cholelithiasis, such as hyperlipidemia, endocrinopathy, cholestasis, or hypercalcemia, should be performed as necessary. Consideration should be given to quarterly to biannual clinical, biochemical, and ultrasonographic monitoring of at-risk asymptomatic patients for development of complications associated with cholelithiasis.

SYMPTOMATIC CHOLELITHIASIS

Symptomatic dogs tend to be younger, more frequently have choledocholiths, and have increased activities of alkaline phosphatase (ALP), alanine aminotransferase (ALT), and gamma glutamyl transferase (GGT) than incidental cases (Allan et al. 2021). Similarly, symptomatic cats tend to have increased ALP and ALT activities, increased bilirubin concentrations, and choledocholiths compared to incidental cases. One retrospective study reported that over 75% of symptomatic cats had a suspected concurrent hepatobiliary disease process and/or biliary tract obstruction contributing to their clinical status; however, only half of these cases had a definitive diagnosis, so causation cannot be proven (Brunet et al. 2023).

TREATMENT

Dissolution of cholelithiasis with ursodeoxycholic acid (UDCA) is attempted in humans meeting specific criteria, and there is evidence to suggest dissolution may have occurred in some dogs (Allan et al. 2021). However, as previously mentioned, the composition of choleliths in humans differs from that of cats and dogs. Bile acid conjugation also differs between humans and companion animals, and this renders a diminished benefit of UDCA as a hydrophilic bile acid in cats and dogs. Therefore, as cats and dogs do not form primary cholesterol stones and have a differing bile acid pool from humans, benefits of UDCA are more likely related to its choleretic effects and multiple hepatoprotective properties rather than dissolution in most cases. Presence of a concurrent hepatobiliary disease process is suspected in most symptomatic dogs, with chronic cholecystitis, mucosal hyperplasia, pericholecystic inflammation, and bactibilia being commonly reported findings (Allan et al. 2021; Kirpensteijn et al. 1993). Similarly in cats, most symptomatic cases are suspected or proven to have concurrent cholangitis, cholecystitis, or both, with or without concurrent biliary tract obstruction (Brunet et al. 2023). Therefore, screening for and appropriately treating concurrent hepatobiliary conditions is recommended in symptomatic cases. In symptomatic but low-risk patients without complete biliary obstruction or rupture, consideration should be given to liver cytology, and to cholecystocentesis for bile cytology and culture. Whilst the risks of cholecystocentesis are low, they are associated with high morbidity and mortality, and may be increased in the presence of cholelithiasis. Cholecystocentesis should always be performed by an experienced ultrasonographer. Surgical intervention is reserved for patients with complete extrahepatic biliary duct obstruction (EHBDO) or rupture, where medical management alone is not feasible. It is essential to be cognizant of complications arising from EHBDO prior to surgical intervention. Patients with complete EHBDO will have depletion of fat-soluble vitamins, notably vitamin K_1, which can result in coagulopathy. It is recommended to assess coagulation status and determine blood type prior to surgical intervention. Discussion of specific surgical options for management of cholelithiasis is beyond the scope of this chapter; however, a noteworthy consideration is that although cats have high mortality rates associated with biliary surgery, with perioperative death reported in 21.7% of cats undergoing cholecystectomy (Simpson et al. 2022), cats with cholelithiasis that undergo cholecystectomy have longer survival times than those that do not (Center et al. 2022). Successful medical management has been reported in cats with biliary tract obstruction, with satisfactory long-term outcomes (Brunet et al. 2023). In patients with EHBDO without biliary rupture where surgical intervention is not feasible (either due to client factors, lack of facilities/expertise, or patient stability), then medical management consisting of appropriate antimicrobial therapy, analgesia, intravenous fluid therapy, and anti-nausea medication can be considered. Patients are typically hyporexic and should voluntary food intake not be achieved despite control of nausea, pain, adequate supportive care, additional methods to increase food palatability such as warming food, and appetite stimulants, then consideration should be given to placement of a feeding tube if inappetence persists for >3–5 days.

SUMMARY

The prognosis of patients with cholelithiasis is good in the absence of EHBDO, biliary rupture, or bile peritonitis, and some asymptomatic patients may never develop clinical signs or complications of their cholelithiasis. Patients with biliary tract obstruction can have favorable long-term outcomes should they survive to discharge, and successful medical management is possible in some cases. Factors that negatively impact survival in patients undergoing extrahepatic biliary surgery include preoperative hyperbilirubinemia and post-extubation hypotension in cats, and the presence of septic bile peritonitis, elevated creatinine, and lower postoperative mean arterial pressure in dogs. Asymptomatic patients should be screened for disease processes that predispose to cholelithiasis, and consideration should be given to routine clinical, biochemical, and ultrasonographic monitoring to assess for development of complications associated with cholelithiasis. There is no evidence to suggest whether treatment with UDCA in asymptomatic patients impacts likelihood of becoming symptomatic, but treatment is unlikely to result in negative clinical consequences in the absence of EHBDO.

GALLBLADDER SLUDGE

Gallbladder sludge is frequently identified in dogs and cats, appearing as echogenic debris within the gallbladder (Center et al. 2022).

CANINE

The clinical relevance of sludge in dogs is currently poorly understood, with no differences in prevalence between healthy dogs, dogs with hepatobiliary disease, and dogs with non-hepatobiliary pathology (Brömel et al. 1998). Sludge occupying over 25% of the gallbladder has been associated with increased gallbladder volume in dogs (Cook et al. 2016), and the presence of sludge is associated with decreased gallbladder emptying (Tsukagoshi et al. 2012), suggesting reduced gallbladder motility or function is associated with sludge development. There is conflicting data on the natural progression of gallbladder sludge in dogs, with some studies reporting patients to remain asymptomatic (Demonaco et al. 2016), and others documenting biliary sludge to occasionally precede GBM (Butler et al. 2022). No risk factors have been identified for progression of sludge to GBM, although non-gravity-dependent sludge has been noted to precede GBM in a moderate proportion of cases, and breeds at risk of GBM are more likely to have non-gravity-dependent sludge (Butler et al. 2022).

Clinicians frequently utilize UDCA in the management of gallbladder sludge; however, evidence of the efficacy of UDCA for this purpose is lacking, and one study found no significant difference in changes in sludge volume between dogs that received UDCA and dogs that did not receive UDCA over a follow-up period greater than one year (Butler et al. 2022). However, given its choleretic and hepatoprotective effects, consideration should be given to administration of UDCA in breeds at risk of mucocele (e.g., Border Terrier, Chihuahua, Miniature Schnauzer, Pomeranian, Shetland Sheepdog), dogs with non-gravity-dependent biliary sludge, and dogs with concurrent hepatobiliary disease processes. It is prudent to recommend ultrasonographic monitoring of affected dogs at high risk of GBM, specifically breeds at increased risk of GBM, dogs with non-gravity-dependent sludge, and dogs with endocrinopathies. Time to development of GBM after initial detection of sludge ranged from seven months to three years in one study (Butler et al. 2022), and therefore ultrasonographic monitoring of at-risk dogs every 6–12 months is likely sufficient.

FELINE

There is a greater evidence base to suggest intraluminal gallbladder content in cats is relevant. The presence of sludge is associated with increased odds of positive bacterial bile culture, and sludge is present in a large proportion of cats with cholangitis and biliary tract obstruction (Policelli Smith et al. 2017); however, some studies report no differences in clinical signs, clinicopathologic variables, or presence of ultrasonographic liver or pancreatic abnormalities between cats with and without sludge (Villm et al. 2022). When identified in the feline patient, intraluminal gallbladder content should prompt investigations for concurrent hepatobiliary disease processes, including cholecystocentesis for bile cytology and culture, and biochemical and ultrasonographic screening for concurrent pancreatopathy and/or enteropathy. In cats with sludge where cholecystitis/cholangitis is suspected, antimicrobial and hepatoprotectant therapy should be administered as appropriate. Cats with concurrent chronic enteropathy, chronic pancreatitis, or dyslipidemia as contributing factors may also benefit from dietary modulation.

GALLBLADDER WALL EDEMA

A striated, triple-layered (hyperechoic-hypoechoic-hyperechoic) appearance of the gallbladder wall on ultrasound is typical of gallbladder wall edema (Figure 18.1b). This feature is commonly referred to as a "double rim sign" or "halo sign." This is nonspecific and can be seen secondary to multiple disease processes, including cholecystitis, pancreatitis, sepsis, immune-mediated hemolytic anemia, acute hemorrhagic diarrhea syndrome, cardiac disease, anaphylaxis, portal hypertension, and dexmedetomidine administration (Turner et al. 2021). An acute onset of clinical signs accompanied by small-volume hemorrhagic peritoneal effusion, elevated ALT activity, and hypothermia should alert the clinician to the possibility of anaphylaxis, and it is important to be cognizant that these patients typically have a good prognosis with appropriate supportive treatment. Cardiac imaging should be performed to exclude pericardial effusion and congestive heart failure, and sampling of any peritoneal effusion is essential to rule out septic peritonitis and biliary rupture. Cholecystocentesis is not recommended in the initial diagnostic workup of patients with gallbladder wall edema, and investigations should instead focus first on ruling out extrahepatic causes.

CHRONIC CHOLECYSTITIS

Chronic cholecystitis in humans is either calculous or acalculous, with the acalculous form theorized to occur secondary to repeated episodes of acute cholecystitis. Chronic cholecystitis is diagnosed based on the histologic finding of lymphoplasmacytic infiltration of the gallbladder mucosa and is usually diagnosed in cholecystectomized dogs. The most frequently reported ultrasonographic features in affected dogs include sludge, mucocele, and cholelithiasis. Typical biochemical abnormalities include elevated ALP and ALT activities, but a considerable proportion of described patients have unremarkable CBC and biochemistry profiles. Chronic cholecystitis has been identified in dogs with cholelithiasis, GBM, gallbladder sludge, and hemocholecysts (Mitsui and Uchida 2023). Toy and Miniature-breed dogs appear to be overrepresented (Mitsui et al. 2021). Clinical signs of patients with chronic cholecystitis often relate to a concurrent active infectious or inflammatory process, cholelithiasis, gallbladder erosion/ulcer, or GBM, with the largest study of dogs with chronic cholecystitis finding 41.5% of cases to have no overt clinical signs (Mitsui et al. 2021). Histochemical detection of bacteria within the gallbladder wall has been documented in approximately one-third of affected dogs, with bacterial antigenic stimulation postulated to play a role in development of chronic cholecystitis, though this theory is unproven. In cases with suspected chronic cholecystitis that fail medical management, cholecystectomy should be considered as both a diagnostic and therapeutic tool.

POLYPOID GALLBLADDER LESIONS

Gallbladder polyps appear as pedunculated echogenic masses protruding into the gallbladder lumen on ultrasound (Figure 18.1c). In dogs, these have been identified concurrent to multiple conditions, including cystic mucinous hyperplasia of the gallbladder (Bargellini et al. 2018), cholecystitis, cholelithiasis, and neoplasia. Differentiation of benign from malignant lesions relies on histology, though cytology may be useful. Clinical signs in dogs with polypoid lesions are usually referable either to the pathology causing the lesion, such as malignancy, or to a concurrent disease process such as cholecystitis, cholelithiasis, or GBM. Cholecystectomy should be performed in cases where malignancy is suspected and in cases where lesions are suspected to be bleeding. Consideration should be given to cholecystectomy for patients with recurrent episodes of cholecystitis and for patients with GBM. In asymptomatic cases where caregivers decline invasive investigations, it is prudent to recommend routine clinical, biochemical, and ultrasonographic monitoring for progression of lesions and development of complications.

HEMOCHOLECYST

Hemocholecyst describes the presence of blood within the gallbladder lumen. Hemocholecysts appear similar to GBM or sludge on ultrasonography (Figure 18.1d) and have been reported in dogs with chronic cholecystitis (Mitsui and Uchida 2023), gallbladder carcinoids, GBM, and leptospirosis (McGregor 2021). Chronic cholecystitis was the most frequent histologic finding in the largest study of dogs with hemocholecysts, with gallbladder rupture present in 35.7% of cases. Despite the histologic finding of chronic cholecystitis, cases commonly presented with a short duration of clinical signs. Echogenic material within the gallbladder lumen in a dog that is unwell, or with a gallbladder mass, or bleeding tendencies, should alert the clinician to the possibility of a hemocholecyst. Treatment relies on management of the underlying disease process, with cholecystectomy recommended in cases where rupture or neoplasia is suspected.

REFERENCES

Allan, F., Watson, P.J., and McCallum, K.E. (2021). Clinical features and outcomes in 38 dogs with cholelithiasis receiving conservative or surgical management. *Journal of Veterinary Internal Medicine* 35 (6): 2730–2742. https://doi.org/10.1111/ JVIM.16284.

Bargellini, P., Orlandi, R., Paloni, C. et al. (2018). Contrast-enhanced ultrasound complements two-dimensional ultrasonography in diagnosing gallbladder diseases in dogs. *Veterinary Radiology & Ultrasound* 59 (3): 345–356. https://doi.org/10.1111/ VRU.12601.

Brömel, C., Barthez, P.Y., Léveillé, R. et al. (1998). Prevalence of gallbladder sludge in dogs as assessed by ultrasonography. *Veterinary Radiology & Ultrasound* 39 (3): 206–221. https://doi.org/10.1111/J.1740-8261.1998.TB00341.X.

Brunet, A., Duperrier-Simond, C., Amoyal, S. et al. (2023). Prevalence and clinical relevance of cholelithiasis in cats: a multicenter retrospective study of 98 cases. *Journal of Veterinary Internal Medicine* 37 (6): 2157–2170. https://doi.org/10.1111/JVIM.16868.

Butler, T., Bexfield, N., Dor, C. et al. (2022). A multicenter retrospective study assessing progression of biliary sludge in dogs using ultrasonography. *Journal of Veterinary Internal Medicine* 36 (3): 976–985. https://doi.org/10.1111/JVIM.16423.

Center, S.A., Randolph, J.F., Warner, K.L. et al. (2022). Clinical features, concurrent disorders, and survival time in cats with suppurative cholangitis-cholangiohepatitis syndrome. *Journal of the American Veterinary Medical Association* 260 (2): 212–227. https://doi.org/10.2460/JAVMA.20.10.0555.

Cook, A.K., Jambhekar, A.V., and Dylewski, A.M. (2016). Gallbladder sludge in dogs: ultrasonographic and clinical findings in 200 patients. *Journal of the American Animal Hospital Association* 52 (3): 125–131. https://doi.org/10.5326/JAAHA-MS-6282.

Demonaco, S.M., Grant, D.C., Larson, M.M. et al. (2016). Spontaneous course of biliary sludge over 12 months in dogs with ultrasonographically identified biliary sludge. *Journal of Veterinary Internal Medicine* 30 (3): 771–778. https://doi.org/10.1111/JVIM.13929.

Kirpensteijn, J., Fingland, R.B., Ulrich, T. et al. (1993). Cholelithiasis in dogs: 29 cases (1980–1990). *Journal of the American Animal Hospital Association* 202 (7): 1137–1142. http://europepmc.org/abstract/MED/8473231.

McGregor, O., O'Brien, K., Harrington, N. et al. (2021). Abdominal ultrasonographic findings and post mortem diagnosis of a haemocholecyst in a case of canine leptospirosis. *Australian Veterinary Practitioner* 51 (2): 97–103.

Mitsui, I., Ohtsuki, S., and Uchida, K. (2021). Chronic cholecystitis of dogs: Clinicopathologic features and relationship with liver. *Animals* 11 (11). https://doi.org/10.3390/ANI11113324/S1.

Mitsui, I. and Uchida, K. (2023). Canine gallbladder erosion/ulcer and hemocholecyst: clinicopathological characteristics of 14 cases. *Animals* 13 (21): 3335. https://doi.org/10.3390/ANI13213335/S1.

Policelli Smith, R., Gookin, J.L., Smolski, W. et al. (2017). Association between gallbladder ultrasound findings and bacterial culture of bile in 70 cats and 202 dogs.

Journal of Veterinary Internal Medicine 31 (5): 1451–1458. https://doi.org/10.1111/JVIM.14792.

Simpson, M., Neville-Towle, J., Lee, K. et al. (2022). Cholecystectomy in 23 cats (2005-2021). *Veterinary Surgery* 51 (1): 109–116. https://doi.org/10.1111/VSU.13741.

Tsukagoshi, T., Ohno, K., Tsukamoto, A. et al. (2012). Decreased gallbladder emptying in dogs with biliary sludge or gallbladder mucocele. *Veterinary Radiology & Ultrasound* 53 (1): 84–91. https://doi.org/10.1111/J.1740-8261.2011.01868.X.

Turner, K., Boyd, C., Stander, N. et al. (2021). Clinical characteristics of two-hundred thirty-two dogs (2006–2018) treated for suspected anaphylaxis in Perth, Western Australia. *Australian Veterinary Association* 99 (12): 505–512. https://doi.org/10.1111/AVJ.13114.

Villm, J., DeMonaco, S., and Larson, M. (2022). Prevalence of gallbladder sludge and associated abnormalities in cats undergoing abdominal ultrasound. *Veterinary Radiology & Ultrasound* 63 (5): 601–608. https://doi.org/10.1111/VRU.13091.

CHAPTER 19 Hepatobiliary Neoplasia

Autumn Dutelle

Department of Veterinary Clinical Sciences, School of Veterinary Medicine, Louisiana State University, Baton Rouge, LA, USA

KEY POINTS

- Massive hepatocellular carcinomas (HCCs) can have a good prognosis with partial or complete surgical resection.
- In cats, bilirubin is a more sensitive biomarker than elevated liver enzymes to detect primary hepatic tumors.
- Biopsy is the gold standard diagnostic method for liver tumors, as it can be difficult to determine if a mass is benign or well-differentiated on cytology.
- A computed tomography (CT) scan is useful for surgical planning, especially for feline hepatobiliary tumors, and can improve intraoperative survival rates.
- Oral targeted therapies, such as toceranib phosphate or sorafenib, may slow the progression of disease, but further clinical trials are needed.

INTRODUCTION

Primary hepatic tumors are rare in dogs and cats. They account for about 1.5% of all canine tumors and 1–3% of our feline tumors (David et al. 2020). In dogs, it is more common for masses in the liver to be from metastatic disease, whereas in cats, primary hepatobiliary tumors are more common. Frequently reported liver infiltrative neoplasms include lymphoma, mast cell tumor, and histiocytic sarcoma.

There are four main histological types or categories of primary liver tumors, which include hepatocellular, bile duct, neuroendocrine, and mesenchymal. These tumors can present in a variety of morphological forms, which include massive, nodular, and diffuse. Massive tumors present as a single large mass that is typically confined to one liver lobe. Nodular forms are often present in multiple liver lobes, while the diffuse form tends to be small to coalescing masses that affect the entirety of the liver (Liptak et al. 2004).

HEPATOCELLULAR TUMORS

Tumors of the hepatic parenchyma come in two main forms, benign and malignant. The benign form is called hepatocellular adenoma or hepatoma, and the malignant form is called hepatocellular carcinoma (HCC). Hepatocellular adenomas are typically an incidental finding, especially in feline patients. They are slow growing and do not spread. They can cause mechanical and space-occupying issues as they grow and have been documented to rupture on occasion.

HCCs are the most common primary malignant tumor in dogs and the second-most common malignant liver tumor in cats (David et al. 2020). They come in all three morphologic forms: massive, nodular, and diffuse. The massive form is the most common presentation. Degenerative vacuolar hepatopathy has been correlated with the development of HCC in dogs. Beagles, Scottish terriers, and Welsh corgis may be predisposed to vacuolar hepatopathy-associated HCC (Leela-arporn et al. 2019a).

BILE DUCT TUMORS

Tumors of the bile duct also come in two main forms, benign and malignant. Biliary cystadenoma, or hepatobiliary cystadenomas, comprise about 30–50% of feline primary liver neoplasms (David et al. 2020; Brandstetter et al. 2023). As the name suggests, they are cystic in appearance and can occur as a massive or nodular form. They are uncommon in dogs.

Bile duct carcinomas (cholangiocarcinomas) are the most common liver tumor in cats and the second most common liver tumor in dogs (David et al. 2020). They can occur in all three morphologic forms: massive, nodular, and diffuse. Both intrahepatic and extrahepatic cholangiocarcinomas are reported. These are aggressive tumors with extensive metastatic potential. In cats, cholangiocarcinoma can metastasize in small patches throughout the abdomen, called carcinomatosis, which can be dry or exudative, resulting in abdominal effusion (David et al. 2020; Brandstetter et al. 2023).

NEUROENDOCRINE NEOPLASMS

Neuroendocrine neoplasms (NENs), historically referred to as carcinoids, were originally thought to arise from the neuroectodermal cells. More recent studies suggest they arise from stem cell precursors. Hepatobiliary NENs can be classified as neuroendocrine carcinomas, which behave aggressively and are typically found in the liver parenchyma. They often metastasize throughout the abdominal cavity and to the pulmonary parenchyma (Balkman 2009). NENs can also be classified as neuroendocrine tumors and are found more often in the gallbladder of older dogs and carry a better prognosis {Kelly et al., 2024, p. 612}

MESENCHYMAL TUMORS

Primary mesenchymal tumors are rare and arise from the connective tissues that make up the liver architecture. Hemangiosarcoma, leiomyosarcomas, and fibrosarcoma are the most common forms, although liposarcomas, rhabdomyosarcomas, osteosarcomas, and malignant mesenchymomas have been documented (Balkman 2009; David et al. 2020). Primary hemangiosarcomas are the most common primary feline mesenchymal liver tumor, while leiomyosarcomas are the most common canine mesenchymal liver tumor. Primary lesions arising from the liver account for only about 4% of canine hemangiosarcomas. Metastatic lesions in the liver are more common, especially for tumors such as hemangiosarcoma and histiocytic sarcomas.

The prognosis for mesenchymal liver tumors often depends on the histological and morphological type, as well as treatment. If the massive form of disease can be surgically resected, the prognosis can be very good. The nodular and diffuse forms can be more difficult to treat and therefore often have a much worse prognosis. Negative prognostic indicators include poorly differentiated tumors, high grades of pleomorphism, infiltrative growth patterns, vascular invasion, and intra-extrahepatic spread (David et al. 2020).

PRESENTING COMPLAINTS

It is common to find a primary liver mass, especially benign ones, as incidental findings. Depending on the size and location, the animal may not be exhibiting clinical signs at home. Yet, malignant tumors are symptomatic in 50–75% of the cases, particularly if the tumor is causing mechanical or functional issues (David et al. 2020). Massive tumors may cause signs associated with a space-occupying mass in the cranial abdomen, such as regurgitation, vomiting, changes in the appetite, and discomfort, especially when lying down. Weight loss is a common clinical sign due to decreased appetite. Some tumors, specifically tumors of the smooth muscle (leiomyomas or leiomyosarcomas), can cause paraneoplastic hypoglycemia leading to weakness and seizures. Obstructive biliary tumors may cause icterus. Primary liver tumors can rupture and lead to hemoabdomen. If liver function is affected by the neoplasm, hepatic encephalopathy may be present.

Occasionally, coughing or respiratory signs can be present if the mass is pressing on the diaphragm and/or metastasized to the thoracic cavity. An animal may present with a full or distended cranial abdomen from the mass or abdominal effusion. On physical exam, a cranial abdominal mass may be palpated in about ¾ of the patients with large masses (David et al. 2020).

DIAGNOSTIC TESTING

To diagnose a cat or dog with a hepatic neoplasm, it is necessary to identify and obtain a sample of the mass. This can be done in a variety of ways, including ultrasound-guided cytology, ultrasound-guided needle biopsy, laparoscopic biopsy, or through an abdominal exploration with subsequent biopsies of abnormal structures.

DIAGNOSTIC IMAGING

Abdominal radiographs can be used as an initial imaging modality if a cranial abdominal mass is palpated on physical exam. A large liver mass may displace the stomach silhouette caudally, and occasionally mineralization is noted in the biliary tree of both cats and dogs with cholangiocarcinoma. An abdominal ultrasound is a better imaging tool, especially for small or subtle masses. The liver parenchyma, as well as the gallbladder and surrounding structures can be visualized with an abdominal ultrasound. A proficient ultrasonographer can discern the liver lobe the mass is arising from in about 58% of cases (Wormser et al. 2016). Further sampling of any abnormal structures can then be guided by the ultrasound. The combination of a patient with thrombocytosis, a >4 cm liver mass, and a heterogenous focal liver lesion was more likely to be malignant than benign (Leela-Arporn et al. 2019b). For multifocal liver masses, an ultrasound score based on liver surface, echogenicity and nodularity of liver parenchyma, gallbladder wall thickness, presence of sludge, and the visibility of the bile ducts has a high predictive accuracy for malignancy (Assawarachan 2019).

CYTOLOGY

Fine needle aspiration via ultrasound guidance can be a relatively non-invasive and inexpensive way to diagnose a liver mass. Performing a CBC for a platelet count is recommended before obtaining cytology to reduce the chance of excessive hemorrhage. A 25G needle has been shown to reduce the hemodilution but may not be practical for larger dogs where a longer needle is required for sampling (Llanos et al. 2023). Please see Chapter 3 for a full discussion of cytopathologic diagnosis of hepatic neoplasms.

BIOPSY

There are three main ways to obtain a liver biopsy sample: ultrasound-guided needle core biopsy, laparoscopic biopsy, and surgical biopsy. Once adequate hemostatic capability is established, a biopsy can be performed. Please see chapter 4 for a discussion of liver biopsy techniques and histology of hepatic cancer.

STAGING TESTS

Additional diagnostic tests, to determine if any metastatic disease or comorbidities are present, are recommended and help us answer the question: "Where is it?"

LABORATORY TESTS

Laboratory diagnostic tests are essential to establish the health of the patient. While there are few specific findings we expect to see with all liver tumors, there are some changes that should be noted and further evaluated if present.

The complete blood count, CBC, may show anemia, leukocytosis, or thrombocytosis. Anemia has been noted in 26–53% of cats and dogs with hepatic tumors in the literature (Liptak et al. 2004; Lapsley et al. 2022; Brandstetter et al. 2023). This could be due to chronic disease process, hemorrhage, or another comorbidity. In a study evaluating surgical resection of canine massive HCCs, leukocytosis was noted in 18–26% of the cases and thrombocytosis in 30–46% of the cases (Liptak et al. 2004; Brandstetter et al. 2023).

On the comprehensive chemistry panel, elevations in the liver enzymes and bilirubin, potassium, or blood urea nitrogen (BUN) may be noted; while a decrease in the proteins, albumin, and blood glucose have been documented in our dog and cat patients. Two different canine studies evaluated chemistry values in relationship to survival times and found that elevations in the ALT, AST, BUN, and GGT were negatively associated with survival times (Liptak et al. 2004; Moyer et al. 2021). Dogs with massive HCCs have concurrent endocrinopathies in 61% of cases, with hyperadrenocorticism being the most common (Leela-Arporn 2019a). In feline patients, hyperbilirubinemia was present in most cases, and significant elevations in ALT levels often correspond to HCCs (Brandstetter et al. 2023).

THORACIC RADIOGRAPHS

Three-view, right and left lateral, and ventral-dorsal views, thoracic radiographs are recommended to evaluate for metastatic disease. While most hepatic tumors typically metastasize throughout the abdomen, some will metastasize to the thoracic cavity, especially to the sternal lymph node. It is also useful to evaluate the other structures on the thoracic films for evidence of comorbidities, which may alter treatment plans or prognosis.

ABDOMINAL ULTRASOUND

As previously discussed, ultrasonography can be useful to determine if a liver tumor is present and can aid in the sampling of it to determine if it is a benign or malignant process. An abdominal ultrasound is also useful for staging the animal because malignant liver tumors often metastasize within the abdominal cavity. Evaluating the lymph nodes, other organs and signs of extra-nodal masses or fluid accumulation is important when staging a patient to help determine the baseline, as well as determine the therapies that are appropriate for the individual patient.

CT SCAN

Computed tomography (CT) is often the preferred imaging modality for liver tumor therapeutic planning purposes (Figures 19.1 and 19.2). Images aid in preoperatively assessing the potential resectability of a mass, which can reduce intraoperative morbidity and mortality. In the Brandstetter

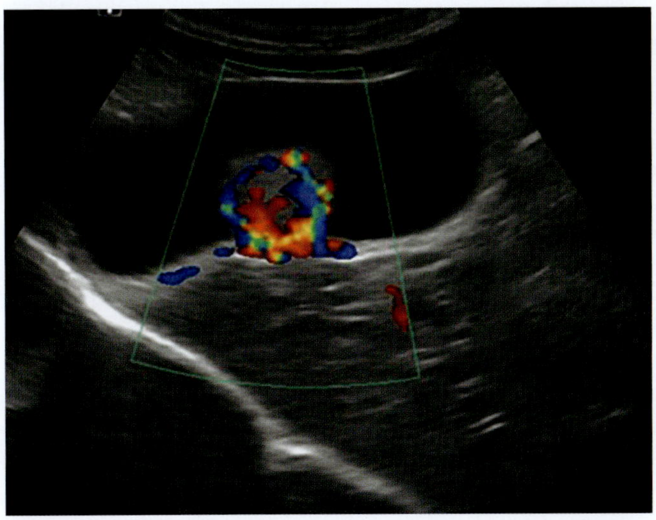

FIGURE 19.1 Sonographic image with color flow doppler of a well vascularized canine gallbladder neuroendocrine neoplasm. Image courtesy of Andrea Johnston

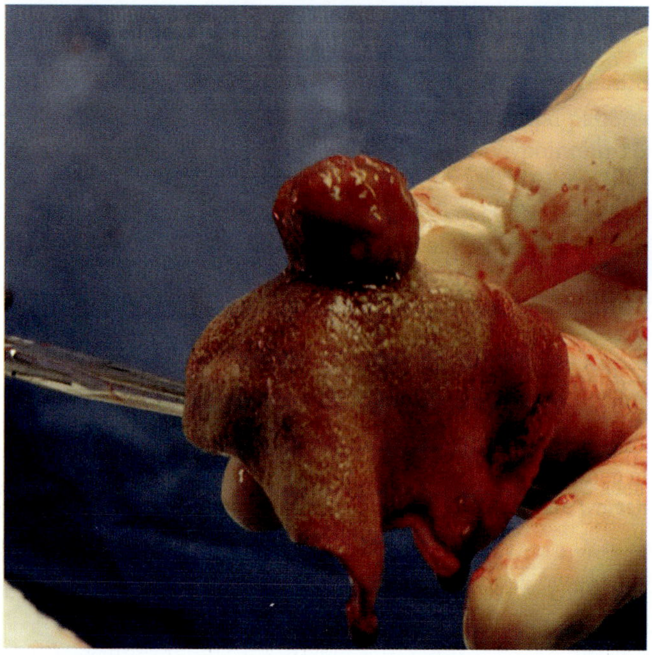

FIGURE 19.2 Gross image of a canine gallbladder neuroendocrine neoplasm. Image courtesy of Andrea Johnston

paper, the intraoperative mortality rate was 23.5% and most of these cats did not receive a CT scan preoperatively (Brandstetter et al. 2023; Smola et al. 2023).

THERAPEUTIC OPTIONS

SURGERY

Surgical resection of massive hepatic tumors is the treatment of choice and has the best prognosis for both canine and feline patients. The completeness of the surgical margin does not seem to affect the overall survival time for the massive HCC (Liptak 2004). In dogs with Massive HCCs, one study found a 4% intraoperative mortality rate with a 28% complication rate. The most common complications included blood loss, compromise to the surrounding vasculature of adjacent liver lobes, transient hypoglycemia, and reduced hepatic function (Liptak et al. 2004). The amount of intra- and postoperative morbidity often depends on the location of the liver mass(es), the ability to plan an approach preoperatively and the experience of the surgeon. The right liver lobes are more difficult to resect due to the surrounding structures, including the vena cava, and a mass in the quadrate liver lobe is a negative prognostic indicator due to the difficulty of surgical resection (Moyer et al. 2021). In our feline patients, the most common intraoperative morbidity is hemorrhage, with an 11% rate (Brandstetter et al. 2023). A recent paper evaluated the time from surgical resection to tumor recurrence for dogs with massive HCC and found them to recur a median of 367 days post resection. They were found on restaging ultrasounds 40% of the time, 29% of the time following presenting with clinical signs, and 25% due to elevated liver enzymes (Lapsley et al. 2022). Recurrence was found earlier if routine staging was performed on every 3-month basis.

Nodular hepatic tumors can be removed if there are only a few nodules and if the nodular masses are able to be safely reached and resected at the time of surgery. Widespread nodular disease affecting multiple liver lobes and the diffuse forms of hepatic neoplasia are unfortunately not amenable to surgical resection.

RADIATION THERAPY

Stereotactic Radiation Therapy (SRT) is a radiation modality that allows for increased doses of radiation to be delivered to precise locations on the body and allows for shorter treatment protocol lengths. The use of SRT in human medicine is a viable option for those diagnosed with inoperable HCCs. The use of this modality was evaluated on dogs with unresectable massive hepatic tumors in a retrospective case series published in Chan et al. (2024). Fourteen dogs were evaluated, and most were treated with 3 × 7–7.5 Gy (daily). Five of nine dogs had stable disease, and three dogs had a partial response and a clinical benefit. One late Grade 5 (death) liver and two later Grade 3 kidney side effects were noted. Median survival time for the group was 164 days (Chan et al. 2024). With the median survival time of clinically managed dogs at 270 days, this is not a recommended therapeutic option currently. Further studies looking at various treatment protocols are recommended to determine the clinical benefit of this modality.

CHEMOTHERAPY

Chemotherapy is generally unrewarding for primary hepatic tumors because they tend to be inherently chemotherapy resistant. Our traditional chemotherapy drugs, typically given at maximally tolerated doses (MTDs), affect cells that are in a state of division by various mechanisms. Adjuvant chemotherapy protocols using Carboplatin, Gemcitabine, Mitoxantrone, and 5-FU show minimal response rates (Ogilvie et al. 1991; Elpiner et al. 2011; David et al. 2020).

CHEMOEMBOLIZATION

For cases of non-resectable massive hepatic tumors, transarterial embolization (TAE) or transarterial chemoembolization (TACE) may be an option if the client lives in an area or is willing to travel to a location that offers this niche modality. An embolizing agent and/or chemotherapy agent (such as drug-eluting doxorubicin beads-DEB-TACE) is delivered into the arteries that feed the massive hepatic tumor via fluoroscopy-aided catheterization. This is a very technical procedure that only a handful of specialists have been certified for. Stable disease occurs in approximately 62% of the patients, while approximately 23% have a partial response. Complications such as hepatic abscesses, septicemia, and cholecystitis/death have been reported. Median survival times are about 337 days for patients presenting with clinical signs that undergo this modality (Rogatko et al. 2021).

ORAL TARGETED THERAPY

Small molecular inhibitors bind to cell surface receptors and are made to typically block a receptor that is responsible for functions such as cell growth, blood vessel formation, or other important signaling in the tumor microenvironment. The use of two kinase inhibitors have been evaluated for the use in canine hepatocellular tumors.

Toceranib phosphate (Palladia trade name) is a receptor transmembrane kinase (RTK) inhibitor that was made to treat canine mast cell tumors. It can target Kit, VEGFR, and PDGFR, which also have functions in the tumor microenvironment. A short-term (60-day) prospective trial looked at dogs with unresectable massive HCC and their response to treatment with oral toceranib at 2–3 mg/kg every other day. Out of six dogs, 50% achieved a partial response, and one dog achieved stable disease. Further prospective trials are needed to confirm the clinical benefit of this medication (Heishima et al. 2019).

Oral sorafenib has been evaluated for the treatment of unresectable advanced HCC in dogs, comparing survival times with a metronomic protocol used in Europe, which includes thalidomide, piroxicam, and cyclophosphamide (Marconato et al. 2020). Seven dogs received sorafenib at a dose of 5 mg/kg twice daily. Median overall survival time for this group was 361 days, where the metronomic chemotherapy group was 27 days. The dogs tolerated the sorafenib well, but inconsistent supply of the drug was a complication of the study design. Further prospective trials are needed to confirm the clinical benefit of this medication (Marconato et al. 2020).

PROGNOSIS

Multiple prognostic markers have been assessed for canine and feline liver cancer (Tables 19.1 and 19.2). Biochemical abnormalities (elevations in ALT, AST, BUN, GGT, and potassium), presence of metastases, large tumor size, and number of masses have been linked to poor overall survival with hepatobiliary cancer (Maeda et al. 2022).

Table 19.1 Canine Primary Liver Tumors Prognostic Indicators

	Positive	Negative
Tumor in quadrate lobe	—	X
Tumor in right side of liver	—	X
Massive form	Good if Surgically Removed MST 850->1460 days if surgically removed; 270 days if medically managed	—
Nodular form	Good if Surgically Removed, see above	Poor if multifocal and non-surgical
Diffuse form	—	X
Neuroendocrine	—	X
Mesenchymal	—	X
HCC	Good if Surgically Removed, see above	—
Bile duct	MST 894 days if intrahepatic tumors removed Good if Surgically Removed	Poor if multifocal and non-surgical or localized or distant metastasis occurring postoperatively (33% patients)
Metastatic disease	—	X

Table 19.2 Feline Primary Liver Tumors Prognostic Indicators

	Positive	Negative
Massive HCC	MST 868 days if surgically removed	—
Bile duct carcinoma	MST 270 days if surgically removed	Poor if non-surgical
Nodular	Good if surgically removed	Poor if multifocal and non-surgical
Diffuse	—	X
Neuroendocrine	—	X
Mesenchymal	—	MST 16 days
Metastatic disease	—	X

REFERENCES

Assawarachan, S. N., Chuchalermporn, P. Maneesaay, P., and Thengchaisri, N. (2019). Evaluation of hepatobiliary ultrasound scores in healthy dogs and dogs with liver diseases. *Veterinary World* 12(8): 1266–1272.

Balkman, C. (2009). Hepatobiliary neoplasia in dogs and cats. *Veterinary Clinics of North America-Small Animal Practice* 39 (3): 617–625.

Brandstetter, V., Schmidt, J. M., Findji, L. et al. (2023). Feline primary nonhematopoietic malignant liver tumours: a multicenter retrospective study (2000–2021). *Veterinary and Comparative Oncology* 21 (2): 191–199.

Chan, Q.Y.P., Morrow, D., and Lurie, D. (2024). Canine primary liver tumors treated with stereotactic body radiation therapy: a case series. *Veterinary Radiology & Ultrasound* 65 (2): 121–129.

David, M.V., Douglas, H.T., and Julius M.L. (2020). *Withrow and MacEwen's Small Animal Clinical Oncology – E-Book*. St. Louis, Missouri: Saunders.

Elpiner, A.K., Brodsky, E.M., Hazzah, T.N. et al. (2011). Single-agent gemcitabine chemotherapy in dogs with hepatocellular carcinomas. *Veterinary and Comparative Oncology* 9 (4): 260–268.

Heishima, K., Iwasaki, R., Kawabe, M. et al. (2019). Short-term administration of single-agent toceranib in six cases of inoperable massive canine hepatocellular carcinoma. *Journal of the American Animal Hospital Association* 55 (1): 35–41

Kelly, N., Y. T. Wu and A. N. Johnston (2024). Gallbladder neuroendocrine neoplasms in dogs and humans. *Veterinary Sciences* 11(8): 371.

Lapsley, J.M., Wavreille, V., Barry, S. et al. (2022). Risk factors and outcome in dogs with recurrent massive hepatocellular carcinoma: a veterinary society of surgical oncology case-control study. *Veterinary and Comparative Oncology* 20 (3): 697–709.

Leela-arporn, R., Ohta, H., Nagata, N. et al. (2019a). Epidemiology of massive hepatocellular carcinoma in dogs: a 4-year retrospective study. *Veterinary Journal* 248: 74–78.

Leela-Arporn, R., Ohta, H., Tamura, M. et al. (2019b). Predictive factors of malignancy in dogs with focal liver lesions using clinical data and ultrasonographic features. *Journal of Veterinary Medical Science* 81 (5): 723–729.

Liptak, J.M., Dernell, W.S., Monnet, E. et al. (2004). Massive hepatocellular carcinoma in dogs: 48 cases (1992–2002). *Journal of the American Veterinary Medical Association* 225 (8): 1225–1230.

Llanos, C., Holmes, E., White, C. et al. (2023). Diagnostic quality of ultrasound-guided fine-needle aspirates samples from the canine liver and spleen is not significantly affected by using 22-, 23-, and 25-gauge needles. *Veterinary Radiology and Ultrasound* 64 (5): 966–972.

Maeda, A., Goto, S., Iwasaki, R. et al. (2022). Outcome of localized bile duct carcinoma in six dogs treated with liver lobectomy. *Journal of the American Animal Hospital Association* 58 (4): 189–193.

Marconato, L., Sabattini, S., Marisi, G. et al. (2020). Sorafenib for the treatment of unresectable hepatocellular carcinoma: preliminary toxicity and activity data in dogs. *Cancers (Basel)* 12 (5): 1272.

Moyer, J., Lopez, D.J., Balkman, C.E. et al. (2021). Factors associated with survival in dogs with a histopathological diagnosis of hepatocellular carcinoma: 94 cases (2007–2018). *Open Veterinary Journal* 11 (1): 144–153.

Ogilvie, G.K., Obradovich, J.E., Elmslie, R.E. et al. (1991). Efficacy of mitoxantrone against various neoplasms in dogs. *Journal of the American Veterinary Medical Association* 198 (9): 1618–1621.

Rogatko, C.P., Weisse, C., Schwarz, T. et al. (2021). Drug-eluting bead chemoembolization for the treatment of nonresectable hepatic carcinoma in dogs: a prospective clinical trial. *Journal of Veterinary Internal Medicine* 35 (3): 1487–1495.

Smola, C., Schwartz, P., Caceres, A. et al. (2023). Computed tomography angiography aids in predicting resectability of isolated liver tumors in dogs. *Journal of the American Veterinary Medical Association* 261 (10): 1–7.

Wormser, C., Reetz J.A., and Giuffrida, M.A. (2016). Diagnostic accuracy of ultrasound to predict the location of solitary hepatic masses in dogs. *Veterinary Surgeons* 45 (2): 208–213.

CHAPTER 20

Nutritional Management of Common Hepatobiliary Disorders

Jonathan Stockman

Department of Molecular Biosciences, School of Veterinary Medicine, University of California Davis, Davis, California, USA

KEY POINTS

- Liver dysfunction leads to significant changes in metabolism.
- Special consideration should be given to preventing energy malnutrition in compromised liver patients or those with a low appetite.
- Enteral tube feeding is often necessary for managing patients with hepatic lipidosis
- Liver disease patients may have increased protein requirements; however, a restriction or change in protein source may be needed to manage patients with hepatic encephalopathy
- Diet change is not necessary for all patients with liver disease; however, diets formulated for liver disease management are indicated in cases of copper-associated hepatitis, hepatic encephalopathy, or urate crystalluria and urolithiasis.

INTRODUCTION

The liver is an important metabolic organ associated with the digestive tract. It produces bile salts, aids in toxin neutralization, and houses various metabolic pathways. The liver is unique in its vascular supply, which includes perfusion by the venous portal system, providing systemic venous blood circulation rather than from an artery. Therefore, there is increased hepatic exposure to insults such as pathogens or toxins.

Liver disease is a relatively common presentation in companion animals and can lead to significant morbidity and mortality. Etiologies of liver disease are many, and include developmental, metabolic, infectious, toxic, and nutritional causes. Advanced disease may result in liver dysfunction and an impairment in the production of plasma proteins and clotting factors, which can complicate clinical management. Disease progression can ultimately lead to hepatic dysfunction/failure, which is defined as a decrease in more than 75% of the functional hepatic mass and the presence of relevant hepatic signs, (Center 1996).

Several liver-associated presentations are common in dogs and cats, including acute or chronic hepatitis, cholangitis, and cholangiohepatitis, vascular diseases (i.e., congenital portosystemic shunts), toxicity, storage diseases (e.g., glycogen or lipid), copper-associated hepatopathy, hepatic lipidosis, and cancer. Typically, patients with liver disease can present with jaundice, hepatic encephalopathy, lethargy, dysrexia, polyuria, polydipsia, vomiting, and diarrhea. Hepatic failure results in alterations in biochemical parameters, including a reduction in blood glucose, cholesterol, albumin, and urea, as well as elevated bilirubin and pre- and post-prandial bile acids.

Dietary intervention and assisted feeding are often necessary in patients with advanced hepatic disease and metabolic complications (Stockman 2025). Adequate nutrition can mitigate complications resulting from liver disease, attenuate progression, reduce the frequency and severity of associated signs, and promote hepatic regeneration. Nutritional support can also prevent the negative energy balance leading to muscle catabolism, decreased lean body mass, and frailty, which are often associated with advanced or severe hepatic pathology.

Clinicians should note that a dietary change is not needed in every patient with chronic liver disease; this depends on the clinical signs and the underlying pathology.

NUTRITIONAL CONSIDERATIONS FOR PATIENTS WITH ADVANCED HEPATIC DISEASE AND FAILURE

Advanced hepatic disease, physical and toxic insults may all lead to hepatic failure if the damage is extensive. Hepatic failure is the clinical manifestation of liver dysfunction and can lead to abnormalities such as hyperglucagonemia, fasting or postprandial hyperglycemia or hypoglycemia, hyperinsulinemia, decreased glycogenesis, etc. The nutritional management of patients with liver failure requires consideration of energy, macronutrient and micronutrient intake as these can affect clinical presentation, organ function, recovery, and disease progression.

ENERGY

Severe illness may lead to negative energy balance and ultimately to a catabolic state, which negatively affects patient prognosis. Despite medical care, severely ill patients often have poor appetite or nausea, causing a reduced food intake (Chan 2012). Deficient energy intake can result from the disease and its effects on liver function or be caused by stress, nausea, altered mentation, or hormonal shifts. The impact of liver disease on nutritional requirements in small animal patients is largely unknown; however, energy intake is often insufficient to prevent catabolism in affected small animal patients (Chan 2012; Chan 2004). The outcomes of a prolonged negative energy balance include frailty, decreased immunity, and impaired tissue repair.

Severe liver disease, such as liver cirrhosis, can further increase energy requirements. A hypermetabolic state may result from systemic vasodilatation and expanded intravascular and cardiac blood volume, ultimately leading to a higher energy expenditure (Tsiaousi et al. 2008). Hyperglucagonemia resulting from decreased hepatic glucagon clearance or increased pancreatic glucagon secretion may contribute to systemic catabolism. Glycogen stores do not last long, and their depletion (within a couple of days) leads to protein (and muscle) catabolism for gluconeogenesis. Hypoglycemia is not a common finding in patients with liver disease despite reduced function. Surprisingly, glucose production is maintained even in severe liver disease with impaired liver function, and peripheral glucose utilization reduction helps conserve blood glucose (Marks and Kathrani 2023; Nadler and Wolfer 1929). Elevated blood glucose is a negative prognostic indicator in critical patients. Hyperglycemia may result from insulin resistance related to systemic inflammation, hyperglucagonemia, or increased hepatic response to glucagon. High blood glucose is a frequent clinical finding in dogs with hepatocutaneous syndrome, along with hypoaminoacidemia, and can result from accelerated hepatic amino acid catabolism and gluconeogenesis (Loftus et al. 2017).

The initial caloric target is most often set to meet the patient's daily resting energy requirements (RER; $70 \times \text{bodyweight(kg)}^{0.75} =$ kcal per day). Additional adjustments may be needed according to body weight and body condition score trends. A catabolic state can result from a failure to meet energy needs and can worsen liver disease. This is often the case in feline hepatic lipidosis, a disease characterized by starvation, causing the mobilization of fatty acids from fat tissues to the liver to be packaged as triglycerides and accumulate in hepatocytes. This ultimately overwhelms the cells, leading to dysfunction. Reversing the negative energy balance often requires a feeding tube placement, as most patients fail to consume sufficient food voluntarily or even with appetite-stimulating medications.

PROTEIN AND AMINO ACIDS

Adequate protein intake is crucial in patients with liver disease. Albumin, clotting factors, lipoproteins, thyroglobulin, and complement proteins are all produced in the liver and are required for immunity, coagulation, endocrine function, and maintaining oncotic pressure. Amino acid metabolism, including the synthesis of nonessential amino acids and the oxidation of amino acids for energy, also requires liver involvement (Charlton 1996).

The molar ratio of the sum of branched-chain amino acids to aromatic amino acids is termed 'Fischer Ratio,' which is often low in patients with liver failure (Rosen et al. 1977). This may lead to aromatic amino acids crossing the blood–brain barrier and possibly contributing to the pathogenesis of hepatic encephalopathy, as they can act similarly to neurotransmitters (Cascino et al. 1982). Supplementation with branch-chain amino acids could restore this ratio and reduce the risk of aromatic amino acids reaching the central nervous system; however, this appears to provide inconsistent benefits and is not often a part of the nutritional management of liver disease in veterinary patients (Konstantis et al. 2022; Marks and Kathrani 2023).

Liver failure can cause elevated blood ammonia because ammonia detoxification relies on the urea cycle, which occurs mostly in the liver. In addition, hyperammonemia may occur due to increased amino acid metabolism, microbial protein fermentation in the large intestine, gluconeogenesis, shunts, or cirrhosis. While ammonia plays an important role in the pathogenesis of hepatic encephalopathy, hyperammonemia is not the sole cause of it. An infusion of ammonium chloride does not result in neural impairment in healthy adult humans (Wilkinson et al. 2011), and hyperammonemia is not always present in dogs suffering from hepatic encephalopathy (Tivers et al. 2014). Therefore, the pathogenesis of hepatic encephalopathy may include additional factors such as inflammatory mediators, neurosteroids, oxidative damage, and potentially a skewed branch-chain to aromatic amino acid ratio as mentioned above (Lidbury et al. 2016).

Dogs with hepatic encephalopathy often improve with a reduced-protein diet. However, a reduced protein intake should not risk a deficiency or protein malnutrition. The National Research Council's (NRC) 2006 publication specifies a recommended allowance (RA) of dietary protein to be used to assess whether protein intake is sufficient.

Protein RA dogs (maintenance) = 3.26 g × body weight (kilogram)^0.75. Protein RA cats (maintenance) = 4.96 g × body weight (kilogram)^0.67 (NRC 2006).

PROTEIN INTAKE REDUCTION IS ONLY INDICATED IN HEPATIC ENCEPHALOPATHY OR URATE UROLITHIASIS

It is hypothesized that increased protein intake above RA helps compensate for the decline in liver-dependent protein metabolism and prevents malnutrition in patients with hyporexia. As discussed below, feeding a non-meat protein, such as vegetarian, egg, or whey protein, can also mitigate the risk of encephalopathy and potentially decrease its severity (Proot et al. 2009). The same protein sources are usually low in purines and, therefore, can reduce the risk of urolithiasis in patients with liver dysfunction.

FAT

Both lipoprotein production and metabolism occur in the liver. Lipoproteins are circulated from peripheral stores back to the liver and vice versa, facilitating lipid transport. Fatty acids are oxidized in the hepatocytes' mitochondria to make ATP and NADH for energy production and acetyl-CoA molecules that may be further metabolized to cholesterol. The liver also produces bile acids from cholesterol, which are conjugated to taurine (and also to glycine in dogs) before secretion from the gallbladder to the small intestine. Hypocholesterolemia may be seen in animals with decreased hepatic function.

Hepatic veterinary therapeutic diets are often formulated to be high fat to increase their energy density for patients with poor appetite or decreased ability to feed. Additionally, dietary fat can increase diet palatability, an important consideration when appetite is poor. Fat also acts as a vehicle for fat-soluble vitamins that can be low in an animal with chronic disease or prolonged hyporexia. Higher fat diets are usually well-tolerated; however, reduced fat diets may be indicated in some cases. Indications for fat reduction include cholestasis and bile duct obstruction, because ingested fat can stimulate the intestinal hormones motilin and cholecystokinin, resulting in contraction of the gall bladder. High-fat diets are also not recommended in patients with hypertriglyceridemia, mucocele, pancreatitis, or chronic enteritis, as they may cause worsened clinical signs and disease severity. Patients with cholestasis can benefit from dietary fat reduction, as they often suffer from diarrhea and steatorrhea caused by decreased fat digestibility.

VITAMINS, MINERALS, AND ANTIOXIDANTS

Hepatic disease, poor appetite, or inability to feed may lead to deficiencies in essential nutrients, including both water-soluble and fat-soluble vitamins. Water-soluble vitamins are often involved in energy metabolism and/or act as coenzymes. Vitamin C is a nonessential vitamin in healthy dogs and cats; however, since its production is primarily in the liver, supplementation may be considered in patients with severe hepatic disease or liver dysfunction (Marks and Kathrani 2023). Conversely, dogs with portosystemic shunts and other forms of chronic liver disease were not found to have a vitamin C deficiency, possibly indicating that vitamin C production is maintained even with liver disease (Hishiyama et al. 2006; Galler et al. 2013). Vitamin C supplementation at a dose of 25 mg per kilogram body weight in dogs is considered safe (Marks and Kathrani 2023). However, being acidic, vitamin C supplementation isn't recommended in patients with acidosis. It is also not recommended in patients with a history of calcium oxalate urolithiasis, or in dogs of breeds considered to be frequent calcium oxalate urolith formers, as vitamin C may be metabolized to oxalic acid. Vitamin C may cause an increase in transition metal oxidation in vitro, contrary to its antioxidant activity, although this was not shown in vivo (Carr and Frei 1999).

As described above, fat-soluble vitamins may be deficient in patients with hepatic disease, particularly in those with poor food intake, fat malabsorption, or cholestasis. The risk of excess fat-soluble vitamins is greater than that of water-soluble vitamins, as fat-soluble vitamins accumulate and can cause toxicity in excess. Water-soluble vitamins have limited body stores, and any excess is usually lost in the urine. One should be particularly careful with vitamin A or D supplementation due to their narrow safety margins.

Healthy animals do not require vitamin K supplementation because it is produced in sufficient amounts by intestinal bacteria. Hepatic vitamin K stores are limited, and severe liver disease and concurrent dysbiosis (caused by the primary disease or antimicrobial use) may lead to reduced vitamin K production and ultimately its depletion. Proteins induced by vitamin K absence or antagonism (PIVKA) may be measured to assess vitamin K status and determine the need for supplementation (Mount et al. 2003). Supplementation of vitamin K can be in the form of vitamin K1 (phylloquinone) or the synthetic form, menadione.

Hepatic stellate cells are the primary store of vitamin A. Therefore, vitamin A depletion is possible in patients with extensive hepatic damage. Vitamin A supplementation was shown to reduce hepatic fibrosis in rodent models for cholestasis (He et al. 2011). However, vitamin A can be hepatotoxic, and clinicians should be cautious with supplementation (Marks and Kathrani 2023).

Vitamin D is often low in people with hepatic disease. Liver damage may impair normal vitamin D activation because its metabolism to 25-hydroxyvitamin-D occurs in the liver. The outcome in people with chronic liver disease was shown to improve with vitamin D supplementation, which was also shown to strengthen the immunologic response to hepatitis C virus (Stokes et al. 2013). It should be noted that the vitamin D status of dogs and cats suffering from liver disease is unknown, and the clinical impact of vitamin D supplementation has not been established in dogs and cats. Vitamin D has a narrow safety range in dogs, and excessive supplementation can cause severe toxicity with hypercalcemia resulting in organ damage. It is strongly recommended that vitamin D therapy is done with the guidance and monitoring of a veterinarian (ideally a boarded specialist in veterinary internal medicine or nutrition), and it is not recommended for all patients.

Vitamin E is often supplemented in patients with liver disease, as it is a prominent antioxidant. It may protect from oxidative stress, especially in conditions characterized by inflammation, such as copper-associated hepatopathy or severe hepatitis. Supplementation doses of vitamin E in the literature are highly variable, and it has a wide safety range compared to other fat-soluble vitamins. Doses range from 10 IU/kg/day to 100–400 IU per dog once or twice daily and 30–50 IU/day in cats (Weingarten and Sande 2015). Very high intake of vitamin E may affect the absorption of other fat-soluble vitamins such as vitamin A and vitamin K.

S-adenosylmethionine (SAMe) is a precursor of glutathione and an important antioxidant. It is often supplemented in liver disease patients, as it is reported to be hepatoprotective. A dose of 20 mg/kg/day, either alone or in combination with silybin showed a beneficial effect on markers of oxidative damage and inflammation in dogs and cats with induced liver injury (Center et al. 2005; Webb et al. 2003). Milk thistle extract (or silymarin) contains silybin, a potent flavonoid that acts as an antioxidant and has several hepatoprotective benefits, including increasing glutathione and inhibiting hepatotoxin binding. While there is limited evidence of the benefit of milk thistle extract supplementation in clinical cases of dogs or cats with liver pathology, experimental studies demonstrated multiple potential benefits to silybin, including antifibrotic, antioxidant, anti-inflammatory, and metabolic effects (Trappoliere et al. 2009). The bioavailability of silybin is greater than that of silymarin and even higher when it is complexed with phosphatidylcholine (i.e., Denamarin Liver Health Supplement for Dogs and Cats, Nutramax Laboratories, Lancaster, SC) (Filburn et al. 2007; Loguercio and Festi 2011). Silybin and silymarin are dosed at 5–15 mg/kg per day by mouth.

Zinc is an essential mineral with various functions, including acting as an antioxidant. Zinc inhibits NADPH oxidase, thereby reducing the production of reactive oxygen species. It is a cofactor of superoxide dismutase (SOD), an enzyme that catalyzes the dismutation of reactive oxygen species and hydrogen peroxide. Zinc induces metallothionein production, a scavenger of reactive oxygen moieties. Intestinal mucosal metallothionein may also act to bind copper in the epithelium and prevent its absorption. Copper bound to metallothionein is then removed from the body in the turnover of intestinal epithelial cells.

As discussed below, copper can have a big role in the pathology of liver disease in dogs and cats because it may accumulate in the liver in patients with cholestatic liver disease or a pathology impairing normal copper excretion.

A high salt intake does not seem to induce high blood pressure in otherwise healthy animals; however, little is known about sodium's impact on portal hypertension that may be present in patients with liver cirrhosis or other liver diseases. Although limited data is available regarding the impact of sodium on blood pressure in dogs and cats, it is generally accepted that high sodium should be avoided in patients with severe cirrhosis, fibrosis, or ascites, due to the risk of exacerbated portal hypertension. Therefore, liver patients are advised to avoid excess dietary salt.

NUTRITIONAL MANAGEMENT OF SPECIFIC LIVER ASSOCIATED DISEASES

HEPATIC VASCULAR SHUNTS, ENCEPHALOPATHY, AND SHUNT-ASSOCIATED URATE UROLITHIASIS

The neurological signs resulting from liver dysfunction often include seizures, abnormal behavior, coma, etc. These vary in presentation and severity and can be temporally associated with mealtimes. Neurological signs can be a presentation in dogs and cats with advanced liver disease and hepatic failure; however, hepatic encephalopathy is most often seen in patients with portosystemic shunts without hepatic failure. The causes for hepatic encephalopathy are only partly known, and several mechanisms may be involved; for example, a liver shunt partially prevents the liver from metabolizing ammonia and other food-associated compounds. Amino acid imbalance can also result in encephalopathic disease as described above. Astrocytes in the central nervous system metabolize ammonia to glutamine, which causes a decrease in expression of glutamate receptors and impacts the cells' osmotic pressure, resulting in cellular edema. The nutritional management of patients with hepatic encephalopathy centers on decreasing ammonia production. However, ammonia level is not always directly associated with the severity of encephalopathic signs (Rothuizen and Van Den Ingh 1982; Lidbury et al. 2016). As previously stated, protein requirements may be elevated in patients with hepatic disease; however, a reduced protein diet with a modified protein source is often necessary to reduce the frequency and severity of encephalopathy. Individual patients vary in protein tolerance and may have different intake thresholds for exhibiting encephalopathic signs. Still, the overall goal is to provide the maximum amount of protein tolerable without neurological signs. An intake of 2.11 g high-quality protein per kilogram body weight was tolerated, met apparent protein requirements, and did not result in encephalopathic disease in most dogs with portosystemic shunts (Laflamme et al. 1993). Diets containing non-meat protein, such as vegetable, egg, or dairy, help reduce metabolites likely involved in the pathogenesis of hepatic encephalopathy, such as ammonia, oxyphenol, and mercaptans (Iqbal et al. 2021; Proot et al. 2009). To prevent protein malnutrition, protein with a high biological value and high digestibility is recommended, particularly in patients who require a low-protein diet to prevent seizures. High digestibility helps reduce the amount of protein ultimately reaching the colon for fermentation, which is an important contributor to the host's ammonia levels.

It can be challenging to nutritionally manage feline patients with congenital portosystemic shunts and hepatic encephalopathy, as most reduced protein diets, such as veterinary therapeutic kidney diets for cats, are inadequate for growth. Some possible approaches can be to compare over-the-counter diets to find a diet formulated for feline growth that is lower in protein, feed a highly digestible veterinary diet with relatively low protein (Hill's Prescription Diet i/d feline dry and canned varieties, Hill's Pet Nutrition, Topeka, KS), or feed a growth diet that includes hydrolyzed soy, a vegetarian protein source (Purina ProPlan Veterinary Diet HA Hydrolyzed dry cat food, Purina ProPlan, St. Louis, MO). It should be noted that veterinary therapeutic diets are reformulated periodically, and clinicians should review nutritional information in updated product guides. A customized diet formulated by a boarded specialist in nutrition may also be used (diplomate of the American College of Veterinary Internal Medicine in Nutrition or the European College of Veterinary and Comparative Nutrition). However, the high metabolic requirements of growing cats increase the risk of nutritional deficiencies if the recipe is not followed precisely or if the available ingredients differ from those used in the formulation; therefore, commercial options are usually preferred.

Manganese and ammonia may synergistically increase oxidative stress and negatively affect astrocytes, according to in vitro studies. Biliary excretion of excess manganese is impaired in advanced hepatic disease and cirrhosis, and manganese can be increased in dogs with congenital shunt abnormalities (Gow et al. 2010). However, reducing dietary manganese was never proven to benefit small animal patients with encephalopathic disease.

Changes in feeding schedule can sometimes help reduce spikes in ammonia production post-prandially. Frequent small meals can help reduce encephalopathic signs (Center 1998). High-fiber diets can assist by increasing gastric emptying time and slowing digestion to attenuate ammonia peaks. Supplementation with soluble fibers or lactulose treatment (a nonabsorbable disaccharide) can expedite intestinal transit and lower intestinal pH, resulting in decreased colonic ammonia production and its absorption.

Urate urolithiasis often accompanies hepatic vascular shunts in dogs and less commonly in cats. Hepatic vascular abnormalities can cause uric acid concentration to increase in the urine. Uric acid is a product of purine degradation and has low water solubility. It is metabolized to allantoin, a water-soluble compound, by hepatic uricase; however, it may increase in patients with liver shunts due to blood being diverted from the liver and the reduction in liver size. Surgical correction of vascular shunts can reduce the risk of urate urolith recurrence. Allopurinol is a synthetic isomer of hypoxanthine, an intermediate metabolite in purine degradation upstream to uric acid that can decrease its production. However, unless purine intake is reduced, this may lead to an increase in the compound xanthine, which can precipitate and form urinary crystals and uroliths. High-purine food items include organ meat and seafood, whereas vegetarian foods, eggs, and dairy are usually low in purines and are preferred in patients with high risk for urate or xanthine urolithiasis.

FELINE HEPATIC LIPIDOSIS

Hepatic lipidosis can be spontaneous or secondary to insufficient energy intake resulting from another disease. Obese cats are at higher risk for feline hepatic lipidosis and may present with a history of significant weight loss in a short time due to dysrexia or anorexia. Assisted feeding is often key to reversing catabolism in patients with hepatic lipidosis because inappetence, nausea,

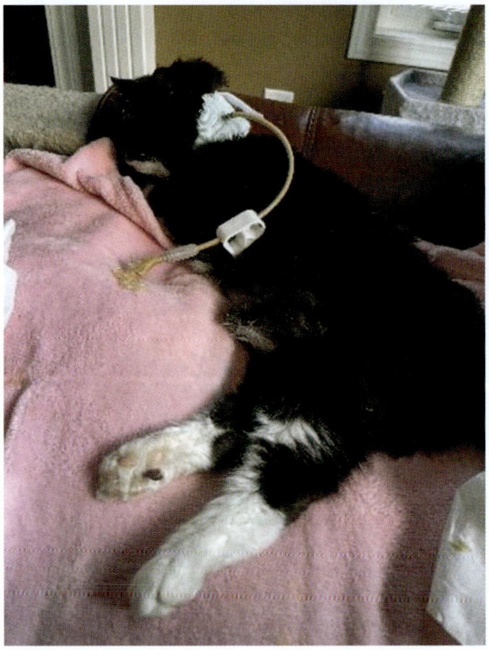

(Credit: Dr. Tammy J Owens, University of Saskatoon, Western School of Veterinary Medicine, Canada)

FIGURE 20.1 An esophagostomy enteral tube in a cat for assisted feeding

or food aversion reduce the likelihood of voluntary food intake (Figure 20.1). Recent data showed that slightly delayed feeding intervention after stabilizing the patient first (for 12–36 hours) may be at least as effective as rapid feeding support (Wallace et al. 2024). Therefore, prioritizing general supportive care (correction of fluids, electrolytes, etc.) may be considered before sedating or anesthetizing the patient for tube placement.

While in the hospital, energy intake should be increased gradually to assess feeding tolerance and to reduce the risk for refeeding syndrome in patients with prolonged anorexia. Typically, feeding amounts are increased daily in 25% increments until reaching the caloric target, which is often the patient's calculated RER. Feeding can include commercial liquid veterinary diets, slurries made from dry or canned veterinary diets mixed in a blender (Table 20.1), or balanced home-prepared formulas. If none of the above options are available, enteral feeding formulas for people can also be used short-term. It should be noted that these products are not balanced for veterinary patients and often do not provide sufficient protein and essential amino acids. All enteral solutions should include arginine, which is of special importance in cats, as a deletion of arginine can cause significant morbidity and mortality even after a single meal. That said, many products are supplemented with arginine or include dairy or soy protein that provides arginine. Clinicians should also avoid products that contain sucrose, a sugar that can lead to fructosuria in cats.

Protein intake should meet or exceed the requirements unless a reduction is indicated to address hepatic encephalopathy, urate urolithiasis, or urate crystalluria. Liquid veterinary diets with soy and milk protein can help mitigate encephalopathic signs (Royal Canin Veterinary Diet Recovery Liquid or Renal Support Liquid (canine and feline), Royal Canin, Aimargues, France). Patients with anorexia may suffer from electrolyte shifts, especially potassium, magnesium, and phosphorus, due to poor intake or resulting from refeeding syndrome. The diet should provide sufficient electrolytes to meet the patient's requirements, and additional enteral potassium can be provided if needed. Most patients with hepatic lipidosis can tolerate fat with no complications. This allows a smaller food volume with higher caloric density. Additional support for liver function can include B vitamins, parenteral vitamin K injections, SAMe, and vitamin E as described above. The B vitamin thiamine is especially important in cats with hepatic lipidosis, as it is important for energy metabolism and may be depleted due to prolonged dysrexia due to limited body stores. Thiamine dosage can range from 10 to 100 mg SQ per day per cat during the refeeding period or 100–200 mg per cat daily via oral supplementation (Marks and Kathrani 2023). L-Carnitine supplementation is often recommended in cats with hepatic lipidosis for several reasons. Carnitine is normally produced in the

Table 20.1 Nutritional Information for Products Prescribed to Dogs with Liver Disease. Information from the USA Product Guides Provided by the Respective Manufacturers for 2024

	AAFCO Dog food nutrient profile (adult) minimums[a]	AAFCO Dog food nutrient profile (growth and reproduction) minimums[a]	Hill's Prescription Diet u/d dry[b]	Hill's Prescription Diet u/d canned[b]	Hill's Prescription Diet l/d dry[b]	Hill's Prescription Diet l/d canned[b]	Royal Canin Veterinary Diet Hepatic dry[c]	Royal Canin Veterinary Diet Hepatic canned[c]	Royal Canin Veterinary Diet Vegetarian dry[c]	Royal Canin Veterinary Diet Vegetarian canned[c]	Purina ProPlan Veterinary Diet HA Hydrolyzed Vegetarian Canine dry[d]	Purina ProPlan Veterinary Diet NF Kidney Function dry[d]	Purina ProPlan Veterinary Diet NF Kidney Function canned[d]
Adequacy statement			Animal feeding tests for adult dogs	Animal feeding tests for adult dogs	Animal feeding tests for adult dogs and puppies	Animal feeding tests for adult dogs and puppies	Intermittent or supplemental feeding	Intermittent or supplemental feeding	Formulated to meet AAFCO profile for adult maintenance	Formulated to meet AAFCO profile for adult maintenance	Formulated to meet AAFCO profile for adult maintenance	Animal feeding tests for adult dogs	Animal feeding tests for adult dogs
Partial ingredient list			Brewers rice, cornstarch, chicken fat, egg product, flaxseed	Water, cornstarch, egg product, chicken fat, pork liver	Brewers rice, chicken, chicken fat, egg product, soybean meal	Water, rice, soybean meal, chicken fat, soybean oil	Brewers rice, brown rice, soy protein isolate, chicken fat, dried beet pulp	Water, brewers rice, corn flour, chicken liver, pork byproducts	Oat groats, brewers rice, potato protein, coconut oil, natural flavors, dried plain beet pulp	Water, soy protein, brewers rice flour, brewers rice, vegetable oil	Cornstarch, hydrolyzed soy protein, coconut oil, partially hydrogenated canola oil, powdered cellulose	Corn, rice, egg, animal fat, sugar	Water, meat byproduct, rice, corn grits, beef, liver
						Nutrients per 1000 kcal							
Crude Protein (g)	45	56.3	32	30	41	44	40.8	45.1	53.4	79.35	57.4	41.5	42.4
Crude Fat (g)	13.8	21.3	48	57	55	54	40.8	27.8	28.6	33.57	28.1	41.7	58.9
Copper (mg)	1.83	3.1	NS	NS	NS	NS	1	1.2	4.22	4.07	3.9	1.9	2.7
Zinc (mg)	20	25	NS	NS	NS	NS	61.4	63.2	70.34	63.07	82.9	43.3	39
Sodium (g)	0.2	0.8	0.51	0.62	0.42	0.5	0.5	0.6	0.84	1.53	0.9	0.8	0.4
Calcium (g)	1.25	3	1.47	1.3	2.47	2.12	1.8	1.8	2.31	1.93	3.4	1.8	1.6
Phosphorus (g)	1	2.5	0.74	0.67	1.57	1.41	1.3	1.2	1.49	1.73	2.4	0.9	0.8

Note: Veterinary therapeutic products may undergo frequent reformulations. always review the most current product guides before prescribing (Stockman 2025/with permission of Elsevier).

[a]Association of American Feed Control Officials, Inc. 2024 Official Publication, Oxford (IN).

[b]Hill's Pet Nutrition, Topeka, KS.

[c]Royal Canin, Aimargues, France.

[d]Purina ProPlan, St. Louis, MO.

NS = not specified.

liver in addition to the dietary supply. It facilitates fatty acid oxidation (beta oxidation) and is often recommended in obese cats during weight loss at an oral dose of 250–500 mg per day per cat (Marks and Kathrani 2023). Taurine supplementation may also be beneficial as an essential nutrient in cats and is likely deficient with prolonged dysrexia. Taurine deficiency in cats can be detrimental and cause heart disease and blindness. While most commercial feline diets include taurine, supplementation is usually safe, and particularly important in cats fed other diets or not yet receiving enteral support. The suggested daily oral taurine dose is 250–500 mg per cat (Marks and Kathrani 2023).

COPPER-ASSOCIATED HEPATITIS

Copper accumulation in hepatocytes can lead to oxidative damage caused by hydroxyl radicals and to chronic inflammation. This disease is often associated with Bedlington terriers, West Highland White terriers, Skye terriers, Labrador retrievers, and Doberman pinchers. A genetic homozygous deletion mutation of a copper transport protein was described in Bedlington terriers, and preliminary data in additional breeds point toward potential additional genetic mutations associated with the disease (Van De Sluis et al. 2002; Pindar and Ramirez 2019). Dogs appear to be less susceptible to hepatic copper accumulation secondary to cholestatic liver disease than cats or people, although this may still occur when dietary copper is high (Webster et al. 2019). Hepatic copper accumulation can occur secondary to cholestasis due to cholangitis in cats.

The NRC 2006 RA for copper in dogs in maintenance is 1.5 mg/1000 kcal, and in cats it is 1.2 mg/1000 kcal (NRC 2006). AAFCO specifies a copper minimum in dogs of 1.83 mg/1000 kcal and 1.25 mg/1000 kcal in adult cats (AAFCO 2024). The association between copper-associated hepatitis and copper amounts or bioavailability in commercial pet food is a hotly debated topic. Several studies documented a gradual increase in copper in canine hepatic liver samples over forty years (Strickland et al. 2018; Johnston et al. 2013). While the cause of this is unclear, banning the use of cupric oxide, a non-bioavailable form of copper, may have contributed to the problem (Center et al. 2021).

Copper quantification and histopathological distribution can help determine if copper restriction and/or chelation therapy is needed (Figure 20.2). The normal amount of hepatic copper in dogs is under 400 ppm dry weight, and in patients suffering from copper-associated hepatitis, it usually exceeds 1000 ppm dry weight. A combination of a low-copper diet with chelation therapy is often needed to reduce high liver copper in patients with primary copper-associated hepatitis.

Dietary copper reduction can be accompanied by zinc supplementation. The amount of copper provided by commercial veterinary therapeutic diets for canine liver disease and feline kidney disease (often utilized in feline liver patients) is listed in Tables 20.1 and 20.2. Alternatively, home-prepared diet recipes can be useful in patients with complex diseases, or if the patient refuses to eat

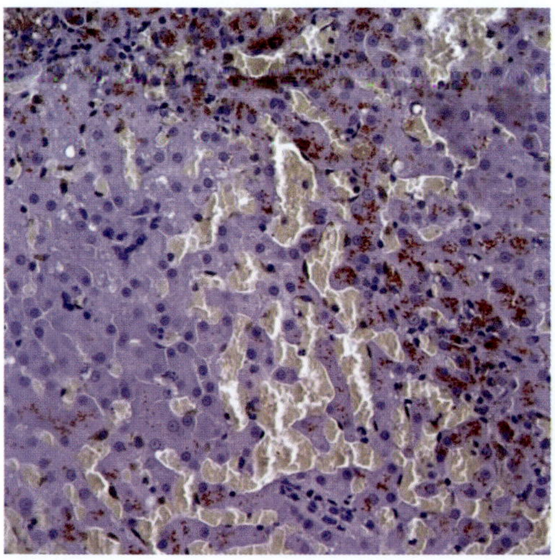

(40× magnification, Credit: Prof. Carmen Fuentealba, Long Island University, Lewyt College of Veterinary Medicine)

FIGURE 20.2 Rubeanic acid–stained hepatic tissue of an adult Doberman Pincher with copper-associated hepatitis

Table 20.2 Nutritional Information for Products Prescribed to Cats with Liver Disease. Information from the USA Product Guides Provided by the Respective Manufacturers for 2024

	AAFCO Cat food nutrient profile (adult) minimums[a]	AAFCO Cat food nutrient profile (growth and reproduction) minimums[a]	Hill's Prescription Diet k/d Early Support Cat Food dry[b]	Hill's Prescription Diet k/d Early Support Cat Food canned[b]	Royal Canin Veterinary Diet Renal Support Early Consult dry cat food[c]	Royal Canin Veterinary Diet Renal Support Early Consult canned cat food[c]	Royal Canin Veterinary Diet Renal Support Liquid[c]	Purina ProPlan Veterinary Diet NF Advanced Care dry cat food[d]	Purina ProPlan Veterinary Diet NF Advanced Care canned cat food[d]
Adequacy statement			Animal feeding tests for adult cats	Animal feeding tests for adult cats	Formulated to meet the nutritional levels for adult cats	Formulated to meet the nutritional levels for adult cats	Intermittent feeding	Intermittent feeding	Intermittent feeding
Partial ingredient list			Chicken, Brewers Rice, Whole Grain Wheat, Corn Protein Meal, Chicken Fat	Water, Chicken, Pork Liver, Carrots, Rice, Pea Protein, Rice Starch	Corn, brewers rice, wheat gluten, corn gluten meal, wheat	Water, pork by-products, chicken liver, brewers rice flour, chicken by-products	Water, maltodextrins, dried milk protein, vegetable oil, soy protein	Brewers rice, tuna, corn, soybean meal, animal fat	Water, meat by-products, chicken hearts, rice, powdered cellulose, pork fat
					Nutrients per 1000 kcal				
Crude Protein (g)	65	75	79	79	73.2	84.1	71.1	69.1	66.9
Crude Fat (g)	22.5	22.5	50	52	36.6	49.5	56.3	41.6	51
Copper (mg)	1.25	3.75 (extruded); 2.1 (canned)	NS	NS	3.9	3.1	2.7	3.8	2.6
Zinc (mg)	18.8	18.8	NS	NS	55.9	53.4	46.7	58.3	32.9
Sodium (g)	0.5	0.5	0.64	0.62	1	0.9	0.9	0.7	0.8
Calcium (g)	1.5	2.5	1.74	1.59	1.8	1.6	1.5	1.7	1.5
Phosphorus (g)	1.25	2	1.26	1.21	1.3	1.2	1.1	0.9	0.9

Note: Veterinary therapeutic products may undergo frequent reformulations. always review the most current product guide before prescribing (Stockman 2025/with permission of Elsevier).

[a]Association of American Feed Control Officials, Inc. 2024 Official Publication, Oxford (IN).

[b]Hill's Pet Nutrition, Topeka, KS.

[c]Royal Canin, Aimargues, France.

[d]Purina ProPlan, St. Louis, MO.

NS = not specified.

a commercial low-copper diet. These diets should be formulated by a board-certified nutritionist (diplomate of the American College of Veterinary Internal Medicine in Nutrition or the European College of Veterinary and Comparative Nutrition) to ensure they are complete and balanced and are indeed reduced in copper.

COMMERCIAL VETERINARY THERAPEUTIC DIETS FOR THE MANAGEMENT OF LIVER DISEASE

While dietary intervention can be helpful in some liver disease patients, others can be maintained on their current diet rather than needing a veterinary therapeutic diet. Therapeutic diets are indicated for hepatic encephalopathy, urate urolithiasis/crystalluria, or copper-associated hepatitis. Few commercial veterinary therapeutic diet options are formulated specifically for canine hepatic disease in dogs, and none are currently available for cats in the USA. Alternatively, diets with vegetarian or vegan protein can be helpful in dogs with hepatic encephalopathy or urate urolithiasis thanks to low purine content and being less encephalopathic. Veterinary renal diets can also be used in patients with hepatic encephalopathy, as they are lower in protein, although they usually include meat protein and internal organs, which are less preferred. Copper content in veterinary hepatic dog diets is usually lower than the NRC 2006 RA (NRC 2006) and the AAFCO minimum (AAFCO 2024). There are no veterinary therapeutic low-copper diets for cats in the USA; however, copper is specified for some veterinary diets, enabling comparisons between possible products (Table 20.2).

Hill's Prescription Diet l/d Liver Care dry and canned dog food (Hill's Pet Nutrition, Topeka, KS) is adequate for adult dogs and growing puppies according to standardized AAFCO feeding protocols. Therefore, this diet can be fed to puppies even though it does not meet the NRC 2006 RA for protein and calcium for growth in dogs, and the adequate intake value of phosphorus for puppies after weaning (NRC 2006). Nutrition-related developmental problems in growing puppies fed this diet are rare; however, a single case report describes angular limb deformity in a Great Dane puppy with a portosystemic shunt (Grant et al. 2021).

Veterinarians often recommend adding additional protein to therapeutic hepatic diets in the form of dairy, whey, egg whites, or chicken breast in hepatic patients who don't require protein reduction. Veterinary hepatic diets have highly digestible and high-quality protein; therefore, it is unlikely that they are protein-deficient, and some underwent feeding trials to substantiate their adequacy. Adding unbalanced food items may cause nutrient dilution and unbalance the overall diet. To prevent this, supplementation of unbalanced foods (human foods, supplements, and treats) should not exceed 10% of the caloric intake. Therefore, high-protein food items added to a veterinary hepatic diet would provide only a small increase in the daily protein amount.

SUMMARY

Hepatic disease is a common clinical presentation with potentially severe consequences. Animals with severe illness require intervention to ensure their requirements are met while addressing their clinical signs and disease complications. Dietary customizations that can benefit the patient's well-being, support liver function, and promote recovery include antioxidants, vitamins, and hepatoprotective supplements. Veterinary hepatic diets for cats are not currently available in the USA; therefore, diets formulated for renal disease or products containing hydrolyzed soy are used instead if protein reduction or a change in protein source is needed, respectively. Veterinary products for canine liver patients are often lower in protein and copper and include non-meat protein. Indications for therapeutic liver diets include copper-associated disease, hepatic encephalopathy, and urate urolithiasis and crystalluria. A diet change to a veterinary hepatic diet is not necessary in other patients.

More data is required to establish protein requirements in small animals with liver disease and the clinical utility of prevalent hepatic supplements.

REFERENCES

Association of American Feed Control Officials, Official Publication. Champaign, IL: AAFCO, 2024.

Cascino, A., Cangiano, C., Fiaccadori, F. et al. (1982). Plasma and cerebrospinal fluid amino acid patterns in hepatic encephalopathy. *Digestive Diseases and Sciences* 27: 828–832.

Carr, A. and Frei, B. (1999). Does vitamin C act as a pro-oxidant under physiological conditions?. *The FASEB Journal* 13: 1007–1024.

Center, S.A. (1996). Acute hepatic injury: hepatic necrosis and fulminant hepatic failure. In: *Strombeck's Small Animal Gastroenterology*, 3e, (ed. W.G. Guilford et al.), 654–704. Philadelphia, Pennsylvania: W. B. Saunders Co.

Center, S.A., Richter, K.P., Twedt, D.C. et al. (2021). Is it time to reconsider current guidelines for copper content in commercial dog foods?. *Journal of the American Veterinary Medical Association* 258: 357–364.

Center, S.A., Warner, K.L., Mccabe, J. et al. (2005). Evaluation of the influence of S-adenosylmethionine on systemic and hepatic effects of prednisolone in dogs. *American Journal of Veterinary Research* 66: 330–341.

Center, S.A. (1998). Nutritional support for dogs and cats with hepatobiliary disease. *The Journal of Nutrition* 128 (12): mS2733–mS2746.

Chan, D.L. (2004). Nutritional requirements of the critically ill patient. *Clinical Techniques in Small Animal Practice* 19: 1–5.

Chan, D.L. (2012). Nutritional requirements in critical illness. In: *Advanced Monitoring and Procedures for Small Animal Emergency and Critical Care* (ed. J.M. Burkitt Creedon and H. Davis), 475–484. New Jersey: Wiley and Sons.

Charlton, M.R. (1996). Protein metabolism and liver disease. *Baillière's Clinical Endocrinology and Metabolism* 10 (4): 617–635.

Filburn, C., Kettenacker, R., and Griffin, D. (2007). Bioavailability of a silybin–phosphatidylcholine complex in dogs. *Journal of Veterinary Pharmacology and Therapeutics* 30: 132–138.

Galler, A., Tran, J., Krammer-Lukas, S. et al. (2013). Blood vitamin levels in dogs with chronic liver disease. *Wien Tierarztl Monatsschr* 100: 133–139.

Gow, A., Marques, A., Yool, D. et al. (2010). Whole blood manganese concentrations in dogs with congenital portosystemic shunts. *Journal of Veterinary Internal Medicine* 24: 90–96.

Grant, C.E., Dodd, S., Abood, S.K. et al. (2021). Commercial diet recommendations and follow-up for a large breed puppy with an intrahepatic portosystemic shunt. *The Canadian Veterinary Journal* 62: 598.

He, H., Mennone, A., Boyer, J.L. et al. (2011). Combination of retinoic acid and ursodeoxycholic acid attenuates liver injury in bile duct–ligated rats and human hepatic cells. *Hepatology* 53: 548–557.

Hishiyama, N., Kayanuma, H., Matsui, T. et al. (2006). Plasma concentration of vitamin C in dogs with a portosystemic shunt. *Canadian Journal of Veterinary Research* 70: 305.

Iqbal, U., Jadeja, R.N., Khara, H.S. et al. (2021). A comprehensive review evaluating the impact of protein source (Vegetarian vs. Meat Based) in hepatic encephalopathy. *Nutrients* 13: 370.

Johnston, A., Center, S., and Mcdonough, S. (2013). Hepatic copper concentrations in Labrador Retrievers with and without chronic hepatitis: 72 cases (1980–2010). *Journal of the American Veterinary Medical Association* 242: 372–380.

Konstantis, G., Pourzitaki, C., Chourdakis, M. et al. (2022). Efficacy of branched chain amino acids supplementation in liver cirrhosis: a systematic review and meta-analysis. *Clinical Nutrition* 41: 1171–1190.

Laflamme, D., Allen, S., and Huber, T. (1993). Apparent dietary protein requirement of dogs with portosystemic shunt. *American Journal of Veterinary Research* 54: 719–723.

Lidbury, J.A., Cook, A.K., and Steiner, J.M. (2016). Hepatic encephalopathy in dogs and cats. *Journal of Veterinary Emergency and Critical Care* 26: 471–487.

Loftus, J.P., Center, S.A., Lucy, J.M. et al. (2017). Characterization of aminoaciduria and hypoaminoacidemia in dogs with hepatocutaneous syndrome. *American Journal of Veterinary Research* 78: 735–744.

Loguercio, C. and Festi, D. (2011). Silybin and the liver: from basic research to clinical practice. *World Journal of Gastroenterology* 17: 2288–2301.

Marks, S.L. and Kathrani, A. (2023). Nutritional management of hepatobiliary diseases. In: *Applied Veterinary Clinical Nutrition*, 2e (ed. A.J. Fascetti, S.J. Delaney, J.A. Larsen et al.), 319–344. NJ: Wiley-Blackwell Publishing.

Mount, M.E., Kim, B.U., and Kass, P.H. (2003). Use of a test for proteins induced by vitamin K absence or antagonism in diagnosis of anticoagulant poisoning in dogs: 325 cases (1987–1997). *Journal of the American Veterinary Medical Association* 222: 194–198.

Nadler, W.H. and Wolfer, J.A. (1929). Hepatogenic hypoglycemia associated with primary liver cell carcinoma. *Archives of Internal Medicine* 44: 700–710.

National Research Council, Ad hoc Committee on Dog and Cat Nutrition. (2006). *Nutrient Requirements of Dogs and Cats*. Washington DC: The National Academies Press.

Pindar, S. and Ramirez, C. (2019). Predicting copper toxicosis: relationship between the ATP7A and ATP7B gene mutations and hepatic copper quantification in dogs. *Human Genetics* 138: 541–546.

Proot, S., Biourge, V., Teske, E. et al. (2009). Soy protein isolate versus meat-based low-protein diet for dogs with congenital portosystemic shunts. *Journal of Veterinary Internal Medicine* 23: 794–800.

Rosen, H.M., Yoshimura, N., Hodgman, J.M. et al. (1977). Plasma amino acid patterns in hepatic encephalopathy of differing etiology. *Gastroenterology* 72: 483–487.

Rothuizen, J. and Van Den Ingh, T. (1982). Arterial and venous ammonia concentrations in the diagnosis of canine hepato-encephalopathy. *Research in Veterinary Science* 33: 17–21.

Stockman, J. (2025). Nutritional management of hepatobiliary diseases in dogs and cats. *Veterinary Clinics of North America: Small Animal Practice* 55 (4): 579–593.

Stokes, C.S., Volmer, D.A., Grünhage, F. et al. (2013). Vitamin D in chronic liver disease. *Liver International* 33: 338–352.

Strickland, J., Buchweitz, J., and Smedley, R. (2018). Hepatic copper concentrations in 546 dogs (1982–2015). *Journal of Veterinary Internal Medicine* 32: 1943–1950.

Tivers, M.S., Handel, I., Gow, A.G. et al. (2014). Hyperammonemia and systemic inflammatory response syndrome predicts presence of hepatic encephalopathy in dogs with congenital portosystemic shunts. *PLoS One* 9: e82303.

Trappoliere, M., Caligiuri, A., Schmid, M. et al. (2009). Silybin, a component of sylimarin, exerts anti-inflammatory and anti-fibrogenic effects on human hepatic stellate cells. *Journal of Hepatology* 50: 1102–1111.

Tsiaousi, E.T., Hatzitolios, A.I., Trygonis, S.K. et al. (2008). Malnutrition in end stage liver disease: recommendations and nutritional support. *Journal of Gastroenterology and Hepatology* 23: 527–533.

Van De Sluis, B., Rothuizen, J., Pearson, P.L. et al. (2002). Identification of a new copper metabolism gene by positional cloning in a purebred dog population. *Human Molecular Genetics* 11: 165–173.

Wallace, O.P., Jablonski, S.A., Thomas, J.S. et al. (2024). Association of time to start of enteral nutrition and outcome in cats with hepatic lipidosis. *Journal of Veterinary Internal Medicine* 8 (6): 3144–3152

Webb, C., Twedt, D., Fettman, M. et al. (2003). S-adenosylmethionine (SAMe) in a feline acetaminophen model of oxidative injury. *Journal of Feline Medicine and Surgery* 5: 69–75.

Webster, C.R.L., Center, S.A., Cullen, J.M. et al. (2019). ACVIM consensus statement on the diagnosis and treatment of chronic hepatitis in dogs. *Journal of Veterinary Internal Medicine* 33: 1173–1200.

Weingarten, M.A. and Sande, A.A. (2015). Acute liver failure in dogs and cats. *Journal of Veterinary Emergency and Critical Care* 25: 455–473.

Wilkinson, D.J., Smeeton, N.J., Castle, P.C. et al. (2011). Absence of neuropsychological impairment in hyperammonaemia in healthy young adults; possible synergism in development of hepatic encephalopathy (HE) symptoms? *Metabolic Brain Disease* 26: 203–212.

Laboratory Assessment of the Exocrine Pancreas

CHAPTER 21

Sue Yee Lim[1] *and Jörg Steiner*[2]

[1] *Department of Small Animal Clinical Sciences, College of Veterinary Medicine & Biomedical Sciences, Texas A&M University College Station, TX, USA*
[2] *Gastrointestinal Laboratory, Department of Small Animal Clinical Sciences, School of Veterinary Medicine and Biomedical Sciences, Texas A&M University, College Station, TX, USA*

KEY POINTS

- Pancreatitis and exocrine pancreatic insufficiency (EPI) are the common disorders of the exocrine pancreas in dogs and cats.
- Quantification of serum pancreatic lipase is useful to aid in the diagnosis of pancreatitis.
- Lipase assays can be broadly divided into immunologic (i.e., pancreatic lipase immunoreactivity [PLI] assays) and catalytic assays (e.g., DGGR-based lipase assays). Some catalytic assays may detect extrapancreatic sources of lipase.
- Measurement of serum trypsin-like immunoreactivity (TLI) is the diagnostic test of choice for the diagnosis of EPI.
- **Pancreatitis:** The diagnostic threshold for the Spec feline pancreas-specific lipase (Spec fPL) assay to be consistent with pancreatitis has changed from ≥ 5.4 µg/L to ≥ 8.8 µg/L in cats.
- **Exocrine pancreatic insufficiency:** The diagnostic threshold for EPI in dogs has changed from ≤ 2.5 µg/L to ≤ 5.5 µg/L.

PANCREATITIS

Pancreatitis is the most common disorder of the exocrine pancreas in both dogs and cats. Antemortem diagnosis is challenging, with histopathology considered the reference standard; however, the development of noninvasive tests, such as serum pancreatic lipase concentration or activity measurements, has made diagnosis easier and increased detection of this disease. Despite their utility, pancreatic lipase results should be interpreted alongside the patient's history, clinical signs, physical examination findings, laboratory data, and diagnostic imaging to reach a comprehensive diagnosis.

SERUM AMYLASE

Amylase is a digestive enzyme produced by the pancreas, but it is not a pancreatic-specific enzyme, as evidenced by measurable serum amylase activities in pancreatectomized dogs (Simpson et al. 1991). Serum amylase activity has a low sensitivity (14–67%) for the diagnosis of pancreatitis in dogs (Steiner et al. 2008; Watson et al. 2010). Additionally, there is no correlation between serum amylase activity and pancreatic histological activity index (Steiner et al. 2008). Consequently, measuring serum amylase activity has a low diagnostic utility for pancreatitis, as a normal level cannot rule out pancreatitis, and an elevated level is often nonspecific. Pancreatic alpha-amylase has been proposed as a more specific amylase biomarker, but further studies are needed to investigate the usefulness of this biomarker (Kim et al. 2024).

Disorders of the Liver, Exocrine Pancreas, and Gastrointestinal Tract in Dogs and Cats, First Edition. Edited by Harry Cridge et al. Published 2026 by John Wiley & Sons, Inc. Companion Website: www.wiley.com/go/cridge/disorders

SERUM PANCREATIC LIPASE

The measurement of serum pancreatic lipase is useful for the diagnosis of pancreatitis in dogs and cats, as this enzyme is specific to pancreatic acinar cells (Steiner et al. 2002). Under physiologic conditions, almost all (~99%) pancreatic lipase is released from the apex of the pancreatic acinar cells into the pancreatic juice for lipid digestion. Less than 1% diffuses through the basolateral aspect of the cells and into the circulation. When the pancreas is inflamed, apical release of pancreatic lipase is blocked, and a large amount is released into the circulation.

There are numerous assays available for measuring serum lipase, and these can be broadly divided into immunologic and catalytic assays. Immunologic assays measure serum pancreatic lipase immunoreactivity (PLI) concentration using antibodies, while catalytic assays measure serum lipase activity. Because there are various types of circulating lipases (e.g., pancreatic, lipoprotein, hepatic), a catalytic assay may measure serum lipase activity without specificity for pancreatic lipase activity, depending on the substrate used and many other factors, such as cofactors or other assay conditions (Lim et al. 2022).

IMMUNOLOGICAL LIPASE ASSAYS

Immunologic assays measuring serum PLI concentration were initially established as a radioimmunoassay (RIA) using polyclonal antibodies against pancreatic lipase and were then commercialized as a send-out enzyme-linked immunosorbent assay (ELISA) test using monoclonal antibodies for dogs and cats (Canine pancreas-specific lipase [Spec cPL] and feline pancreas-specific lipase [Spec fPL], IDEXX Laboratories, Westbrook, Maine). The Spec cPL and fPL assays have been analytically validated and show good linearity, accuracy, and precision and are not affected by lipemia, hemolysis, or icterus (Huth et al. 2010; Wu et al. 2023). Because these immunologic assays specifically measure pancreatic lipase, they are not affected by extrapancreatic lipases. This is demonstrated in dogs with EPI, which have negligible serum PLI concentrations due to substantial loss of exocrine pancreatic function (Steiner et al. 2006). Additionally, the administration of heparin, which induces release of lipoprotein and hepatic lipase into the circulation, did not increase serum PLI concentrations in dogs and cats (Steiner et al. 2006; Lim et al. 2020). The Spec cPL and fPL assays are generally considered to be sensitive and specific for the diagnosis of pancreatitis in dogs and cats (Lim et al. 2022). The reported values vary widely across studies depending on the cut-off values used, criteria used to diagnose pancreatitis (i.e., histopathology, clinical signs, ultrasonographic findings), the type (i.e., acute, chronic), and the severity of pancreatitis (i.e., mild, moderate, severe). A normal serum PLI concentration ($\leq$ 200 µg/L for dogs, $\leq$ 4.4 µg/L for cats) indicates that pancreatitis is highly unlikely, and other diseases causing similar signs to pancreatitis should be investigated. Serum PLI concentrations $\geq$ 400 µg/L or $\geq$ 8.8 µg/L are consistent for pancreatitis in dogs and cats, respectively. The diagnostic threshold (i.e., cut-off value) and reference interval for cats were recently reevaluated due to the relatively low historical cut-off value for pancreatitis ($\geq$ 5.4 µg/L), which may lead to diagnosing cats with subclinical pancreatitis (Wu et al. 2023). The specificity of Spec fPL for the diagnosis of pancreatitis in cats is 98% with the revised cutoff (Wu et al. 2023). Future studies investigating the sensitivity of this higher cutoff are needed.

Physiologically, serum PLI concentrations of kittens are similar to those in adult cats (Stavroulaki et al. 2022). There is no available information regarding aging dogs and cats. In healthy dogs, feeding does not alter serum PLI concentrations, but in a small subset of dogs with GI disease, serum PLI concentration may be altered (Steiner et al. 2014; Melco et al. 2024). Hence, it is ideally recommended to fast for at least eight hours prior to testing, although some clinicians will submit pancreatic lipase testing in non-fasted dogs, particularly when there is concern for decreased compliance/failure to return when a repeat blood draw is recommended. Obesity can affect serum PLI concentration, as 20% of healthy overweight and 50% of diabetic overweight cats had concentrations indicative of pancreatitis, although the presence of subclinical pancreatitis cannot be ruled out (Jørgensen et al. 2025). Several studies have reported increased serum PLI concentrations in patients with renal, gastrointestinal, cardiac, or endocrine diseases; neoplasia; infections; intervertebral disc disease; and portal hypertension (Cridge et al. 2022; Lim et al. 2022). Specifically looking at dogs with renal disease, serum PLI concentrations have been shown to increase in dogs with acute kidney injury needing dialysis, but this may represent concurrent pancreatitis (Takada et al. 2018). In contrast, serum PLI concentrations were not increased in dogs and cats with experimentally induced chronic kidney disease (CKD) (Xenoulis et al. 2021; Steiner et al. 2010a). This is important because the likelihood of developing CKD increases with age in cats with pancreatitis, and gastrointestinal signs associated with chronic uremia may be indistinguishable from those of pancreatitis (Dulude et al. 2024).

In addition to the send-out Spec cPL and fPL assays, rapid semiquantitative immunologic point-of-care tests (POCT; SNAP cPL and fPL, IDEXX Laboratories, Westbrook, Maine) that can be used pet-side are available. The reported sensitivities and specificities of the SNAP cPL test range from 74 to 100% and 59 to 78%, respectively (Mccord et al. 2012; Haworth et al. 2014; Cridge et al. 2018). A study in healthy and sick cats that did not have pancreatitis showed an overall specificity of 89% for the SNAP fPL test (Xenoulis et al. 2023). Because the **SeN**sitivity of the SNAP test is generally higher than its specificity, using the SPin and **SN**out rule, a normal test rules **OUT** the presence of pancreatitis, while an abnormal test suggests the presence of pancreatitis, which should be confirmed with the quantitative Spec PL send-out tests. The recent change in reference interval and diagnostic threshold of the Spec fPL assay (Wu et al. 2023) did not change the overall interpretation of the SNAP fPL test (Schnauss et al. 2019; Xenoulis et al. 2023).

Currently, there are various additional commercial send-out and pet-side immunoassays with different geographical availability. In Europe, in-house ELISAs measuring serum PLI concentrations were established using antibodies (polyclonal for dogs, not reported for cats) against recombinant pancreatic lipase (Laboklin GmbH & Co KG) (Torner et al. 2020; Aupperle-Lellbach et al. 2020). In an initial publication, both assays failed analytical validation (Hofel et al. 2015). While changes to these assays were not disclosed, a subsequent publication by authors from the manufacturing laboratory reported partial analytical validation of these PLI assays to show good repeatability but has dilutional linearities that were outside the standard metrics of an acceptable assay (80–120%) (Aupperle-Lellbach et al. 2020; Torner et al. 2020). The sensitivities of these assays are 75–91% and 57–82%, and the specificities are 63–82% and 74% in dogs and cats, respectively. Future analytical and diagnostic evaluations of these assays are needed before their routine use can be recommended.

Two other POCT immunoassays (VetScan cPL Rapid Test; Zoetis; Vcheck cPL 2.0 and fPL 2.0; Bionote USA Inc.) were developed for the measurement of serum PL concentrations in companion animals. The VetScan cPL measures serum PL concentration using polyclonal antibodies against pancreatic lipase in dogs. A dedicated assay reader provides quantitative results. The manufacturer reports that it is affected by hemolysis, but not icterus, lipemia, or anticoagulants. A partial analytical validation showed that the test had suboptimal linearity, repeatability, and reproducibility (Steiner et al. 2019a). In addition, less than half of the test samples adhered to the manufacturer's specifications of being within 60 μg/L of its measured Spec cPL concentration (Steiner et al. 2019a).

The Vcheck cPL 2.0 and fPL 2.0 assays measure serum PL concentration using antibodies against pancreatic lipase in dogs and cats. Partial analytical validation data are available for the original versions of this assay (Vcheck cPL and fPL) (Cridge et al. 2020; Steiner et al. 2019b; Jakus et al. 2023). A recent publication on the Vcheck cPL assay reported good repeatability and acceptable linearity at low concentrations. However, at high concentrations, linearity was not maintained (Jakus et al. 2023). Additionally, despite using the reference intervals established for Spec cPL and fPL, the results were not comparable, as method comparison showed that the Vcheck cPL consistently measured higher concentrations than the Spec cPL (Bilic-Zulle 2011). As with all new assays, all these assays should undergo robust analytical validation before they can be recommended for use in a clinical setting.

CATALYTIC LIPASE ASSAYS

Catalytic lipase assays measure serum lipase activity by quantifying the rate of the hydrolysis of a substrate by lipase enzymes (Lim et al. 2022). The hydrolytic products usually result in a color change that corresponds with the lipolytic activity of a sample. Serum lipase activity, commonly included in chemistry profiles, uses substrates such as 1,2-diglyceride that measure various types of lipases and can be increased in many extrapancreatic diseases in addition to pancreatitis. A newer substrate (1,2-o-dilauryl-rac-glycero-3-glutaric acid-[6'-methylresorufin] ester or simply DGGR) was introduced as being more pancreatic lipase specific than 1,2-diglyceride (Graca et al. 2005; Panteghini et al. 2001). There is a misconception that all assays utilizing DGGR as a substrate perform equally. However, this is not the case, as there are no two assays using the same substrate that are comparable because, in addition to substrate, assay performance depends on specific cofactors, such as bile acids and colipase, assay conditions, and the analyzer. This explains why the various studies on sensitivity and specificity of DGGR-based lipase assays demonstrate limited agreement. Every lipase activity assay, even if using the same substrate, must undergo individual analytical as well as clinical validation before routine clinical use. Some DGGR-based assays have been shown to have good dilutional linearity, repeatability, and reproducibility, while others have not been tested (Graca et al. 2005; Goodband et al. 2018). The assay is variably affected by hemolysis and lipemia but is unaffected by sample freezing, glycerol, and anticoagulants (Goodband et al. 2018; Graca et al. 2005). Some DGGR-based lipase assays are affected by lipoprotein and/or hepatic lipase as shown by heparin induction or by pancreatic lipase-related protein 2, a lipase synthesized and secreted by many different tissues, including the exocrine pancreas and other non-pancreatic organs (Graca et al. 2005; Lim et al. 2020). The sensitivities and specificities range widely from 41 to 91 and 64 to 100%, respectively, in dogs and 37–67% and 63–100%, respectively, in cats (Cridge et al. 2018; Hope et al. 2021; Oppliger et al. 2013; Oppliger et al. 2016). Some studies have concluded that the DGGR-based lipase assay can be used interchangeably with the Spec PL assays due to its high correlation (Spearman, Pearson) and/or agreement (Kappa's Cohen), but it must be cautioned that these analyses are not suitable for comparison of laboratory methods that measure the same analyte but for comparison of subjective clinical findings (Oppliger et al. 2013; Goodband et al. 2018; Bilic-Zulle 2011).

In a study of critically ill dogs with elevated DGGR-lipase activity >3x upper reference interval (URI), only one-third had a clinical diagnosis of acute pancreatitis (Prummer et al. 2020). Apart from pancreatitis, other conditions associated with elevated DGGR-lipase activities are renal, endocrine, or immune-mediated diseases and upper respiratory obstruction (Prummer et al. 2020; Quigley et al. 2001; Linari et al. 2021). Specifically, looking at dogs with acute kidney injury, more than half developed elevated DGGR-lipase activity (>3x URI) during hospitalization, but only one-third had a clinical and sonographic diagnosis of acute pancreatitis. Again, this hyperlipasemia could be due to the effect of extrapancreatic lipases on the DGGR-based lipase assay or the presence of concurrent pancreatitis that was not evident on ultrasound (Bendeler et al. 2023).

Until recently, the DGGR-based lipase assay is only available as a send-out laboratory test (Precision PSL, Antech). A new DGGR-based lipase assay (Catalyst Pancreatic Lipase Test, IDEXX Laboratories, Westbrook, Maine) that is compatible with commonly used in-house chemical analyzers is currently available. Data provided by the manufacturer shows this DGGR-based lipase activity assay to be the first DGGR-based assay that is specific for the measurement for pancreatic lipase and thus the diagnosis of pancreatitis (JMS, personal communication). The assay is currently undergoing external validation.

TRYPSIN AND TRYPSINOGEN

Briefly, trypsinogen is synthesized exclusively by the pancreatic acinar cells and is activated to trypsin in the duodenum. Trypsin may escape into the circulation during pancreatitis. The trypsin-like immunoreactivity (TLI) assay measures concentrations of trypsinogen and trypsin in serum. Serum TLI concentration has low sensitivities of 30–40% for the diagnosis of pancreatitis in dogs and cats (Steiner et al. 2008; Gerhardt et al. 2001). Therefore, its usefulness for the diagnosis of pancreatitis is limited. In dogs with experimentally induced pancreatitis, serum TLI concentrations increases but declines earlier when compared to serum pancreatic lipase activity. This might be due to its shorter half-life and explains why serum TLI concentration is only elevated in a small subset of patients presenting with clinical signs of pancreatitis. Additionally, there is no correlation between serum TLI concentration with the histopathological severity of pancreatitis in dogs (Steiner et al. 2008). Serum TLI concentration could also be increased in asymptomatic dogs and cats for unknown reasons. In conclusion, serum TLI concentration is not a suitable marker for pancreatitis in either dogs or cats suspected of having pancreatitis.

EXOCRINE PANCREATIC INSUFFICIENCY

Exocrine pancreatic insufficiency (EPI) is the second most common exocrine pancreatic disorder in dogs and cats. It is caused by deficiency in exocrine pancreatic enzymes resulting in malabsorption of nutrients. Clinical signs of EPI may include steatorrhea, weight loss, flatulence, diarrhea, and abdominal pain. Clinical signs in cats are more subtle and may be demonstrated by weight loss alone. Early diagnosis may be challenging, as clinical signs may not manifest until >90% of exocrine pancreatic function has been destroyed. Serum TLI concentration is considered the reference standard for diagnosis of EPI in both dogs and cats.

TRYPSIN AND TRYPSINOGEN

Trypsinogen (a zymogen) is synthesized exclusively by the pancreatic acinar cells and is activated to trypsin in the duodenum. The serum concentration of these enzymes (trypsinogen and trypsin) can be measured using a TLI assay. Although serum PLI and TLI concentrations are both reduced in dogs with EPI, there remains a small overlap for serum PLI concentration between healthy dogs and dogs with EPI (Steiner et al. 2006). Conversely, serum TLI concentration is reduced in dogs and cats with experimental or naturally occurring EPI; with no overlap between healthy dogs and EPI dogs (Simpson et al. 1991; Williams and Batt 1988; Steiner and Williams 2000; Williams and Batt 1983). Therefore, measuring serum TLI concentration serves as an indirect assessment of the pancreatic enzyme secretory capacity and remains as the gold standard for diagnosing EPI in dogs and cats, due to its high sensitivity and specificity (Williams and Batt 1988; Steiner and Williams 2000).

Serum canine TLI (cTLI) and feline TLI (fTLI) concentrations were initially measured with two different RIA assays using rabbit anti-trypsin polyclonal antibodies (Steiner et al. 1996; Steiner and Williams 2000; Williams and Batt 1983). Currently, serum cTLI is measured using a commercial solid phase, enzyme-labeled, chemiluminescent immunometric assay (Immulite 2000 analyzer, Siemens Healthineers) that is widely used by veterinary diagnostic laboratories worldwide. This assay uses mouse anti-TLI monoclonal antibodies. The fTLI RIA assay is only available through the Texas A&M Gastrointestinal Laboratory. An in-house ELISA for fTLI was established in Europe (Laboklin GmbH & Co KG) and partially analytically validated (Torner et al. 2021).

Feeding does not cause clinically important increases in serum TLI concentrations in healthy animals (Williams and Batt 1988; Steiner and Williams 1999; Saver et al. 2021). However, the effect of feeding on serum TLI concentrations can be influenced by gastrointestinal disease in dogs (Melco et al. 2024). Therefore, withholding food for at least eight hours (or overnight) is currently recommended to standardize testing procedures. Serum TLI concentrations of kittens are similar to those in adult cats (Stavroulaki et al. 2022). There is no available information regarding puppies or aging dogs and cats. A drug history should also be obtained, as serum TLI concentration can increase with immunosuppressive doses of dexamethasone (Lucena et al. 1999). Serum TLI concentration is not affected by oral pancreatic extracts. As such, there is no need to withdraw pancreatic enzyme replacement therapy (PERT) prior to testing. Similarly, response to treatment (including PERT) is assessed by clinical signs, as serum TLI concentration is not expected to improve with adequate PERT.

The interpretation of any test result should be done in relation to the clinical presentation of the patient (Figure 21.1). A low serum TLI concentration (< 5.5 μg/L in dogs, < 8 μg/L in cats) with consistent clinical signs is diagnostic for EPI. Recently, the cTLI cut-off value was reevaluated after dogs showing clinical signs consistent with EPI were identified but did not meet the previous stringent cutoff of < 2.5 μg/L. Based on a recent retrospective study, this cut-off value was adjusted to < 5.5 μg/L, resulting in a sensitivity of 95.7% and specificity of 83% for the diagnosis of EPI in dogs (Wu 2024). This shift could be attributed to better recognition and earlier testing for EPI in dogs (Figure 21.2) and cats. Some dogs and cats have an incidentally elevated serum TLI concentration. The clinical significance of this elevation is unknown in an asymptomatic dog or cat. Elevated TLI may be associated with pancreatitis or renal insufficiency. Serum TLI concentrations may be increased in 30–40% of dogs and cats with pancreatitis as trypsin from residual pancreatic acinar cells escapes into the circulation (Steiner et al. 2008; Gerhardt et al. 2001). Therefore, concurrent pancreatitis in a patient with EPI may cause a false negative test result (Lankisch 1982; Watson et al. 2010). An elevated serum TLI concentration can

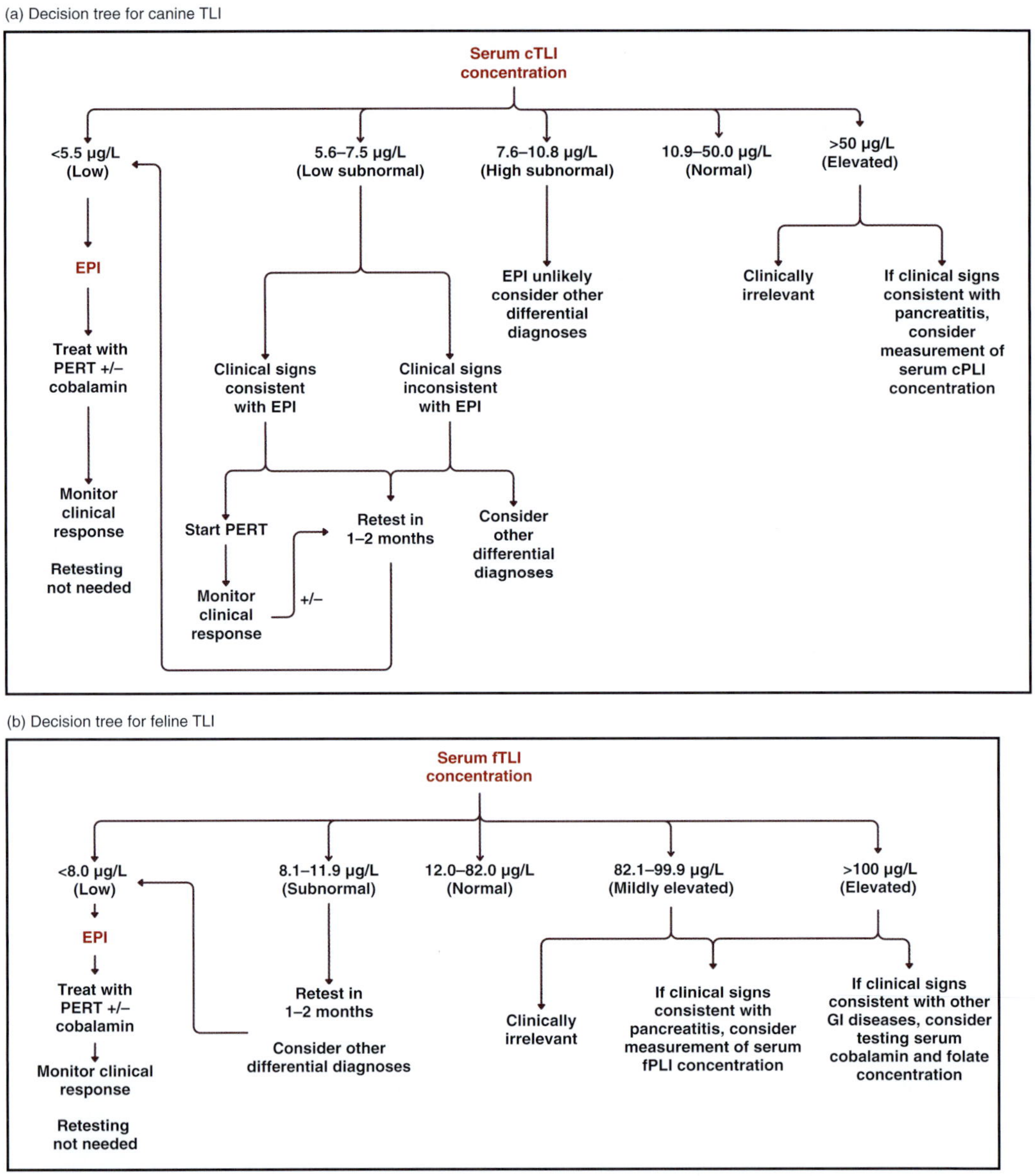

FIGURE 21.1 (a) Decision tree for canine trypsin-like immunoreactivity (cTLI), exocrine pancreatic insufficiency (EPI); pancreatic enzyme replacement therapy (PEI); canine pancreatic lipase immunoreactivity (cPLI). (b) Decision tree for feline trypsin-like immunoreactivity (fTLI), exocrine pancreatic insufficiency (EPI); pancreatic enzyme replacement therapy (PERT); feline pancreatic lipase immunoreactivity (fPLI)

be confirmed with a Spec PL, as this test is more reliable for diagnosing pancreatitis. Experimentally, serum TLI concentration has been shown to increase in 1 of 3 dogs with acute kidney injury and 2 of 3 cats with CKD (Hulsebosch et al. 2016; Xenoulis et al. 2021). Therefore, the diagnosis of EPI in dogs and cats with concurrent renal insufficiency may be missed. Serum TLI concentrations are not increased in dogs with diabetes (Hamilton et al. 2021).

In patients with clinical signs consistent with EPI but with a discordant serum TLI concentration (Figures 21.2a and b), it is important to consider the presence of concurrent diseases (e.g., pancreatitis, renal insufficiency) or medications (e.g., dexamethasone) that might cause a false negative test result. If no confounding factors are present and the patient has a serum TLI concentration at the lower end of the subnormal range, a therapeutic trial with pancreatic extracts can be started and the patient is monitored closely for clinical improvement. Repeating a serum TLI concentration in 1–2 months after initial blood sampling can be helpful to determine if serum TLI concentration has further decreased, supporting a diagnosis of EPI.

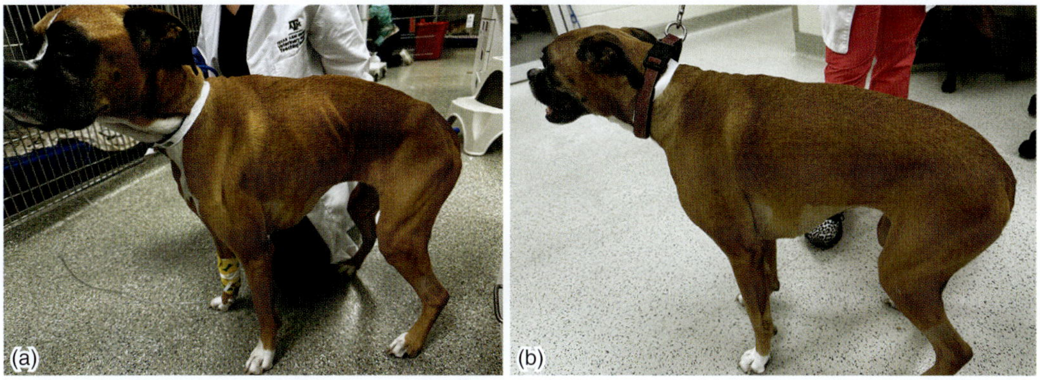

FIGURE 21.2 (a) A 7-year-old female spayed boxer dog presenting with severe rapid weight loss (7 kg in 6 months) despite consuming 12 times the daily caloric requirements. Serum cTLI concentration was 7.1 μg/L (low subnormal) at presentation. (b) This patient was started on pancreatic enzyme replacement therapy, probiotics, and cobalamin supplementation and gained 4 kg in 3 weeks. Incidentally, the pancreas of this patient could not be definitively identified on abdominal computed tomography (obtained at the time of initial presentation for other reasons)

FECAL ELASTASE

Fecal elastase-1 is currently the test of choice for the diagnosis of EPI in people (Nelson 2024). It measures pancreatic elastase-1 in feces. This enzyme is produced in pancreatic acinar cells and is secreted with pancreatic juice into the intestines. It is minimally degraded by endogenous or bacterial proteases, concentrates as it passes through the intestines (colonic concentration is 20× of duodenal concentration) (Spillmann 2001), and its fecal concentration correlates somewhat with pancreatic output. However, it has been shown that this test has low specificity, leading to an overdiagnosis of EPI in certain patients. This was demonstrated in a recent meta-analysis, which found that in groups of patients with a low probability of having EPI (such as those with irritable bowel syndrome), fecal elastase-1 was falsely positive in 1 out of 10 people (Vanga et al. 2018). Additionally, 2 out of 10 healthy individuals over the age of 60, without gastrointestinal disease or diabetes mellitus, were diagnosed with EPI based on low fecal elastase-1 concentrations (Herzig et al. 2011). A canine-specific fecal elastase-1 ELISA was established and analytically validated (Spillmann 2001). However, similar to the test in people, this assay has a low positive predictive value of 50–60% (Spillmann 2001). The high rate of false positives has also been demonstrated in another study, which documented that 1 in 4 dogs with normal serum cTLI concentrations had a low fecal elastase-1 (Steiner et al. 2010b). The qualitative point-of-care test (Pancreas Elastase 1 Quick™ Canine rapid test, ScheBo Biotech AG, Giessen, Germany) is commercially available and is positive when fecal elastase-1 < 10 μg/g feces, but the POCT version has not been analytically validated in the primary literature. Thus, it is recommended that a diagnosis of EPI based on the measurement of fecal elastase-1 is confirmed by measurement of serum cTLI concentration before initiating therapy.

OTHERS

Other tests have been used historically for the diagnosis of EPI, including fat absorption, fecal proteolytic activity, and chymotrypsin activity using oral N-benzoyl-L-tyrosyl p-aminobenzoic acid (BT-PABA). These cumbersome and less sensitive tests have been replaced largely by the availability of highly species-specific TLI assays. This has improved the diagnostic capabilities of EPI, leading to its prompt treatment and reversal of clinical signs. However, for exotic species for which there is no TLI assay, fecal proteolytic activity on a casein agar is a reasonable alternative. Lastly, cobalamin and folate should be measured in patients with suspected EPI, as many dogs and cats with EPI are hypocobalaminemic (Xenoulis et al. 2016; Chang et al. 2022).

REFERENCES

Aupperle-Lellbach, H., Torner, K., Staudacher, M. et al. (2020). Histopathological findings and canine pancreatic lipase immunoreactivity in normal dogs and dogs with inflammatory and neoplastic diseases of the pancreas. *Journal of Veterinary Internal Medicine* 34 (3): 1127–1134. https://doi.org/10.1111/jvim.15779.

Bendeler, K.S., Howard, J., Francey, T. et al. (2023). Hyperlipasemia in dogs with acute kidney injury treated with and without hemodialysis. *Journal of Veterinary Internal Medicine* 37 (3): 1067–1076. https://doi.org/10.1111/jvim.16693.

Bilic-Zulle, L. (2011). Comparison of methods: Passing and Bablok regression. *Biochemia Medica* 21 (1): 49–52. https://doi.org/10.11613/bm.2011.010.

Chang, C.H., Lidbury, J.A., Suchodolski, J.S. et al. (2022). Effect of oral or injectable supplementation with cobalamin in dogs with hypocobalaminemia caused by chronic enteropathy or exocrine pancreatic insufficiency. *Journal of Veterinary Internal Medicine* 36 (5): 1607–1621. https://doi.org/10.1111/jvim.16528.

Cridge, H., Lim, S.Y., Algül, H. et al. (2022). New insights into the etiology, risk factors, and pathogenesis of pancreatitis in dogs: potential impacts on clinical practice. *Journal of Veterinary Internal Medicine* 36 (3): 847–864. https://doi.org/10.1111/jvim.16437.

Cridge, H., Mackin, A.J., Lidbury, J.A. et al. (2020). Comparative repeatability of pancreatic lipase assays in the commercial and in-house laboratory environments. *Journal of Veterinary Internal Medicine* 34 (3): 1150–1156. https://doi.org/10.1111/jvim.15763.

Cridge, H., Macleod, A.G., Pachtinger, G.E. et al. (2018). Evaluation of SNAP cPL, Spec cPL, VetScan cPL Rapid Test, and Precision PSL assays for the diagnosis of clinical pancreatitis in dogs. *Journal of Veterinary Internal Medicine* 32 (2): 658–664. https://doi.org/10.1111/jvim.15039.

Dulude, M.D., Ford, S.L., and Lynch, H. (2024). Association between pancreatitis and chronic kidney disease in cats: a retrospective review of 154 cats presented to a specialty hospital between October 1, 2017, and October 1, 2022. *Journal of the American Veterinary Medical Association* 262 (5): 640–648. https://doi.org/10.2460/javma.23.11.0615.

Gerhardt, A., Steiner, J.M., Williams, D.A. et al. (2001). Comparison of the sensitivity of different diagnostic tests for pancreatitis in cats. *Journal of Veterinary Internal Medicine* 15 (4): 329–333.

Goodband, E.L., Serrano, G., Constantino-Casas, F. et al. (2018). Validation of a commercial 1,2-o-dilauryl-rac-glycero glutaric acid-(6'-methylresorufin) ester lipase assay for diagnosis of canine pancreatitis. *Veterinary Record Open* 5 (1): e000270. https://doi.org/10.1136/vetreco-2017-000270.

Graca, R., Messick, J., Mccullough, S. et al. (2005). Validation and diagnostic efficacy of a lipase assay using the substrate 1,2-o-dilauryl-rac-glycero glutaric acid-(6' methyl resorufin)-ester for the diagnosis of acute pancreatitis in dogs. *Veterinary Clinical Pathology* 34 (1): 39–43. https://doi.org/10.1111/j.1939-165X.2005.tb00007.x.

Hamilton, K., O'kell, A.L., and Gilor, C. (2021). Serum trypsin-like immunoreactivity in dogs with diabetes mellitus. *Journal of Veterinary Internal Medicine* 35 (4): 1713–1719. https://doi.org/10.1111/jvim.16208.

Haworth, M.D., Hosgood, G., Swindells, K.L. et al. (2014). Diagnostic accuracy of the SNAP and Spec canine pancreatic lipase tests for pancreatitis in dogs presenting with clinical signs of acute abdominal disease. *Journal of Veterinary Emergency and Critical Care* 24 (2): 135–143. https://doi.org/10.1111/vec.12158.

Herzig, K.H., Purhonen, A.K., Rasanen, K.M. et al. (2011). Fecal pancreatic elastase-1 levels in older individuals without known gastrointestinal diseases or diabetes mellitus. *BMC Geriatrics* 11: 4. https://doi.org/10.1186/1471-2318-11-4.

Hofel, E., Rieker, T., Suchodolski, J.S. et al. (2015). Measurement of canine and feline pancreatic lipase immunoreactivity - analytical comparison of new commercial assays with established assays. *Tierärztliche Praxis Ausgabe K: Kleintiere / Heimtiere* 43 (6): 399–408. https://doi.org/10.15654/TPK-140821.

Hope, A., Bailen, E.L., Shiel, R.E. et al. (2021). Retrospective study evaluation of DGGR lipase for diagnosis, agreement with pancreatic lipase and prognosis in dogs with suspected acute pancreatitis. *Journal of Small Animal Practice* 62 (12): 1092–1100. https://doi.org/10.1111/jsap.13379.

Hulsebosch, S.E., Palm, C.A., Segev, G. et al. (2016). Evaluation of canine pancreas-specific lipase activity, lipase activity, and trypsin-like immunoreactivity in an experimental model of acute kidney injury in dogs. *Journal of Veterinary Internal Medicine* 30 (1): 192–199. https://doi.org/10.1111/jvim.13806.

Huth, S.P., Relford, R., Steiner, J.M. et al. (2010). Analytical validation of an ELISA for measurement of canine pancreas-specific lipase. *Veterinary Clinical Pathology* 39 (3): 346–353. https://doi.org/10.1111/j.1939-165X.2010.00245.x.

Jakus, P., Strage, E., Abrahamsson, J. et al. (2023). Partial validation of the Vcheck canine pancreatic lipase assay. *Veterinary Clinical Pathology* 52 (2): 271–275. https://doi.org/10.1111/vcp.13207.

Jørgensen, F.K., Bjornvad, C.R., Krabbe, B. et al. (2025). Evaluation of laboratory findings indicating pancreatitis in healthy lean, obese, and diabetic cats. *Journal of Veterinary Internal Medicine* 39 (1): e17236. https://doi.org/10.1111/jvim.17236.

Kim, K., Kim, H.H., Joo, J.B. et al. (2024). Evaluation of the clinical usefulness of pancreatic alpha amylase as a novel biomarker in dogs with acute pancreatitis: a pilot study. *Veterinary Quarterly* 44 (1): 1–7. https://doi.org/10.1080/01652176.2024.2326007.

Lankisch, P.G. (1982). Exocrine pancreatic function tests. *Gut* 23 (9): 777–798. https://doi.org/10.1136/gut.23.9.777.

Lim, S.Y., Steiner, J.M., and Cridge, H. (2022). Understanding lipase assays in the diagnosis of pancreatitis in veterinary medicine. *Journal of the American Veterinary Medical Association* 260 (11): 1249–1258. https://doi.org/10.2460/javma.22.03.0144.

Lim, S.Y., Xenoulis, P.G., Stavroulaki, E.M. et al. (2020). The 1,2-o-dilauryl-rac-glycero-3-glutaric acid-(6'-methylresorufin) ester (DGGR) lipase assay in cats and dogs is not specific for pancreatic lipase. *Veterinary Clinical Pathology* 49 (4): 607–613. https://doi.org/10.1111/vcp.12906.

Linari, G., Dondi, F., Segatore, S. et al. (2021). Evaluation of 1,2-O-dilauryl-rac-glycero glutaric acid-(6'-methylresorufin) ester (DGGR) and 1,2-diglyceride lipase assays in dogs with naturally occurring hypercortisolism. *Journal of Veterinary Diagnostic Investigation* 33 (5): 817–824. https://doi.org/10.1177/10406387211021345

Lucena, R., Ginel, P.J., Novales, M. et al. (1999). Effects of dexamethasone administration on serum trypsin-like immunoreactivity in healthy dogs. *American Journal of Veterinary Research* 60 (11): 1357–1359.

Mccord, K., Morley, P.S., Armstrong, J. et al. (2012). A multi-institutional study evaluating the diagnostic utility of the spec cPL and SNAP(R) cPL in clinical acute pancreatitis in 84 dogs. *Journal of Veterinary Internal Medicine* 26 (4): 888–896. https://doi.org/10.1111/j.1939-1676.2012.00951.x.

Melco, A., Pritchard, J.C., Hetzel, S.J. et al. (2024). The effect of feeding on serum concentrations of cobalamin, folate, trypsin-like immunoreactivity, and pancreatic lipase immunoreactivity in dogs with signs of chronic gastrointestinal disease. *Journal of Veterinary Internal Medicine* 38 (3): 1465–1474. https://doi.org/10.1111/jvim.17064.

Nelson, H.A. (2024). Preanalytical and analytical factors affecting elastase quantitation in stool. *Clinical Biochemistry* 131–132: 110811. https://doi.org/10.1016/j.clinbiochem.2024.110811.

Oppliger, S., Hartnack, S., Riond, B. et al. (2013). Agreement of the serum Spec fPL and 1,2-o-dilauryl-rac-glycero-3-glutaric acid-(6'-methylresorufin) ester lipase assay for the determination of serum lipase in cats with suspicion of pancreatitis. *Journal of Veterinary Internal Medicine* 27 (5): 1077–1082. https://doi.org/10.1111/jvim.12150.

Oppliger, S., Hilbe, M., Hartnack, S. et al. (2016). Comparison of serum Spec fPL(™) and 1,2-o-dilauryl-rac-glycero-3-glutaric acid-(6'-methylresorufin) ester assay in 60 cats using standardized assessment of pancreatic histology. *Journal of Veterinary Internal Medicine* 30 (3): 764–770. https://doi.org/10.1111/jvim.13924.

Panteghini, M., Bonora, R., and Pagani, F. (2001). Measurement of pancreatic lipase activity in serum by a kinetic colorimetric assay using a new chromogenic substrate. *Annals of Clinical Biochemistry* 38 (4): 365–370. https://doi.org/10.1258/0004563011900876.

Prummer, J.K., Howard, J., Grandt, L.M. et al. (2020). Hyperlipasemia in critically ill dogs with and without acute pancreatitis: Prevalence, underlying diseases, predictors, and outcome. *Journal of Veterinary Internal Medicine* 34 (6): 2319–2329. https://doi.org/10.1111/jvim.15902.

Quigley, K.A., Jackson, M.L., and Haines, D.M. (2001). Hyperlipasemia in 6 dogs with pancreatic or hepatic neoplasia: evidence for tumor lipase production. *Veterinary Clinical Pathology* 30 (3): 114–120. https://doi.org/10.1111/j.1939-165x.2001.tb00418.x.

Saver, A.T., Steiner, J.M., Hetzel, S.J. et al. (2021). Effect of withholding food on serum concentrations of cobalamin, folate, trypsin-like immunoreactivity, and pancreatic lipase immunoreactivity in healthy dogs. *American Journal of Veterinary Research* 82 (5): 367–373. https://doi.org/10.2460/ajvr.82.5.367.

Schnauss, F., Hanisch, F., and Burgener, I.A. (2019). Diagnosis of feline pancreatitis with SNAP fPL and Spec fPL. *Journal of Feline Medicine and Surgery* 21 (8): 700–707. https://doi.org/10.1177/1098612X18796624.

Simpson, K.W., Simpson, J.W., Lake, S. et al. (1991). Effect of pancreatectomy on plasma activities of amylase, isoamylase, lipase and trypsin-like immunoreactivity in dogs. *Research in Veterinary Science* 51 (1): 78–82. https://doi.org/10.1016/0034-5288(91)90035-m.

Spillmann, T. (2001). An immunoassay for canine pancreatic elastase 1 as an indicator for exocrine pancreatic insufficiency in dogs. *Journal of Veterinary Diagnostic Investigation* 13 (6): 468–474. https://doi.org/10.1177/104063870101300603.

Stavroulaki, E.M., Kokkinaki, K.C.G., Saridomichelakis, M.N. et al. (2022). Serial measurement of serum pancreatic lipase immunoreactivity, feline trypsin-like immunoreactivity, and cobalamin concentrations in kittens. *Veterinary Sciences* 9 (9): 469. https://doi.org/10.3390/vetsci9090469.

Steiner, J.M., Berridge, B.R., Wojcieszyn, J. et al. (2002). Cellular immunolocalization of gastric and pancreatic lipase in various tissues obtained from dogs. *American Journal of Veterinary Research* 63 (5): 722–727. https://doi.org/10.2460/ajvr.2002.63.722.

Steiner, J.M., Guadiano, P., Gomez, R.R. et al. (2019a). Partial analytical validation of the VetScan cPL rapid test. *Veterinary Clinical Pathology* 48 (4): 683–690. https://doi.org/10.1111/vcp.12796.

Steiner, J.M., Liu, J., Drexel, J. et al. (2019b). Partial analytical validation of a new in-clinic CPLI test (VCheck cPL). In: *Proceedings of the 44th World Small Animal Veterinary Association Congress*, 681. Toronto, Canada (16–19 July 2019): WSAVA.

Steiner, J.M., Medinger, T.L., and Williams, D.A. (1996). Development and validation of a radioimmunoassay for feline trypsin-like immunoreactivity. *American Journal of Veterinary Research* 57 (10): 1417–1420.

Steiner, J.M., Newman, S., Xenoulis, P. et al. (2008). Sensitivity of serum markers for pancreatitis in dogs with macroscopic evidence of pancreatitis. *Veterinary Therapeutics: Research in Applied Veterinary Medicine*, 9 (4): 263–273.

Steiner, J.M., Finco, D.R., and Williams, D.A. (2010a). Serum lipase activity and canine pancreatic lipase immunoreactivity (cPLI) concentration in dogs with experimentally induced chronic renal failure. *Veterinary Research* 3 (3): 58–63.

Steiner, J.M., Rehfeld, J.F., and Pantchev, N. (2010b). Evaluation of fecal elastase and serum cholecystokinin in dogs with a false positive fecal elastase test. *Journal of Veterinary Internal Medicine* 24 (3): 643–646. https://doi.org/10.1111/j.1939-1676.2010.0489.x.

Steiner, J.M., Ruaux, C.G., and Williams, D.A. (2014). Influence of feeding on serum canine pancreatic lipase immunoreactivity concentrations. *Veterinary medicine (Auckland, N.Z.)* 5: 139–142. https://doi.org/10.2147/VMRR.S69576.

Steiner, J.M., Rutz, G.M., and Williams, D.A. (2006). Serum lipase activities and pancreatic lipase immunoreactivity concentrations in dogs with exocrine pancreatic insufficiency. *American Journal of Veterinary Research* 67 (1): 84–87. https://doi.org/10.2460/ajvr.67.1.84.

Steiner, J.M. and Williams, D.A. (1999). Influence of feeding on serum feline trypsin-like immunoreactivity. *American Journal of Veterinary Research* 60 (7): 895–897.

Steiner, J.M. and Williams, D.A. (2000). Serum feline trypsin-like immunoreactivity in cats with exocrine pancreatic insufficiency. *Journal of Veterinary Internal Medicine* 14 (6): 627–629. https://doi.org/10.1892/0891-6640(2000)014<0627:sftiic>2.3.co;2.

Takada, K., Palm, C.A., Epstein, S.E. et al. (2018). Assessment of canine pancreas-specific lipase and outcomes in dogs with hemodialysis-dependent acute kidney injury. *Journal of Veterinary Internal Medicine* 32 (2): 722–726. https://doi.org/10.1111/jvim.15047.

Torner, K., Grassinger, J.M., Weber, C.N. et al. (2021). Signalment and clinical data of cats with exocrine pancreatic insufficiency diagnosed using feline trypsin-like immunoreactivity in routine diagnostics. *Veterinary Sciences* 8 (8): 155. https://doi.org/10.3390/vetsci8080155.

Torner, K., Staudacher, M., Tress, U. et al. (2020). Histopathology and feline pancreatic lipase immunoreactivity in inflammatory, hyperplastic and neoplastic pancreatic diseases in cats. *Journal of Comparative Pathology* 174: 63–72. https://doi.org/10.1016/j.jcpa.2019.10.195.

Vanga, R.R., Tansel, A., Sidiq, S. et al. (2018). Diagnostic performance of measurement of fecal elastase-1 in detection of exocrine pancreatic insufficiency: systematic review and meta-analysis. *Clinical Gastroenterology and Hepatology* 16 (8): 1220–1228 e4. https://doi.org/10.1016/j.cgh.2018.01.027.

Watson, P.J., Archer, J., Roulois, A.J. et al. (2010). Observational study of 14 cases of chronic pancreatitis in dogs. *Veterinary Record* 167 (25): 968–976. https://doi.org/10.1136/vr.c4912.

Williams, D.A. and Batt, R.M. (1983). Diagnosis of canine exocrine pancreatic insufficiency by the assay of serum trypsin-like immunoreactivity. *Journal of Small Animal Practice* 24 (9): 583–588. https://doi.org/10.1111/j.1748-5827.1983.tb00404.x.

Williams, D.A. and Batt, R.M. (1988). Sensitivity and specificity of radioimmunoassay of serum trypsin-like immunoreactivity for the diagnosis of canine exocrine pancreatic insufficiency. *Journal of the American Veterinary Medical Association* 192 (2): 195–201.

Wu, Y., Chuang, W.H., Lidbury, J.A. et al. (2024). Re-evaluation of the reference interval and cut-off value for canine trypsin-like immunoreactivity assay. In: *Research Communications of the 34th ECVIM-CA Congress, ECVIM 2024*, 3584. Lyon, France (5–7 September 2024).

Wu, Y.A., Steiner, J.M., Huisinga, E. et al. (2023). Analytical validation of an ELISA for the measurement of feline pancreas-specific lipase and re-evaluation of the reference interval and decision threshold for diagnosing pancreatitis. *Veterinary Clinical Pathology* 52 (3): 482–492. https://doi.org/10.1111/vcp.13283.

Xenoulis, P.G., Moraiti, K.T., Finco D.R. et al. (2021). Serum feline pancreatic lipase immunoreactivity and trypsin-like immunoreactivity concentrations in cats with experimentally induced chronic kidney disease. *Journal of Veterinary Internal Medicine* 35 (6): 2821–2827. https://doi.org/10.1111/jvim.16296.

Xenoulis, P.G., Moraiti, K.T., Spanou, V.M. et al. (2023). Specificity of a pancreatic lipase point-of-care test and agreement with pancreatic lipase immunoreactivity in cats without clinical evidence of pancreatitis. *Journal of Feline Medicine and Surgery* 25 (7): https://doi.org/10.1177/1098612X231183299.

Xenoulis, P.G., Zoran, D.L., Fosgate, G.T. et al. (2016). Feline exocrine pancreatic insufficiency: a retrospective study of 150 cases. *Journal of Veterinary Internal Medicine* 30 (6): 1790–1797. https://doi.org/10.1111/jvim.14560.

Diagnostic Imaging of the Exocrine Pancreas

CHAPTER 22

Angela Marolf

Department of Veterinary Clinical Sciences, College of Veterinary Medicine, The Ohio State University, Columbus, OH, USA

KEY POINTS

- Ultrasound changes associated with pancreatitis include enlargement, hypoechoic parenchyma, surrounding hyperechoic mesentery/fat, with or without free fluid.
- Ultrasound changes associated with pancreatic neoplasia can overlap with pancreatitis but include a hypoechoic to mixed echoic nodule/mass in any location of the pancreas.
- Computed tomography (CT) utilizes intravenous contrast to evaluate the pancreatic parenchyma and eliminates superimposition of adjacent structures.
- CT imaging features of acute pancreatitis include pancreatic enlargement, changes in pancreatic parenchymal contrast enhancement, peripancreatic/mesenteric inflammation, fluid, and portal vein thrombosis (PVT). CT has an enhanced ability to detect PVT relative to ultrasound, which may alter therapeutic management.

INTRODUCTION

The pancreas is in the cranial and mid abdomen caudal to the liver. Imaging of the pancreas can be challenging due to its thin, lobulated shape and proximity to gas and fluid-filled structures like the stomach and duodenum, which can become superimposed over the pancreas and hinder its evaluation. The canine and feline pancreas is composed of right and left lobes connected by a body. The right lobe lies along the medial side of the duodenum and courses cranially to unite with the body. The body lies near the pylorus and portal vein with the left limb extending laterally near the left kidney and spleen. Pancreatic ductal anatomy is different between dogs and cats. The major duct in dogs is the accessory duct which empties onto the minor duodenal papilla. In cats, the major duct is the pancreatic duct which empties onto the major duodenal papilla along with the common bile duct.

Imaging can help diagnose different pancreatic disorders. In the past, abdominal radiography was commonly performed in dogs and cats suspected of pancreatic disease. Today, ultrasound is the most used modality; however, computed tomography (CT) is increasingly utilized in pancreatic imaging. Magnetic resonance (MR) imaging has been used less commonly.

RADIOGRAPHIC IMAGING OF THE PANCREAS

The normal pancreas is usually unidentified in the cranial abdominal on standard radiographs. For dogs and cats with clinical signs associated with pancreatic diseases, abdominal radiographs are a first line diagnostic to evaluate the gastrointestinal tract for presence of mechanical intestinal obstruction or other causes of vomiting, diarrhea, or inappetence. Acute pancreatitis or other pancreatic

Disorders of the Liver, Exocrine Pancreas, and Gastrointestinal Tract in Dogs and Cats, First Edition. Edited by Harry Cridge et al. Published 2026 by John Wiley & Sons, Inc. Companion Website: www.wiley.com/go/cridge/disorders

diseases may have the following radiographic changes: cranial abdominal decreased serosal detail, a focal mass effect between the stomach and colon, and mild gas dilation of the duodenum.

ULTRASOUND IMAGING OF THE PANCREAS

For dogs and cats, the normal sonographic appearance of the pancreas is typically isoechoic to mildly hypoechoic to the surrounding mesentery and hypoechoic to the adjacent spleen with smooth margins (Mattoon and Nyland 2015). The pancreas should measure less than 10 mm in thickness in normal dogs and cats; however, there can be variation in thickness of the individual right and left lobes and body (Penninck et al. 2013; Etue et al. 2001). Normal measurements of the pancreatic duct are available for dogs and cats with a general guideline of slightly less than 1.0 mm diameter (Penninck et al. 2013; Etue et al. 2001). Overlying gas within the stomach and duodenum or operator experience can limit imaging of the pancreas.

The use of ultrasound guided fine needle aspiration or biopsy can be beneficial for obtaining samples for cytological or histological diagnosis of abnormal tissue identified on imaging. Dogs and cats will usually need heavy sedation for pancreatic aspirates due to its proximity to other gastrointestinal structures. The complications associated with this procedure are low with a good diagnostic yield (Cordner et al. 2015).

ACUTE PANCREATITIS

Pancreatitis is the most common exocrine pancreatic disease in dogs and cats (Newman et al. 2006; De Cock et al. 2007). Ultrasound findings in dogs and cats with acute pancreatitis can include pancreatic parenchymal changes such as enlargement, irregular margins, and hypoechoic parenchyma. Additionally, peripancreatic changes often accompany acute pancreatitis and include hyperechoic surrounding mesenteric fat, peripancreatic fluid, and common bile duct dilation (Penninck 2015). Pancreatic duct dilation is possible. One or more of the above findings can occur, and milder forms of pancreatitis may have slight enlargement of a segment of the pancreas, i.e., focal increased thickness in one lobe with normal to mildly hypoechoic pancreatic parenchyma. More severe acute pancreatitis manifests as marked thickening of a segment or the entire pancreas, markedly hypoechoic pancreatic parenchyma with hyperechoic mesentery and free fluid. Secondary extrahepatic biliary duct obstruction may be due to compression by the thickened pancreas (Figure 22.1).

Contrast-enhanced ultrasound has been used to evaluate dogs with acute pancreatitis. This technique showed altered perfusion patterns in dogs with pancreatitis compared to healthy dogs (Rademacher et al. 2016). Serial ultrasound examinations may be beneficial in dogs with suspected acute pancreatitis as initial examination may identify only minimal to no changes in the pancreas and peripancreatic tissues. As disease progresses, imaging changes to the pancreas may become more apparent (Leoni et al. 2020).

Elastography is a newer noninvasive imaging technique which assesses tissue stiffness with diseased tissues having different stiffness values compared to healthy tissues (Sigrist et al. 2017). Dogs with acute pancreatitis were assessed with elastography and showed changes to their pancreas compared to control dogs (Lopes et al. 2020).

CHRONIC PANCREATITIS

Chronic pancreatitis is difficult to identify with ultrasound imaging in dogs or cats. Possible sonographic changes associated with chronic pancreatitis include normal to small size with a heterogenous echogenicity and/or nodular margins. Mineralization may be present and may lead to acoustic shadowing.

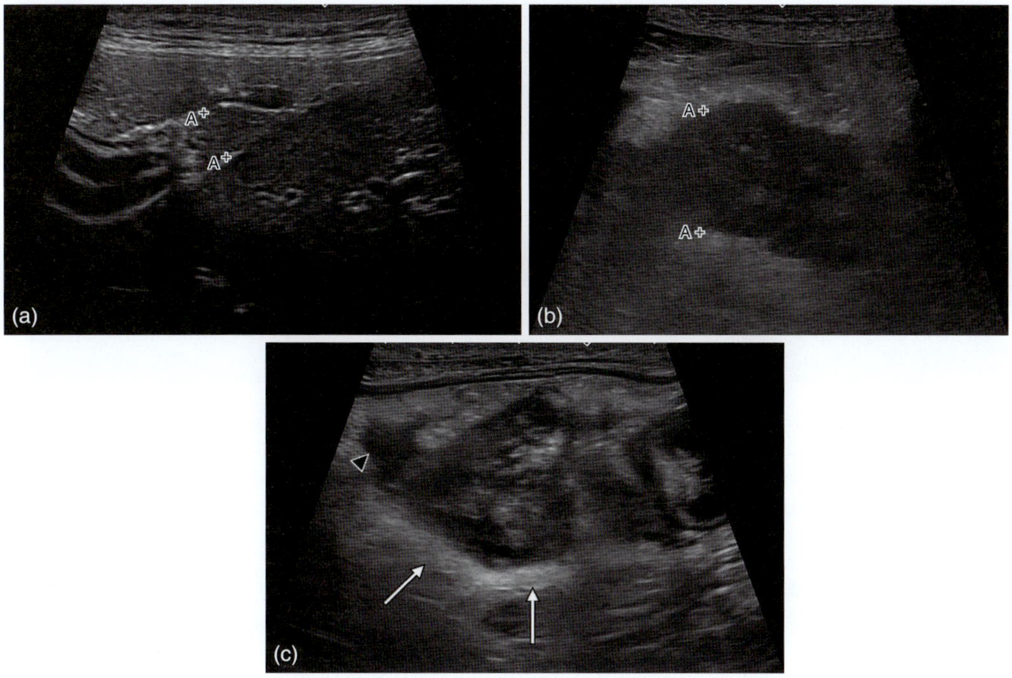

FIGURE 22.1 (a) Sagittal plane image of the normal right limb of the pancreas in a dog. Note the portion of visible pancreas within the calipers with smooth margins and is slightly hypoechoic to the adjacent falciform fat. A portion of the liver is to the right of the pancreas and duodenum is left and dorsal. (b) Transverse plane image of the left limb of the pancreas in a dog with acute pancreatitis. Note the hypoechoic parenchyma (calipers), irregular margins, and hyperechoic surrounding mesentery. The caliper measurement was 2.2 cm in thickness. (c) Transverse plane image of the right limb of the pancreas in a dog with more severe pancreatitis. Note the markedly hypoechoic parenchyma, internal hyperechogenicities, surrounding hyperechoic mesentery (arrow), and a small pocket of free fluid (arrowhead)

PANCREATIC FLUID ACCUMULATIONS (E.G., ABSCESSES/PSEUDOCYSTS)

Sequelae, such as abscess and pseudocyst formation, may develop because of pancreatitis. Both are fluid collections with pseudocysts developing a fibrotic capsule. Abscesses are an infected fluid collection. Both structures will contain hypoechoic to anechoic fluid with distal acoustic enhancement and varying degrees of thickened walls. Aspiration, cytological analysis, and culture of the contents are necessary for definitive diagnosis and for further therapeutic recommendations. Leakage or rupture of the abscess or pseudocyst is possible during or after aspiration, so attempts to completely drain the fluid should be made.

PANCREATIC NEOPLASIA

Pancreatic neoplasia is less common than pancreatitis (Bennett et al. 2001). Various kinds of masses can arise in the exocrine pancreas including nodular hyperplasia, adenocarcinoma, lymphoma, and metastatic tumors. Distinguishing pancreatitis from pancreatic neoplasia with ultrasound may be challenging due to the overlapping features of both diseases. Regional lymphadenopathy can occur with both diseases, and peripancreatic tissue changes are often similar (Bennett et al. 2001). Involvement of adjacent organs such as stomach, duodenum, spleen, and lymph nodes can occur in inflammatory or granulomatous disease and neoplasia, and other primary neoplasia can involve the pancreas such as liver or bile duct neoplasia (Bennett et al. 2001). Often, pancreatic neoplasia is focal in nature, varies in size and location, and can be of hypo to mixed echogenicity. Fine-needle aspiration or biopsy of the involved organs is required for definitive diagnosis (Figure 22.2a).

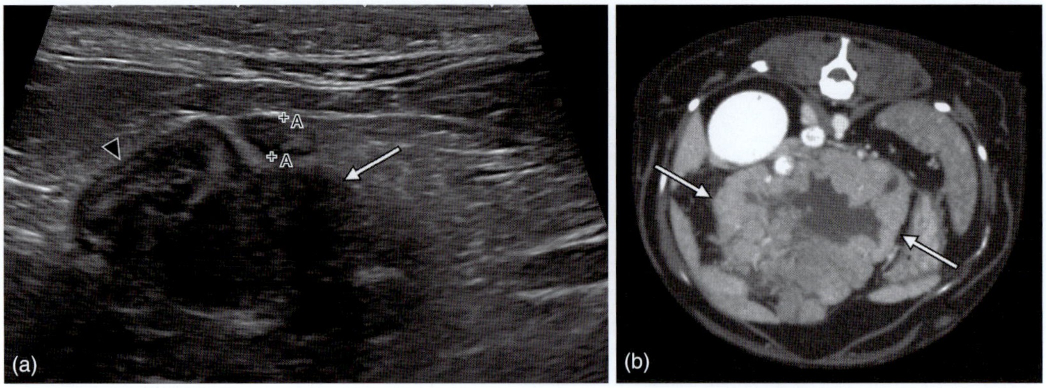

FIGURE 22.2 (a) Transverse plane ultrasound image of a cat with a hypoechoic mass (arrow) within the right pancreas adjacent to the duodenum (arrowhead). The oblong structure measured with calipers is the pancreaticoduodenal lymph node. (b) CT transverse plane venous phase image of a dog with a mass within the body of the pancreas (arrows). Note the internal fluid and contrast-enhancing rim

COMPUTED TOMOGRAPHIC IMAGING OF THE PANCREAS

With CT imaging of the pancreas, intravenous iodinated contrast is helpful to assess the pancreatic parenchyma. On CT imaging the pancreas is iso- to hypoattenuating compared to the liver and spleen with homogeneous parenchymal enhancement and smooth margins (Cáceres et al. 2006; Park et al. 2020). Normal CT size measurements of the right and left lobe and body of the pancreas have been established in dogs and cats (Cáceres et al. 2006; Seacrest et al. 2018). CT imaging is advantageous as the entire pancreas can be evaluated due to lack of superimposition of other organs. This global view of the pancreas and portal vein ensures complete evaluation in dogs and cats with suspected pancreatitis or other pancreatic disease. CT is becoming more readily used for assessment of pancreatitis in dogs (French et al. 2019). Intravenous iodinated contrast can assess the pancreatic parenchyma for contrast enhancement alterations. The common bile duct can be traced to its entrance on the major duodenal papilla, allowing for identification of extrahepatic biliary duct dilation. Additionally, the adjacent vasculature, particularly the portal vein, can be viewed for evidence of thrombosis.

ACUTE PANCREATITIS AND SEQUELAE

CT imaging features of acute pancreatitis include parenchymal changes such as enlargement, irregular margins, and alterations in parenchymal enhancement. Peripancreatic changes such as mesenteric fat stranding, free fluid, lymphadenopathy, and portal vein thrombosis can be seen. A more heterogeneous enhancement pattern is often associated with areas of decreased pancreatic perfusion or necrosis. Heterogeneous pancreatic contrast enhancement has been linked with portal vein thrombosis indicating more severe pancreatitis and a poorer prognosis in dogs (French et al. 2019). Dogs with milder forms of pancreatitis often have mild thickening of the pancreas with normal homogeneous contrast enhancement. Evaluation of pancreatic perfusion with CT in dogs with pancreatitis can provide additional information and has identified differences in pancreatic perfusion between dogs with acute pancreatitis and healthy dogs (von Stade et al. 2023). Sequelae are readily identified with CT imaging; abscesses and pseudocysts are hypoattenuating, and the walls surrounding pseudocysts and abscesses may contrast enhance. Chronic pancreatitis has not been well described in CT imaging; however, similar imaging features would be expected as in ultrasound such as normal to small size, irregular margins, heterogenous attenuation, and contrast enhancement with or without mineralization (Figure 22.3).

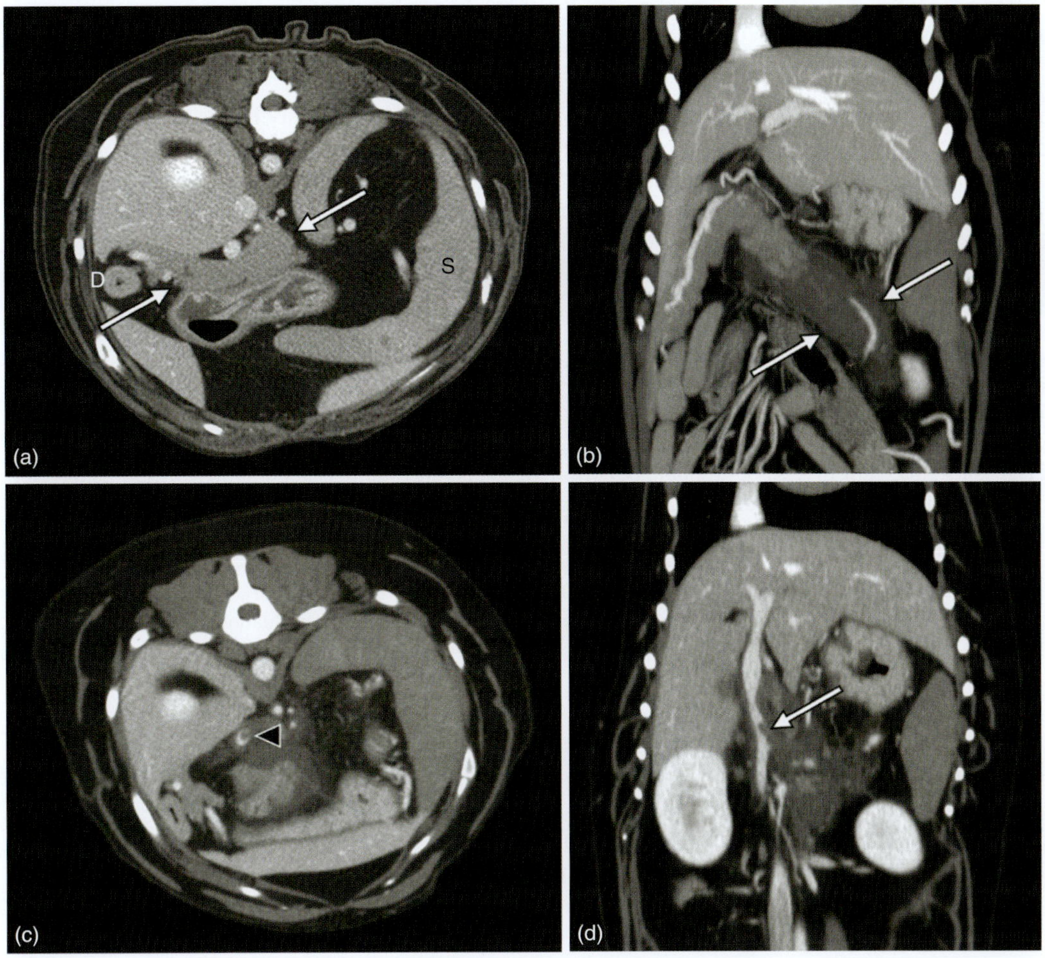

FIGURE 22.3 (a) CT transverse plane venous phase image of the body and right lobe of the normal pancreas of a dog (arrows). Note the smooth margins, thin appearance, and homogeneous contrast enhancement. S = spleen, and D = duodenum. (b) CT dorsal plane reconstruction in venous phase including the right limb, body, and left limb of a dog with acute pancreatitis. Note the left lobe of the pancreas (arrows) is enlarged, hypoattenuating, and heterogeneously contrast-enhancing with surrounding irregular fat stranding. (c) CT transverse plane in venous phase image of dog with acute pancreatitis and portal vein thrombosis. Note the enlarged, irregular, and heterogeneously contrast-enhancing body of the pancreas and the filling defect within the portal vein (arrowhead). (d) CT dorsal plane reconstruction in venous phase of the same dog as in (c). Note the non-enhancing, enlarged, and heterogeneously enhancing pancreas and filling defect in the adjacent portal vein (arrow)

PANCREATIC NEOPLASIA

Pancreatic nodules and masses are more easily identified with CT imaging. CT angiography can be helpful in diagnosing pancreatic neoplasia due to altered contrast enhancement of the nodule or mass compared to the adjacent parenchyma. CT features of exocrine pancreatic carcinomas include a solitary mass, heterogeneous contrast enhancement often with a fluid-filled center (Dunn et al. 2024). Lymphadenopathy and other peripancreatic changes can be identified with CT imaging; however, aspirate or biopsy is still recommended for definitive diagnosis (Dunn et al. 2024) (Figure 22.2b).

MRI IMAGING OF THE PANCREAS

On magnetic resonance imaging (MRI), the normal pancreas is uniformly hyperintense relative to the liver on T1-weighted images and is iso- to hypointense on T2 fat-saturated images. When evaluating for pancreatitis, in both humans and cats, MRI images are assessed for pancreatic parenchymal hyperintensity (on T2 fat-saturated images), contrast enhancement, pancreatic duct dilatation, and peripancreatic abnormalities (Balci et al. 2009; Marolf et al. 2013). Recently, evaluation of MRI in dogs and cats indicated feasibility of this modality in assessing the biliary tract and pancreas (Rahmani et al. 2023; Rahmani et al. 2024).

SUMMARY

Diagnostic imaging is integral in evaluating dogs and cats with suspected pancreatic disease, both for ruling out other causes of presenting clinical signs and to demonstrate pancreatic pathology. Ultrasound is most utilized and there can be overlap in imaging features of different disease processes in the pancreas. CT has high accuracy in diagnosing pancreatic diseases and should be considered when ultrasound is not definitive, further characterization of the disease process is needed, or clinical signs are worsening in the face of treatment.

REFERENCES

Balci, N.C., Bieneman, B.K., Bilgin, M. et al. (2009). Magnetic resonance imaging in pancreatitis. *Top Magn Reason Imaging* 20 (1): 25–30.

Bennett, P.F., Hahn, K.A., Toal, R.L. et al. (2001). Ultrasonographic and cytopathological diagnosis of exocrine pancreatic carcinoma in the dog and cat. *Journal of the American Animal Hospital Association* 37: 466–473.

Cáceres, A.V., Zwingenberger, A.L., Hardam, E. et al. (2006). Helical computed tomographic angiography of the normal canine pancreas. *Veterinary Radiology & Ultrasound* 47 (3): 270.

Cordner, L.P., Sharkey, L.C., Armstrong, P.J. et al. (2015). Cytologic findings and diagnostic yield in 92 dogs undergoing fine needle aspiration of the pancreas. *Journal of Veterinary Diagnostic Investigation* 27 (2): 236–240.

De Cock, H.E., Forman, M.A., Farver, T.B. et al. (2007). Prevalence and histopathologic characteristics of pancreatitis in cats. *Veterinary Pathology* 44 (1): 39.

Dunn, A., Rao, S., Husbands, B. et al. (2024). Computed tomographic features of exocrine pancreatic carcinomas in dogs and cats. *Veterinary Radiology & Ultrasound* 65 (4): 400–407.

Etue, S.M., Penninck, D.G., Labato, M.A. et al. (2001). Ultrasonography of the normal feline pancreas and associated anatomic landmarks: a prospective study of 20 cats. *Veterinary Radiology & Ultrasound* 42 (4): 330.

French, J.M., Twedt, D.C., Rao, S. et al. (2019). Computed tomographic angiography and ultrasonography in the diagnosis and evaluation of acute pancreatitis in dogs. *Journal of Veterinary Internal Medicine* 33 (1): 79.

Leoni, F.P., Pelligra, T., Citi, S. et al. (2020). Ultrasonographic monitoring in 38 dogs with clinically suspected acute pancreatitis. *Veterinary Sciences* 7 (4): 180.

Lopes, M.A., Feliciano, M.A., Uscategui, R.A. et al. (2020). Pancreatic evaluation in dogs using different ultrasonographic techniques-preliminary results. *Acta Veterinaria* 70 (2): 255–266.

Marolf, A.J., Kraft, S.L., Dunphy, T.R. et al. (2013). Magnetic resonance (MR) imaging and MR cholangiopancreatography findings in cats with cholangitis and pancreatitis. *Journal of Feline Medicine and Surgery* 15 (4): 285–294.

Mattoon, J.S. and Nyland, T.G. (2015). Pancreas. In: *Small Animal Diagnostic Ultrasound* (ed. J.S. Mattoon and T.G. Nyland), 3e, 439. St. Louis Missouri: Elsevier Publishing.

Newman, S.J., Steiner, J.M., Woosley, K. et al. (2006). Histologic assessment and grading of the exocrine pancreas in the dog. *Journal of Veterinary Diagnostic Investigation* 18 (1): 115.

Park, J.Y., Bugbee, A., Sharma, A. et al. (2020). Feline pancreatic ducts are consistently identified on CT and more likely to be dilated in the body of pancreas in cats with elevated feline pancreatic lipase immunoreactivity. *Veterinary Radiology & Ultrasound* 61 (3): 255.

Penninck, D.G. (2015). Gastrointestinal tract. In: *Atlas of Small Animal Ultrasonography* (ed. D.G. Penninc and M-a d'Anjou), 2e, 259. Ames, Iowa: Blackwell Publishing.

Penninck, D.G., Zeyen, U., Taeymans, O.N. et al. (2013). Ultrasonographic measurement of the pancreas and pancreatic duct in clinically normal dogs. *American Journal of Veterinary Research* 74 (3): 433.

Rademacher, N., Schur, D., Gaschen, F. et al. (2016). Contrast-enhanced ultrasonography of the pancreas in healthy dogs and in dogs with acute pancreatitis. *Veterinary Radiology & Ultrasound* 56 (1): 58–64.

Rahmani, V., Peltonen, J., Amarilla, S. et al. (2023). Feasibility of magnetic resonance cholangiopancreatography in dogs—a post-mortem study. *Animals* 13 (15): 2517.

Rahmani, V., Peltonen, J., Hmelnikov, D. et al. (2024). Three-dimensional magnetic resonance cholangiography is superior to two-dimensional single-shot magnetic resonance cholangiography for visualization and image quality of the feline and canine biliary tract: a postmortem study. *Veterinary Radiology & Ultrasound* 54 (4): 377–384.

Seacrest, S., Sharma, A., and Bugbee, A. (2018). Triple phase computed tomography of the pancreas in healthy cats. *Veterinary Radiology & Ultrasound* 59 (2): 163–168.

Sigrist, R.M., Liau, J., Kaffas, A.E. et al. (2017). Ultrasound elastography: review of techniques and clinical applications. *Theranostics* 7 (5): 1303–1329.

von Stade, L., Rao, S., and Marolf, A. (2023). Computed tomographic evaluation of pancreatic perfusion in 10 dogs with acute pancreatitis. *Veterinary Radiology & Ultrasound* 64 (5): 823–833.

CHAPTER 23 Cytology of the Exocrine Pancreas

Francisco O. Conrado[1] *and Leslie C. Sharkey*[2]

[1]*Department of Comparative Pathobiology, Cummings School of Veterinary Medicine Tufts University, North Grafton, MA, USA*
[2]*Department of Clinical Sciences, Cummings School of Veterinary Medicine Tufts University, North Grafton, MA, USA*

KEY POINTS

- Cytologic sampling of the pancreas is low risk in dogs and cats.
- Cytologic diagnosis of nodular hyperplasia, pancreatitis, and pancreatic neoplasms is reliable.
- Infectious etiologies can be identified cytologically in the pancreas.
- Optimal interpretation of pancreatic cytology is in the context of clinical and imaging findings.

INTRODUCTION

Diagnosing pancreatic disease is complicated by nonspecific clinical signs, lack of accurate biomarkers, and the skill required for accurate imaging and sampling (Mansfield 2015). Fine-needle aspiration (FNA) biopsies are considered diagnostically valuable and low-risk (Cordner et al. 2010). While histopathology remains the reference standard for characterization of pancreatic pathology, there are inconsistencies between microscopic lesions and clinical disease. The potential multifocal distribution of inflammatory lesions requires comprehensive sampling to ensure identification of pathologic processes; however, false negatives still occur, particularly in cats. Cytopathology can be leveraged to distinguish inflammatory from hyperplastic and neoplastic lesions, although differentiation of benign and well-differentiated malignant disturbances of growth can be problematic, as can determination of primary pathologic process among comorbidities (Newman et al. 2005; Bazelle and Watson 2014).

SAMPLE COLLECTION

Ultrasound-guided FNA is frequently used to obtain pancreatic tissue samples for cytopathologic evaluation. While non-aspiration techniques can reduce blood contamination, aspiration should be considered for pancreatic FNA to ensure adequate cellularity (Cordner et al. 2015; Crain et al. 2015). Indications for sampling include the presence of nodules or masses, organomegaly, or changes in echogenicity. However, different pancreatic lesions often appear sonographically similar and findings can be operator-dependent, necessitating microscopic analysis for enhanced interpretation (Hecht and Henry 2007). Impression smears of surgically excised biopsies are also suitable preparations for cytopathologic evaluation. When effusion is present, peritoneal fluid analysis can complement interpretation (Bennett et al. 2001; Armstrong and Williams 2012).

Disorders of the Liver, Exocrine Pancreas, and Gastrointestinal Tract in Dogs and Cats, First Edition. Edited by Harry Cridge et al. Published 2026 by John Wiley & Sons, Inc. Companion Website: www.wiley.com/go/cridge/disorders

NORMAL CYTOLOGIC FINDINGS

Pancreatic cytology samples contain clustered exocrine epithelial cells in a background of blood or proteinaceous fluid. Acinar cells are small-to-medium polygonal cells, with low-to-moderate nuclear-to-cytoplasmic (N:C) ratios, and small-to-moderate amounts of pale basophilic cytoplasm filled with eosinophilic zymogen granules (Figure 23.1a). Nuclei are round, basally located, and contain stippled to reticulated chromatin with occasional small, prominent nucleoli. Minimal anisocytosis and anisokaryosis are observed. Less frequently, ductal epithelial cells occur, ranging from cuboidal cells with higher N:C ratios to columnar cells, which may have cilia (Bjorneby and Kari 2002). Scattered leukocytes and mesothelial cells may be present.

ABNORMAL CYTOLOGIC FINDINGS

INFLAMMATION AND TISSUE INJURY

Damage to pancreatic parenchyma triggers the release of digestive enzymes, leading to necrosis and inflammation (Figure 23.1b). Necrosis is often accompanied by saponification of surrounding fat, characterized by the presence of inflammation and calcium deposits appearing as bright refractile structures using polarized light. Chronic injury can result in fibrosis.

Pancreatitis

Pancreatitis is the most common pancreatic condition, with middle-aged to older animals more frequently diagnosed. Miniature Schnauzers, Boxers, Border Collies, Cocker Spaniels, Cavalier King Charles Spaniels, and various terriers may be predisposed (Watson et al. 2007). Pancreatitis has been identified in more than 50% of necropsied cats (De Cock et al. 2007). Pancreatitis is broadly classified as acute or chronic based on the onset and duration of clinical signs, or histologically based on the type of inflammatory cells, presence of fibrosis, and degree of atrophy.

Acute pancreatitis (AP) can be severe and rapidly progressive with high risk of systemic complications including disseminated intravascular coagulation (DIC) or multiple organ dysfunction syndrome. Aspiration is indicated in cases with mass-like lesions or lack of response to treatment. Cytologic findings in AP typically include a neutrophil-predominant mixed inflammatory infiltrate with fewer macrophages and lymphocytes. Hemorrhage, characterized by hemosiderin-laden macrophages and hematoidin crystals may be present. Acinar cells can have degenerative changes including swelling, cytoplasmic pallor or foaminess (hydropic change), and loss of zymogen granules. Varying degrees of necrosis affect the pancreatic parenchyma and surrounding adipose tissue, appearing as amorphous blue–gray material interspersed with necrotic cells. Dystrophic mineralization results in the presence of calcified material (Figure 23.1c). Hyperplastic changes can occur in the acinar cells, which can exhibit significant atypia in the context of inflammation, warranting caution to avoid overinterpretation as neoplasia (Figure 23.1d).

Chronic pancreatitis (CP) tends to have a milder or even subclinical presentation (Bazelle and Watson 2014). It is defined by the presence of permanent pancreatic changes, primarily fibrosis and atrophy, often with lymphocytic infiltrates. Extensive pancreatic atrophy (>80–90%) can lead to exocrine pancreatic insufficiency (EPI) and diabetes mellitus (DM). Cytologic characterization of CP is anecdotal, suggesting low-cellularity samples with hyperplastic acinar cells, lymphocytes, plasma cells, macrophages, and possibly the presence of matrix reflecting fibrosis (Figure 23.1e). Neutrophils and necrosis suggest concurrent acute inflammation.

Infectious Causes

Pancreatic abscesses are an uncommon but serious complication of pancreatitis. Miniature Schnauzers may be predisposed (Anderson et al. 2008). These can present as single or multiple masses, or even diffusely affect the pancreas. Ultrasound typically reveals cavitary lesions with

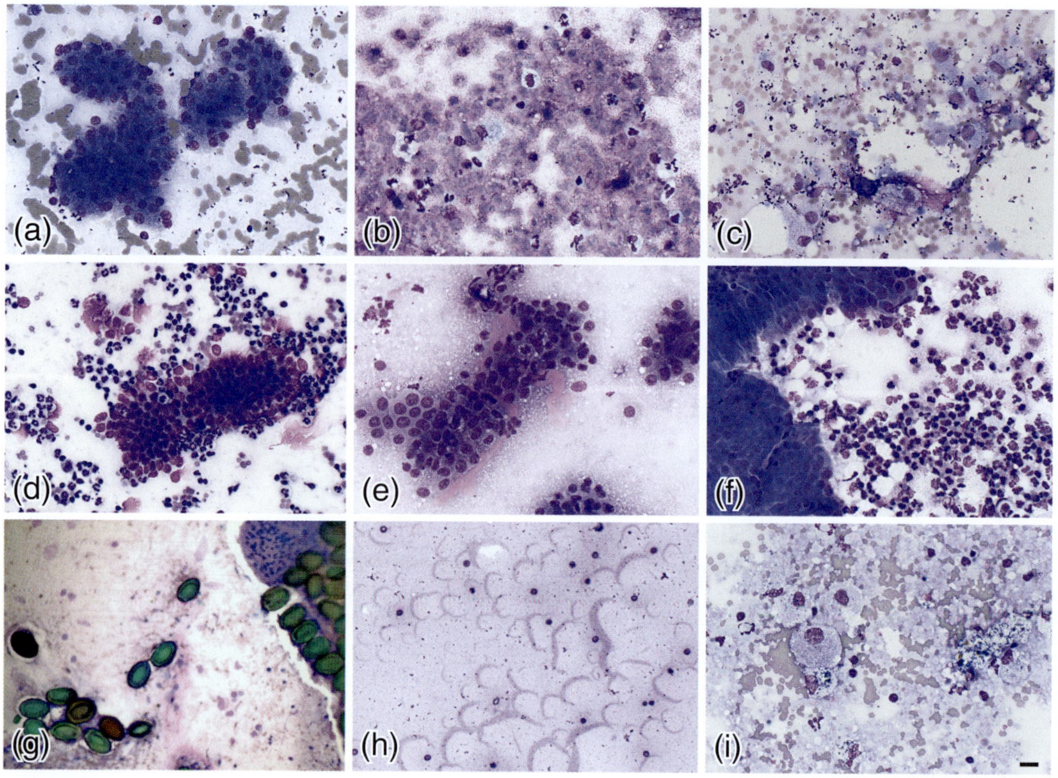

FIGURE 23.1 Photomicrographs of pancreatic cytology. (a) Unremarkable exocrine epithelial cells from a feline pancreas. (b) Mixed inflammation and abundant necrotic debris in a pancreatic mass from a dog. (c) Mixed inflammation and crystalline mineralized material from a cat with pancreatitis. (d) Mixed (predominantly neutrophilic) inflammation and mild epithelial atypia/hyperplasia in a cat. (e) Mild epithelial atypia and evidence of fibrosis (bright pink, streaming, extracellular matrix) in a pancreatic mass from a cat. (f) Marked, septic neutrophilic inflammation and mild epithelial atypia in a pancreatic abscess from a cat. (g) Numerous yellow–brown, oval, *Eurytrema procyonis* fluke ova in a pancreatic nodule from a cat (courtesy of Dr. Tara Piech). (h) Low-cellularity, proteinaceous fluid from a pancreatic cyst in a dog (note the basophilic protein crescents in the background). (i) Proteinaceous fluid with evidence of macrophagic inflammation and chronic hemorrhage (hemosiderin pigment and hematoidin crystals) in a pancreatic cyst from a cat. Wright Giemsa, 500× magnification. Bar = 20 μm. *Source*: With permission of Dr. Francisco O. Conrado and Dr. Tara Piech (g).

variably thick walls and heterogeneous contents. Cytologically, pancreatic abscesses are characterized by abundant degenerate neutrophils with vacuolated macrophages and lymphocytes, against a background of cellular debris (Figure 23.1f). The presence of acinar cells supports pancreatic origin. While bacteria may be observed, cultures are often negative (Johnson and Mann 2006; Anderson et al. 2008). Possible sources of infection include the bloodstream, gastrointestinal tract, and biliary tree (Nemoto et al. 2017). Differentiating pancreatic abscesses from AP can be challenging without identifying organisms.

Pancreatic flukes (*Eurytrema procyonis*) infect foxes, raccoons, and rarely domestic cats in the eastern United States (Hoffman et al. 2017). They tend to localize in the tail of the pancreas, with adult flukes showing a predilection for the pancreatic and bile ducts and the gallbladder. While often asymptomatic, heavy fluke burdens can lead to inflammation, hyperplasia, fibrosis, and in severe cases, pancreatitis, pancreatic atrophy, and EPI. However, significant pancreatic damage is rare in cats (Vyhnal et al. 2008; Köster et al. 2017). Cytologic diagnosis can be challenging, as adult flukes are often fragmented. However, the presence of suckers within cellular parenchymal fragments can be helpful. Fluke eggs are readily identifiable by their green to brown staining, 40–50 × 30–40 μm diameter, and single operculum (Figure 23.1g).

While primary infections of the pancreas are rare, the pancreas can be involved as part of systemic diseases, including multiple systemic infections. Pancreatic necrosis has been observed in cats with systemic calicivirus infection (Pesavento et al. 2004).

CYSTIC LESIONS

Cystic lesions of the pancreas include congenital cysts, acquired retention cysts, or pseudocysts. Cystic neoplasms are rare (Yoshimura et al. 2013). Congenital cysts, primarily seen in cats with polycystic kidney disease or hepatic cysts, are thin-walled hypoechoic structures containing thin, clear fluid (Coleman et al. 2005; Lafuente et al. 2018). Pseudocysts, the most common type, are typically a consequence of pancreatitis (VanEnkevort et al. 1999; Branter and Viviano 2010). Sonographically, they are more irregular with thicker walls and more echogenic contents than true cysts. Lacking a true epithelial lining, pseudocysts are walled by granulation tissue and contain fluid that varies from clear to turbid and bloody. Cysts are cytologically generic, characterized by low cellularity with occasional macrophages and neutrophils (Bjorneby and Kari 2002) (Figure 23.1h). Crystalline debris, cholesterol crystals, and hemorrhage may be present (Figure 23.1i). Aspiration of these lesions can facilitate differentiation from abscesses and cystic neoplasms, which account for a significant proportion of pancreatic tumors in cats (Yoshimura et al. 2013; Törner et al. 2019). Pseudocyst fluid lipase activity might be elevated compared to serum (VanEnkevort et al. 1999).

HYPERPLASIA

Pancreatic acinar nodular hyperplasia (NH) is a frequent incidental finding in older animals and is not considered preneoplastic (Newman et al. 2005). NH is asymptomatic, with multiple, variably sized (usually 1–2 cm) nodules discovered incidentally on ultrasound examinations (Hecht et al. 2007). Aspiration typically yields highly cellular samples with cohesive clusters of well-differentiated acinar cells often mixed with larger cells with higher N:C ratios, increased cytoplasmic basophilia, and fewer granules (Figure 23.2a, b). Slight increases in anisocytosis and anisokaryosis, occasional binucleation, and rare mitotic figures can also be observed. Histopathology may be required in some cases to completely exclude a well-differentiated neoplasm. Ultrasonographic features suggestive of NH are integrated with cytologic features to aid diagnostic interpretation (Newman et al. 2005).

NEOPLASIA

Pancreatic Adenoma

Pancreatic adenomas are rare, benign exocrine tumors that are often incidental (Seaman 2004). While most arise from acinar cells, ductular origin is described. Adenomas are small (usually <1 cm), single, encapsulated masses that can cause compression and atrophy of the surrounding pancreatic tissue; some are cystic. Acinar adenomas display acinar formations with uniform cells and intervening fibrovascular stroma and parallel cytologic findings. Ductal adenomas form tubular and ductular structures composed of cuboidal to columnar cells, sometimes exhibiting pseudostratification and cyst formation. Mild anisocytosis, anisokaryosis, and rare mitotic figures may be observed. However, it is important to note that these neoplastic cells can closely resemble those seen in normal pancreatic tissue, hyperplastic nodules, and even some well-differentiated adenocarcinomas (Figure 23.2c).

Pancreatic Carcinoma

Pancreatic adenocarcinoma, while uncommon in dogs and cats, is the most frequently diagnosed exocrine pancreatic tumor and has a poor prognosis. The incidence increases with age, with no breed or sex predilection. Clinical signs are nonspecific. While pancreatitis-like abnormalities may be seen on routine bloodwork, markedly elevated serum lipase activity (e.g., >10 000 IU/mL) raises suspicion for pancreatic carcinoma. DM can be a concurrent finding, particularly in cats (Linderman et al. 2013). Ultrasonography typically reveals solitary or multiple hypoechoic, occasionally cystic masses. In cats, a mass > 2 cm is likely to be malignant (Hecht et al. 2007). For detailed imaging findings and additional information, see Chapters 22 and 31.

Histologically, pancreatic carcinoma encompasses several subtypes, including ductal, acinar, hyalinizing, mixed exocrine-endocrine, undifferentiated, colloidal (or mucinous non-cystic), and squamous cell carcinoma (SCC). Ductal and acinar adenocarcinomas are most prevalent in dogs and cats. Well-differentiated tumors closely resemble normal pancreatic tissue histologically, with uniform cells, preserved zymogen granulation, and high N:C ratios. Poorly differentiated tumors exhibit lower N:C ratios, enlarged nuclei with coarse chromatin, increased pleomorphism, and frequent mitoses. Canine hyalinizing pancreatic adenocarcinoma is characterized by distinctive aggregates of eosinophilic hyaline material within the stroma and ductal lumens, the exact composition of which remains unclear (Dennis et al. 2008). While rare, several other subtypes of pancreatic carcinoma are reported in cats, including colloidal carcinoma, characterized by abundant mucin production, and SCC, likely of pancreatic duct origin (Gebbie et al. 2012).

Cytologic evaluation of pancreatic masses generally correlates well with histopathology, although further study is warranted to clarify the relationship. Distinguishing well-differentiated adenocarcinomas from adenomas and hyperplasia is complicated by overlapping cellular features (Figure 23.2d), while poorly differentiated tumors are easier to identify. Aspirates of pancreatic

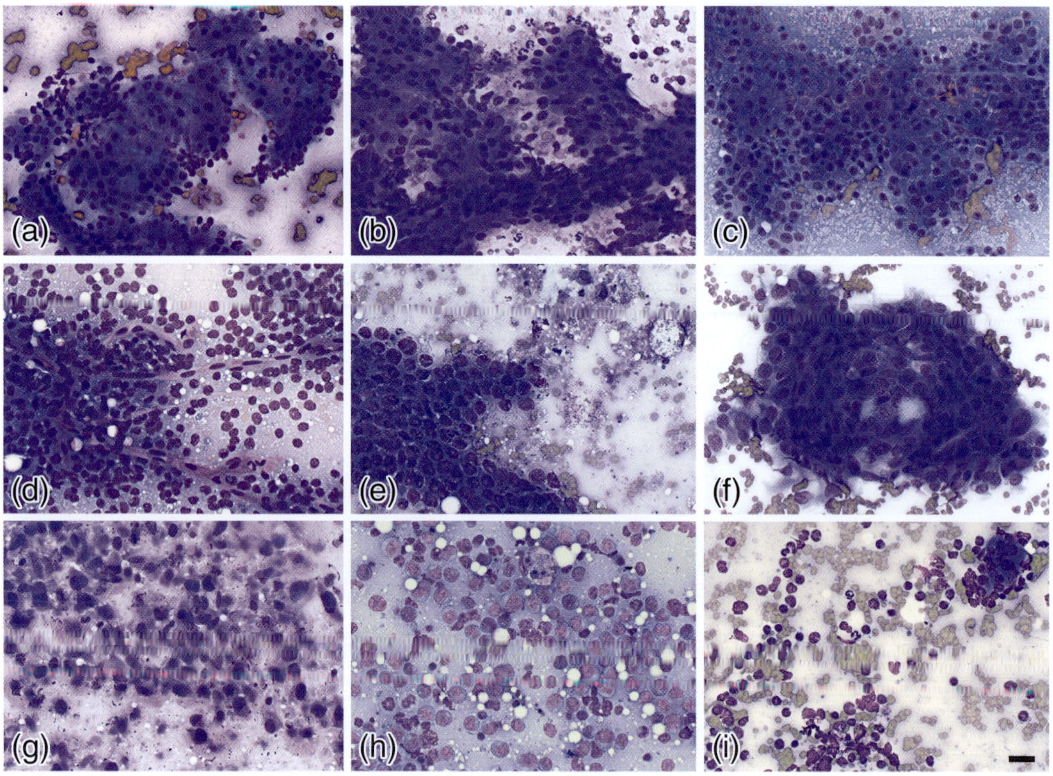

FIGURE 23.2 Photomicrographs of pancreatic cytology. (a) Hyperplastic epithelium from a mildly enlarged pancreas in a dog. (b) Hyperplastic epithelium associated with mild neutrophilic inflammation (upper right corner) in a cat. (c) Mildly to moderately atypical epithelium (hyperplasia vs. adenoma) from a markedly thickened and irregular pancreas in a cat. (d) Well-differentiated carcinoma with abundant capillaries in a pancreatic mass from a cat. (e) Carcinoma with associated necrosis (amorphous basophilic material on the center and upper right corner) in a 2.0-cm pancreatic mass from a cat. (f) Anaplastic carcinoma in a pancreatic mass from a cat (note the pronounced anisocytosis and anisokaryosis). (g) Necrotic pancreatic adenocarcinoma in a dog (note the poor preservation of the cells, loss of cellular detail, and blue-gray cytoplasmic discoloration consistent with necrosis). (h) Large-cell lymphoma in the pancreas of a dog (no pancreatic tissue seen on cytology). (i) Intermediate-cell lymphoma in the pancreas of a cat (note the small cluster of mildly atypical pancreatic epithelium on the upper right corner). Wright Giemsa, 500× magnification. Bar = 20 μm. *Source*: With permission of Francisco O. Conrado

adenocarcinomas are typically highly cellular and sometimes display cellular crowding or disorganization. Epithelial cells form clusters, rows, and/or sheets, sometimes exhibiting acinar or tubular structures. Increased cytoplasmic basophilia and occasional vacuolization may also be seen (Figure 23.2e). Well-differentiated acinar adenocarcinomas may retain zymogen granules, while poorly differentiated carcinomas often lack specific features confirming pancreatic origin (Figure 23.2f). Nuclear chromatin is reticular to coarsely clumped, and nuclear margins may be irregular, with prominent, variably shaped nucleoli seen. Neoplastic cells can demonstrate marked pleomorphism, with pronounced anisocytosis, anisokaryosis, karyomegaly, and increased N:C ratios. Abnormal mitotic figures further support malignancy. The background often contains inflammation, hemorrhage, and/or necrosis (Figure 23.2g).

Nonepithelial Tumors

Nonepithelial pancreatic tumors are rare in small animals (Hecht et al. 2007; Cordner et al. 2015). Lymphoma (Figure 23.2h, i), fibrosarcoma, hemangiosarcoma, liposarcoma, malignant nerve sheath tumor, carcinosarcoma, and malignant melanoma, and multicentric neoplasms like histiocytic sarcoma and histiocytosis are described (Hayden et al. 1993; Lamb et al. 1995; Bjorneby and Kari 2002; Yamamoto et al. 2012; Rissi et al. 2019).

REFERENCES

Anderson, J.R., Cornell, K.K., Parnell, N.K. et al. (2008). Pancreatic abscess in 36 dogs: a retrospective analysis of prognostic indicators. *Journal of the American Animal Hospital Association* 44 (4): 171–179. https://doi.org/10.5326/0440171.

Armstrong, P.J. and Williams, D.A. (2012). Pancreatitis in Cats. *Topics in Companion Animal Medicine* 27 (3): 140–147. https://doi.org/10.1053/j.tcam.2012.09.001.

Bazelle, J. and Watson, P. (2014). Pancreatitis in cats: is it acute, is it chronic, is it significant? *Journal of Feline Medicine and Surgery* 16 (5): 395–406. https://doi.org/10.1177/1098612X14523186.

Bennett, P., Hahn, K.A., Toal, R.L. et al. (2001). Ultrasonographic and cytopathological diagnosis of exocrine pancreatic carcinoma in the dog and cat. *Journal of the American Animal Hospital Association* 37 (5): 466–473. https://doi.org/10.5326/15473317-37-5-466.

Bjorneby, J.M. and Kari, S. (2002). Cytology of the pancreas. *Veterinary Clinics of North America: Small Animal Practice* 32 (6): 1293–1312. https://doi.org/10.1016/S0195-5616(02)00046-3.

Branter, E.M. and Viviano, K.R. (2010). Multiple recurrent pancreatic cysts with associated pancreatic inflammation and atrophy in a cat. *Journal of Feline Medicine and Surgery* 12 (10): 822–827. https://doi.org/10.1016/j.jfms.2010.06.005.

Coleman, M., Robson, M., and Harvey, C. (2005). Pancreatic cyst in a cat. *New Zealand Veterinary Journal* 53 (2): 157–159. https://doi.org/10.1080/00480169.2005.36495.

Cordner, A.P., Armstrong, P.L., Newman, S.J. et al. (2010). Effect of pancreatic tissue sampling on serum pancreatic enzyme levels in clinically healthy dogs. *Journal of Veterinary Diagnostic Investigation* 22 (5): 702–707. https://doi.org/10.1177/104063871002200505.

Cordner, A.P., Sharkey, L.C., Armstrong, P.J. et al. (2015). Cytologic findings and diagnostic yield in 92 dogs undergoing fine-needle aspiration of the pancreas. *Journal of Veterinary Diagnostic Investigation* 27 (2): 236–240. https://doi.org/10.1177/1040638715574862.

Crain, S.K., Sharkey, L.C., Cordner, A.P. et al. (2015). Safety of ultrasound-guided fine-needle aspiration of the feline pancreas: a case-control study. *Journal of Feline Medicine and Surgery* 17 (10): 858–863. https://doi.org/10.1177/1098612X14557910.

De Cock, H.E.V., Forman, M.A., Farver, T.B. et al. (2007). Prevalence and histopathologic characteristics of pancreatitis in cats. *Veterinary Pathology* 44 (1): 39–49. https://doi.org/10.1354/vp.44-1-39.

Dennis, M.M., O'Brien, T.D., Wayne. T. et al. (2008). Hyalinizing pancreatic adenocarcinoma in six dogs. *Veterinary Pathology* 45 (4): 475–483. https://doi.org/10.1354/vp.45-4-475.

Gebbie, R., Hardcastle, M.R., Hunter, S.A. et al. (2012). Transcoelomic spread and metastasis of a squamous cell carcinoma of presumed pancreatic duct origin in a cat. *New Zealand Veterinary Journal* 60 (2): 154–159. https://doi.org/10.1080/00480169.2011.639056.

Hayden, D.W., Waters, D.J., Burke, B.A. et al. (1993). Disseminated malignant histiocytosis in a golden retriever: clinicopathologic, ultrastructural, and immunohistochemical findings. *Veterinary Pathology* 30 (3): 256–264. https://doi.org/10.1177/030098589303000306.

Hecht, S. and Henry, G. (2007). Sonographic evaluation of the normal and abnormal pancreas. *Clinical Techniques in Small Animal Practice* 22 (3): 115–121. https://doi.org/10.1053/j.ctsap.2007.05.005.

Hecht, S., Penninck, D.G., and Keating, J.H. (2007). Imaging findings in pancreatic neoplasia and nodular hyperplasia in 19 cats. *Veterinary Radiology & Ultrasound* 48 (1): 45–50. https://doi.org/10.1111/j.1740-8261.2007.00203.x.

Hoffman, D.A., Piech, T.L., Taylor, H.L. et al. (2017). What is your diagnosis? pancreatic aspirate from a cat. *Veterinary Clinical Pathology* 46 (3): 540–541. https://doi.org/10.1111/vcp.12501.

Johnson, M.D. and Mann, F.A. (2006). Treatment for pancreatic abscesses via omentalization with abdominal closure versus open peritoneal drainage in dogs: 15 cases (1994–2004). *Journal of the American Veterinary Medical Association* 228 (3): 397–402. https://doi.org/10.2460/javma.228.3.397.

Köster, L.S., Shell, L., Ketzis, J. et al. (2017). Diagnosis of pancreatic disease in feline platynosomosis. *Journal of Feline Medicine and Surgery* 19 (12): 1192–1198. https://doi.org/10.1177/1098612X16685676.

Lafuente, S., Fresno, L., Anselmi, C. et al. (2018). Complete laparoscopic excision of a hepatic cyst and omentopexy in a Persian cat. *Journal of Feline Medicine and Surgery Open Reports* 4 (2): 2055116918817631. https://doi.org/10.1177/2055116918817631.

Lamb, C., Simpson, K.W., Boswood, A. et al. (1995) Ultrasonography of pancreatic neoplasia in the dog: a retrospective review of 16 cases. *Veterinary Record* 137 (3): 65–68. https://doi.org/10.1136/vr.137.3.65.

Linderman, M.J., Brodsky, E.M., de Lorimier, L-P. et al. (2013). Feline exocrine pancreatic carcinoma: a retrospective study of 34 cases. *Veterinary and Comparative Oncology* 11 (3): 208–218. https://doi.org/10.1111/j.1476-5829.2012.00320.x.

Mansfield, C. (2015). Practical interpretation and application of exocrine pancreatic testing in small animals. *Clinics in Laboratory Medicine* 35 (3): 535–554. https://doi.org/10.1016/j.cll.2015.05.004.

Nemoto, Y., Haraguchi, T., Shimokawa Miyama, T. et al. (2017). Pancreatic abscess in a cat due to staphylococcus aureus infection. *Journal of Veterinary Medical Science* 79 (7): 1146–1150. https://doi.org/10.1292/jvms.17-0026.

Newman, S.J., Steiner, J.M., Woosley, K. et al. (2005). Correlation of age and incidence of pancreatic exocrine nodular hyperplasia in the dog. *Veterinary Pathology* 42 (4): 510–513. https://doi.org/10.1354/vp.42-4-510.

Pesavento, P.A., Maclachlan, N.J., Dillard-Telm, L. et al. (2004). Pathologic, immunohistochemical, and electron microscopic findings in naturally occurring virulent systemic feline calicivirus infection in cats. *Veterinary Pathology* 41 (3): 257–263. https://doi.org/10.1354/vp.41-3-257.

Rissi, D.R., Brown, C.A., Gendron, K. et al. (2019). Pancreatic Langerhans cell histiocytosis in a cat. *Journal of Veterinary Diagnostic Investigation* 31 (6): 859–863. https://doi.org/10.1177/1040638719874857.

Seaman, R.L. (2004). Exocrine pancreatic neoplasia in the cat: a case series. *Journal of the American Animal Hospital Association* 40 (3): 238–245. https://doi.org/10.5326/0400238.

Törner, K., Aupperle-Lellbach, H., Staudacher, A. et al. (2019). Primary solid and cystic tumours of the exocrine pancreas in cats. *Journal of Comparative Pathology* 169: 5–19. https://doi.org/10.1016/j.jcpa.2019.04.002.

VanEnkevort, B.A., O'Brien, R.T., and Young, K.M. (1999). Pancreatic pseudocysts in 4 dogs and 2 cats: ultrasonographic and clinicopathologic findings. *Journal of Veterinary Internal Medicine* 13 (4): 309–313. https://doi.org/10.1111/j.1939-1676.1999.tb02186.x.

Vyhnal, K.K., Vyhnal, K.K., Barr, S.C. et al. (2008). *Eurytrema procyonis* and pancreatitis in a cat. *Journal of Feline Medicine and Surgery* 10 (4): 384–387. https://doi.org/10.1016/j.jfms.2008.01.001.

Watson, P.J., Roulois, A.J.A., Scase, T. et al. (2007). Prevalence and breed distribution of chronic pancreatitis at post-mortem examination in first-opinion dogs. *Journal of Small Animal Practice* 48 (11): 609–618. https://doi.org/10.1111/j.1748-5827.2007.00448.x.

Yamamoto, R., Suzuki, K., Uchida, K. et al. (2012). Pancreatic carcinosarcoma in a cat. *Journal of Comparative Pathology* 147 (2–3): 223–226. https://doi.org/10.1016/j.jcpa.2012.01.022.

Yoshimura, H., Matsuda, Y., Kawamoto, Y. et al. (2013). Acinar cell cystadenoma of the pancreas in a cat. *Journal of Comparative Pathology* 149 (2–3): 225–228. https://doi.org/10.1016/j.jcpa.2013.01.006.

Histopathology of the Exocrine Pancreas

CHAPTER 24

Victoria Watson, DVM, PhD, Diplomate ACVP

Department of Pathobiology & Diagnostic Investigations, College of Veterinary Medicine, Michigan State University, East Lansing, MI, USA

KEY POINTS

- The primary microscopic features of acute pancreatic necrosis are necrosis at the periphery of the lobule which progresses inwards, neutrophils or suppurative inflammation, and peripancreatic fat necrosis and saponification.
- Histopathologic patterns of chronic pancreatitis include Interstitial (periductular) and parenchymal (lobular) patterns.
- The distribution of lesions is often variable and multifocal; therefore, a normal biopsy may not rule out pancreatitis in other lobules.
- Exocrine pancreatic insufficiency can lead to complete loss of the acinar structure of lobules, complete absence of lobules, to only ducts and islets present.
- Exocrine pancreatic neoplasia is rare and can vary from focal to affecting multiple lobules, and carcinomatosis may occur.

INTRODUCTION

The pancreas in dogs and cats spans within the mesentery along the greater curvature of the stomach and follows the descending part of the duodenum. The pancreas is composed of the left lobe (along the greater curvature of the stomach), body (adjacent to the pylorus), and right lobe (medial to the descending duodenum). Further division of the pancreas into lobules creates a cobblestone appearance. As shown in Figure 24.1a, these lobules are separated by connective tissue and contain acinar glands, intercalated ducts, and intralobular ducts (Eurell and Frappier 2006). Intralobular ducts form interlobular ducts, which then come together to create the pancreatic and accessory pancreatic ducts (Eurell and Frappier 2006). The primary secretory epithelial cells in the pancreas are the acinar epithelial cells and the ductal epithelial cells (Eurell and Frappier 2006; Pawlina 2024). The acinar cells are triangular and contain abundant hypereosinophilic granules called zymogen granules, which contain the proenzymes (Eurell and Frappier 2006; Pawlina 2024). The ductal epithelial cells secrete bicarbonate and water. While the exocrine structures are the focus of this section, there is multifocally interspersed endocrine tissue forming the pancreatic islets as well. Here, we will review the gross and microscopic appearances of major diseases of the pancreas in dogs and cats, including acute pancreatic necrosis and acute pancreatitis, zinc toxicity, chronic pancreatitis, pancreatic atrophy, and exocrine pancreatic neoplasia.

ACUTE PANCREATIC NECROSIS AND INFLAMMATION

Acute pancreatic necrosis (APN) and acute pancreatitis are often used interchangeably; however, there are some differences in the microscopic features of these two entities. Clinically both APN and acute pancreatitis are defined by a sudden onset of clinical signs and are considered inflammatory

Disorders of the Liver, Exocrine Pancreas, and Gastrointestinal Tract in Dogs and Cats, First Edition. Edited by Harry Cridge et al. Published 2026 by John Wiley & Sons, Inc. Companion Website: www.wiley.com/go/cridge/disorders

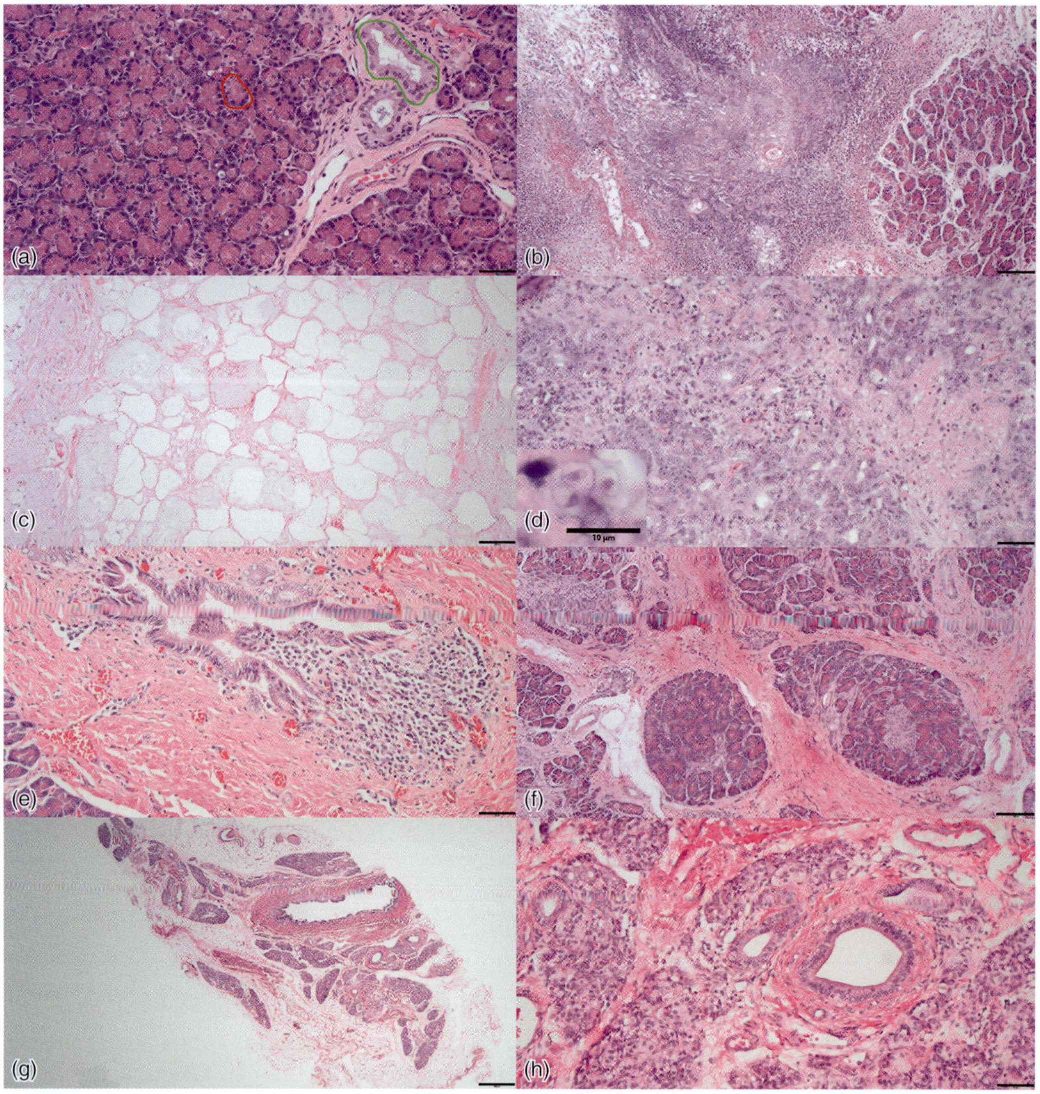

FIGURE 24.1 Representative photomicrographs of normal pancreas, pancreatitis, and pancreatic atrophy. (a) Normal appearance of lobules and interlobular septum (bar = 50 μm, 200 ×). The red circle surrounds an acinus composed of acinar epithelial cells with zymogen granules and the green circle surrounds an interlobular duct lined by columnar epithelial cells. (b) Acute pancreatic necrosis with suppurative pancreatitis (bar = 100 μm, 100 ×). (c) The photomicrograph shows the microscopic appearance of peripancreatic fat necrosis or saponification (bar = 100 μm, 100 ×). (d) Although rare, acute pancreatitis can occur in cats with toxoplasmosis (bar = 50 μm, 200 ×). The inset shows the protozoal zoites of *T. gondii* (bar = 10 μm, 1000 ×). (e) The microscopic features of periductular fibrosis and lymphocytic inflammation in a Cocker spaniel (bar = 100 μm, 100 ×). (f) Chronic pancreatitis with separation of lobules with abundant fibrosis and lobular atrophy secondary to fibrosis (bar = 100 μm, 100 ×). (g, h) The pancreas from a 12-month-old German Shepherd with exocrine pancreatic insufficiency. (g) Low magnification photomicrograph of a section of pancreatic lobules (bar = 500 μm, 20 ×). (h) A higher magnification photomicrograph demonstrates that the remaining cells in the pancreatic lobules are islets and ductular epithelium; there are no recognizable acinar cells (bar = 50 μm, 200 ×). Courtesy of Dr. Victoria Watson of Michigan State University Veterinary Diagnostic Laboratory

processes induced by blocked secretion of enzymes from the pancreatic acinar cell, subsequent fusion of pancreatic proenzymes with lysosomes (co-localization), and inappropriate activation of proenzymes to enzymes (Mansfield 2012a). The initiating factor(s) leading to this blocked secretion and co-localization, among other mechanisms, is not clear. APN and inflammation may lead to systemic inflammatory response syndrome (SIRS) secondary to vascular lesions and cytokine storm (Mansfield 2012b; Hietaranta et al. 1999).

ACUTE PANCREATIC NECROSIS

APN is initially identified via ultrasound-guided aspirate or biopsy, gross examination, or microscopically as peripancreatic fat necrosis (also termed saponification due to breakdown of fat into smaller components and combining with calcium), and mineralization. Necrosis then extends into the outer acinar cells, which lose cellular detail. Necrosis extends to invade the lobules from the periphery to the center (Figure 24.1b). Due to this pattern of periphery being first affected, there is even more evidence for the role of hypoperfusion or hypoxia in the mechanism of APN. The role of high lipid diets or acute ingestion of lipid-containing food may be associated with increased lipid peroxidation leading to membrane breakage and cellular necrosis. Moreover, overweight dogs and dogs with hypertriglyceridemia are more likely to develop APN (Hess et al. 1999).

On postmortem examination, the abdomen may contain serosanguinous fluid. Petechiae and ecchymoses may be noted on the serosal surface of abdominal organs, including the pancreas. Saponification of fat appears grossly as small (often less than 5 mm), white, firm foci within the peripancreatic mesenteric fat.

Microscopic examination of the pancreas often reveals acinar cell necrosis, interlobular edema, vascular thrombosis, and neutrophilic or histiocytic inflammation along the margin between necrosis and remaining parenchyma. Necrosis is characterized by hypereosinophilic, shrunken acinar cells, and nuclear changes like nuclear burst or fragmentation (karyorrhexis) and nuclear shrinkage or condensation (pyknosis). As necrosis progresses, there is a complete loss of cellular and nuclear structure. Higher numbers of vascular thrombi and regions of ischemia have been linked to an increased risk of fatality (Hess et al. 1999). Microscopic features of saponification of fat are loss of normal clear adipocytes and replacement with pale amphophilic material, representing fat necrosis (Figure 24.1c) and calcium deposition.

ZINC TOXICITY

Zinc toxicity is a specific and rare cause of APN due to the buildup of zinc in the pancreas, the normal excretory pathway of zinc. In the United States, zinc toxicity is most often due to ingestion of pennies minted after 1982 or other zinc-containing metals (Foote et al. 2020; Mikszewski et al. 2003). A retrospective study published in 2023 identified evidence of pancreatitis in 5.5% and suspicion of pancreatitis in 29% of dogs ($n = 55$) with zinc toxicosis (Henke et al. 2023).

Microscopic features of zinc toxicity include acinar cell degeneration and necrosis, characterized by loss of zymogen granules, cytoplasmic microvesicular vacuolation, cellular shrinkage, and karyorrhectic to pyknotic nuclei – leading to acinar atrophy (Foote et al. 2020; Maxie 2016). Additional lesions, depending on clinical course, may include interlobular edema (acute) or fibrosis (more chronic).

ACUTE PANCREATITIS

In acute pancreatitis, inflammation may be variable throughout the pancreas and peripancreatic mesenteric fat. This has clinical relevance since a single pancreatic biopsy is unlikely to represent a complete picture of what is going on within the pancreas as a whole. Grossly, the pancreas is similar to that described in APN; there is peripancreatic and interlobular edema, and the pancreatic parenchyma contains multiple regions of hemorrhage. Microscopically, pancreatitis starts within the center of lobules or surrounding intralobular or interlobular ducts. The primary inflammatory cell type in acute pancreatitis is the neutrophil. Neutrophilic inflammation can lead to overactive respiratory bursts and release of reactive oxygen species exacerbating the inflammation and pancreatic damage. The pancreatic damage is noted microscopically as ductal necrosis, edematous expansion of interlobular parenchyma, and multifocal hemorrhages in areas of necrosis. As the disease continues, the neutrophilic inflammation, necrosis, edema, and hemorrhage can extend to obscure a large portion of the pancreas.

Pancreatitis in cats has been linked to obesity, diabetes mellitus, acute abdominal trauma, and many other disease processes (Maxie 2016; Jørgensen et al. 2025). Cats with obesity or diabetes mellitus may have subclinical pancreatitis (Jørgensen et al. 2025). Although there is anecdotal evidence for *Toxoplasma gondii* and *Bartonella* species being a cause of pancreatitis, studies show conflicting data. A 2009 study demonstrated no correlation of pancreatitis with increased serum antibodies to *T. gondii* or *Bartonella* species in cats with pancreatitis diagnosed by elevated feline pancreatic lipase immunoreactivity (fPLI) (Bayliss et al. 2009; Dubey and Carpenter 1993). The association of *T. gondii* and pancreatitis is therefore somewhat controversial. The author has seen one case of *T. gondii* associated with necrotizing pancreatitis in a 5-year-old cat with systemic toxoplasmosis (Figure 24.1d). It is however reasonable to consider performing toxoplasma titers in cats with suspected pancreatitis, or where histopathologic features are evident.

Postmortem studies have also identified dogs with a mixture of acute and chronic changes (Newman et al. 2004, 2006). For example, dogs may have a mixture of necrosis and neutrophils – suppurative inflammation with concurrent lymphocytic inflammation. The examples of acute and chronic are 1. necrosis + neutrophils = suppurative inflammation and 2. lymphocytic inflammation, respectively. Likewise, the pancreatic sections with suppurative inflammation may also have evidence of fibrosis. These findings are generally multifocal and do not diffusely affect the pancreas.

CHRONIC PANCREATITIS

Chronic pancreatitis is defined by microscopic evidence of irreversible damage leading to loss of function. The patterns of chronic pancreatitis include chronic interstitial pancreatitis originating in or around the interlobular ducts and parenchymal pancreas. The causes are thought to be recurrent acute pancreatitis or APN, autoimmune pancreatitis, or genetic predisposition. In human patients, interlobular fibrosis, lymphoplasmacytic periductal inflammation, and sclerosis are associated with autoimmune pancreatitis (Zamboni et al. 2004). Similar lesions are identified in spaniels, particularly Cocker and Cavalier King Charles spaniels, which may indicate those breeds have some form of autoimmune pancreatitis (Figure 24.1e).

In cats and dogs with chronic pancreatis, the organ is diffusely atrophied and multinodular. Nodules are often representative of nodular hyperplasia or fibrosis. Fibrosis is consistently present and may be within the interlobular septa, acini, or both (Figure 24.1f). When present around ducts, fibrosis can lead to some degree of obstruction. In addition to fibrosis, the microscopic features include loss of parenchyma, lymphocytic inflammation, or a mixture of lymphocytes and plasma cells (Watson 2012). These microscopic features often lead to loss of exocrine tissue and function.

There are few published studies using scoring or grading systems, including a study in humans with 16 categories to establish 4 grades (Zamboni et al. 2004) with mild, moderate, and severe designations, and two grading schemes in dogs (Newman et al. 2006; Watson et al. 2007). One grading scheme evaluated any nonneoplastic pancreatic lesions (Newman et al. 2006) and the other investigated lesions of chronic pancreatitis in deceased dogs, which received a postmortem examination (Watson et al. 2007). The first grading scheme, by Newman et al. (2006), graded the presence of neutrophilic inflammation, lymphocytic inflammation, necrosis (pancreatic and peripancreatic mesenteric fat), edema, fibrosis, atrophy, and nodular formation. This study obtained 101 pancreases for review and most of the findings were in Grade 1 designation (mild). The most common findings were mild lymphocytic inflammation, most often in the periductular interstitium, and nodular hyperplasia; however, this study examined many sections of pancreas, obtaining a section every 2 cm, and the lesions were not diffusely present in all sections. It is not clinically nor financially applicable to obtain so many samples in a diagnostic setting either in live animals or deceased animals, so comparing these findings to clinical cases and other studies may be difficult. The second postmortem study, done by Watson et al. (2007) specifically looked at the prevalence of chronic pancreatis in 200 postmortem examined dogs and they utilized robust detailed parameters, including an "other" group for lesions interpreted to be secondary to other disease process(es). The most interesting finding in the Watson et al. studies is the variation in lesion distribution related to breed; Cavalier King Charles spaniels, Cocker spaniels, and boxers were more likely to have interlobular lesions, while terriers and collies were more likely to have lobular lesions with minimal or no involvement with the interlobular septa (Watson 2012; Watson et al. 2007). Cocker spaniels have been further studied by this group of authors and the common lesions of chronic pancreatitis in that breed are damage to interlobular ducts, periductular fibrosis, and lymphocytic inflammation (Coddou et al. 2024; Watson et al. 2011). Chronic pancreatitis with a high degree of fibrosis can lead to dysfunction of endocrine islets (diabetes mellitus) and exocrine tissue (exocrine pancreatic insufficiency [EPI]).

EXOCRINE PANCREATIC INSUFFICIENCY

EPI can be either primary (atrophy) or secondary (pancreatic damage), and the microscopic features of the two types varies. Pancreatic acinar atrophy (PAA) is considered a complex inheritance in German Shepherds (Tsai et al. 2013; Moeller et al. 2002), but has been less frequently diagnosed in rough-coated collies and other breeds (Batchelor et al. 2007). PAA is associated with lymphocytic inflammation in the early stages of disease; however, when biopsies are performed, the disease has usually progressed to complete exocrine atrophy. Any remaining pancreatic exocrine acini and lobules do not retain glandular organization and only few disorganized acinar cells remain; the only remaining pancreatic tissue is composed of pancreatic ducts and islets (Figure 24.1g, h). While fibrosis is not a feature of PAA, it is one of the common lesions in secondary pancreatic insufficiency.

EPI in older animals is most often associated with pancreatic damage due to repeated pancreatitis or chronic changes following pancreatic necrosis. EPI in these dogs is often a slow progression as the damage to the pancreas increases and more fibrosis is laid down replacing normal parenchyma or obstructing ducts. Chronic pancreatitis with fibrosis leading to EPI is seen in Cavalier King Charles spaniels, and Cocker spaniels.

PANCREATIC HYPERPLASIA AND NEOPLASIA

Nodular expansion of the exocrine pancreas occurs with hyperplasia and neoplasia. Hyperplastic nodules are relatively common, reported in 80% of 101 dogs in one study, both in dogs with ($n = 76$) pancreatic lesions and without ($n = 25$) (Newman et al. 2005). Hyperplasia appears often as pale tan to grey, firm, small nodules expanding the normal pancreas. Microscopically, the hyperplastic acinar cells have hypereosinophilic or poorly stained cytoplasm, and there may be loss of normal glandular appearance (Figure 24.2a). Cytoplasmic vacuolation (Figure 24.2a inset) is common and pancreatic islets are often unaffected. The primary way to differentiate hyperplastic nodules from adenomas is examination of the margins. At the margins of hyperplastic nodules, there is no compression of adjacent tissue. Adenomas are benign and often subclinical (i.e., only found on autopsy). Adenomas which arise from ductular epithelium have a tubular, sometimes cystic pattern, whereas more solid adenomas arise from acinar epithelial cells.

Exocrine pancreatic adenocarcinomas are uncommon. The gross appearance of pancreatic adenocarcinomas may be a solitary mass or may be multiple masses throughout the pancreas and carcinomatosis may also be present throughout the mesentery and serosal surfaces of abdominal organs. Microscopically, pancreatic adenocarcinomas are sorted into four patterns – acinar (Figure 24.2b), tubular: small (Figure 24.2c) or large, and hyalinizing (Figure 24.2d) – however, a single carcinoma may have more than one pattern. Acinar pancreatic adenocarcinomas are usually more solid and neoplastic acinar cells may retain zymogen granules. Hyalinizing pancreatic adenocarcinomas contain homogenous, eosinophilic material, which stains with periodic acid-Schiff (PAS) reaction. All pancreatic adenocarcinomas are likely to have invasion into blood vessels and lymphatics as they are highly metastatic. A rare paraneoplastic syndrome, which can occur with pancreatic adenocarcinomas, leads to alopecia

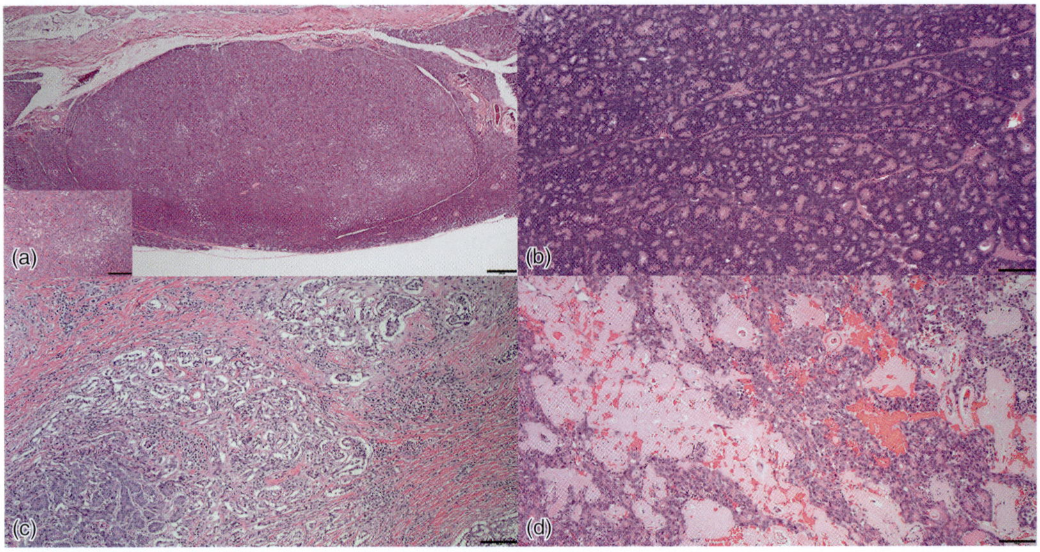

FIGURE 24.2 Representative photomicrographs of nodular hyperplasia and pancreatic adenocarcinomas. (a) A low magnification view of a hyperplastic nodule (bar = 200 μm, 40 ×) and the inset shows the dense cellularity of the nodule and cytoplasmic vacuolation (bar = 100 μm, 100 ×). (b) The appearance of an acinar pancreatic adenocarcinoma. (c) A small tubular type. (d) The hyalinizing type with eosinophilic, homogenous, glassy material (bar = 100 μm, 100 ×). Courtesy of Dr. Victoria Watson of Michigan State University Veterinary Diagnostic Laboratory

and atrophic epidermal stratum corneum along the ventral aspect, limbs, and face of cats. Another rare entity in humans, termed pancreatitis, panniculitis, and polyarthritis (PPP) syndrome has been published in a Cavalier King Charles spaniel with a pancreatic adenocarcinoma (Hagelskamp et al. 2024). It is important to note that inflammatory lesions and high serum pancreatic lipase concentrations can occur in conjunction with pancreatic neoplasia.

REFERENCES

Batchelor, D.J., Noble, P.J., Cripps, P.J. et al. (2007). Breed associations for canine exocrine pancreatic insufficiency. *Journal of Veterinary Internal Medicine* 21: 207–214.

Bayliss, D.B., Steiner, J.M., Sucholdolski, J.S. et al. (2009). Serum feline pancreatic lipase immunoreactivity concentration and seroprevalences of antibodies against *Toxoplasma gondii* and *Bartonella* species in client-owned cats. *Journal of Feline Medicine and Surgery* 11: 663–667.

Coddou, M.F., Blacklaws, B., and Watson, P.J. (2024). Clinical manifestations of chronic pancreatitis in English cocker spaniels. *Journal of Veterinary Internal Medicine* 38: 2129–2137.

Dubey, J.P. and Carpenter, J.L. (1993). Histologically confirmed clinical toxoplasmosis in cats: 100 cases (1952–1990). *Journal of the American Veterinary Medical Association* 203: 1556–1566.

Eurell, J.A. and Frappier, B.L. (2006). *Dellmann's Textbook of Veterinary Histology*, 6e. Ames, IA: Blackwell Publishing.

Foote, K., Gilroy, C., Burton, S. et al. (2020). Zinc toxicosis - Associated hemolytic anemia and pancreatic disease in 2 dogs. *The Canadian Veterinary Journal* 61: 147–152.

Hagelskamp, A., White, A.G., Gallman, J. et al. (2024). Pancreatitis, panniculitis, and polyarthritis syndrome in a dog with hyalinizing pancreatic adenocarcinoma. *Journal of Veterinary Diagnostic Investigation* 36: 886–890.

Henke, C.S., Beal, M.W., Walton, R.A.L. et al. (2023). Retrospective evaluation of the clinical course and outcome of zinc toxicosis due to metallic foreign bodies in dogs (2005–2021): 55 cases. *Journal of Veterinary Emergency and Critical Care (San Antonio)* 33: 676–684.

Hess, R.S., Kass, P.H., Shofer, F.S. et al. (1999). Evaluation of risk factors for fatal acute pancreatitis in dogs. *Journal of the American Veterinary Medical Association* 214: 46–51.

Hietaranta, A., Kemppainen, E., Puolakkainen, P. et al. (1999). Extracellular phospholipases A2 in relation to systemic inflammatory response syndrome (SIRS) and systemic complications in severe acute pancreatitis. *Pancreas* 18: 385–391.

Jørgensen, F.K., Bjornvad, C.R., Krabbe, B. et al. (2025). Evaluation of laboratory findings indicating pancreatitis in healthy lean, obese, and diabetic cats. *Journal of Veterinary Internal Medicine* 39: e17236.

Mansfield, C. (2012a). Acute pancreatitis in dogs: advances in understanding, diagnostics, and treatment. *Topics in Companion Animal Medicine* 27: 123–132.

Mansfield, C. (2012b). Pathophysiology of acute pancreatitis: potential application from experimental models and human medicine to dogs. *Journal of Veterinary Internal Medicine* 26: 875–887.

Maxie, M.G. (2016). *Jubb, Kennedy, and Palmer's Pathology of Domestic Animals*, 6e. St. Louis, Missouri: Elsevier.

Mikszewski, J.S., Saunders, H.M., and Hess, R.S. (2003). Zinc-associated acute pancreatitis in a dog. *Journal of Small Animal Practice* 44: 177–180.

Moeller, E.M., Steiner, J.M., Clark, L.A. et al. (2002). Inheritance of pancreatic acinar atrophy in German Shepherd Dogs. *American Journal of Veterinary Research* 63: 1429–1434.

Newman, S., Steiner, J., Woosley, K. et al. (2004). Localization of pancreatic inflammation and necrosis in dogs. *Journal of Veterinary Internal Medicine* 18: 488–493.

Newman, S.J., Steiner, J.M., Woosley, K. et al. (2005). Correlation of age and incidence of pancreatic exocrine nodular hyperplasia in the dog. *Veterinary Pathology* 42: 510–513.

Newman, S.J., Steiner, J.M., Woosley, K. et al. (2006). Histologic assessment and grading of the exocrine pancreas in the dog. *Journal of Veterinary Diagnostic Investigation* 18: 115–118.

Pawlina, W. (2024). *Histology: A Text and Atlas: With Correlated Cell and Molecular Biology*, 9e. Lippincott Williams & Wilkins, a Wolters Kluwer business.

Tsai, K.L., Starr-Moss, A.N., Venkataraman, G.M. et al. (2013). Alleles of the major histocompatibility complex play a role in the pathogenesis of pancreatic acinar atrophy in dogs. *Immunogenetics* 65: 501–509.

Watson, P. (2012). Chronic pancreatitis in dogs. *Topics in Companion Animal Medicine* 27: 133–139.

Watson, P.J., Roulois, A., Scase, T. et al. (2011). Characterization of chronic pancreatitis in English Cocker Spaniels. *Journal of Veterinary Internal Medicine* 25: 797–804.

Watson, P.J., Roulois, A.J., Scase, T. et al. (2007). Prevalence and breed distribution of chronic pancreatitis at post-mortem examination in first-opinion dogs. *Journal of Small Animal Practice* 48: 609–618.

Zamboni, G., Lüttges, J., Capelli, P. et al. (2004). Histopathological features of diagnostic and clinical relevance in autoimmune pancreatitis: a study on 53 resection specimens and 9 biopsy specimens. *Virchows Archiv* 445: 552–563.

CHAPTER 25 Acute Pancreatitis in Dogs

Harry Cridge

Department of Small Animal Clinical Sciences, College of Veterinary Medicine, Michigan State University, East Lansing, MI, USA

KEY POINTS

- Underlying risk factors for pancreatitis should be investigated in each dog, particularly when recurrent disease is noted.
- Diagnosis of pancreatitis is based on an overall clinical assessment, including integration of data from the dog's history, physical examination, bloodwork (including pancreatic lipase), and imaging. An incomplete clinical diagnosis may result in a misdiagnosis.
- Treatment of pancreatitis is based on five pillars, (i) analgesia, (ii) anti-emetics, (iii) fluid therapy, (iv) nutrition, and (v) targeted therapeutics (e.g., fuzapladib sodium).

INTRODUCTION

Pancreatitis is the most common disorder of the exocrine pancreas in dogs and includes both acute and chronic forms. Traditionally, the disorder was defined histopathologically; however, limitations associated with the cost, invasiveness, and anesthetic stability of patients have prevented the routine use of biopsies in clinical practice. Given this, acute pancreatitis (AP) and chronic pancreatitis (CP) are often defined clinically (Cridge et al. 2021).AP is taken to represent dogs with a rapid onset of severe clinical signs. In contrast, CP is typically taken to represent more long-standing or waxing-and-waning forms of mild disease. It is important to note, however, that acute on CP is common.

While Miniature Schnauzers and terrier breeds are predisposed to pancreatitis, any dog can go on to develop the disease. Increasing frequency of diagnosis is noted when an animal reaches middle to older age.

ETIOLOGY AND RISK FACTORS

The etiology of pancreatitis is complex and poorly understood, with most of our understanding originating from experimental models (non-canine species) and observations in clinical disease. Ultimately for a dog to develop pancreatitis, it needs to have an underlying risk factor, an inciting cause, or a combination of both. These overcome the bodies local defense mechanisms and trigger a sequence of steps ("acinar events") that occur inside the pancreatic acinar cells, such as co-localization, where inactive digestive enzymes (zymogens) come together with lysosomes triggering their premature activation. These acinar events then trigger pancreatic inflammation and necrosis, the degree of which likely determines whether a dog develops clinically evident disease and its severity (Cridge et al. 2022a).

Most cases of pancreatitis in dogs are thought to be idiopathic; however, this is likely due to the limited evaluation for underlying causes that takes place in most clinical cases. Indeed, many risk factors for pancreatitis have been proposed (see Table 25.1).

Evaluating for these risk factors is important, particularly, in dogs with recurrent disease. Thus, the author recommends that "repeat offenders" not only have the original diagnosis confirmed but

Disorders of the Liver, Exocrine Pancreas, and Gastrointestinal Tract in Dogs and Cats, First Edition. Edited by Harry Cridge et al. Published 2026 by John Wiley & Sons, Inc. Companion Website: www.wiley.com/go/cridge/disorders

Table 25.1 Potential Risk Factors for Pancreatitis

Category	Potential risk factors
Diet	High-fat diet
	Ingestion of food human/table scraps
	Ingestion of trash/unusual food items
Endocrinopathies	Cushing's disease
	Diabetes mellitus
	Hypothyroidism
Lipid disorders	Hypertriglyceridemia (primary or secondary)
Drugs/toxins	Phenobarbital
	Potassium bromide
	Others: L-asparaginase, azathioprine, TMS, organophosphates, furosemide, zinc, clomipramine, meglumine, atovaquone/proguanil

Note: Additional risk factors are possible (e.g., hypercalcemia, obesity, etc.), but the most common/most investigated are listed in Table 25.1. *Source*: Adapted from Cridge et al. (2022a); Cridge et al. (2022b).

also have screening for dietary and drug factors, endocrinopathies, hypertriglyceridemia (often not included on a routine chemistry), and hypercalcemia, to identify an underlying risk factor, where possible.

CLINICAL DIAGNOSIS OF AP

CLINICAL SIGNS AND PHYSICAL EXAMINATION FINDINGS

The clinical presentation of pancreatitis is broad (Cridge et al. 2022b). Dogs with clinically severe disease often present with significant vomiting, dehydration, and cranial abdominal pain (Hess et al. 1998). Cranial abdominal pain may be evidenced by the so-called "prayer-posture" (Figure 25.1). However, dogs with more mild-to-moderate disease, or with acute on chronic flare ups, often present with more subtle clinical signs such as inappetence, lethargy, or nausea (Cridge et al. 2022b). Other possible clinical signs include diarrhea, weight loss, polyuria/polydipsia, respiratory compromise, borborygmi, and trembling (Cridge et al. 2022b).

Given the broad clinical spectrum of pancreatitis, it is important to maintain pancreatitis on the list of differential diagnoses for any dog with gastrointestinal upset or nonspecific lethargy and inappetence.

ROUTINE BLOODWORK

It is recommended to perform a minimum database (complete blood count [CBC], serum chemistry including triglycerides, and urinalysis) in all dogs with suspected pancreatitis. This is because of the broad and nonspecific clinical signs of the disease and the need to rule out alternative differential diagnoses.

The CBC may reveal dehydration (increased packed cell volume and total protein), a left shift in neutrophils, and potentially thrombocytopenia. Thrombocytopenia is typically mild and due to consumption or challenging blood draw (spurious), but severe thrombocytopenia may represent disseminated intravascular coagulation.

The serum chemistry may reveal azotemia (prerenal > renal), mild hypoalbuminemia (negative acute phase protein, although this is often masked by concurrent dehydration), and potentially hyperbilirubinemia (concerning for potential extrahepatic bile duct obstruction). Regional inflammation, portal drainage of the pancreas, and cholestasis may result in mild-to-moderate

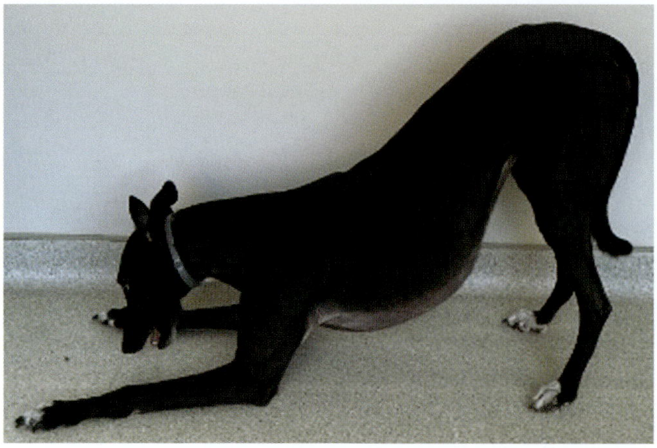

FIGURE 25.1 A 4-year-old female spayed Greyhound demonstrates the "prayer-posture" characteristic for cranial abdominal pain. Photo by Harry Cridge

increases in liver enzyme activities, with alkaline phosphatase (ALP) activity usually greater than alanine aminotransferase (ALT) activity. These biochemical changes are nonspecific and are also seen in other differential diagnoses for pancreatitis. Thus, a minimum database alone cannot diagnosis pancreatitis. Serum electrolytes should be measured and may warrant supplementation (i.e., hypokalemia) alongside intravenous fluid therapy.

Serum triglycerides are not included on many routine biochemical profiles; however, measurement of fasting triglyceride status is of critical importance in cases of pancreatitis. As marked hypertriglyceridemia (>600–800 mg/dL) can predispose to pancreatitis (Xenoulis et al. 2010).A urine sample should be collected upon initial presentation to allow for measurement of pre-rehydration urine specific gravity (USG). A USG >1.030 in conjunction with dehydration, may represent a prerenal azotemia, in contrast isosthenuria (1.008–1.012) may represent acute kidney injury.

PANCREATIC LIPASE TESTING

In health <99% of pancreatic lipase enters the systemic circulation. Therefore, detection of significant amounts of pancreatic lipase in the bloodstream is indicative of pancreatic acinar cell damage, most commonly due to pancreatitis. Given this, pancreatic lipase is one of the few biochemical parameters specific to exocrine pancreatic damage, and therefore it has gained a significant role in the diagnostic approach to suspected pancreatitis cases. This contrasts with nonspecific lipase and amylase, which are poorly sensitive or specific for the diagnosis of pancreatitis

Many different commercial pancreatic lipase assays exist, but they are broadly broken down into catalytic and immunological assays. Catalytic assays (e.g., DGGR Lipase/Precision PSL/Catalyst PL) measure lipase activity using an enzymatic reaction. In contrast, immunologic assays (e.g., Spec cPL/VetScan cPL/Vcheck cPL) measure lipase concentration via the specific binding of an antibody to pancreatic lipase (Lim et al. 2022). Because several lipases are structurally similar, catalytic assays may detect extrapancreatic lipases (Lim et al. 2022; Lim et al. 2020). It is important to enquire about the analytical specificity of a catalytic assay prior to use, as it is thought to vary between manufactures, even when the same substrate (e.g., DGGR) is used. All assays should be analytically and clinically validated prior to routine clinical use.

Elevated pancreatic lipase assay concentration/activity can also be seen in dogs with secondary pancreatic injury, thus necessitating integration of lipase data with imaging to ensure that the veterinarian has identified and is treating the most significant disease first.

For a more comprehensive assessment of pancreatic lipase assays please see "Chapter 21."

DIAGNOSTIC IMAGING

Diagnostic imaging is an integral component of the diagnostic approach to dogs with suspected pancreatitis. It plays two predominant roles (i) to rule out other differential diagnoses with similar clinical signs, and (ii) to help confirm a diagnosis of pancreatitis as part of an overall clinical assessment.

The dual role of imaging means that imaging modalities such as abdominal X-rays, which aren't sensitive or specific for pancreatitis, still maintain a crucial role in the diagnostic approach to these patients. Abdominal radiographs are readily available and provide an important tool to help rule out gastrointestinal obstructions/foreign bodies, which may require surgical management. Potential abnormalities that can be seen on radiographs in cases of pancreatitis include loss of serosal detail in the cranial abdomen (due to peritoneal fluid), an increased pyloroduodenal angle, and mild gas dilation in the duodenum (Hess et al. 1998), but these are not sensitive or specific for a diagnosis of pancreatitis.

Abdominal ultrasound is generally accepted to be the imaging modality of choice for dogs with suspected pancreatitis. Ultrasonographic findings reflect the presence of pancreatic edema that develops in pancreatitis. Thus, the pancreas becomes enlarged and hypoechoic and is often surrounded by a bright (hyperechoic) mesentery. The greater the number of sonographic abnormalities, the greater the diagnostic specificity for pancreatitis (Cridge et al. 2020). Regional inflammation may also cause gastric or duodenal thickening, which typically resolves with time (Murakami et al. 2019; Hardwick et al. 2022). Other changes may include evidence of extrahepatic bile duct obstruction (intrahepatic and bile duct dilation), ascites, and ileus. If free fluid is noted on abdominal ultrasound, it should be sampled, where possible and safe (i.e., no thrombocytopenia), to rule out septic processes or bile peritonitis.

Importantly there can be discrepant results noted between abdominal ultrasound and pancreatic lipase testing. This can be frustrating for clinicians but can be easily explained by the different timelines for onset and resolution of lipase and ultrasound abnormalities after onset of pancreatitis. Pancreatic lipase has a short half-life and likely reflects current disease status; in contrast, ultrasonographic evidence of pancreatitis can persist well after resolution of clinical and biochemical abnormalities (Mitchell et al. 2024). Therefore, when discrepant results are noted, repeating each modality may provide additional insight into disease onset or resolution.

Computed tomography (CT) may be used in some practices when gas-shadowing precludes evaluation of the pancreas or when a portal vein thrombus is suspected (French et al. 2019).

For a more comprehensive overview of diagnostic imaging for dogs with suspected pancreatitis please see "Chapter 22."

ADDITIONAL COMMENTS

As mentioned previously, histopathology is rarely indicated in the diagnostic approach to AP. Indeed, the multifocal nature of pancreatic inflammation can make pancreatic biopsies hard to interpret even when they are performed (Cridge et al. 2021; Newman et al. 2004). Histopathology is only considered by the author when an abdominal exploration is being performed for another reason or when neoplasia or pancreatic abscess (as part of surgical resection) is highly suspected. Cytology may be a suitable alternative to biopsies, but additional studies are needed to determine the degree of diagnostic agreement between pancreatic cytology and histopathology.

FIVE PILLARS OF AP TREATMENT

ANALGESIA

All dogs with pancreatitis should be considered to have a component of abdominal pain, even when it is not overtly evident on physical examination. Opioids are considered the analgesic of choice for pancreatitis, with full mu agonists (e.g., fentanyl, methadone) considered for severe pain, and other opioids (e.g., buprenorphine) considered for more mild disease. The use of lidocaine and ketamine continuous rate infusions may provide additional analgesia in markedly painful dogs and may reduce opioid requirement.

If a dog suddenly becomes more painful on abdominal palpation, it is important to repeat abdominal imaging to evaluate for complications such as peripancreatic fluid accumulations or thrombus formation or presence of concurrent disease.

Oral analgesics for pancreatitis are currently limited, and many clinicians provide gabapentin as an outpatient analgesic. Additional studies are needed to optimize outpatient pain management in AP. Nonsteroidal anti-inflammatory drugs are considered contraindicated due to renal and gastrointestinal adverse effects.

ANTI-EMETICS

Maropitant citrate (Cerenia®) and ondansetron (Zofran®) are commonly utilized either alone or in combination for the management of vomiting and nausea associated with pancreatitis. Adequate anti-emetics are crucial to not only control the clinical signs of disease but also to increase the chances of an animal returning to voluntary food intake.

FLUID THERAPY

Fluid therapy is important to correct dehydration and maintain pancreatic perfusion. It is the author's opinion that there is often a focus on aggressive fluid rehydration in dogs with pancreatitis, which can sometimes lead to overhydration. Indeed, in human medicine more "moderate" fluid therapy protocols are now preferred over more "aggressive" fluid resuscitation (de-Madaria et al. 2022). Fluid therapy should be adjusted to the individual dogs' needs based on their level of dehydration and ongoing losses. Frequent changes in fluid rates are often needed during hospitalization to adapt to the dogs' changing needs.

Moderate-to-severe dehydration requires inpatient management and intravenous fluid therapy, whereas more mild cases can be managed with subcutaneous fluids on an outpatient basis. Significant electrolyte derangements (i.e., marked hypokalemia) should also be corrected alongside fluid therapy.

NUTRITION

The role of nutrition in pancreatitis has significantly evolved over the past several years. Traditionally, it was recommended to rest the pancreas to avoid pancreatic stimulation; however, we now know that the principles that underpinned the "rest-the-gut" hypothesis are of reduced relevance in clinical disease. We now also know that withholding nutrition can have negative effects on enterocytes and the gut-barrier function in experimental models, and that early enteral nutrition is well tolerated in both dogs and cats with pancreatitis (Mansfield et al. 2011; Klaus et al. 2009). Therefore, early enteral feeding is strongly encouraged in cases of pancreatitis.

The duration of inappetence prior to hospitalization can assist a clinician in determining whether supportive care and appetite stimulation may be a suitable therapeutic plan or whether placement of a feeding tube is indicated (typically when >3 days of inappetence has been noted). Warming food, utilizing multiple flavors and textures of foods, hand feeding, and control of nausea can all promote voluntary food intake. If a feeding tube is required, the author prefers nasogastric (or nasoesophageal) tubes over esophageal feeding tubes as they can be placed noninvasively and under brief sedation. Feeding tube placement should be confirmed via radiographs prior to use.

It is common practice to start feeding at one-fourth to one-third of the dog's resting energy requirement (RER) and to slowly titrate the number of kcal per day up to a maximum of 100% RER over a period of several days. RER (kcal/day) = 70 × body weight (kg)$^{0.75}$. Enteral feedings should be spaced out and initially provide no more than 5–10 mL/kg of body weight at a time.

Low-fat gastrointestinal diets are often initiated as the preferred nutritional source. Low-fat diets should be continued long-term when hypertriglyceridemia (particularly >600–800 mg/dL) is present or when recurrent bouts of pancreatitis are observed. If a prescription low-fat diet is cost prohibitive to the owner, or where concurrent disease necessitates nutritional prioritization, alternate diets may be fed, while still avoiding high-fat diets, provided the owner is aware of the potential relationship between dietary fat content and potential risk for development of pancreatitis.

TARGETED THERAPEUTICS

Fuzapladib sodium (Panoquell-CA1) is a novel therapeutic that has been shown to improve the clinical signs associated with the acute onset of pancreatitis in dogs (Steiner et al. 2023). The drug works by inhibiting activation of leukocyte function-associated antigen 1 (LFA-1), thereby reducing the extravasation of neutrophils into the tissues and thus reducing inflammation. More data may help to determine the optimal usage of this drug and aid in case selection, but at this time the author uses this drug where financially feasible. The medication is currently available in Japan and the United States and is given intravenously q24h for three days.

CONFLICT OF INTEREST

Dr. Cridge receives speaker honoraria and research support from CEVA Animal Health, who market and distribute fuzapladib sodium (Panoquell-CA1) within the United States.

REFERENCES

Cook, A.K., Breitschwerdt, E.B., Levine, J.F. et al. (1993). Risk factors associated with acute pancreatitis in dogs: 101 cases (1985–1990). *Journal of the American Veterinary Medical Association* 203: 673–679.

Cridge, H., Lim, S.Y., Algul, H. et al. (2022a). New insights into the etiology, risk factors, and pathogenesis of pancreatitis in dogs: potential impacts on clinical practice. *Journal of Veterinary Internal Medicine* 36: 847–864.

Cridge, H., Scott, N., and Steiner, J.M. (2022b). Risk factors and clinical presentation in dogs with increased serum pancreatic lipase concentrations-a descriptive analysis. *Animals (Basel)* 12 (12): 1581.

Cridge, H., Sullivant, A.M., Wills, R.W. et al. (2020). Association between abdominal ultrasound findings, the specific canine pancreatic lipase assay, clinical severity indices, and clinical diagnosis in dogs with pancreatitis. *Journal of Veterinary Internal Medicine* 34: 636–643.

Cridge, H., Twedt, D.C., Marolf, A.J. et al. (2021). Advances in the diagnosis of acute pancreatitis in dogs. *Journal of Veterinary Internal Medicine* 35: 2572–2587.

de-Madaria, E., Buxbaum, J.L., Maisonneuve, P. et al. (2022). Aggressive or moderate fluid resuscitation in acute pancreatitis. *New England Journal of Medicine* 387: 989–1000.

French, J.M., Twedt, D.C., Rao, S. et al. (2019). Computed tomographic angiography and ultrasonography in the diagnosis and evaluation of acute pancreatitis in dogs. *Journal of Veterinary Internal Medicine* 33: 79–88.

Hardwick, J.J., Reeve, E.J., Hezzell, M.J. et al. (2022). Prevalence of ultrasonographic gastrointestinal wall changes in dogs with acute pancreatitis: a retrospective study (2012–2020). *Journal of Veterinary Internal Medicine* 36: 947–956.

Hess, R.S., Saunders, H.M., Van Winkle, T.J. et al. (1998). Clinical, clinicopathologic, radiographic, and ultrasonographic abnormalities in dogs with fatal acute pancreatitis: 70 cases (1986–1995). *Journal of the American Veterinary Medical Association* 213: 665–670.

Klaus, J.A., Rudloff, E., and Kirby, R. (2009). Nasogastric tube feeding in cats with suspected acute pancreatitis: 55 cases (2001–2006). *Journal of Veterinary Emergency and Critical Care (San Antonio)* 19: 337–346.

Lim, S.Y., Steiner, J.M., and Cridge, H. (2022). Understanding lipase assays in the diagnosis of pancreatitis in veterinary medicine. *Journal of the American Veterinary Medical Association* 260: 1249–1258.

Lim, S.Y., Xenoulis, P.G., Stavroulaki, E.M. et al. (2020). The 1,2-o-dilauryl-rac-glycero-3-glutaric acid-(6'-methylresorufin) ester (DGGR) lipase assay in cats and dogs is not specific for pancreatic lipase. *Veterinary Clinical Pathology* 49: 607–613.

Mansfield, C.S., James, F.E., Steiner, J.M. et al. (2011). A pilot study to assess tolerability of early enteral nutrition via esophagostomy tube feeding in dogs with severe acute pancreatitis. *Journal of Veterinary Internal Medicine* 25: 419–425.

Mitchell, L., Wang, S., Lawver, J. et al. (2024). Serial monitoring of pancreatic lipase immunoreactivity, C-reactive protein, abdominal ultrasonography, and clinical severity in dogs with suspected pancreatitis. *Journal of Veterinary Internal Medicine* 38: 987–994.

Murakami, M., Heng, H.G., Lim, C.K. et al. (2019). Ultrasonographic features of presumed gastric wall edema in 14 dogs with pancreatitis. *Journal of Veterinary Internal Medicine* 33: 1260–1265.

Newman, S., Steiner, J., Woosley, K. et al. (2004). Localization of pancreatic inflammation and necrosis in dogs. *Journal of Veterinary Internal Medicine* 18: 488–493.

Steiner, J.M., Lainesse, C., Noshiro, Y. et al. (2023). Fuzapladib in a randomized controlled multicenter masked study in dogs with presumptive acute onset pancreatitis. *Journal of Veterinary Internal Medicine* 37 (6): 2084–2092.

Xenoulis, P.G., Suchodolski, J.S., Ruaux, C.G. et al. (2010). Association between serum triglyceride and canine pancreatic lipase immunoreactivity concentrations in miniature schnauzers. *Journal of Veterinary Internal Medicine* 46: 229–234.

Chronic Pancreatitis in Dogs

CHAPTER 26

Penny Watson

Emeritus Fellow – Emmanuel College, University of Cambridge, Cambridge, UK

KEY POINTS

- Chronic pancreatitis (CP) is a common condition in dogs which is under-recognized because of nonspecific clinical signs and low sensitivity of noninvasive diagnostic tests.
- CP can have a significant impact on the quality of life of affected dogs causing chronic pain. Treatment is focused on a low-fat diet, analgesia, and management of any exocrine or endocrine insufficiency that develops.
- A subset of dogs with CP, particularly English Cocker Spaniels, suffer from an autoimmune disease, which also affects tear ducts, salivary ducts, kidneys, and anal sacs and may respond to immunosuppressive medication.

INTRODUCTION

Chronic pancreatitis (CP) is common, yet it's rarely diagnosed, due to nonspecific signs and the poor performance of available tests. Nonetheless, CP significantly effects quality of life and increased awareness is important to facilitate treatment.

CP is a continuing inflammatory disease characterized by pancreatic parenchyma destruction, leading to pain and progressive impairment of exocrine and/or endocrine function (Etemad and Whitcomb 2001). The gold standard for diagnosis of CP in humans is histological. However, most dogs (and humans) do not have biopsies performed, as it's invasive, doesn't change treatment, and it isn't indicated unless neoplasia is suspected.

PREVALENCE, SIGNALMENT, AND CAUSES

Postmortem studies reveal a high prevalence of CP in dogs of 34–70% (Newman et al. 2004; Watson et al. 2007). While the higher figure is likely an overestimation for general practice, CP is clearly common. In addition, up to 40% of dogs presenting with fatal acute pancreatitis have underlying chronic changes on histology (Hess et al. 1998). The cause of CP in most dogs is unknown. An autoimmune disease has been identified in English cocker spaniels (ECSs) which may also affect other breeds. This is similar to IgG4-related disease in humans and is characterized by immune-mediated attack on pancreatic ducts and ≥1 of tear ducts, kidneys (causing protein-losing nephropathy [PLN]), salivary glands, and anal sacs. The bile duct is rarely affected in dogs (Coddou et al. 2020, 2024).

SIGNALMENT

Any age or breed of dog can be affected, but diagnosis is more common in middle-aged to older dogs. In the United States, dogs of non-sporting/toy breeds are most affected with Labradors, boxers, collies, and miniature schnauzers overrepresented. Median reported body weight is 19.3 kg

Disorders of the Liver, Exocrine Pancreas, and Gastrointestinal Tract in Dogs and Cats, First Edition. Edited by Harry Cridge et al. Published 2026 by John Wiley & Sons, Inc. Companion Website: www.wiley.com/go/cridge/disorders

(Bostrom et al. 2013). Boxers and collies are overrepresented in the United Kingdom, where spaniel breeds also have a high prevalence, particularly ECS and cavalier king Charles spaniels (Watson et al. 2007, 2011).

DIAGNOSIS

CLINICAL PRESENTATION

The symptomatology of CP is nonspecific. Dogs with low-grade disease show waxing and waning mild-to-moderate gastrointestinal (GI) signs, lethargy, and abdominal pain (Watson et al. 2010). Typically, the owner describes episodes of anorexia and depression with or without vomiting. Diarrhea may occur, usually 1–2 days after the beginning of an episode, or more consistently if exocrine pancreatic insufficiency (EPI) is developing. Hematochezia is common. In the author's experience, abdominal pain, particularly post prandially, is frequent, with owners and veterinarians underestimating subtle signs such as stretching after eating or increased sleeping. Pain has a low prevalence, but lethargy is commonly seen in retrospective studies (Bostrom et al. 2013; Kuzi et al. 2023) likely due to an underestimation of the behavioral effects of chronic pain. Analgesic trials are utilized to unmask behavioral signs of pain. Some dogs with CP present with polydipsia/polyuria (PU/PD), which may be a response to abdominal pain/nausea. Dogs with acute-on-chronic disease show signs which are very similar to acute pancreatitis.

Differential diagnoses for mild cases include chronic enteropathy (CE), hypoadrenocorticism, or low-grade hepatic or renal disease. Some dogs present with concurrent diabetes mellitus (DM) and/or EPI. A dog with DM and EPI likely has end stage CP.

On examination, dogs with low-grade CP show few signs apart from focal pain on meticulous cranioventral abdominal palpation. There may be weight loss, poor body condition, or a dry coat consistent with EPI. ECSs with CP should be assessed for keratoconjunctivitis sicca (KCS), dry mouth (in the absence of dehydration), and anal sac disease. Blood pressure measurement is wise in ECSs as hypertension is common with their PLN.

CLINICAL PATHOLOGY

Once CP is suspected, diagnosis is made presumptively based on pancreas-specific blood tests and abdominal ultrasound, together with ruling out other differentials. Unfortunately, both clinical pathology and imaging have lower sensitivities for CP when compared with acute disease, likely due to loss of tissue and a relative lack of inflammation and edema.

Canine pancreatic-specific lipase (cPLI) likely has the highest sensitivity and specificity for CP, although published studies of small numbers of dogs with histological disease show only a sensitivity of 42–58% (Watson et al. 2010; Goodband et al. 2018). The latter study suggested DGGR lipase had a similar sensitivity for CP (57%).

It is important to perform a full complete blood count (CBC) biochemistry, and urinalysis in affected dogs. There may be primary (autoimmune) or secondary renal compromise and liver enzymes, and bilirubin may be elevated. It is not uncommon for acute-on-chronic pancreatitis to result in transient extrahepatic biliary tract obstruction. On CBC, neutrophilia and anemia of chronic disease are common. Urine should be checked for glucosuria, proteinuria, and specific gravity. If EPI is suspected, trypsin-like immunoreactivity (TLI) should be measured, but this can be falsely elevated to within the reference interval (RI) during bouts of pancreatic inflammation (Watson et al. 2010). It is best measured when the dog is clinically stable. Serum cobalamin should be measured due to potential lack of intrinsic factor.

DIAGNOSTIC IMAGING

Radiographs are of limited utility in CP, except for ruling out intestinal obstruction in acute-on-chronic presentations. Pancreatic ultrasound has a high specificity but low sensitivity for CP. One study revealed a sensitivity of 56% for finding pancreatic abnormalities on ultrasound (Watson et al. 2010). Findings vary from a normal pancreas to hyper- or hypoechoic. Inflammatory mass lesions (which can mimic neoplasia) may be found in ECSs, and adhesions may alter the anatomic relationship to the duodenum (Watson et al. 2011).

HISTOLOGY

Pancreatic biopsies should be avoided unless there is a suspicion of neoplasia due to their invasiveness and the potential (albeit low) for complications (Pratschke et al. 2014). If a laparotomy is performed for another reason, the pancreas should be examined visually and biopsies may be taken from the tip of lobe(s), particularly if the pancreas is grossly abnormal.

OVERALL CRITERIA FOR DIAGNOSIS OF CP

In conclusion, if a dog has repeated episodes of compatible clinical signs, elevated pancreas-specific enzymes and an abnormal pancreatic ultrasound, presumptive CP can be diagnosed with a high degree of suspicion. In an ECS, these findings combined with KCS and proteinuria gives a high degree of suspicion of autoimmune pancreatitis, and invasive biopsies are not justified to confirm this.

TREATMENT

Treatment of CP is supportive and symptomatic, with immunosuppression in suspected autoimmune cases. Dogs with acute-on-chronic episodes are treated as for acute pancreatitis (Chapter 25). Emergency management is unaffected by underlying disease chronicity. Awareness of possible underlying CP, however, affects long-term management including identifying developing EPI and/or DM.

For dogs with low-grade, chronic disease and for long-term management after an acute crisis, treatment focuses on analgesia, diet, and management of exocrine and/or endocrine insufficiency.

ANALGESIA AND DIET

Chronic pain is a significant factor for many dogs. Feeding a low-fat diet may reduce post-prandial pain, but many dogs require intermittent or long-term analgesia. It is helpful to consider treatment using a "pain pyramid" approach (Figure 26.1). Finding effective oral analgesics for long-term use can be challenging. Classical nonsteroidal anti-inflammatory drugs are not advisable due to the risk of concurrent GI inflammation and renal disease. The author commences with oral acetaminophen at 15 mg/kg PO q8h. This analgesic is commonly used in the United Kingdom, where there is an oral preparation licensed for dogs (Bello and Dye 2023). The pharmacokinetics in dogs are well understood and it appears safe although its use should be avoided in liver disease, and it should never be used in cats. Toxic doses are reported to be >150 mg/kg (Hjelle and Grauer 1986). Codeine is combined with acetaminophen in the UK canine formulation and some human drugs.

Oral acetaminophen alone is unlikely to be sufficient in all but the mildest cases and transmucosal buprenorphine could be added for flare-ups. Other drugs to consider are detailed in Figure 26.1. Drugs should be added incrementally and then removed, if possible, as pain lessens. The owner is crucial in documenting responses to analgesia using validated canine chronic pain measures (Self 2024; Mathews et al. 2014).

TREATMENT OF SUSPECTED AUTOIMMUNE CP

ECSs and other dogs with suspected IgG4-RD should be treated symptomatically together with topical cyclosporine for KCS and treatment for proteinuria and hypertension with angiotensin-converting enzyme inhibitors or receptor blockers. If symptomatic treatment is not effective in controlling proteinuria or recurrent bouts of pancreatitis, consideration should be given to trial treatment with immunosuppression (prednisolone or cyclosporine). The author favors cyclosporine in dogs with proteinuria. Immunosuppression is effective in humans, but there is no published efficacy in dogs.

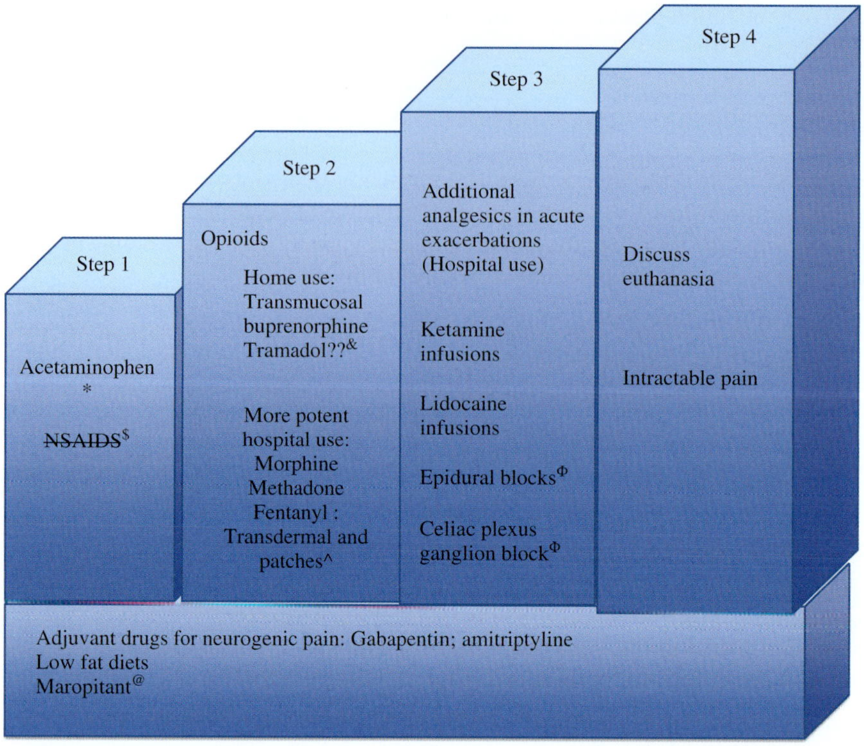

FIGURE 26.1 Analgesic ladder for dogs and cats with chronic pancreatitis (CP), based on the human analgesic ladder in Sebastiano et al. (2005), which is based on the World Health Organization analgesic ladder for cancer pain. (Reproduced from Watson (2018) with permission of John Wiley & Sons). Note each step in the ladder can be added to the previous step for multimodal analgesia. *Preferred non-opioid drug in dogs, provided liver function is normal. Not to be used in cats. $Nonsteroidal anti-inflammatories – higher risk of GI side effects in pancreatitis and only to be used when renal function is normal. Avoid in ECS with immune-mediated pancreatitis and proteinuria. &Efficacy of tramadol in dogs is very uncertain. Transmucosal buprenorphine would be preferred. ^Animals can be sent home with Fentanyl patches but great care must be taken about human contact particularly with children. @Substance P has been implicated in the neuropathic pain of CP, so maropitant may have a role in multimodal analgesia, although recent meta-analysis questioned this (Kinobe and Miyake, 2020). ᶲOnly to be administered by suitably trained individuals (Self 2024; Kinobe and Miyake 2020; and Sebastiano et al. 2005)

TREATMENT OF LONG-TERM SEQUELAE: EPI AND DM

Dogs with CP should be assessed for signs of EPI and given pancreatic enzymes as necessary. Evidence suggests that dogs, like humans, are diagnosed with CP late in the course of disease after a prolonged subclinical period, where exocrine function is already compromised. It is therefore wise to take a proactive approach, supplementing enzymes in most cases (and certainly dogs with weight loss, steatorrhea, or poor coat quality), even if TLI is normal. This mimics advice in people where enzyme supplementation is started when CP is diagnosed. Cobalamin should be supplemented as necessary.

Dogs developing DM secondary to CP should receive standard treatment for DM. Advice specific to end stage CP is to avoid high fiber diabetic diets, many of which are calorie restricted and thus not applicable to dogs with incipient exocrine insufficiency. A manufactured low-fat diet is appropriate in these cases. If enzymes are added to food after treatment for DM has commenced, the insulin dose will likely need to be increased due to more efficient digestion. Dogs with CP do not appear to have a worse outcome than other diabetic dogs.

REFERENCES

Bello, A.M. and Dye, C. (2023). Current perceptions and use of paracetamol in dogs among veterinary surgeons working in the United Kingdom. *Veterinary Medicine and Science* 9 (2): 679–686. https://doi.org/10.1002/vms3.1058.

Bostrom, B.M., Xenoulis, P.G., Newman, S.J.et al. (2013). Chronic pancreatitis in dogs: a retrospective study of clinical, clinicopathological, and histopathological findings in 61 cases. *The Veterinary Journal* 195 (1): 73–79. https://doi.org/10.1016/j.tvjl.2012.06.034.

Coddou, M.F., Blacklaws, B., and Watson, P.J. (2024). Clinical manifestations of chronic pancreatitis in English cocker spaniels. *Journal of Veterinary Internal Medicine* 38 (4): 2129–2137. https://doi.org/10.1111/jvim.17100.

Coddou, M.F., Constantino-Casas, F., Scase, T. et al. (2020). Chronic inflammatory disease in the pancreas, kidney and salivary glands of English cocker spaniels and dogs of other breeds shows similar histological features to human IgG4-related disease. *Journal of Comparative Pathology* 177: 18–33. https://doi.org/10.1016/j.jcpa.2020.03.008.

Etemad, B., and Whitcomb, D.C. (2001). Chronic pancreatitis: diagnosis, classification, and new genetic developments. *Gastroenterology* 120 (3): 682–707. https://doi.org/10.1053/gast.2001.22586.

Goodband, E.L., Serrano, G., Constantino-Casas, F. et al. (2018). Validation of a commercial 1,2-o-dilauryl-rac-glycero glutaric acid-(6'-methylresorufin) ester lipase assay for diagnosis of canine pancreatitis. *Veterinary Record Open* 5 (1): e000270–e000275. https://doi.org/10.1136/vetreco-2017-000270.

Hess, R.S., Saunders, H.M., Van Winkle, T.J. et al. (1998). Clinical, clinicopathologic, radiographic, and ultrasonographic abnormalities in dogs with fatal acute pancreatitis: 70 cases (1986–1995). *Journal of the American Veterinary Medical Association* 213 (5): 665–670.

Hjelle, J.J. and Grauer, G.F. (1986). Acetaminophen-induced toxicosis in dogs and cats. *Journal of the American Veterinary Medical Association* 188 (7): 742–746.

Kinobe, R.T. and Miyake, Y. (2020). Evaluating the anti-inflammatory and analgesic properties of maropitant: a systematic review and meta-analysis. *The Veterinary Journal* 259: 105471. https://doi.org/10.1016/j.tvjl.2020.105471.

Kuzi, S., Adlersberg, D., Aroch, I. et al. (2023). Utility of 1,2-o-dilauryl-rac-glycero glutaric acid-(6′-methylresorufin)-ester-lipase for monitoring dogs with chronic pancreatitis. *Journal of Veterinary Internal Medicine* 37 (2): 437–445. https://doi.org/10.1111/jvim.16638.

Mathews, K., Kronen, P.W., Lascelles, D. et al. (2014). Guidelines for recognition, assessment and treatment of pain. *Journal of Small Animal Practice* 55 (6): E10–E68. https://doi.org/10.1111/jsap.12200.

Newman, S., Steiner, J., Woosley, K. et al. (2004). Localization of pancreatic inflammation and necrosis in dogs. *Journal of Veterinary Internal Medicine* 18 (4): 488–493.

Pratschke, K.M., Ryan, J., McAlinden, A. et al. (2014). Pancreatic surgical biopsy in 24 dogs and 19 cats: postoperative complications and clinical relevance of histological findings. *Journal of Small Animal Practice* 56 (1): 60–66. https://doi.org/10.1111/jsap.12262.

Sebastiano, P.D., Weigand, M.A., Köninger, J. et al. (2005). Conservative treatment of pain in chronic pancreatitis: guidelines for clinical routine. In: *Clinical Pancreatology for Practising Gastroenterologists and Surgeons* (ed. J.E. Dominguez-Munoz), 273–279. Blackwell Publishing Malden Massachusetts.

Self, I. (2024). Analgesia in acute and chronic pancreatitis. In: *Canine Hepatobiliary and Exocrine Pancreatic Diseases. Veterinary Internal Medicine Series* (ed. P. Watson, Feldman, E.C., and Fracassi, F.), 139–141. Florida: Edra Publishing.

Watson, P.J., Archer, J., Roulois, A.J. et al. (2010). Observational study of 14 cases of chronic pancreatitis in dogs. *Veterinary Record* 167 (25): 968–976. https://doi.org/10.1136/vr.c4912.

Watson, P.J., Roulois, A.J.A., Scase, T. et al. (2007). Prevalence and breed distribution of chronic pancreatitis at post-mortem examination in first-opinion dogs. *Journal of Small Animal Practice* 48 (11): 609–618. https://doi.org/10.1111/j.1748-5827.2007.00448.x.

Watson, P.J., Roulois, A., Scase, T. et al. (2011). Characterization of chronic pancreatitis in English cocker spaniels. *Journal of Veterinary Internal Medicine* 25 (4): 797–804. https://doi.org/10.1111/j.1939-1676.2011.0744.x.

Watson, (2018). Chronic Pancreatitis. In: *Chronic Disease Management for Small Animals* (ed. W. Dunbar Gram, R.W. Milner, and R. Lobetti), 181–186. Hoboken: Wiley-Blackwell.

CHAPTER 27 Pancreatitis Complications

Melissa Bucknoff

Department of Small Animal Clinical Sciences, College of Veterinary Medicine, University of Florida, Gainesville, FL, USA

KEY POINTS

- Nonspecific supportive and symptomatic therapies are the mainstay of treatment, though more targeted therapies (e.g., leukocyte function-associated antigen (LFA-1) activation inhibitors) may be utilized in dogs to limit clinical signs associated with acute pancreatitis (AP).
- Recurrent AP may result in development of chronic pancreatitis (CP), which could lead to exocrine pancreatic insufficiency (EPI).
- Complications of pancreatitis include fluid accumulations, extrahepatic bile duct obstruction (EHBDO), ileus, and other systemic complications.
- Thromboprophylaxis should be considered in dogs and cats with severe AP particularly when multiple risk factors are present.

INTRODUCTION

Acute pancreatitis (AP) can be an unforgiving disease with clinical signs ranging from mild to severe. Stable patients can quickly destabilize and need to be monitored closely. In severe cases, acute abdominal signs are almost always present. Initial assessment focuses on hemodynamic stability and ruling out surgical disease (i.e., septic peritonitis). Treatment targets supportive/symptomatic care. Local and systemic complications contribute to morbidity and mortality. Clinicians should anticipate, promptly recognize, and manage complications accordingly (Table 27.1).

LOCAL COMPLICATIONS

Acute pancreatic necrosis is a feature in severe pancreatitis cases. Pancreatic blood flow alterations, intra-acinar trypsin activation, neutrophilic invasion, reactive oxygen species, and pancreatic infarcts contribute to pathologic necrosis (Cridge et al. 2022). Degree of necrosis correlates with more complications, systemic inflammatory response syndrome (SIRS), multiple organ dysfunction syndrome (MODS), and disseminated intravascular coagulation (DIC). More severe pancreatic necrosis can increase risk of thromboemboli locally and at distant sites.

Pancreatic fluid accumulations occur variably in cats and dogs, usually due to pseudocyst formation or walled-off necrosis. Sterile processes predominate, though ultrasound-guided fluid sampling is recommended to determine treatment. In dogs with AP-associated pancreatic fluid, aspiration was safe and uncomplicated in all cases (Talbot 2022). Septic fluid accumulations are uncommon but may be an indication for surgery. Medical management carries a better prognosis, especially in septic cases. Human medical evidence suggests pancreatic abscessation takes several weeks to develop following acute inflammation (Bittner et al. 1987). Incidence of pancreatitis-associated pancreatic abscessation in animals is currently unknown. Routine use of antibiotics is discouraged for pancreatitis, unless guided by cytological evidence, culture, and sensitivity testing.

Disorders of the Liver, Exocrine Pancreas, and Gastrointestinal Tract in Dogs and Cats, First Edition. Edited by Harry Cridge et al. Published 2026 by John Wiley & Sons, Inc. Companion Website: www.wiley.com/go/cridge/disorders

Table 27.1 Complications of Pancreatitis

Local	Systemic
Pancreatic necrosis	SIRS
Pancreatic fluid accumulations	MODS
Pancreatic abscess	DIC/thromboembolic complications
Pancreatitis-associated EHBDO	AKI
Regional thromboembolic disease	Cardiac injury
Gastrointestinal dysmotility	Aspiration pneumonitis/pneumonia
	ALI/ARDS
	Effusions
	GI bacterial translocation
	Ionized hypocalcemia
	Hyperglycemia

ALI, acute lung injury; *ARDS,* acute respiratory distress syndrome; *DIC,* disseminated intravascular coagulation; *EHBDO,* extrahepatic bile duct obstruction; *GI,* gastrointestinal; *MODS,* multiple organ dysfunction syndrome; *SIRS,* systemic inflammatory response syndrome.

Extrahepatic bile duct obstruction (EHBDO) can develop from pancreatic inflammation causing common bile duct compression. Medical management appears feasible in most dogs and survival is better without need for surgical or percutaneous gallbladder decompression (Lim et al. 2024). A feline study reported EHBDO as the most common indication for surgically managing severe AP and carried a good prognosis (Son et al. 2010). Short-term anti-inflammatory corticosteroids (prednisone/prednisolone: 1 mg/kg/day) may be beneficial for reducing inflammation and bile duct compression and may prevent the need for surgical decompression of the bile duct. However, if rupture is present or highly suspected surgery is indicated. Corticosteroid use must always be weighed heavily against risks.

Gastrointestinal ileus occurs due to pancreatic proximity and inflammation. Antiemetics and promotility agents are mainstays of supportive care. Opioid analgesics may worsen signs; however, it should also be noted that inadequate analgesia (pain relief) may also contribute to ileus. Therefore, dose escalation and de-escalation can be trialed in cases of gastrointestinal ileus secondary to pancreatitis. A multimodal approach prioritizing opioid-sparing techniques is advocated. Early enteral nutrition is recommended to reduce gastrointestinal complications.

SYSTEMIC COMPLICATIONS

Severe AP catalyzes SIRS and can progress to MODS. Organs with extensive capillary beds are most vulnerable (i.e. lung, liver, pancreas). Increased vascular permeability compromises subendothelial glycocalyx integrity resulting in vascular leak, tissue edema, and effusions. While potentially reversible, progressive organ dysfunction negatively impacts survival (Hackett 2011). Comorbid complications include HL, chronic enteropathy, renal disease, DM, and preexisting hepatobiliary inflammation (Forman et al. 2021). Treatment is tailored individually utilizing a body-systems approach to manage new organ dysfunction. The conditionally approved fuzapladib sodium for acute AP treatment in dogs is a novel LFA-1 activation inhibitor, preventing extravasation of neutrophils from capillary beds. Activated neutrophil extravasation into pancreatic and extrapancreatic tissues perpetuates inflammation (Spillman 2023). Sequelae, like acute respiratory distress syndrome (ARDS), occur partly by such mechanisms. Reducing inflammation severity may reduce morbidity and limit complications, although additional studies are needed to further investigate this hypothesis.

Coagulation derangement is well-documented with AP (Nielsen et al. 2019). Systemic inflammation activates coagulation leading to microthrombi and DIC, and consumptive coagulopathy may worsen prognosis in dogs (Fabrès et al. 2019). Pancreatitis is a risk factor for thrombosis in dogs and cats (Goggs et al. 2019). Thromboembolic complications can be devastating. Thromboemboli are often identified in multiple organs post-mortem. The left pancreatic lobe is closely associated with the splenic vein. Inflammation can alter flow, compress the vessel, and activate local endothelial cells causing global hypercoagulability. Splenic and/or portal vein thrombosis contribute to morbidity and length of hospitalization. Pulmonary thromboembolism (PTE) can cause respiratory distress, syncope, or sudden death. CT angiography is ideal for diagnosing PTE, though patient stability must be considered. Thromboprophylaxis should be considered in dogs with severe AP, especially in acute necrotizing cases, and cats with high risk for thrombosis (i.e. AP and sepsis or AP and cardiomegaly) (Goggs et al. 2019).

Ionized hypocalcemia is common, though hypercalcemia has been reported in dogs. Hypocalcemia is likely due to pancreatic/peripancreatic fat saponification, though other mechanisms may exist. Ionized hypocalcemia is a negative prognostic indicator in cats and possibly dogs (Fabrès et al. 2019). Calcium supplementation is often reserved for severe clinical cases (i.e. tetany, seizures) due to concern for exacerbating free radical production and cellular injury.

Acute kidney injury (AKI) due to a combination of hypovolemia, cytokine-induced ischemia, inflammation, and oxidative stress is frequent with AP (Gori et al. 2019). Creatinine and urine production should be closely monitored. Specific biomarkers of AKI may differentiate prerenal and renal azotemia and serve as early indicators in non-azotemic patients. Cystatin C is highly specific for proximal tubular injury and may be a better indicator of AKI in cats than dogs (de Oliveira Paes-Leme et al. 2021), though its utility in pancreatitis has yet to be investigated. Mortality rates are usually higher in patients that develop AKI. Management strategies include goal-directed fluid therapy and avoiding fluid overload. Renal replacement therapy may be considered in some cases.

Myocarditis is an underappreciated cardiovascular complication of AP. While not treated specifically, cardiac arrhythmias should be treated as indicated guided by continuous electrocardiography (ECG) monitoring. Echocardiography can identify altered myocardial contractility, guiding need for positive inotropic agents. Cardiac biomarkers (troponin I, N-terminal pro-B-type natriuretic peptide) have not correlated with degree of myocardial injury (Cridge et al. 2023).

Respiratory complications may arise due to ARDS, PTE, aspiration pneumonitis, or pneumonia. Vomiting, regurgitation, or profound sedation can lead to aspiration of sterile gastric contents. Antibiotics are not always indicated but may be required if aspiration pneumonia develops, particularly if gastric acid suppressants were administered (a neutral gastric pH increases the risk of viable bacterial populations being present in aspirated material secondary to vomiting). Three-view thoracic radiography and/or point-of-care ultrasound should be performed in patients with new respiratory signs or fever.

Transient hyperglycemia can occur, though sometimes diabetic ketoacidosis develops. Pancreatitis-associated insulin resistance or depletion may require short-term insulin therapy until returning to normoglycemia with clinical improvement. Some cases require long-term treatment.

CHRONIC PANCREATITIS

After surviving an AP episode, patients can return to normal or develop episodic flare-ups. No clinical test exists to predict if AP will result in CP, although risk factors may include breed disposition and comorbidities, such as DM, hyperlipidemia, HL, chronic enteropathy, and cholangitis/cholangiohepatitis. It is likely that recurrent episodes of acute or acute-on-chronic pancreatitis are underestimated in the literature due to limited long-term follow-up studies in pancreatitis patients.

Bittner, R., Block, S., Büchler, M. et al. (1987). Pancreatic abscess and infected pancreatic necrosis: different local septic complications in acute pancreatitis. *Digestive Diseases and Sciences* 32 (10): 1082–1087.

Cridge, H., Lim, S.Y., Algül, H. et al. (2022). New insights into the etiology, risk factors, and pathogenesis of pancreatitis in dogs: potential impacts on clinical practice. *Journal of Veterinary Internal Medicine* 36: 847–864.

Cridge, H., Langlois, D.K., Steiner, J.M. et al. (2023). Cardiovascular abnormalities in dogs with acute pancreatitis. *Journal of Veterinary Internal Medicine* 37 (1): 28–36.

de Oliveira Paes-Leme, F., Souza, E.M., Paes, P.R.O. et al. (2021). Cystatin C and IRIS: advances in the evaluation of kidney function in critically ill dogs. *Frontiers in Veterinary Science* 8: 1–5. https://doi.org/10.3389/fvets.2021.721845.

Fabrès, V., Dossin, O., Reif, C. et al. (2019). Development and validation of a novel clinical scoring system for short-term prediction of death in dogs with acute pancreatitis. *Journal of Veterinary Internal Medicine* 33: 499–507.

Forman, M.A., Steiner, J.M., Armstrong, P.J. et al. (2021). ACVIM consensus statement on pancreatitis in cats. *Journal of Veterinary Internal Medicine* 35: 703–723.

Goggs, R., Blais, M.C., Brainard, B.M. et al. (2019). American college of veterinary emergency and critical care (ACVECC) consensus on the rational use of antithrombotics in veterinary critical care (CURATIVE) guidelines: small animal. *Journal of Veterinary Emergency and Critical Care* 29: 12–36.

Gori, E., Lippi, I., Guidi, G. et al. (2019). Acute pancreatitis and acute kidney injury in dogs. *The Veterinary Journal* 245: 77–81.

Hackett, T.B. (2011). Introduction to multiple organ dysfunction and failure. *Veterinary Clinics of North America Small Animal Practice* 41 (4): 703–707.

Lim, S.Y., Cridge, H., Twedt, D.C. et al. (2024). Management of acute-onset pancreatitis in dogs: a narrative review. *Journal of the American Veterinary Association* 262 (9): 1231–1240.

Nielsen, L., Holm, J., Rozanski, E. et al. (2019). Multicenter investigation of hemostatic dysfunction in 15 dogs with acute pancreatitis. *Journal of Veterinary Emergency and Critical Care* 29 (3): 264–268.

Son, T.T., Thompson, L., Serrano, S. et al. (2010). Surgical intervention in the management of severe acute pancreatitis in cats: 8 cases (2003–2007). *Journal of Veterinary Emergency and Critical Care* 20 (4): 426–435.

Spillman, T. (2023). Pancreatitis: etiology, pathogenesis, and pathophysiologic consequences. In: *Textbook of Veterinary Internal Medicine* (ed. S.J. Ettinger, E.C. Feldman, and E. Cote), 1859–1861. St. Louis: Elsevier.

Talbot, C.T. (2022). Medical and surgical management of pancreatic fluid accumulations in dogs: a retrospective study of 15 cases. *Journal of Veterinary Internal Medicine* 36: 919–926.

CHAPTER 28 Pancreatitis in Cats

Betty Chow[1] *and Marnin Forman*[2]

[1] *VCA Animal Specialty and Emergency Center, Los Angeles, CA, USA*
[2] *Cornell University Veterinary Specialists, Stamford, CT, USA*

KEY POINTS

- Chronic pancreatitis (CP) in cats is a common condition that is likely under-recognized due to non-specific clinical signs, and less sensitive and specific non-invasive diagnostic tests.
- Evaluation for comorbidities is paramount, particularly in cases with persistent clinical signs or responding poorly to management.
- Treatment is often supportive care and includes addressing other comorbidities such as chronic enteropathies and long-term sequelae for CP, such as diabetes mellitus and exocrine pancreatic insufficiency.

INTRODUCTION

Pancreatitis, an inflammatory disorder of the pancreas, is commonly diagnosed in cats. With histopathology, it is classified as acute pancreatitis (AP), chronic pancreatitis (CP), or a component of both (acute-on-chronic pancreatitis), although from a clinical perspective, classification is based on severity of clinical signs (mild/moderate, severe, or subclinical pancreatitis) (Watson 2015) and occurrence (acute, recurrent/chronic). For CP, diagnosis is more challenging, and treatment options are less defined than AP. Comorbidities (i.e., chronic enteropathies [CE] and hepatobiliary disease) are present in approximately 50% of cats and complications of CP (i.e., endocrine and exocrine impairment) are common (Forman et al. 2021). This chapter reviews the current knowledge of pancreatitis in cats, including its pathophysiology, clinical presentation, diagnosis, and treatment.

PATHOPHYSIOLOGY

The pancreas is composed of a left and right limb that are united by the body. In cats, in contrast to dogs, there is typically one major pancreatic duct that joins the common bile duct just prior to entering the duodenum at the ampulla of Vater. A small percentage (20%) of cats have a secondary minor, or accessory, pancreatic duct that enters the duodenum separately (Griffin 2020).

Although often idiopathic, multiple conditions (including infectious etiologies, cancers, adverse drug reactions, trauma) can cause AP in cats. The etiology of CP in cats is debated, but may result from recurrent AP, or may be de-novo "chronic" from the outset (Watson 2015). Autoimmune pancreatitis (AIP) occurs uncommonly in humans and can be categorized as type 1 (systemic immune-mediated disease) and type 2 (associated with CE). Although the presence of antibodies against the pancreas has not been established in cats, a positive response to immunosuppressive therapy in some cats may suggest an immune-mediated etiology (Forman et al. 2021). In addition, inflammation in adjacent abdominal organs, such as the gastrointestinal tract or the hepatobiliary system, termed "triaditis", may also cause inflammation within the pancreas (Simpson 2015).

In a study of 115 cats undergoing post-mortem, CP was commonly detected (50% had only CP), with AP only detected in a small percentage (15%). Many of the cats diagnosed with CP on

Disorders of the Liver, Exocrine Pancreas, and Gastrointestinal Tract in Dogs and Cats, First Edition. Edited by Harry Cridge et al. Published 2026 by John Wiley & Sons, Inc. Companion Website: www.wiley.com/go/cridge/disorders

histopathology did not have clinical signs attributed to CP (subclinical pancreatitis). The clinical significance is unclear and may be from misclassification based on histopathology or an earlier stage of disease (De Cock et al. 2007).

CLINICAL PRESENTATION

Pancreatitis has no age, sex, or breed predisposition. Although there has been a correlation between older cats and CP (De Cock et al. 2007), no age cutoff has been established. Clinical presentations in cats with AP or CP are often nonspecific. Common presenting signs include lethargy, inappetence, vomiting, diarrhea, or weight loss. Physical examination may reveal dehydration, hypothermia or pyrexia, icterus, pallor, and abdominal discomfort, the latter may be under-recognized in cats. Less common findings may include tachypnea, dyspnea, and cranial organomegaly or abdominal mass (Ferreri et al. 2003). Often, cats with CP will have lower grade but more chronic clinical signs that can wax and wane over time. Cats with CP may present with acute marked clinical signs or an acute increase in chronic signs. Differentiating AP from an acute flare-up of CP may be difficult clinically, and while it may not be important for initial treatment, recognizing the potential sequelae of CP, such as the development of exocrine pancreatic insufficiency (EPI) and diabetes mellitus (DM) is important. It can also influence long-term management decisions. It is important to recognize other common comorbidities of CP that can cause overlapping clinical signs, such as "triaditis" (Černá et al. 2020). The prevalence of triaditis varies between studies and has been reported in 50–56% of cats diagnosed with pancreatitis, and 32–50% of cats with cholangitis (Simpson 2015). In a prospective study aiming to evaluate the prevalence of triaditis in symptomatic and asymptomatic cats, 34% of cats had concurrent lesions of chronic inflammatory enteropathy (CIE), 6.4% of cats had both CIE and pancreatitis, and 17% of cats had triaditis. Triaditis was identified in only symptomatic cats (Fragkou et al. 2016). Triaditis is more common in cats with CP, since these cats are more likely to have concurrent diseases than cats with AP (100% vs. 83%, respectively). Other comorbidities associated with both AP and CP include hepatic lipidosis, less commonly reported nephritis, and immune-mediated hemolytic anemia.

DIAGNOSTIC EVALUATION

Reaching a diagnosis of pancreatitis in cats is challenging. Histopathology is the only confirmatory test for the diagnosis (Watson 2015); however, it has limitations and is not performed routinely. A clinical diagnosis classification scheme for pancreatitis in cats has been proposed that incorporates clinical, laboratory, and imaging findings, and when available, cytopathologic findings (see below). CP cannot be distinguished from AP based on clinical or laboratory findings. Although it is often inferred from pancreatic ultrasound findings, this approach has limitations. Practically, CP is diagnosed based on recurrent episodes of pancreatitis with supported laboratory testing, typically persistent elevations in pancreatic enzymes. CP can be distinguished from recurrent AP with normalization of clinical signs, abnormal imaging findings, and pancreatic enzyme elevations between episodes; however, since many cats with AP have concurrent CP, and therefore a distinction may not be possible (Forman et al. 2021).

A complete blood count, serum biochemistry panel, urinalysis, and in some cases thyroid or fecal testing are important in the evaluation of any sick patient. Hematologic abnormalities in cats with CP are less common than in AP. An inflammatory leukogram, characterized by a neutrophilia with a left shift or a neutropenia, is uncommon. A non-regenerative anemia, secondary to chronic disease or inflammation, can be present. Serum biochemical abnormalities, including elevations of hepatic enzyme activities and kidney biomarkers are common, but are variable and likely secondary to comorbidities, including hepatobiliary disease (i.e., cholangitis, hepatic lipidosis), CE, chronic kidney disease, and/or hyperthyroidism. Hyperglycemia with glucosuria may be seen in cats with suspected CP, since DM can be a common complication, although these are also frequently observed in physiologically stressed cats, particularly in a hospital environment, and should be evaluated further (i.e., fructosamine testing or continuous blood glucose monitoring). Unlike dogs and humans, hyperlipidemia with increased serum triglyceride and/or cholesterol concentrations has not been associated with CP (or AP) in cats.

A wide range of serum pancreatic-directed testing is available to evaluate cats with suspected CP. These tests are routinely available and included in standard biochemistry panels, add-on tests, or GI panels, which also evaluate for evidence of CE and EPI. The ideal biomarker for CP in cats has not been determined. In humans, and likely in cats, biomarkers are more accurate with severe, more extensive, and AP than in chronic and low-grade pancreatitis. Considerations of which pancreatic-directed testing is performed include diagnostic accuracy, diagnostic turnaround time (in-clinic vs. referral laboratory testing, regionally availability), and expectation of pancreatitis at the pre-diagnostic stage.

The ideal biomarker for pancreatitis would be able to detect acinar cell damage and pancreatitis, be synthesized by acinar cells, not be secreted by non-acinar cells (i.e., enterocytes), and not be rapidly cleared from the bloodstream. Pancreatic acinar cells synthesize a wide variety of digestive enzymes; however, many are not only secreted by the acinar cells but also long-lasting in the bloodstream.

Enzymatic activity of serum amylase and lipase, measured by older generation testing (using 1,2-diglyceride as a substrate), has poor diagnostic sensitivity and lacks tissue specificity, with minimal utility as biomarkers for CP in cats. Feline Trypsin-like immunoreactivity (fTLI) also has poor diagnostic sensitivity and specificity for CP; however, decreased serum fTLI concentrations remain the gold standard diagnostic test for EPI, a late-term CP complication. Increased serum fTLI concentrations can be detected in cats with AP, CE, or decreased glomerular filtration rate (Stockham 2008).

Pancreatic lipase is useful as a biomarker and can be measured by a specific assay, serum pancreatic lipase immunoreactivity (fPLI). This marker was initially measured using a radioimmunoassay, then a highly specific, analytically validated, commercial ELISA (Spec fPL) was developed. A reference interval for the Spec fPL test was determined in healthy cats to be 0.7 – 3.5 μg/L and an fPLI concentration of ≥ 5.4 μg/L to be consistent with pancreatitis. With a fPLI of 5.4 μg/L as the diagnostic cutoff, the sensitivity was 79.4%, specificity was 79.7%, and positive and negative predictive values were 69% and 87%, respectively (Forman et al. 2021). This reference interval is no longer utilized. In a large, retrospective study, there was a significantly lower proportion of false-positive results than false-negative results; supporting an increased Spec fPL result indicates that pancreatitis is a probable diagnosis; however, a normal value does not rule out pancreatitis (Lee et al. 2020). The Spec fPL reference interval was updated after a new validation study, with a value of ≤ 4.4 μg/L determined as the normal interval, ≥ 8.9 μg/L as consistent with pancreatitis, and 4.5–8.8 μg/L as the equivocal interval (Wu et al. 2023). In-clinic assays are available for the immunologic measurement of pancreatic lipase, including the SNAP fPL. This provides rapid information on the likelihood of pancreatitis. The SNAP fPL is designed to prioritize sensitivity and rule out pancreatitis. The updated Spec fPL reference interval did not impact this test.

A catalytic assay for measuring serum lipase activity using the substrate 1,2-o-dilauryl-rac-glycero-3-glutaric acid-(6′-methylresorufin)-ester (DGGR) has also been analytically validated. The DGGR-based lipase assay had a good agreement with Spec fPL concentration with a Cohen's kappa coefficient of 0.7 (Oppliger et al. 2014). Using post-mortem pancreatic histopathology as a gold standard, the sensitivity and specificity for the DGGR assay (cutoff value >26 U/L) were 36.8 and 100%, respectively; however, when considering lymphocytic infiltration up to 10% as normal, the sensitivity increased at the expense of the specificity, at 66.7% and 78.6%, respectively. This study also detected a similar trend in diagnostic accuracy for the Spec fPL test (cutoff value ≥ 5.4 μg/L), with improved sensitivity, 61.1% and 69.0%, when considering higher amounts of pancreatic lymphocytic infiltration as normal (Oppliger et al. 2016). An alternate DGGR assay (Catalyst PL, IDEXX Laboratories) has recently been released to the market (US) and appears to be highly specific to lipase of pancreatic origin, although peer-reviewed publications are needed to further evaluate the assay.

Although survey abdominal radiography is beneficial in screening for differential diagnoses (i.e., GI foreign bodies and constipation), it has limited diagnostic accuracy and is neither sensitive nor specific for diagnosing pancreatitis in cats. Radiographic signs are more common with AP than

CP, including peritoneal loss of detail in the cranial abdomen or a mass effect (Stieger-Vanegas and Frank 2018).

In cats with suspected CP, abdominal ultrasound remains the primary imaging modality and should be considered part of the minimum database. Ultrasound can also detect abnormalities in the gastrointestinal tract, biliary system, liver, and kidneys, which can be more clinically relevant to the presenting clinical signs. Optimal ultrasound images of the pancreas are often obtained by experienced ultrasonographers with high frequency (>7.5 MHz) transducers. The left lobe's thickness is 5–9 mm and is located between the stomach's caudal curvature and the transverse colon's cranial border and is reported to be more readily visible than the right. The right lobe's thickness is 3–6 mm and is identified by tracing the body to the right of the portal vein and medial to the duodenum. The pancreatic duct diameter is usually visualized as a small hypoechoic tubular structure centrally located within the left lobe. The pancreatic duct diameter will increase in older healthy cats. In cats less than 10 years, the mean duct diameter is 0.8 +/− 0.25 mm, and in cats greater than 10 years of age, the mean is 1.3 +/− 0.4 mm in diameter, with dilation of up to 2.5 mm seen as an incidental geriatric change (Griffin 2020). Many ultrasound studies that evaluate cats diagnosed with pancreatitis do not distinguish between AP, CP, or acute-on-chronic pancreatitis. Ultrasound lacks sensitivity and specificity in differentiating normal from AP or CP (Ferreri et al. 2003). AP in cats can have normal or equivocal sonographic findings or pancreatomegaly with hypoechoic echogenicity, hyperechoic surrounding mesentery, irregular capsular margin, and focal to diffuse abdominal effusion. The sensitivity of these findings ranges from 11 to 67%, and sensitivity is considered to be severity- and operator-dependent and impacted by ultrasound resolution. The most accurate ultrasound abnormalities for diagnosing pancreatitis have not been determined. The greatest agreement between the fPLI and DGGR lipase activity is with hypoechoic and heteroechoic echogenicity and pancreatomegaly (Oppliger et al. 2014). Ultrasonographic findings of CP in cats have not been well researched or established. If a cat with CP is evaluated during a worsening of clinical signs, both AP and CP are likely present, which can result in an overlap of AP and CP abnormalities. Findings in cats with CP may include hyperechoic or heteroechoic pancreas, irregular capsular margin, dilated common bile duct (in some cases, biliary stones are detected), and, less frequently, peripancreatic fluid or pancreatomegaly. Pancreatic nodules, masses, or fluid accumulations (updated term for pseudocyst) are not infrequently detected. Pancreatic nodular hyperplasia (i.e., parenchymal nodules up to 1 cm in diameter and pancreatic enlargement) can be an incidental finding in older cats. Pancreatic neoplasms are rare in cats but are being detected with increased frequency with improvements in pancreatic imaging and sampling. Cytology or histopathology is helpful to characterize nodules, masses, and fluid accumulation, including screening for cancer or infectious complications (Griffin 2020). (see Chapter 22).

Advanced imaging of the pancreas, with computed tomography (CT) and less frequently, magnetic resonance imaging (MRI), is a routine and in many cases, first-line, imaging modality for pancreatitis in people; however, it is not used routinely as a diagnostic test in cats. Findings distinguishing AP from CP in cats have not been defined with CT or MRI (see Chapter 22).

Sampling of the pancreas is not routinely performed to diagnosis AP or CP; however, it should be considered in cases of pancreatic nodules or masses, particularly if singular and >1 cm, or fluid accumulations are visualized, or to confirm a diagnosis of CP with inconclusive diagnostic results. Despite historical concerns over inducing inflammation or seeding neoplasms, ultrasound-guided fine-needle aspiration (FNA) cytology of the pancreas in cats can be safely performed with little or no risk for complications and is quick and inexpensive (Crain et al. 2015). A 20–25-gauge, 1.5- to 3-inch long needle is typically utilized. Ideally, multiple samples within the lesion are aspirated. Non-diagnostic samples are uncommon, with a cytologic recovery rate of 67%; however, aspirates in cats with CP are often poorly cellular. Cytologic findings with CP include reactive fibroblasts and mixed inflammatory cells (neutrophils, lymphocytes, and plasma cells). Fluid analysis is often classified as high-protein transudate or exudate (Andreasen et al. 2010). Neoplastic cells, infected necrosis, or microbial agents can be identified with increased diagnostic yields for bacterial identification with concurrent bacterial cultures.

Pancreatic histopathology remains the gold standard for diagnosing pancreatitis in cats and is the only proven technique to distinguish AP from CP (De Cock et al. 2007; Ferreri et al. 2003). A pancreatic histology scoring system in cats has been developed and then modified. However, known limitations limit frequent utilization, including invasiveness in obtaining biopsies, debate on diagnostic inflammatory cell thresholds, and the patchy distribution of lesions throughout the pancreas that necessitate multiple biopsies (De Cock et al. 2007). Macroscopic lesions of CP can be subtle or non-apparent and include micropancreatic with a nodular appearance. Microscopic lesions of CP are characterized by lymphocytic or lymphoplasmacytic inflammation and fibrosis, which can be extensive and cause cystic dilation and acinar atrophy. Microscopic evidence of concurrent AP is often detected, and cancers or microbial agents are less commonly detected. The clinical significance of histologically mild pancreatitis, particularly if based on lymphocytic infiltration, has been questioned, and this may be a variant of normal in older cats (De Cock et al. 2007).

TREATMENT

Cats diagnosed with CP can present variably. This chapter will focus on cats presenting with low-to-moderate grade chronic clinical signs, often waxing and waning over time, and diagnostic testing does not indicate a complication of CP or comorbid disease. Many cats with CP will present with acute, moderate-to-severe clinical signs that are attributed to AP and need to be managed with intensive, often in-patient care, focusing on fluid therapy (correction of fluid and electrolyte imbalances), analgesia (opioids), control of vomiting and apparent nausea (anti-emetics), and nutritional support (appetite stimulation and/or assisted feeding). In severe and complicated cases, additional treatments, including blood pressure support, blood product transfusions, antibiotics, glucocorticoids, and potentially surgery, are needed. Addressing risk factors, treating complications, and managing comorbidities are integral for the successful management, improvement in outcomes, and potentially prevention of recurrence of AP. Alternatively, some cats with CP will present with subtle-to-mild clinical signs attributed to CP, but a clinically important comorbid or alternative disease needs to be prioritized. This can include diabetic ketoacidosis, CE, GI obstruction, renal disease, hepatobiliary disease (including bacterial cholangitis), neoplasia, or cardiac disease (Forman et al. 2021).

The primary focus of treatment of CP without comorbidities is supportive and symptomatic. Adverse clinical signs, including vomiting, inappetence, and, less frequently, diarrhea, are often intermittent, mild, and of short duration. On examination, these patients are hydrated to <5% dehydrated, which allows for outpatient management. A longer duration of severe clinical signs, moderate to marked dehydration, evidence of hypoperfusion, metabolic acidosis, or prerenal azotemia would warrant hospitalization and more aggressive therapy. Subcutaneous fluid therapy is frequently administered to correct dehydration. The ideal crystalloid fluids have not been determined, with Lactated Ringer's or a similar solution often being the first choice. Anti-emetics are often utilized to address vomiting and apparent nausea, reduce fluid and electrolyte loss, encourage return to normal appetite, and reduce the potential for secondary esophagitis and aspiration pneumonia. The ideal antiemetic has not been determined. Maropitant citrate (Cerenia®), a neurokinin 1 (NK 1) receptor antagonist, is highly effective and FDA-approved for vomiting in cats at a dose of 1 mg/kg SC q24h and is also commonly prescribed extra-label to be administered IV or PO also at a dose of 1 mg/kg q24h. Additional potential benefits of maropitant are visceral analgesia and anti-inflammatory action. Dolasetron (Anzemet®) and ondansetron (Zofran®) are 5HT3 receptor antagonists that can be used as a first-line antiemetic, or an additive antiemetic in addition to maropitant, at a dose of 0.4–1.0 mg/kg IV, PO, SC q6–12h (extra-label). Since marked, antiemetic-resistant vomiting is not expected with CP, alternative differentials should be considered if combination therapy is prescribed (Forman et al. 2021).

Many cats with CP may have episodic inappetence, which can result in weight loss from malnutrition, impaired gastrointestinal barrier and immune function. Appetite stimulants often effectively restore voluntary food intake in cats with CP. The transdermal formulation of mirtazapine (Mirataz®) is highly effective and FDA-approved for cats for the treatment of weight loss at a dose of approximately 2 mg per cat on the ear pinna once daily for 14 days. Mirtazapine also has anti-emetic activity. Adverse side effects (vocalization, tremors, agitation, vomiting, abnormal gait/ataxia) have been reported. More adverse effects were detected with oral administration and higher doses (i.e., 3.75 mg/day). Capromorelin (Elura®) is an effective appetite stimulant that is an FDA-approved treatment for the management of weight loss in cats with CKD, a common comorbidity with CP. The dosing is 2 mg/kg orally once daily. Adverse side effects have been reported, including vomiting, hypersalivation, and behavioral changes, and there have been anecdotal reports of cases of bradycardia and unexplained death shortly after capromorelin administration.

Analgesia may be indicated in some cats with CP. Pain is difficult to evaluate in cats and is likely underestimated, especially in cats with AP. The frequency of pain in cats with CP is unknown. In the authors' experience, it is less frequent. Abdominal pain can contribute to persistent inappetence, and pain management may be indicated in CP cats with unexplained inappetence. The ideal analgesic in cats with CP has not been determined. Buprenorphine (Buprenex®) 0.005–0.02 mg/kg IV, SQ, or oral transmucosal q8–12h is often adequate for outpatient analgesia in cats with CP. As a first-line analgesic or an additive analgesic, gabapentin 5–10 mg/kg PO q8–12h is also commonly considered. As new analgesics are developed and evaluated, pain management recommendations for cats with CP will likely be updated.

There is limited scientific and clinical data guiding the optimal nutritional management for cats with CP, once voluntary food intake has been restored. Cats are more prone to carbohydrate intolerance and have higher dietary protein and fat requirements. Unlike dogs and humans, they have a higher tolerance for dietary fat. The role of dietary fat is less certain in cats and should be assessed on an individual basis. Excessive fat restriction should be avoided to maintain caloric density. Practically, initial dietary decisions are often individualized to the patient and focused on palatability and comorbidities (i.e., chronic kidney disease, DM, EPI, CE). Highly digestible enteral diets are currently recommended for long-term management. A novel protein or hydrolyzed protein diet should be considered if a concurrent enteropathy is suspected with CP. Multiple small meals per day may maximize digestion in cats with EPI (Cridge et al. 2024).

Initial experiences with immune-modulating therapies suggest these treatments may be an important and targeted therapy to treat CP; however, additional research is needed. Historically, there has been a reluctance to use corticosteroids for the treatment of pancreatitis due to concerns that glucocorticoids may be a risk factor for the development of pancreatitis; however, studies in dogs and humans have not established a definitive relationship. In a study in healthy cats, prednisolone (median dose 1.28 mg/kg PO q24h) did not significantly increase DGGR-lipase activity or fPLI concentrations (Pacheva 2023). Once-daily cyclosporin (5–7.9 mg/kg PO q24h) resulted in a decrease in fPLI concentrations in cats with CP in one study (Hoeyrup 2020) but not in another (Wu 2022), which reported a transient reduction (noted after 10 days but not 21 days of treatment) in fPLI concentrations only with twice-daily cyclosporin (5 mg/kg PO q12h). Prednisolone (2 mg/kg PO q12h) did not significantly decrease fPLI concentrations in that study. Long-term clinical trials are needed, particularly if clinical improvement is detected. Currently, immune-modulating therapies are not routinely recommended for treating CP in cats. If these therapies are utilized, screening for occult infections (i.e., bacterial cholangitis, UTI, regional infectious causes of pancreatitis) and comorbidities (i.e., cancers, cardiomyopathies) that might be adversely affected by therapy is important.

PROGNOSIS/COMPLICATIONS

The prognosis of CP in cats is highly variable. Given the large percentage of subclinical CP in cats, its prognosis likely depends on the severity and prognosis of other comorbidities or potential sequelae. Pancreatitis may contribute to both a combination of impaired insulin secretion as well as insulin resistance. Clinical or histopathological evidence of pancreatitis may be present in over half of the cats with DM, although similar findings have also been found in control cats. In a study evaluating cats with diabetes ketosis/ketoacidosis, approximately one-third of cats had concurrent pancreatitis (Bruskiewicz et al. 1997). Evaluation for comorbidities should be considered in cats with DM, particularly in cats where there is poorly controlled DM, or with chronic or recurrent episodes of clinical illness or diabetic ketosis/ketoacidosis. In a large study evaluating EPI in cats, 58% had other comorbidities, including DM (9%) and pancreatitis (11%) (Xenoulis et al. 2016). Due to the large functional reserve of the pancreas, DM and EPI may not develop until 80–90% of the exocrine and endocrine tissue has been lost. Therefore, earlier recognition of CP would be beneficial. Early diagnosis and management of comorbidities is likely paramount to the short- and long-term outcome of cats with CP.

REFERENCES

Andreasen, C.B., Jergens A.E., and Meyer D.J. (2010). Oral cavity, gastrointestinal tract, and associated structures. In: *Canine and Feline Cytology: A Color Atlas and Interpretation Guide* (ed. R.E. Raskin, M.D.). St. Louis: Saunders Elsevier.

Bruskiewicz, K.A., Nelson, R.W., Feldman, E.C. et al. (1997). Diabetic ketosis and ketoacidosis in cats: 42 cases (1980–1995). *Journal of the American Veterinary Medical Association* 211: 188–192.

Černá, P., Kilpatrick, S., and Gunn-Moore, D.A. (2020). Feline comorbidities: what do we really know about feline triaditis? *Journal of Feline Medicine and Surgery* 22: 1047–1067.

Crain, S.K., Sharkey, L.C., Cordner, A.P. et al. (2015). Safety of ultrasound-guided fine-needle aspiration of the feline pancreas: a case-control study. *Journal of Feline Medicine and Surgery* 17: 858–863.

Cridge, H., Parker, V.J., and Kathrani, A. (2024). Nutritional management of pancreatitis and concurrent disease in dogs and cats. *Journal of the American Veterinary Medical Association* 262: 834–840.

De Cock, H.E.V., Forman, M.A., Farver, T.B. et al. (2007). Prevalence and histopathologic characteristics of pancreatitis in cats. *Veterinary Pathology* 44: 39–49.

Ferreri, J.A., Hardam, E., Kimmel, S.E. et al. (2003). Clinical differentiation of acute necrotizing from chronic nonsuppurative pancreatitis in cats: 63 cases (1996–2001). *Journal of the American Veterinary Medical Association* 223: 469–474.

Forman, M.A., Steiner, J.M., Armstrong, P.J. et al. (2021). ACVIM consensus statement on pancreatitis in cats. *Journal of Veterinary Internal Medicine* 35: 703–723.

Fragkou, F.C., Adamama-Moraitou, K.K., Poutahidis, T. et al. (2016). Prevalence and clinicopathological features of triaditis in a prospective case series of symptomatic and asymptomatic cats. *Journal of Veterinary Internal Medicine* 30: 1031–1045.

Griffin, S. (2020). Feline abdominal ultrasonography: what's normal? What's abnormal? The pancreas. *Journal of Feline Medicine and Surgery* 22: 241–259.

Hoeyrup, S. (2020). ECVIM. Effects of cyclosporine treatment on supranormal feline serum pancreatic lipase immunoreactivity concentrations. Abstract. *ECVIM-CA Congress.*

Lee, C., Kathrani, A., and Maddison, J. (2020). Retrospective study of the diagnostic utility of Spec fPL in the assessment of 274 sick cats. *Journal of Veterinary Internal Medicine* 34: 1406–1412.

Oppliger, S., Hartnack, S., Reusch, C.E. et al. (2014). Agreement of serum feline pancreas-specific lipase and colorimetric lipase assays with pancreatic ultrasonographic findings in cats with suspicion of pancreatitis: 161 cases (2008–2012). *Journal of Veterinary Internal Medicine* 244: 1060–1065.

Oppliger, S., Hilbe, M., Hartnack, S. et al. (2016). Comparison of serum spec fPL(™) and 1,2-o-dilauryl-rac-glycero-3-glutaric acid-(6'-methylresorufin) ester assay in 60 cats using standardized assessment of pancreatic histology. *Journal of Veterinary Internal Medicine* 30: 764–770.

Pacheva, B. (2023). ACVIM. Effects of prednisolone on DGGR-lipase activity (LIPC Roche) and pancreatic lipase immunoreactivity (SpecfPL) in cats. Abstract. *ACVIM Forum.*

Simpson, K.W. (2015). Pancreatitis and triaditis in cats: causes and treatment. *Journal of Small Animal Practice* 56: 40–49.

Stieger-Vanegas S.M. and Frank P.M. (2018). The peritoneal space. In: *Textbook of Veterinary Diagnostic Radiology* (ed. D.E. Thrall.), St. Louis, MO: Elsevier.

Stockham, S. (2008). *Fundamentals of Veterinary Clinical Pathology*, Ames: Blackwell Publishing.

Watson, P. (2015). Pancreatitis in dogs and cats: definitions and pathophysiology. *Journal of Small Animal Practice* 56: 3–12.

Wu, L. (2022). ACVIM. A randomized non-controlled open-label trial in cats comparing cyclosporine and prednisolone for treating chronic pancreatitis. Abstract. *ACVIM Forum.*

Wu, Y.-A., Steiner, J.M., Huisinga, E. et al. (2023). Analytical validation of an ELISA for the measurement of feline pancreas-specific lipase and re-evaluation of the reference interval and decision threshold for diagnosing pancreatitis. *Veterinary Clinical Pathology* 52: 482–492.

Xenoulis, P.G., Zoran, D.L., Fosgate, G.T. et al. (2016). Feline exocrine pancreatic insufficiency: a retrospective study of 150 cases. *Journal of Veterinary Internal Medicine* 30: 1790–1797.

Exocrine Pancreatic Insufficiency in Dogs

CHAPTER 29

Patrick C. Barko and David A. Williams

Department of Veterinary Clinical Medicine, College of Veterinary Medicine, University of Illinois at Urbana-Champaign, Urbana-Champaign, IL, USA

KEY POINTS

- Exocrine pancreatic insufficiency (EPI) is a malabsorptive syndrome caused by insufficient synthesis and secretion of digestive enzymes from the exocrine pancreas.
- German Shepherd Dogs (GSDs) and several other breeds are predisposed to EPI, but dogs of any breed can be affected.
- Pancreatic acinar atrophy (PAA) is the most common cause of EPI in dogs.
- The clinical presentation of EPI in dogs is typically characterized by chronic weight loss with a normal or increased appetite, and chronic diarrhea.
- A diagnosis of EPI is confirmed by documenting subnormal serum concentrations of canine trypsin-like immunoreactivity (cTLI).
- Oral Pancreatic Enzyme Replacement Therapy (PERT) is an essential therapy for EPI in dogs and must be given with every meal. Nearly all dogs with EPI require lifelong PERT.
- Cobalamin deficiency is common in dogs with EPI. Parenteral and oral cobalamin supplementation are equally efficacious in correcting cobalamin deficiencies and will likely be required for life.
- Adjunctive therapies, including dietary modification, probiotics, and antimicrobial drugs (tylosin), can be useful in dogs with an inadequate response to PERT.
- Dog with EPI can have an excellent prognosis with appropriate monitoring and management with PERT.

INTRODUCTION

Exocrine pancreatic insufficiency (EPI) is a malabsorptive syndrome caused by insufficient synthesis and secretion of digestive enzymes by pancreatic acini (Cridge et al. 2023; Westermarck and Wiberg 2012). Normally, the exocrine pancreas synthesizes and secretes digestive enzymes, including lipase, amylase, and proteases, into the duodenum via the pancreatic ducts. These enzymes are essential for digestion and absorption of dietary nutrients (triglycerides, starches, and proteins) in the small intestine. Insufficient secretion of these enzymes results in maldigestion and malabsorption of dietary nutrients, leading to the hallmark clinical signs of EPI, including weight loss, polyphagia, and diarrhea. The exocrine pancreas has a remarkable functional reserve capacity, and clinical signs are typically not observed until >90% of pancreatic acinar function has been lost. Additionally, digestive enzymes from other tissues (e.g., gastric lipase) contribute to macronutrient digestion. Owing to these factors, the presence and severity of clinical signs vary significantly among affected individuals. EPI is diagnosed by observing compatible clinical signs of gastrointestinal dysfunction (e.g., weight loss, diarrhea) and measuring subnormal serum concentrations of canine-specific trypsin-like immunoreactivity (cTLI). Pancreatic enzyme replacement therapy (PERT) is the core therapy for EPI, but

Disorders of the Liver, Exocrine Pancreas, and Gastrointestinal Tract in Dogs and Cats, First Edition. Edited by Harry Cridge et al. Published 2026 by John Wiley & Sons, Inc. Companion Website: www.wiley.com/go/cridge/disorders

adjunct treatments such as cobalamin supplementation and dietary modification are required for an optimal response to PERT in many dogs. The prognosis for EPI with PERT and appropriate supportive care is good, with most dogs experiencing resolution of clinical signs and good quality of life.

ETIOPATHOGENESIS, GENETICS, AND PATHOPHYSIOLOGY

A variety of lesions can cause EPI in dogs, including pancreatic acinar atrophy (PAA), chronic pancreatitis (CP), pancreatic duct obstruction (mass, surgical complication, trauma), pancreatic neoplasia, and exocrine pancreatic hypoplasia/aplasia. Of these, PAA is likely the most common underlying cause of EPI in dogs. PAA is associated with progressive and selective loss of pancreatic acinar cells and their replacement by adipose and connective tissue with minimal inflammation or fibrosis, leading to a loss of functional acinar tissue (Figure 29.1) (Wiberg 2004; Westermarck et al. 1993). Immunohistochemical investigations of GSDs and rough-coated collies have revealed lymphocytic infiltration of the exocrine pancreas by $CD4^+$ and $CD8^+$ T-cells in dogs with subclinical PAA (Wiberg et al. 2000). In these dogs with subclinical PAA, indirect immunofluorescence staining revealed weak reactions of serum antibodies with pancreatic acinar cells. These findings suggest an immune-mediated component to the pathogenesis of PAA. CP is probably the second most common cause of EPI in dogs (Watson 2003; Watson et al. 2010). Other potential causes of EPI are rare.

Early studies of EPI in GSDs were suggestive of an autosomal recessive pattern of inheritance, however a test breeding of unrelated two GSDs with EPI resulted in only two of the six offspring eventually developing PAA, contradicting this hypothesis and suggesting a more complex mode of inheritance (Westermarck 1980; Moeller et al. 2000; Westermarck et al. 2010). A genome-wide association study of 100 GSDs with PAA identified several single-nucleotide polymorphisms mapping to the dog leukocyte antigen (DLA) complex on chromosome 12 (Tsai et al. 2012). A previous

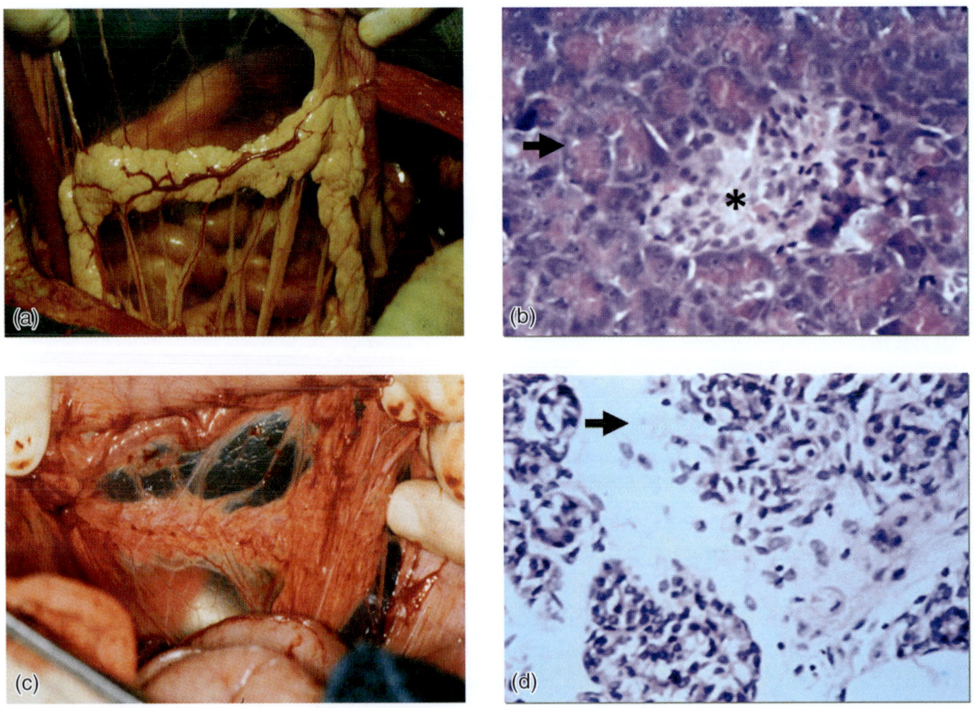

FIGURE 29.1 Gross and histologic findings of exocrine pancreatic insufficiency (EPI). Gross (a) and microscopic (b) images of a healthy dog reveal a normal pancreatic tissue with exocrine pancreatic cells organized into functional secretory acini (arrow) surrounding islet cells (asterisk). In EPI due to pancreatic acinar atrophy (PAA), pancreatic mass is grossly reduced compared to normal (c), acinar cells are atrophied, and the exocrine pancreas consists solely of residual adipose and non-acinar pancreatic tissue (d, arrow)

study revealed upregulation of *DLA-88* expression in the pancreata of GSDs with PAA (Clark et al. 2005). Other studies have identified duplication of DLA-DBQ1 as a risk allele for EPI in both GSDs and Pembroke Welsh Corgis (Tsai et al. 2013; Evans et al. 2015). Collectively, these genetic, histopathologic, and immunologic investigations suggest that PAA has an immune-mediated pathogenesis with polygenetic risk factors, which may be associated with immune dysregulation related to disease-associated DLA alleles, especially in pre-disposed breeds.

Regardless of its underlying etiopathogenesis, clinical signs of EPI are caused by defective dietary nutrient absorption due to a failure to digest dietary proteins, starches, and fat. In addition to malnutrition due to caloric deficit, specific deficiencies of selected micronutrients can develop, together leading to poor body condition despite normal or even increased appetite. The presence of unabsorbed dietary macromolecules in the intestinal lumen causes osmotic diarrhea, steatorrhea, and enteric microbiota dysbiosis (EMD). In dogs with EPI, EMD is characterized by small intestinal bacterial overgrowth (SIBO), lower microbiota diversity, and decreased abundance of important commensal bacteria such as *Peptacetobacter hiranonis* (previously known as *Clostridium hiranonis*) (Williams et al. 1987; Simpson et al. 1990; Isaiah et al. 2017; Blake et al., 2019). EMD can plausibly contribute to the pathophysiology of diarrhea, flatulence, and abdominal discomfort, changes in appetite, and other clinical signs in affected animals due to excessive gas production from anaerobic microbial metabolism, exacerbation of cobalamin deficiency, and induction of intestinal mucosal inflammatory responses.

DIAGNOSIS OF EXOCRINE PANCREATIC INSUFFICIENCY

DIAGNOSTIC CRITERIA

A diagnosis of EPI is achieved by observation of chronic clinical signs of gastrointestinal dysfunction such as weight loss and diarrhea; exclusion of metabolic, systemic, and gastrointestinal disorders associated with similar clinical signs; and diagnostically subnormal serum cTLI concentrations (Williams and Batt 1983). Observing a positive response to PERT further supports a diagnosis of EPI, whereas inadequate responses to therapy suggest the presence of a concurrent disease process, such as chronic enteropathy. Findings from historical clinical signs, physical examination, clinicopathology, and diagnostic imaging cannot distinguish dogs with EPI from those with other chronic gastrointestinal disorders. It is important to exclude EPI early in the diagnostic evaluation of all dogs with signs of gastrointestinal dysfunction, before clinical signs become extreme. Early diagnosis also allows appropriate prompt initiation of PERT and avoids unnecessary and expensive investigation of alternative diagnoses.

CLINICAL PRESENTATION

Associations with EPI have been reported for several breeds, including German Shepherd Dogs (GSDs), rough-coated collies, Cavalier King Charles spaniels, Pembroke Welsh corgis, cairn terriers, chows, cocker spaniels, Eurasian dogs, and West Highland white terriers (Westermarck 1980; Moeller et al. 2000; Westermarck et al. 1989; Wiberg et al. 1999b; Batchelor et al. 2007a; Proschowsky and Fredholm 2007). However, dogs of any breed can be affected by EPI. While dogs of any age can be affected, those with PAA are likely to develop EPI at a younger age than those with CP (Batchelor et al. 2007a). EPI can be subclinical, especially in the early stages of PAA. In patients with clinically overt EPI, diarrhea (>90%), weight loss (>80%), and polyphagia (>50%) are the most reported clinical signs in a recent retrospective study (Soetart et al. 2019). Less frequently reported signs include vomiting, urgency to defecate, coprophagia, polyuria, and dermatologic problems. Whereas most dogs with EPI have normal or increased appetite, anorexia is seen occasionally and may reflect a concurrent disorder such as chronic enteropathy. Dogs with EPI due to non-PAA causes such as CP and neoplasia may present with historical clinical signs atypical for EPI, such as anorexia and abdominal pain. Dogs with EPI secondary to CP may also have diabetes mellitus and associated clinical signs and lab abnormalities. Physical examination of dogs with EPI typically reveals poor body condition, though dogs earlier in the progression of EPI may not have significantly altered body condition. Results from routine clinicopathologic investigation, including complete blood counts, serum biochemistry panels, and urinalyses, are typically unremarkable in uncomplicated EPI. In one study of 34 dogs with EPI, abdominal ultrasound revealed decreased mean pancreatic thickness compared to healthy dogs; however, 68% of dogs with EPI had no ultrasonographic pancreatic lesions, and the pancreas could not be identified in 35% of dogs (Pelligra et al. 2022). In the same study, 85% of dogs with EPI had ultrasonographic abnormalities of the small intestines, suggestive of a chronic enteropathy. Thus, a normal ultrasonographic appearance of the pancreas does not exclude a diagnosis of EPI, and concurrent small lesions are commonly identified.

TRYPSIN-LIKE IMMUNOREACTIVITY

Serum canine trypsin-like immunoreactivity (cTLI) is the diagnostic "gold standard" for EPI in dogs (Williams and Batt 1983; Williams and Batt 1988). Serum concentrations of cTLI are directly correlated to the mass of functioning pancreatic acinar tissue and are highly sensitive and specific for diagnosing EPI. Recently, reference intervals for the serum cTLI assay have been revised due to upward drift of the commercially available assay. The authors encourage the reader to utilize the most up-to-date reference intervals for serum cTLI from their reference laboratory. At the time of writing, serum cTLI concentrations <5.6 μg/L are considered diagnostic for EPI (Wu et al., 2024). Serum cTLI concentrations between 5.6 and 10.8 μg/L are subnormal, but not unequivocally diagnostic for EPI. Serial monitoring of serum cTLI, a therapeutic PERT trial, or both can aid in the assessment of these equivocal, subnormal serum cTLI results. Persistently equivocal, subnormal cTLI concentrations, consistent with subclinical EPI (sEPI), have been identified in apparently healthy dogs of predisposed breeds such as GSDs, and some of these dogs may ultimately progress to develop clinically overt EPI (Wiberg et al. 1999a; Wiberg et al. 2002). Serum cTLI concentrations can increase after feeding and should ideally be measured after fasting for at least six hours (Saver et al. 2021). Very rarely, cases of suspected isolated lipase deficiency have been reported in dogs (Viviano and Ziglioli 2013). In these patients, serum cTLI may be within normal limits, and measurement of serum canine pancreatic lipase can aid in diagnosis (although some healthy dogs have serum pancreatic lipase concentrations below the detectable limit of some assays). Serum cTLI is not impacted by oral administration of pancreatic enzymes, meaning PERT can be initiated as a therapeutic trial before a diagnosis of EPI is confirmed when there is a strong clinical suspicion for EPI.

ANCILLARY DIAGNOSTICS

Micronutrient deficiencies are common and ancillary diagnostics to assess the nutritional state of dogs with EPI are often recommended. Cobalamin (vitamin B12) deficiency is common in dogs with EPI and a negative prognostic indicator for treatment outcomes (Soetart et al. 2019; Batchelor et al. 2007b). Thus, measurement of serum cobalamin is recommended whenever EPI is strongly suspected or confirmed. Hyperfolatemia, likely secondary to small intestinal microbiota dysbiosis, is also common in dogs with EPI, whereas hypofolatemia is not, and when the latter is present, it is indicative of an additional associated enteropathy exacerbating malabsorption in the upper small intestine (Soetart et al. 2019). Serum cobalamin and folate concentrations should be routinely measured in dogs with EPI to evaluate for micronutrient deficiencies, EMD/SIBO, and concurrent enteropathies. Serum concentrations of lipid-soluble vitamins (A, D, or E) may be decreased in dogs with EPI compared with healthy dogs, presumably due to dietary fat malabsorption (Rutz et al. 2004; Barko and Williams 2018). Vitamin K deficiency has been reported in humans and cats with EPI, but not dogs (Barnes et al. 2020; Estes-Doetsch et al. 2024). As the clinical impact of lipid-soluble vitamin deficiencies has not been investigated in dogs with EPI, the authors do not recommend routine measurement of vitamins A, D, or E. However, it is reasonable to consider measuring them in dogs with an inadequate response to therapy to determine if supplementation is indicated as an adjunctive therapy. A quantitative PCR-based canine fecal microbiota dysbiosis index (DI) has recently been developed to aid in the diagnosis of EMD in dogs (Texas A&M Gastrointestinal Laboratory,

College Station, TX, United States) (AlShawaqfeh et al. 2017). A previous study identified higher DI, consistent with EMD, in dogs with EPI compared with healthy controls (Blake et al. 2019). The authors recommend testing the fecal microbiota DI in dogs with persistent diarrhea following initiation and optimization of PERT and dietary therapy. In theory, increased DI in these patients could justify treatments targeting enteric microbiota (e.g., probiotics, prebiotics, fecal microbiota transplantation, antibiotics). However, the clinical efficacy of integrating fecal DI into therapeutic decisions has not been proven.

TREATMENT

PANCREATIC ENZYME REPLACEMENT THERAPY

PERT is an essential therapy for almost all dogs with EPI, since extra-pancreatic sources of digestive enzymes alone are very rarely sufficient to maintain normal health. A previous study found that failure to receive PERT is an independent, negative prognostic factor for dogs with EPI (Soetart et al. 2019). There are several different formulations of pancreatic enzymes, including powdered pancreatic enzyme extracts, enteric-coated preparations, and raw pancreas. For most dogs with EPI, powdered pancreatic enzyme extracts of porcine origin are the first-line approach to PERT. These enzymes are widely available, can be purchased in bulk (enzymediane.com), and provide a convenient means to titrate the dose to effect for individual patients. Starting doses for PERT vary according to the manufacturer and potency of the enzyme preparation but generally start at ½–1 tsp per cup of food (or per 10 kg of body weight) per meal. Following a positive clinical response, the enzyme dose can be gradually reduced in ¼–½ tsp increments every 5–7 days to identify the lowest effective dose and thereby reduce the cost associated with long-term treatment. If there is an inadequate initial response, or diarrhea returns upon dose reduction, incremental increases in the enzyme dose should be made to effect. It is the authors' experience that doses >2 teaspoons of pancreatic enzyme powder per dog per meal are unnecessary in most cases. Other causes of poor treatment response (e.g., hypocobalaminemia, concurrent chronic enteropathy, enteric microbiota dysbiosis) should be investigated in patients that do not respond to initial attempts at PERT. Except in extremely rare circumstances, dogs with EPI will require PERT with every meal for the remainder of their lives.

Alternative forms of PERT have been used successfully in dogs, including enteric-coated formulations and raw pancreas. In theory, enteric coatings protect the pancreatic enzymes from inactivation by gastric acid and proteases. Enteric coatings are usually formulated for humans and owing to differences in human and canine gastrointestinal physiology, it cannot be assumed that their properties are suitable for use in dogs. Results from clinical trials of enteric-coated enzymes are mixed. One controlled trial identified significantly greater weight gain in dogs receiving the enteric-coated formulation compared with an identical, non-enteric-coated enzyme (Mas et al. 2012). A more recent study failed to identify differences in efficacy between enteric-coated and non-coated enzyme preparations in dogs (Parambeth et al. 2018). The authors do not routinely recommend enteric-coated enzyme formulations, but they can be considered in refractory cases when increasing doses of non-enteric-coated enzymes have been ineffective and other causes of poor treatment response have been excluded. Raw or fresh-frozen pancreas (bovine, porcine) contains digestive enzymes and may be fed to animals with EPI as an alternative to commercial pancreatic enzyme products. Dosing of raw pancreas is less consistent than with commercial extracts, but 1–3 ounces (30–90 g) of raw pancreas can be considered equivalent to one tsp of powdered extract. The authors recommend cutting the fresh, raw pancreas into small pieces, measuring the portions for each meal, and freezing the raw pancreas until fed. Raw pancreas products are effective and may be less costly than commercial powdered extracts. Raw pancreas can contain bacteria and other infectious agents that may pose a risk to the health of the animal and owner (Davies et al. 2019). Thus, raw pancreas should only be considered when commercial enzyme extracts are not available, should be obtained from properly inspected sources, and handled in a sanitary manner (Westermarck and Wiberg 2006).

Regardless of the nature of the enzyme preparation, PERT is almost always well-tolerated. Oral bleeding has been reported in some dogs with EPI receiving PERT in the form of dried extract (Rutz et al. 2002). Should oral bleeding or irritation occur, a reduction in the enzyme dose to the minimum required to control clinical signs of EPI is recommended and is usually followed by resolution of the oral lesions. Feeding a highly digestible (low fiber) diet may allow even further reductions in enzyme dose. Despite anecdotal claims to the contrary, there is no evidence that pre-incubation of the enzymes with food prevents oral mucosal bleeding, nor does it enhance the efficacy of treatment (Pidgeon and Strombeck 1982).

DIETARY MODIFICATION

Responses to dietary therapy in dogs with EPI receiving PERT are highly variable, and no single approach to dietary therapy has been shown to be consistently efficacious (Westermarck and Wiberg 2006). Nonetheless, dietary modification is considered an important adjunctive therapy for dogs with EPI that do not respond adequately to PERT. In the initial phase of treating EPI, the authors recommend continuing the current diet, provided it is nutritionally balanced and contains moderate fat content. If clinical signs of gastrointestinal dysfunction persist following optimization of PERT dosing (see above), therapeutic diet trials are recommended. Low-fat diets were traditionally recommended for dogs with EPI, but they have not been associated with improved outcomes and can exacerbate malnutrition due to poor calorie density and fat-soluble vitamin absorption (Batchelor et al. 2007b). Therefore, low-fat diets are not recommended for treating EPI in dogs. High-fiber diets are also not recommended due to their lower caloric density and the effect of dietary fiber on reducing pancreatic lipase activity (Westermarck and Wiberg 2006; Dutta and Hlasko 1985). Highly digestible, low-residue diets with moderate fat content are a reasonable first-line approach to dietary therapy in dogs with EPI. Hydrolyzed protein and novel antigen diets can also be considered on a trial-and-error basis when other diets have not proved to be effective or there a clinical suspicion of a concurrent chronic enteropathy (Tolbert et al. 2022).

MANAGING COBALAMIN DEFICIENCY

Cobalamin deficiency is common in dogs with EPI and is an independent risk factor for poor treatment outcomes (Soetart et al. 2019; Batchelor et al. 2007b). Additionally, cobalamin deficiency can contribute to clinical signs of gastrointestinal dysfunction (Kather et al. 2020). Therefore, cobalamin supplementation is a necessary adjunctive therapy in many dogs with EPI. Ideally, cobalamin supplementation would only be initiated in patients with a documented deficiency. The authors recommend initiating cobalamin supplementation when serum cobalamin concentrations are <300 ng/L. When possible, serial measurements of serum cobalamin concentrations would be used to validate the efficacy of supplementation. Owing to the presumed safety of cobalamin supplementation and high prevalence of hypocobalaminemia in dogs with EPI, supplementation should be initiated in all dogs in which serum cobalamin cannot be measured. Both parenteral and oral cobalamin supplementation have been found to be effective at normalizing serum cobalamin concentrations in dogs with hypocobalaminemia (Toresson et al. 2018). Various dosing strategies for cobalamin supplementation have been described. More information about cobalamin supplementation in EPI is found in a recent review (Cridge et al. 2023).

OTHER ADJUNCTIVE THERAPIES

Several therapeutic approaches have been proposed to manage patients with an inadequate response to treatment following optimization of PERT dosing and failure of dietary therapy. EMD and SIBO can persist following treatment with PERT (Isaiah et al. 2017; Blake et al. 2019). Thus, adjunct therapies targeting enteric microbiota are often recommended in cases with an inadequate response to PERT. These include probiotics, prebiotics, and antimicrobial drugs. Prebiotics and probiotics have the potential to ameliorate EMD associated with EPI and improve gastrointestinal function. Anecdotally, some dogs with EPI appear to respond to pre- and probiotics, but there are no clinical studies documenting their clinical impact in affected dogs. Fiber and prebiotic supplementation, other than those already formulated in balanced diets, should be instituted cautiously, due to the possibility of excessive supplementation contributing to gastrointestinal problems (Dutta and Hlasko 1985). Tylosin, a macrolide antibiotic, has historically been prescribed as an adjunctive therapy for EPI in dogs. A single study established an impact of tylosin in ameliorating SIBO in dogs with EPI, but there are no controlled clinical trials establishing its efficacy to improve fecal quality in dogs with EPI and persistent diarrhea following PERT (Westermarck et al. 1993). Emerging evidence supports potentially deleterious effects of antimicrobial drugs, including tylosin, on gastrointestinal microbiomes of dogs (Manchester et al. 2019). Therefore, the authors do not recommend routine use of antimicrobial therapy in dogs with EPI and reserve tylosin and other antimicrobial drugs for cases in which optimization of PERT, cobalamin supplementation, and dietary modification have failed to improve fecal quality. Tylosin is administered initially at 25 mg/kg once daily by mouth for 2–4 weeks. If improvement in stool quality is observed, the dose can be tapered downward in 25–30% increments every 1–2 weeks to find the lowest effective dose. If clinical signs return upon discontinuation, tylosin can be reinitiated at the most recently effective dose and given indefinitely. Fecal microbiota transplantation (FMT) is an emerging approach to manage chronic intestinal disorders associated with microbiota dysbiosis, but there are no reports of its use to treat dogs with EPI.

Owing to the potential for deficiencies in lipid-soluble vitamins in dogs with EPI, supplementation with vitamins A, D, and E can be considered as an adjunctive therapy in dogs with documented deficiencies. There are no studies documenting the clinical impact or risk of adverse effects of lipid-soluble vitamin supplementation in dogs with EPI. However, vitamins A, D, and E can participate in regulating gastrointestinal physiology, and it is plausible that deficiencies contribute to clinical signs of gastrointestinal dysfunction (Kunisawa and Kiyono 2013; Bakdash et al. 2015; Sun 2010). While supplementation with vitamin E is unlikely to cause serious adverse effects, the risk of toxic accumulation of vitamins A and D is significant, and so supplementation should be considered only in patients with documented deficiencies, ideally following consultation with a veterinary nutritionist. Serial measurements of serum lipid-soluble vitamin concentrations should be monitored during therapy to monitor for toxic accumulation. Various other medications and dietary supplements have been reportedly used to treat EPI in dogs. Owing to the inactivation of lipase in the acidic conditions of the stomach, gastric acid-suppressant medications (proton pump inhibitors, H2 antagonists) have been recommended for some dogs with EPI and an inadequate response to PERT. However, there is no documented clinical benefit of antacid therapy in dogs with EPI (Batchelor et al. 2007b). Additionally, administration of omeprazole, a proton pump inhibitor, is associated with changes to the enteric microbiome that could contribute to EMD/SIBO that promote gastrointestinal dysfunction in dogs (Garcia-Mazcorro et al. 2012). Slippery elm is a nutraceutical compound that is commonly administered by owners of dogs with EPI, based on anecdotal reports of efficacy from internet forums. Slippery elm may have prebiotic and other properties that could benefit gastrointestinal function, but there are no controlled clinical trials demonstrating its efficacy or safety in dogs with EPI.

PROGNOSIS

The prognosis for dogs with EPI is generally good, with most dogs experiencing a normal life expectancy and high quality of life with PERT and other appropriate adjunct therapies. In most dogs with EPI a combination of PERT, a high-quality diet and cobalamin supplementation are all that is required to normalize fecal quality and restore healthy body condition. Nearly 100% of dogs with EPI require lifelong therapy with PERT. A retrospective study identified complete remission of clinical signs in 60% and partial remission in 17% of dogs with EPI treated with PERT, indicating a satisfactory response to therapy in most dogs (Batchelor et al. 2007b). Among dogs with inadequate responses to PERT, diarrhea appears to be the most commonly persistent problem (Batchelor et al. 2007b; German 2012; Wiberg et al. 1998). For these dogs, successful individualized adjunctive therapies, commonly based on careful dietary modification, will often be found by trial and error. Improvement in stool quality is anticipated within 1–2 weeks of initiating treatment, whereas poor body condition can take weeks or months to improve.

REFERENCES

AlShawaqfeh, M.K., Wajid, B., Minamoto, Y. et al. (2017). A dysbiosis index to assess microbial changes in fecal samples of dogs with chronic inflammatory enteropathy. *FEMS Microbiology Ecology* 93.

Bakdash, G., Vogelpoel, L.T., van Capel, T.M. et al. (2015). Retinoic acid primes human dendritic cells to induce gut-homing, IL-10-producing regulatory T cells. *Mucosal Immunology* 8: 265–278.

Barko, P.C. and Williams, D.A. (2018). Serum concentrations of lipid-soluble vitamins in dogs with exocrine pancreatic insufficiency treated with pancreatic enzymes. *Journal of Veterinary Internal Medicine* 32: 1600–1608.

Barnes, A.J., Gates, K., and Kuntz, J. (2020). Fat-soluble vitamin deficiency and subsequent coagulopathy in a cat with exocrine pancreatic insufficiency. *Veterinary Record Case Reports* 8: e001019.

Batchelor, D.J., Noble, P.J., Cripps, P.J. et al. (2007a). Breed associations for canine exocrine pancreatic insufficiency. *Journal of Veterinary Internal Medicine* 21: 207–214.

Batchelor, D.J., Noble, P.J., Taylor, R.H. et al. (2007b). Prognostic factors in canine exocrine pancreatic insufficiency: prolonged survival is likely if clinical remission is achieved. *Journal of Veterinary Internal Medicine* 21: 54–60.

Blake, A.B., Guard, B.C., Honneffer, J.B. et al. (2019). Altered microbiota, fecal lactate, and fecal bile acids in dogs with gastrointestinal disease. *PLoS One* 14: e0224454.

Clark, L.A., Wahl, J.M., Steiner, J.M. et al. (2005). Linkage analysis and gene expression profile of pancreatic acinar atrophy in the German shepherd dog. *Mammalian Genome* 16: 955–962.

Cridge, H., Williams, D.A., and Barko, P.C. (2023). Exocrine pancreatic insufficiency in dogs and cats. *Journal of the American Veterinary Medical Association* 1: 1–10.

Davies, R.H., Lawes, J.R., and Wales, A.D. (2019). Raw diets for dogs and cats: a review, with particular reference to microbiological hazards. *Journal of Small Animal Practice* 60: 329–339.

Dutta, S.K. and Hlasko, J. (1985). Dietary fiber in pancreatic disease: effect of high fiber diet on fat malabsorption in pancreatic insufficiency and in vitro study of the interaction of dietary fiber with pancreatic enzymes. *American Journal of Clinical Nutrition* 41: 517–525.

Estes-Doetsch, H., Roberts, K., Newkirk, M. et al. (2024). Fat-soluble vitamin deficiency and exocrine pancreatic insufficiency among adults with chronic pancreatitis: Is routine monitoring necessary for all patients? *Nutrition in Clinical Practice* 39: 129–140.

Evans, J.M., Tsai, K.L., Starr-Moss, A.N. et al. (2015). Association of DLA-DQB1 alleles with exocrine pancreatic insufficiency in Pembroke Welsh corgis. *Animal Genetics* 46: 462–465.

Garcia-Mazcorro, J.F., Suchodolski, J.S., Jones, K.R. et al. (2012). Effect of the proton pump inhibitor omeprazole on the gastrointestinal bacterial microbiota of healthy dogs. *FEMS Microbiology Ecology* 80: 624–636.

German, A.J. (2012). Exocrine pancreatic insufficiency in the dog: breed associations, nutritional considerations, and long-term outcome. *Topics in Companion Animal Medicine* 27: 104–108.

Isaiah, A., Parambeth, J.C., Steiner, J.M. et al. (2017). The fecal microbiome of dogs with exocrine pancreatic insufficiency. *Anaerobe* 45: 50–58.

Kather, S., Grützner, N., Kook, P.H. et al. (2020). Review of cobalamin status and disorders of cobalamin metabolism in dogs. *Journal of Veterinary Internal Medicine* 34: 13.

Kunisawa, J. and Kiyono, H. (2013). Vitamin-mediated regulation of intestinal immunity. *Frontiers in Immunology* 4: 189.

Manchester, A.C., Webb, C.B., Blake, A.B. et al. (2019). Long-term impact of tylosin on fecal microbiota and fecal bile acids of healthy dogs. *Journal of Veterinary Internal Medicine* 33: 2605–2617.

Mas, A., Noble, P-J.M., Cripps, P.J. et al. (2012). A blinded randomised controlled trial to determine the effect of enteric coating on enzyme treatment for canine exocrine pancreatic efficiency. *BMC Veterinary Research* 8: 127.

Moeller, E.M., Steiner, J.M., Clark, L.A. et al. (2000). Inheritance of pancreatic acinar atrophy in American German shepherd dogs. *Journal of Veterinary Internal Medicine* 14: 377.

Parambeth, J.C., Fosgate, G.T., Suchodolski, J.S. et al. (2018). Randomized placebo controlled clinical trial of an enteric coated micro-pelleted formulation of a pancreatic enzyme supplement in dogs with exocrine pancreatic insufficiency. *Journal of Veterinary Internal Medicine* 32: 1591–1599.

Pelligra, T., Puccinelli, C., Marchetti, V. et al. (2022). Ultrasonographic findings of exocrine pancreatic insufficiency in dogs. *Veterinary Sciences* 9 (8):407.

Pidgeon, G. and Strombeck, D.R. (1982). Evaluation of treatment for pancreatic exocrine insufficiency in dogs with ligated pancreatic ducts. *American Journal of Veterinary Research* 43: 461–464.

Proschowsky, H.F. and Fredholm, M. (2007). Exocrine pancreatic insufficiency in the Eurasian dog breed - Inheritance and exclusion of two candidate genes. *Animal Genetics* 38: 171–173.

Rutz, G.M., Steiner, J.M., and Williams, D.A. (2002). Oral bleeding associated with pancreatic enzyme supplementation in three dogs with exocrine pancreatic insufficiency. *Journal of the American Veterinary Medical Association* 221: 1714, 1716–1718.

Rutz, G.M., Steiner, J.M., Bauer, J.E. et al. (2004). Effects of exchange of dietary medium chain triglycerides for long-chain triglycerides on serum biochemical variables and subjectively assessed well-being of dogs with exocrine pancreatic insufficiency. *American Journal of Veterinary Research* 65: 1293–1301.

Saver, A.T., Steiner, J.M., Hetzel, S.J. et al. (2021). Effect of withholding food on serum concentrations of cobalamin, folate, trypsin-like immunoreactivity, and pancreatic lipase immunoreactivity in healthy dogs. *American Journal of Veterinary Research* 82: 367–373.

Simpson, K.W., Batt, R.M., Jones, D. et al. (1990). Effects of exocrine pancreatic insufficiency and replacement therapy on the bacterial flora of the duodenum in dogs. *American Journal of Veterinary Research* 51: 203–206.

Soetart, N., Rochel, D., Drut, A. et al. (2019). Serum cobalamin and folate as prognostic factors in canine exocrine pancreatic insufficiency: an observational cohort study of 299 dogs. *The Veterinary Journal* 243: 15–20.

Sun, J. (2010). Vitamin D and mucosal immune function. *Current Opinion in Gastroenterology* 26: 591–595.

Tolbert, M.K., Murphy, M., Gaylord, L. et al. (2022). Dietary management of chronic enteropathy in dogs. *Journal of Small Animal Practice* 63 (6): 425–434. https://doi.org/10.1111/JSAP.13471.

Toresson, L., Steiner, J.M., Razdan, P. et al. (2018). Comparison of efficacy of oral and parenteral cobalamin supplementation in normalising low cobalamin concentrations in dogs: a randomised controlled study. *The Veterinary Journal* 232: 27–32.

Tsai, K.L., Noorai, R.E., Starr-Moss, A.N. et al. (2012). Genome-wide association studies for multiple diseases of the German shepherd dog. *Mammalian Genome* 23: 203–211.

Tsai, K.L., Starr-Moss, A.N., Venkataraman, G.M. et al. (2013). Alleles of the major histocompatibility complex play a role in the pathogenesis of pancreatic acinar atrophy in dogs. *Immunogenetics* 65: 501–509.

Viviano, K.R. and Ziglioli, V. (2013). Suspected isolated pancreatic enzyme deficiencies in dogs. *Journal of Veterinary Internal Medicine* 27: 588–591.

Watson, P.J. (2003). Exocrine pancreatic insufficiency as an end stage of pancreatitis in four dogs. *Journal of Small Animal Practice* 44: 306–312.

Watson, P.J., Archer, J., Roulois, A.J. et al. (2010). Observational study of 14 cases of chronic pancreatitis in dogs. *Veterinary Record* 167: 968–976.

Westermarck, E. (1980). The hereditary nature of canine pancreatic degenerative atrophy in the German shepherd dog. *Acta Veterinaria Scandinavica* 21: 389–394.

Westermarck, E. and Wiberg, M. (2012). Exocrine pancreatic insufficiency in the dog: historical background, diagnosis, and treatment. *Topics in Companion Animal Medicine* 27: 96–103.

Westermarck, E. and Wiberg, M.E. (2006). Effects of diet on clinical signs of exocrine pancreatic insufficiency in dogs. *Journal of the American Veterinary Medical Association* 228: 225–229.

Westermarck, E., Batt, R.M., Vaillant, C. et al. (1993). Sequential study of pancreatic structure and function during development of pancreatic acinar atrophy in a German shepherd dog. *American Journal of Veterinary Research* 54: 1088–1094.

Westermarck, E., Myllys, V., and Aho, M. (1993). Effect of treatment on the jejunal and colonic bacterial flora of dogs with exocrine pancreatic insufficiency. *Pancreas* 8: 559–562.

Westermarck, E., Pamilo, P., and Wiberg, M. (1989). Pancreatic degenerative atrophy in the collie breed: a hereditary disease. *Zentralbl Veterinarmed A* 36: 549–554.

Westermarck, E., Saari, S.A.M., and Wiberg, M.E. (2010). Heritability of exocrine pancreatic insufficiency in German Shepherd dogs. *Journal of Veterinary Internal Medicine* 24: 450–452.

Wiberg, M., Lautala, H., and Westermarck, E. (1998). Response to long-term enzyme replacement treatment in dogs with exocrine pancreatic insufficiency - PubMed. *Journal of the American Veterinary Medical Association* 213: 86–90.

Wiberg, M.E. (2004). Pancreatic acinar atrophy in German shepherd dogs and rough-coated collies. Etiopathogenesis, diagnosis and treatment. A review. *Veterinary Quarterly* 26: 61–75.

Wiberg, M.E. and Westermarck, E. (2002). Subclinical exocrine pancreatic insufficiency in dogs. *Journal of the American Veterinary Medical Association* 220: 1183–1187.

Wiberg, M.E., Nurmi, A.K., and Westermarck, E. (1999a). Serum trypsinlike immunoreactivity measurement for the diagnosis of subclinical exocrine pancreatic insufficiency. *Journal of Veterinary Internal Medicine* 13: 426–432.

Wiberg, M.E., Saari, S.A.M., and Westermarck, E. (1999b). Exocrine pancreatic atrophy in German shepherd dogs and rough-coated collies: an end result of lymphocytic pancreatitis. *Veterinary Pathology* 36: 530–541.

Wiberg, M.E., Saari, S.A.M., Westermarck, E. et al. (2000). Cellular and humoral immune responses in atrophic lymphocytic pancreatitis in German shepherd dogs and rough-coated collies. *Veterinary Immunology and Immunopathology* 76: 103–115.

Williams, D.A. and Batt, R.M. (1983). Diagnosis of canine exocrine pancreatic insufficiency by the assay of serum trypsin-like immunoreactivity. *Journal of Small Animal Practice* 24: 547–604.

Williams, D.A. and Batt, R.M. (1988). Sensitivity and specificity of radioimmunoassay of serum trypsin-like immunoreactivity for the diagnosis of canine exocrine pancreatic insufficiency. *Journal of the American Veterinary Medical Association* 192: 195–201.

Williams, D.A., Batt, R.M., and McLean, L. (1987). Bacterial overgrowth in the duodenum of dogs with exocrine pancreatic insufficiency. *Journal of the American Veterinary Medical Association* 191: 201–206.

Wu, Y.A., Chuang, W.H., Lidbury, J. et al. (2024). Research communications of the 34th ECVIM-CA congress (Re-evaluation of the reference interval and cut-off value for canine trypsin-like immunoreactivity assay). *Journal of Veterinary Internal Medicine* 38: 3537–3694.

Exocrine Pancreatic Insufficiency in Cats

CHAPTER 30

Panagiotis G. Xenoulis

Clinic of Medicine, Faculty of Veterinary Science, University of Thessaly, Karditsa, Greece
Department of Small Animal Clinical Sciences, School of Veterinary and Biomedical Sciences, Texas A&M University, College Station, TX, USA

INTRODUCTION

Exocrine pancreatic insufficiency (EPI) is caused by inadequate production of digestive enzymes from pancreatic acinar cells, leading to maldigestion and subsequent clinical signs such as weight loss and diarrhea. EPI has previously been considered rare in the cat, but it is now recognized that most cases of feline EPI escaped diagnosis in the past due to the lack of sensitive and specific diagnostic tests, low awareness of the disease, and its coexistence with other gastrointestinal (GI) conditions that cause similar clinical signs. The literature on feline EPI is sparse, consisting of 10 cases of confirmed or suspected EPI published between 1975 and 2009, as well as 2 small case series that included a total of 36 cases (Thompson et al. 2009). More recently, a retrospective, survey-based study that evaluated 150 cats with EPI diagnosed based on low TLI concentrations was published (Xenoulis et al. 2016).

EPIDEMIOLOGY

The true prevalence of feline EPI is unknown. Of 180 648 cats that entered the Veterinary Medical Data Base from the early 1980s to the early 1990s, only 11 (0.006%) were diagnosed with EPI (Steiner 2012). However, since the introduction of the feline trypsin-like immunoreactivity (fTLI) assay in 1995 (Steiner et al. 1996), diagnosis has increased. In a recent study, the Gastrointestinal Laboratory's database at Texas A&M University was searched over a period of 2008–2010, and 1,094 of 46,529 serum samples from cats submitted for fTLI measurement had concentrations diagnostic for EPI (2.4%) (Xenoulis et al. 2016). Similarly, at the author's institution, in a series of 100 cats with signs of a chronic enteropathy, 2 cats (2%) were diagnosed with concurrent EPI. Therefore, it appears that EPI is not as uncommon as previously suspected.

ETIOLOGY AND PATHOPHYSIOLOGY

No studies have specifically investigated the causes of EPI in cats. Chronic pancreatitis leading to gradual destruction of acinar cells has been traditionally cited as almost the sole cause of EPI in cats. However, this was based on a small number of case reports of cats diagnosed with EPI (Steiner 2012; Williams 1996). Although chronic pancreatitis is still believed to be the most common cause of feline EPI, other etiologies may also exist. In recent studies, several cats were diagnosed with EPI at a young age, making chronic pancreatitis less likely and suggesting that different etiologies may exist in those cases (Xenoulis et al. 2016). Other less common or rare etiologies for EPI include

Disorders of the Liver, Exocrine Pancreas, and Gastrointestinal Tract in Dogs and Cats, First Edition. Edited by Harry Cridge et al. Published 2026 by John Wiley & Sons, Inc. Companion Website: www.wiley.com/go/cridge/disorders

pancreatic acinar atrophy, pancreatic hypoplasia or aplasia, pressure atrophy due to pancreatic duct obstruction, and *Eurytrema procyonis* infestation (Steiner 2012). Pancreatic acinar atrophy, the most common cause of EPI in dogs, has been reported in a small number of cats with EPI but may be underdiagnosed. In dogs, isolated pancreatic lipase deficiency has been reported as a cause of EPI (while other pancreatic enzymes are normally produced) (Xenoulis et al. 2007), but this has not been reported in cats.

The exocrine pancreas has an exceptional functional reserve, and clinical signs of EPI are believed to develop only when >90% of the secretory capacity of the exocrine pancreas is lost (Steiner 2012). Regardless of the cause, insufficient production and secretion of pancreatic enzymes in the small intestine leads to maldigestion of nutrients. The large amount of undigested nutrients in the intestine may lead to osmotic diarrhea, while decreased absorption of nutrients causes weight loss.

Of major importance is the pathophysiologic association between pancreatic function and cobalamin absorption. The intrinsic factor is a cobalamin-binding protein that facilitates cobalamin absorption in the ileum. In contrast to dogs, in whom the intrinsic factor is also produced in the stomach, the intrinsic factor in cats is produced exclusively in the exocrine pancreas. Therefore, EPI leads to reduced production and secretion of intrinsic factor, resulting in decreased intestinal absorption of cobalamin. This results in hypocobalaminemia and cobalamin deficiency (Ruaux 2013).

In cases in which EPI is a result of chronic pancreatitis, destruction of the endocrine portion of the pancreas may lead to concurrent diabetes mellitus. Additionally, many cats with EPI have concurrent chronic enteropathy (chronic inflammatory enteropathy or small cell lymphoma), hepatic disease, and/or pancreatic inflammation.

SIGNALMENT

There is no significant breed or sex predisposition (Xenoulis et al. 2016). The median age of cats with EPI is about 8 years, but the age range is wide: from 3 months to 19 years (Xenoulis et al. 2016). This is important because EPI has been traditionally considered a disease of middle-aged to older cats. EPI should be considered in any age of cat.

CLINICAL SIGNS

The clinical signs of EPI in cats are nonspecific and are also often seen in other more common diseases (e.g., hyperthyroidism, chronic enteropathies, pancreatitis, chronic kidney disease), making recognition of EPI challenging. Weight loss was by far the most common clinical sign and was present in more than 90% of 150 cats in one study (Figure 30.1) (Xenoulis et al. 2016). In the same study, weight loss was the only clinical sign in 5% of the cats. Loose stools (Figure 30.2) occurred in only 62% of those cats, with two-thirds of them having occasional watery diarrhea. This is in contrast with the typical EPI dog, where loose stools are reported in the vast majority of cases (95% in one study) (Batchelor et al. 2007). Other clinical signs include poor haircoat (50%), polyphagia (42%), anorexia (42%), lethargy (40%), vomiting (19%), and greasy soiling of the haircoat (Figure 30.3) (Xenoulis et al. 2016). As most cats reported with EPI also had concurrent diseases (e.g., concurrent chronic enteropathy), the clinical signs caused by EPI are blurred and some of the reported clinical signs (e.g., anorexia, depression, vomiting) are not typical of EPI and are more likely to be associated with concurrent diseases. There has been one report of a cat with EPI that developed D-lactic acidosis, presumably due to increased bacterial fermentation in the intestine as a result of bacterial overgrowth, who presented with clinical signs of weakness, lethargy, and ataxia. This is considered to be rare.

It is clear that the clinical presentation of many cats with EPI differs from the typical presentation seen in dogs. Clinical signs are more subtle and less specific in cats, and therefore, EPI should be suspected in cases with unexplained weight loss or anorexia even when diarrhea or polyphagia are not present. EPI should also be suspected in cats with chronic enteropathies that do not respond

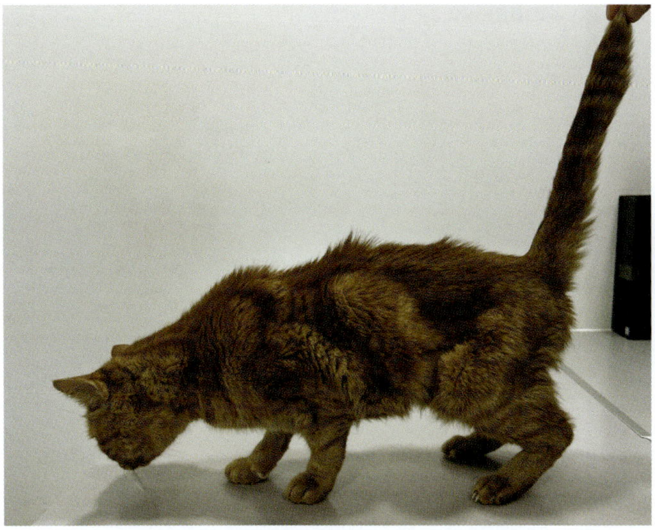

FIGURE 30.1 This cat was diagnosed with EPI and chronic inflammatory enteropathy. The cat is thin (body condition score 2/9). This cat had a normal appetite

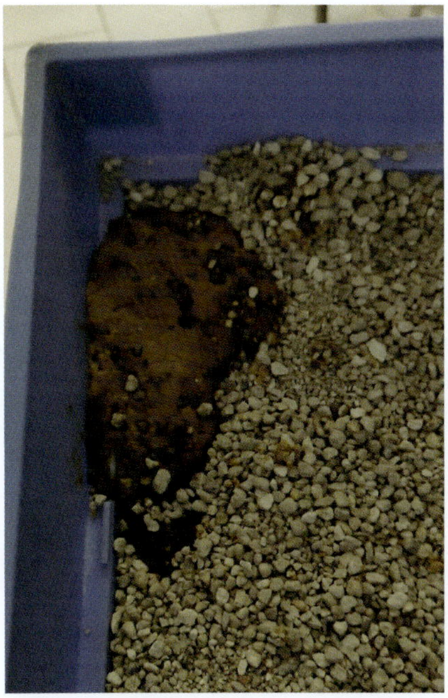

FIGURE 30.2 Feces from the cat in Figure 30.1

to appropriate treatment. Alternatively, all cats diagnosed with a chronic inflammatory enteropathy or small cell lymphoma could be screened for concurrent EPI.

DIAGNOSIS

EPI is initially suspected based on clinical presentation (see above). Cats with GI inflammatory diseases may also have EPI. Cats with GI diseases (e.g., IBD) that do not respond to appropriate treatment may have concurrent EPI that remains undiagnosed. Therefore, in a cat diagnosed with a chronic enteropathy or other GI disease that continues to lose weight or have loose stools despite appropriate treatment, EPI should be in the differential diagnosis list. The author currently

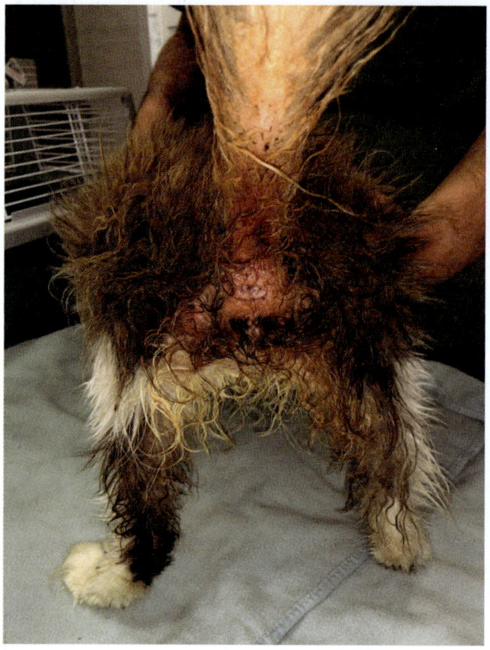

FIGURE 30.3 Cat with chronic inflammatory enteropathy and EPI. Note the greasy soiling of the haircoat

recommends testing for EPI in all cats diagnosed with a chronic inflammatory enteropathy or small cell lymphoma as part of their diagnostic evaluation.

ROUTINE CLINICAL PATHOLOGY

Results of a complete blood count and serum biochemical profile are usually normal or show nonspecific changes. However, due to concurrent diseases, several hematological and biochemical changes may be present, reflecting those diseases (e.g., anemia, increased liver enzyme activities, hyperglycemia, hypoalbuminemia). None of these findings are specific for EPI.

SERUM COBALAMIN

Serum cobalamin concentrations are decreased in the majority of cats with EPI (80–100%) (Xenoulis et al. 2016). There is evidence that tissue cobalamin is depleted before hypocobalaminemia develops, and therefore, even normocobalaminemic cats could still have cellular cobalamin deficiency. Although common in cats with EPI, hypocobalaminemia is not specific for EPI because it is commonly present in cats with other conditions (such as chronic inflammatory enteropathies, small cell lymphoma, hyperthyroidism) (Ruaux 2013).

SERUM TLI CONCENTRATIONS

EPI is a functional disease and requires a functional diagnosis (Steiner 2012). The gold standard for the diagnosis is measurement of serum fTLI concentration (85–100% specificity; sensitivity unknown but considered to be high) (Xenoulis et al. 2016; Ruaux 2013). Ideally, fasting samples should be obtained for serum fTLI measurement. The TLI assays are species-specific, and assays developed and validated for dogs or humans are not appropriate for use in cats. The TLI assays detect the trypsinogen produced by the exocrine pancreas that circulates in the blood. In case of EPI, due to significant reduction of the functional capacity of the exocrine pancreas, serum trypsinogen concentrations are reduced, and these are reflected as subnormal serum fTLI concentrations. Currently, the only validated assay for fTLI is offered by the Gastrointestinal Laboratory at Texas A&M University. The reference range of this assay is 12 to 82 μg/L; values $\leq$ 8 μg/L are considered diagnostic for EPI. Some cats with GI clinical signs have serum fTLI concentrations in the questionable range

(8–12 μg/L). These cats should be retested a few weeks or months later to check whether fTLI concentrations have normalized or are in the diagnostic range for EPI. Because trypsinogen is excreted by the kidney, serum fTLI concentrations may be falsely increased in cats with decreased kidney function (Steiner et al. 2002). Therefore, a diagnosis of EPI may be hampered in some cats with azotemia due to chronic kidney disease. In cats in whom EPI is suspected and who are azotemic, reevaluation of serum fTLI concentrations after improvement of azotemia may be needed.

IMAGING AND PATHOLOGY

Imaging modalities (radiographs, ultrasound, computed tomography) are not helpful for the diagnosis of EPI in cats because they do not reflect the functional capacity of the pancreas. However, imaging can be useful for the diagnosis or exclusion of concurrent diseases or diseases that can cause similar clinical signs. Gross appearance of a small pancreas and histopathology are also not useful for a diagnosis of EPI because they do not reflect the functional capacity of the pancreas.

TREATMENT

ENZYME REPLACEMENT THERAPY

As in dogs, the mainstay of treatment in cats with EPI is pancreatic enzyme supplementation. There are several commercial products (dried extracts of porcine pancreas) available, but no studies have evaluated the efficacy of different products and preparations in this species. In a recent study, no difference was identified with regard to the specific product or type of pancreatic enzyme used for the treatment of feline EPI, and therefore, all products might be equally effective (Xenoulis et al. 2016). Although older studies in dogs supported the use of powdered products while enteric-coated products were considered less effective, a recent prospective, placebo-controlled study showed that enteric-coated products may be more efficacious (Mas et al. 2012). Raw pancreas from beef, pork, or game may also be used (Steiner 2012). The author's personal preference is powdered or enteric-coated products.

Regardless of the product used, pancreatic enzymes should be added to each meal and thoroughly mixed with food. The dose for each product has not been established, and it is titrated for each cat based on response to treatment. An initial dose of one teaspoon of pancreatic enzyme powder per meal seems appropriate (Steiner 2012). Enteric-coated products could be used at an initial dose of 300 mg of pancreatin per day (divided in each meal). Response to treatment is expected to be quick, with resolution of loose stools usually within the first week. After resolution of clinical signs, gradual reduction to the lowest effective dose should be attempted. If raw pancreas is used, about 50 g per meal is appropriate as initial dose, with dose adjustments as needed. Raw pancreas should be kept frozen in portions of 50 g until use (for several months without losing efficacy). However, it should be made clear to the owners that feeding raw pancreas may be associated with a small risk of infectious and parasitic disease transmission (e.g., bovine spongiform encephalitis, Aujeszky disease, and parasites such as *Echinococcus* spp.) (Steiner 2012).

Due to their ability to break down protein and fat, pancreatic enzymes can cause oral or esophageal irritation and ulcers if they remain long enough in contact with the oral or esophageal mucosa. Therefore, powdered pancreatic enzymes should be mixed thoroughly with food, while administration of tablets or capsules should be followed by food or water consumption to reduce the risk for stomatitis and esophagitis (Steiner 2012).

COBALAMIN SUPPLEMENTATION

Cobalamin supplementation is also of major importance and has been shown to favorably affect response to treatment both in EPI cats and cats with chronic enteropathies, two conditions that often coexist (Xenoulis et al. 2016; Ruaux et al. 2005). Cobalamin deficiency can lead to intestinal inflammation and villus atrophy, disturbance of various biochemical pathways, and malabsorption of nutrients such as folate (Ruaux 2013). In cats with GI disease and severe hypocobalaminemia, cobalamin supplementation led to significant increases in body weight and improvement of vomiting and diarrhea (Ruaux et al. 2005). In a study of 150 cats with EPI, cobalamin supplementation favorably affected the response to treatment, even in cats with normal serum cobalamin concentrations (Xenoulis et al. 2016). Finally, hypocobalaminemia associated with certain GI diseases in dogs has been shown to be a negative prognostic factor, and hypocobalaminemia in dogs with EPI was associated with shorter survival (Soetart et al. 2019; Volkmann et al. 2017).

The exact serum cobalamin concentration that indicates cellular cobalamin deficiency and designates the need for cobalamin supplementation is currently unknown and hampered by the fact that normal serum cobalamin concentrations vary greatly among laboratories. The use of markers of cobalamin deficiency, such as serum methylmalonic acid (MMA) concentrations, is more useful but not routinely available (Worhunsky et al. 2013).

In addition to cats with hypocobalaminemia, in whom cobalamin supplementation is clearly indicated, some normocobalaminemic cats with EPI (especially those in the lower range of the reference interval) could benefit from cobalamin supplementation, possibly because these cats have cellular cobalamin deficiency (Xenoulis et al. 2016; Ruaux 2013; Worhunsky et al. 2013). Due to the fact that virtually all cats with EPI either have or are prone to develop cobalamin deficiency due to lack of intrinsic factor, it might be recommended that cats with EPI should be supplemented with cobalamin regardless of their serum cobalamin concentration.

Due to lack of intrinsic factor and the resulting impaired cobalamin absorption by the GI tract, parenteral cobalamin supplementation is typically recommended (Steiner 2012; Ruaux 2013). Studies on the kinetics of parenteral cobalamin supplementation in cats with or without GI disease indicate that the serum half-life of cobalamin is 5 and 13 days, respectively (Simpson et al. 2001). Protocols on cobalamin supplementation in cats with GI disease have been published, and efficacy may be variable depending upon the underlying GI disease, the frequency of administration, and the formulation used (Steiner 2012; Ruaux 2013). In a recent study (Chang et al. 2024), both parenteral and oral administration of cyanocobalamin were found to be effective in cats with EPI. Hydroxycobalamin is also likely equally effective. The recommended doses are 250 μg per cat, SC or IM, every one week for six weeks and an additional dose four weeks after the sixth injection. Oral dose is 250 μg per cat daily for 12 weeks. Monthly rechecks of serum cobalamin concentrations are recommended. Many cats will require long-term cobalamin supplementation despite enzyme replacement treatment for EPI.

ANTIBIOTICS AND INTESTINAL MICROBIOTA MODIFICATION

Antibiotic use was not found to affect response to treatment in cats with EPI in one study (Xenoulis et al. 2016). Antibiotics have been used in the past in dogs with EPI to control concurrent intestinal dysbiosis, although no clear benefit has been shown in some studies. However, disturbances of the microbiota in cats with EPI have not been fully described or confirmed, and therefore, antibiotic use is of unknown benefit in these cases. In addition, antibiotic use is known to induce long-lasting intestinal dysbiosis in cats. Therefore, the author currently does not recommend the use of antibiotics in cats with EPI.

Probiotics may also be able to control intestinal dysbiosis, but no studies are available. Fecal microbiota transplantation (FMT) is gaining ground as a means of intestinal microbiota modification but studies in cats with EPI are lacking.

DIETARY RECOMMENDATIONS

No evidence-based dietary recommendations can be made for cats with EPI. A good quality, high protein maintenance diet would seem appropriate in most cases unless concurrent diseases are present that make necessary the use of specific clinical diets. As many cats with EPI and concurrent chronic enteropathy have significant weight loss, diets with high caloric density should be selected if possible. Some cats with concurrent chronic enteropathy may benefit from hypoallergenic diets (protein restricted or hydrolyzed), and so concurrent diseases may need to be prioritized when selecting a diet.

OTHER TREATMENTS

Some authors recommend using a proton-pump inhibitor (e.g., omeprazole or pantoprazole) concurrently with pancreatic enzyme replacement therapy to reduce gastric acidity and decrease enzyme inhibition in the stomach. However, the benefits of such treatment are unknown, and most cats seem to respond well without such intervention. Cats that do not respond well to pancreatic enzyme and cobalamin supplementation may be put on a proton-pump inhibitor to see if this will change the response to treatment.

There have been occasional reports of cats with EPI that presented with coagulopathy that responded to vitamin K_1 supplementation. Although believed to be very rare, if bleeding diathesis is noted in an EPI cat, coagulation parameters should be measured, and vitamin K supplementation should be initiated.

PROGNOSIS

Overall response to treatment is considered good in 60% of cases, and cats with EPI that are treated appropriately typically have an excellent prognosis and a good quality of life (Xenoulis et al. 2016). Only 13% of cases have been reported to have a poor response to treatment. The reason that some cats do not respond well to treatment for EPI is not clear. Lack of or partial response to treatment might be due to lack of cobalamin administration or the presence of inadequately managed concurrent diseases (e.g., chronic enteropathies, liver disease). All cats that do not respond to appropriate treatment should be reevaluated for wrong diagnosis or important concurrent disease.

REFERENCES

Batchelor, D.J., Noble, P.J.M., Cripps, P.J. et al. (2007). Breed associations for canine exocrine pancreatic insufficiency. *Journal of Veterinary Internal Medicine* 21: 207–214.

Chang, C.H., Lidbury, J., Suchodolski, J.S. et al. (2024). Effect of oral or subcutaneous administration of cyanocobalamin in hypocobalaminemic cats with chronic gastrointestinal disease or exocrine pancreatic insufficiency. *Journal of Veterinary Internal Medicine* 38 (5): 2464–2479.

Mas, A., Noble, P.J., Cripps, P.J., et al. (2012). A blinded randomised controlled trial to determine the effect of enteric coating on enzyme treatment for canine exocrine pancreatic efficiency. *BMC Veterinary Research* 8: 127.

Ruaux, C.G. (2013). Cobalamin in companion animals: diagnostic marker, deficiency states and therapeutic implications. *The Veterinary Journal* 196: 145–152.

Ruaux, C.G., Steiner, J.M., and Williams, D.A. (2005). Early biochemical and clinical responses to cobalamin supplementation in cats with signs of gastrointestinal disease and severe hypocobalaminemia. *Journal of Veterinary Internal Medicine* 19: 155–160.

Simpson, K.W., Fyfe, J., Cornetta, A. et al. (2001). Subnormal concentrations of serum cobalamin (Vitamin B 12) in cats with gastrointestinal disease. *Journal of Veterinary Internal Medicine* 15: 26–32.

Soetart, N., Rochel, D., Drut, A. et al. (2019). Serum cobalamin and folate as prognostic factors in canine exocrine pancreatic insufficiency: an observational cohort study of 299 dogs. *The Veterinary Journal* 243: 15–20.

Steiner, J.M. (2012). Exocrine pancreatic insufficiency in the cat. *Topics in Companion Animal Medicine* 27: 113–116.

Steiner, J.M., Finco, D.R., and Williams, D.A. (2002). Serum feline trypsin-like immunoreactivity (fTLI) in cats with experimentally induced chronic renal failure. *Journal of Veterinary Internal Medicine* 16: 385.

Steiner, J.M., Medinger, T.L., and Williams, D.A. (1996). Development and validation of a radioimmunoassay for feline trypsin-like immunoreactivity. *American Journal of Veterinary Research* 57: 1417–1420.

Thompson, K.A., Parnell, N.K., Hohenhaus, A.E. et al. (2009). Feline exocrine pancreatic insufficiency: 16 cases (1992–2007). *Journal of Feline Medicine and Surgery* 11 (12): 935–940.

Volkmann, M., Steiner, J.M., Fosgate, G.T. et al. (2017). Chronic diarrhea in dogs - retrospective study in 136 cases. *Journal of Veterinary Internal Medicine* 31: 1043–1055.

Williams, D.A. (1996). The pancreas. In: *Small Animal Gastroenterology* (eds. D.R. Strombeck, W.G. Guilford, S.A. Center et al.), 381–410. Philadelphia: W.B. Saunders.

Worhunsky, P., Toulza, O., Rishniw, M. et al. (2013). The relationship of serum cobalamin to methylmalonic acid concentrations and clinical variables in cats. *Journal of Veterinary Internal Medicine* 27: 1056–1063.

Xenoulis, P.G., Fradkin, J.M., Rapp, S.W. et al. (2007). Suspected isolated pancreatic lipase deficiency in a dog. *Journal of Veterinary Internal Medicine* 21: 1113–1116.

Xenoulis, P.G., Zoran, D.L., Fosgate, G.T. et al. (2016). Feline exocrine pancreatic insufficiency: a retrospective study of 150 cases. *Journal of Veterinary Internal* 30: 1790–1797.

Neoplasia and Uncommon Disorders of the Exocrine Pancreas

CHAPTER 31

Sue Yee Lim

Department of Small Animal Clinical Sciences, College of Veterinary Medicine & Biomedical Sciences, Texas A&M University, College Station, TX, USA

KEY POINTS

- Exocrine pancreatic neoplasia is rare in dogs and cats.
- The prognosis remains poor, with many patients presenting with local and/or distant metastasis at the time of diagnosis.
- Exocrine pancreatic neoplasia is often accompanied by pancreatic inflammation, which can lead to elevated serum pancreatic lipase concentrations or activities.
- A pancreatic mass may be malignant, benign, or inflammatory and can be challenging to differentiate antemortem. Ultrasound-guided fine needle aspirate or surgical biopsy may assist in diagnosis.

EXOCRINE PANCREATIC NEOPLASIA

Exocrine pancreatic neoplasia is rare in dogs and cats and has an incidence rate of about 1% in both species (Priester 1974; Cony et al. 2023). In contrast, exocrine pancreatic neoplasia is the fourth leading cause of cancer death worldwide in people (Cronin et al. 2022). The exocrine pancreas comprises acinar cells arranged in clusters called acini, which have an empty center where ductal epithelium forms ducts. Pancreatic exocrine neoplasia can arise from the acinar cells or ductal epithelium. Pancreatic adenocarcinoma (including ductal adenocarcinoma) is most common and accounts for 85% of all pancreatic neoplasia in people (Rawla et al. 2019). Interestingly, pancreatic acinar carcinoma is more common in dogs and cats (Selmic 2020; Aupperle-Lellbach et al. 2019; Linderman et al. 2013; Cony et al. 2023). Pancreatic exocrine carcinomas show aggressive biological behavior even in the early stages in people, dogs, and cats (Aupperle-Lellbach et al. 2019; Selmic 2020; Linderman et al. 2013; Torner et al. 2020). However, it is associated with few clinical signs that are often nonspecific and thus are not diagnosed until late in the disease when most have regional or distant spread (Cronin et al. 2022; Selmic 2020). As such, pancreatic exocrine carcinoma carries a poor prognosis in people, dogs, and cats.

RISK FACTORS

The exact cause of exocrine pancreatic carcinoma in people is not known, although certain risk factors such as tobacco smoking, dietary factors, alcohol, obesity, diabetes mellitus, chronic pancreatitis, and genetics have been identified (Rawla et al. 2019). There is no comparable information available for dogs and cats, as this disease is rare in these species. In people, KRAS mutations are seen in pancreatic ductal carcinoma, but these mutations have not been found in dogs and cats (Crozier et al. 2016). Exocrine pancreatic carcinomas are seen in older patients with an average of 10 years in dogs and 12 years in cats (Aupperle-Lellbach et al. 2019; Dunn et al. 2024;

Disorders of the Liver, Exocrine Pancreas, and Gastrointestinal Tract in Dogs and Cats, First Edition. Edited by Harry Cridge et al. Published 2026 by John Wiley & Sons, Inc. Companion Website: www.wiley.com/go/cridge/disorders

Pinard et al. 2021; Linderman et al. 2013). Although exceedingly rare, there is one report of a necropsy-confirmed pancreatic carcinoma in a kitten (<1 year) (Cony et al. 2023). Historically, more females have been reported than males, but recent studies have not shown a clear sex predilection (Priester 1974; Aupperle-Lellbach et al. 2019; Dunn et al. 2024; Pinard et al. 2021). One study reported more male than female cats (Linderman et al. 2013). There is no clear breed predisposition other than Airedale terriers (Priester 1974).

PRESENTING HISTORY AND CLINICAL SIGNS

Exocrine pancreatic carcinoma may be accompanied by concurrent pancreatic inflammation. (Aupperle-Lellbach et al. 2019; Torner et al. 2020). Therefore, dogs and cats may present for suspected pancreatitis with nonspecific clinical signs such as lethargy, hyporexia or anorexia, vomiting, weight loss, and diarrhea (Dunn et al. 2024; Pinard et al. 2021; Aupperle-Lellbach et al. 2020; Torner et al. 2020; Linderman et al. 2013; Seaman 2004). On physical examination, a patient may have a palpable cranial abdominal mass with a variable level of abdominal pain, dehydration, distended abdomen from mass effect or peritoneal effusion, and/or jaundice. Dogs may present with panniculitis and polyarthritis, which are associated with pancreatitis or pancreatic carcinoma in people (Arbelaez-Cortes et al. 2014; Gear et al. 2006). Cats may present with alopecia of the ventral trunk and limbs, which is a distinctive paraneoplastic syndrome in cats with pancreatic adenocarcinoma or cholangiocarcinoma (Tasker et al. 1999).

CLINICOPATHOLOGIC FINDINGS

A minimum database (CBC, chemistry, and urinalysis) is recommended for all sick patients. Changes seen on the minimum database are often nonspecific and may be similar to patients with pancreatitis (Seaman 2004; Pinard et al. 2021; Linderman et al. 2013). On CBC, we may see hemoconcentration indicating dehydration, while a non-regenerative mild anemia may be more common in cats with chronic disease. There may be an inflammatory leukogram (leukocytosis with neutrophilia and toxic changes seen on smear evaluation) or leukopenia (more common in cats). A patient may have azotemia, elevated liver enzymes (ALT, ALP), hyperlipasemia, and hyperbilirubinemia. A urinalysis is needed to differentiate pre-renal from renal azotemia and may demonstrate bilirubinuria.

Serum pancreatic lipase concentrations (as measured by Spec PL assay or PLI in-house ELISAs) or activities (as measured by DGGR-lipase assays) can also be elevated in patients with exocrine pancreatic carcinoma due to concurrent pancreatitis (Aupperle-Lellbach et al. 2020; Aupperle-Lellbach et al. 2019; Torner et al. 2020). In a small study in dogs, pancreatic lipase-producing tumors of the pancreas (adenocarcinoma, carcinoma) and liver (hepatocellular carcinoma) resulted in marked hyperlipasemia beyond what is typically observed in patients with pancreatitis (Quigley et al. 2001). With the exception of one dog with documented peripancreatic inflammation, it is unclear whether other patients in this study have accompanying pancreatitis. Serum trypsin-like immunoreactivity concentrations may be elevated in some patients with concurrent pancreatitis or may be low in patients developing exocrine pancreatic insufficiency as a sequela of their exocrine pancreatic carcinoma (Linderman et al. 2013; Bright 1985). Serum C-reactive protein concentrations may also be elevated due to nonspecific local and systemic inflammation.

DIAGNOSTIC IMAGING FINDINGS

Diagnostic imaging is important for the diagnosis of exocrine pancreatic carcinoma in dogs and cats. On radiographs, a mass effect may be identified in the cranial abdomen with loss of serosal details due to the presence of inflammation and/or effusion (Seaman 2004; Linderman et al. 2013; Hecht et al. 2007). There could be accompanying hepatomegaly (reactive or metastasis). Although rare, distant pulmonary metastasis, sternal lymphadenopathy, and pleural effusion have been reported in cats (Linderman et al. 2013).

Ultrasound is a useful and noninvasive diagnostic imaging modality for pancreatic disease. Ultrasonographic findings are dependent on the biological nature of the neoplasia. In dogs, exocrine pancreatic carcinoma can appear as a distinct heterogeneous mass (up to 6 cm) with occasional cavitated centers (Pinard et al. 2021). The right pancreatic limb is most affected, with variable distribution in the left limb or pancreatic body. Small pancreatic nodules seen on B-mode ultrasound can be differentiated from insulinoma with contrast-enhanced ultrasound (Vanderperren et al. 2014). Pancreatic adenocarcinomas are poorly enhanced (hypovascular) lesions, while insulinomas are uniformly contrast-enhanced (hypervascular) lesions (Vanderperren et al. 2014). Dogs can also have multiple smaller nodules throughout their pancreas, and this must be differentiated from nodular hyperplasia, which is a common benign finding of no clinical significance in older dogs. Patients with diffuse non-mass forming exocrine pancreatic carcinoma can have a normal-appearing pancreas, hypoechoic and enlarged (most often diagnosed primarily as pancreatitis or pancreatic edema on imaging), or mildly enlarged with rounded borders (Pinard et al. 2021). In cats, exocrine pancreatic carcinoma can appear as a single mass (ranging from 0.4 to 12 cm) or as multifocal nodules (ranging from 0.5 to 2 cm) (Linderman et al. 2013; Hecht et al. 2007; Cony et al. 2023). The left pancreatic limb is most commonly affected, with variable distribution in the right limb or pancreatic body (Linderman et al. 2013; Cony et al. 2023). There is a tendency for neoplastic lesions to manifest as a single large lesion >2 cm, although this is often not sufficient to assist in prioritizing differentials (Hecht et al. 2007). Cats can also have dilated bile and/or pancreatic ducts due to the location of the lesion (Hecht et al. 2007). Similar to dogs, it can be challenging to differentiate multinodular pancreatic carcinoma from benign nodular hyperplasia (Hecht et al. 2007; Torner et al. 2020).

Like people, most dogs and cats diagnosed with exocrine pancreatic carcinoma have local and distant metastasis at the time of diagnosis (Cronin et al. 2022; Pinard et al. 2021; Hecht et al. 2007). Common sites include the liver, regional lymph nodes, and small intestines (Aupperle-Lellbach et al. 2019; Pinard et al. 2021; Hecht et al. 2007). Liver metastasis can appear as generalized hepatomegaly with diffuse nodules that may appear hypoechoic, heterogenous, or targetoid (Pinard et al. 2021; Linderman et al. 2013). Its biological behavior cannot be predicted from B-mode ultrasound appearance. Less common sites include the spleen, diffuse carcinomatosis, adipose tissue, lungs, diaphragm, and brain (Chang et al. 2007; Pinard et al. 2021; Monteiro and O'Brien 2004; Cony et al. 2023). Interestingly, pulmonary metastasis without local spread has been reported in dogs (Pinard et al. 2021).

Computed tomography and magnetic resonance imaging are used frequently in people, especially because exocrine pancreatic carcinoma is a disease with a high rate of local invasion and distant metastasis. In a multicenter study, CT features of exocrine pancreatic carcinomas in dogs and cats mirrored their findings on ultrasound and included a well-defined, heterogeneously contrast-enhancing mass, often with a non-enhancing fluid to soft tissue attenuating center (Dunn et al. 2024). The right pancreatic limb was most affected, followed by the left limb and pancreatic body. Masses on the right pancreatic limb are more commonly associated with extrahepatic bile duct obstruction. Other concurrent peripancreatic findings include fat-stranding, soft tissue nodules, and peritoneal effusion (Dunn et al. 2024). Magnetic resonance imaging findings of exocrine pancreatic neoplasia have not been reported in veterinary medicine.

PATHOLOGY AND SAMPLING

Grossly, exocrine pancreatic carcinoma in dogs and cats can present as a large mass (reported up to 8 cm in dogs and 12 cm in cats), multinodular (Figure 31.1a), or diffuse (Aupperle-Lellbach et al. 2019; Torner et al. 2020; Cony et al. 2023). Pancreatic cystic adenomas in cats can appear as large masses (up to 6 cm) but have a multicystic smooth cut surface (Torner et al. 2020). Exocrine pancreatic carcinoma can be accompanied by varying degrees of hemorrhage, necrosis, and inflammation (Van Wettere 2022). The lesion is usually firmer than the surrounding pancreas due to the proliferation of fibrous connective tissue (Van Wettere 2022). The affected pancreas

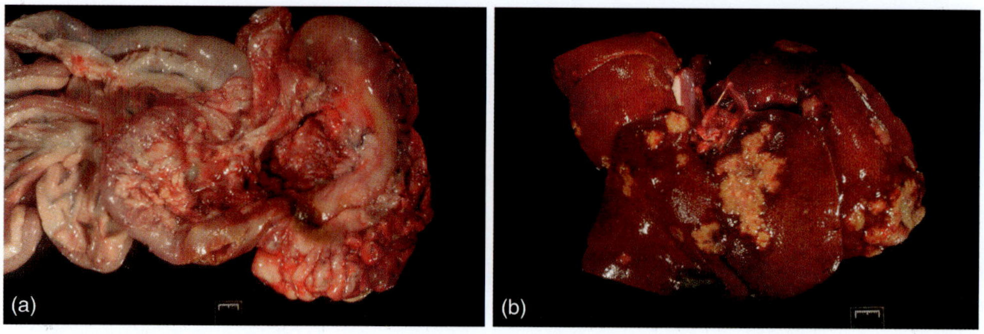

FIGURE 31.1 Pancreatic adenocarcinoma with metastasis to the liver and regional lymph nodes in a 7-year-old female spayed Shih Tzu. (a) The pancreas is diffusely enlarged, firm to hard, and multinodular with loss of normal architecture. (b) Throughout all liver lobes are numerous, multifocal, pale tan, firm, elevated nodules with a depressed center. Images courtesy of Dr. Raquel Rech (DVM, MS, PhD, DACVP) and Dr. Chi-Hsuan Sung (DVM, PhD)

may invade adjacent tissue and metastasize locally to the liver (Figure 31.1b) and surrounding lymph nodes (pancreaticoduodenal, hepatic). Seeding into the peritoneal cavity is suspected when there are multiple nodules over the mesentery, omentum, and serosa of abdominal organs. On histopathology, vascular invasion is also common (Aupperle-Lellbach et al. 2019; Torner et al. 2020).

Ultrasound-guided fine needle aspirates of the pancreas for cytology can be performed safely even in sick patients (Cordner et al. 2015). In one study, diagnosis of exocrine pancreatic carcinoma (along with other tumors, including lymphoma, neuroendocrine tumor, and sarcoma) could be achieved with cytology (Cordner et al. 2015). Benign lesions such as exocrine pancreatic hyperplasia can also be identified (Cordner et al. 2015). Exocrine pancreatic neoplasia in dogs and cats is often accompanied by pancreatic inflammation (Torner et al. 2020; Aupperle-Lellbach et al. 2019). However, pancreatic cytology has its limitations, as epithelial cells can show atypical (or dysplastic) features in the presence of overwhelming inflammation, and this atypia may be confused for features of malignancy. In short, the presence of neoplastic cells without overwhelming inflammation is suggestive of exocrine pancreatic neoplasia, but the presence of inflammation without neoplastic cells does not rule out neoplasia. Percutaneous ultrasound-guided Tru-Cut biopsy, surgical incisional/excisional biopsy, or laparoscopic biopsy is more useful but often unattainable in sick and unstable patients. Additional studies are ongoing to determine the degree of correlation between fine needle aspirates of the pancreas and histopathologic features.

TREATMENT AND PROGNOSIS

Pancreatic exocrine carcinoma carries a poor prognosis in people, dogs, and cats. Accounting for euthanasia at the time of initial diagnosis, dogs and cats with pancreatic carcinoma have short survival times (1–30 days in dogs, 97–165 days in cats) (Pinard et al. 2021; Linderman et al. 2013; Aupperle-Lellbach et al. 2019). Cats with effusion at the time of diagnosis had a shorter mean survival time (30 days) when compared to those without effusion (165 days) (Linderman et al. 2013). Because the effusion was sampled in only 25% of patients, it is unknown if these effusions represent carcinomatosis (Linderman et al. 2013). In dogs and cats, tumor size is not associated with survival (Linderman et al. 2013; Pinard et al. 2021). In dogs, tumor location and lymph node metastasis are also not associated with survival (Pinard et al. 2021). A variant of exocrine pancreatic carcinoma termed hyalinizing pancreatic adenocarcinoma is reported to have low-grade malignancy with some dogs surviving >15 months after diagnosis (Dennis et al. 2008). Although mitotic rate or degree of differentiation was not statistically significant with respect to survival or disease progression, cats with well-differentiated tumors have been reported to survive up to 330 days without adjuvant chemotherapy (Linderman et al. 2013).

The benefits of therapy with surgery or radiation and adjuvant chemotherapy remain unknown in dogs and cats alike (Pinard et al. 2021; Linderman et al. 2013). Surgical therapy includes exploratory, with biopsy for inoperable lesions and pancreaticoduodenectomy for operable lesions. The median survival time for cats undergoing surgery is longer (165 days) than for cats without (30 days) (Linderman et al. 2013). Radiation therapy includes stereotactic radiation therapy (20 Gy) to the center of the pancreatic mass (Pinard et al. 2021). Chemotherapy protocols vary widely (Linderman et al. 2013). The median survival time for cats receiving chemotherapy as part of their therapy is longer (165 days) than for cats without (7 days) (Linderman et al. 2013). However, survival is still low with only 3 out of 32 cats in the study surviving beyond a year. All these cats received some form of chemotherapy and/or surgery (Linderman et al. 2013). The median survival time for cats receiving NSAIDs (meloxicam, piroxicam) is longer (165 days) than for cats without (26 days) (Linderman et al. 2013).

LESS COMMON EXOCRINE PANCREATIC LESIONS

Exocrine pancreatic adenomas are rare in dogs and cats. Like exocrine pancreatic carcinoma, they can arise from the acinar cells or ductal epithelium. However, in contrast with carcinomas, adenomas are usually solitary small lesions. Histologically, adenomas can be challenging to differentiate from hyperplastic nodules, although hyperplastic nodules tend to be numerous. Rarely, exocrine pancreatic adenoma can be cystic. Other cystic lesions of the pancreas include pancreatic fluid accumulations (e.g., pseudocyst or pancreatic cyst). Pancreatic pseudocyst is seen in people as a sequela of acute pancreatitis. It occurs infrequently in dogs and cats (VanEnkevort et al. 1999; Hines et al. 1996). It is a fluid-filled fibrous sac that is non-epithelialized and can contain blood, cellular debris, and pancreatic enzymes. It can form within the pancreas or adjacent to the pancreas. Pancreatic cysts are congenital abnormalities that are believed to result from cystic dilation of pancreatic ducts. They can also occur as a component of congenital polycystic disease affecting the liver and kidneys and have been reported in Cairn terriers, West Highland White terriers, and Persian cats. Unlike pseudocysts, true cysts are lined with epithelial cells. Although usually benign without clinical significance, the large pancreatic cyst can cause clinical signs due to its mass effect. This was reported in a five-month-old puppy with a 16 cm cyst originating from the left pancreatic limb causing abdominal pain, bilateral pelvic limb weakness, reluctance to walk, intermittent vomiting, and diarrhea, which resolved with surgical removal of the cyst (Healy et al. 2022). Ectopic splenic tissues have been reported in dogs and cats and should not be mistaken for neoplasia. Grossly, they appear to be firm, well-demarcated, dark red, spherical lesions. When examined microscopically, they are composed of normal splenic tissues.

REFERENCES

Arbelaez-Cortes, A., Vanegas-Garcia, A.L., Restrepo-Escobar, M. et al. (2014). Polyarthritis and pancreatic panniculitis associated with pancreatic carcinoma: review of the literature. *Journal of Clinical Rheumatology* 20 (8): 433–436. https://doi.org/10.1097/RHU.0000000000000181.

Aupperle-Lellbach, H., Torner, K., Staudacher, M. et al. (2019). Characterization of 22 canine pancreatic carcinomas and review of literature. *Journal of Comparative Pathology* 173: 71–82. https://doi.org/10.1016/j.jcpa.2019.10.008.

Aupperle-Lellbach, H., Torner, K., Staudacher, M. et al. (2020). Histopathological findings and canine pancreatic lipase immunoreactivity in normal dogs and dogs with inflammatory and neoplastic diseases of the pancreas. *Journal of Veterinary Internal Medicine* 34 (3): 1127–1134. https://doi.org/10.1111/jvim.15779.

Bright, J.M. (1985). Pancreatic adenocarcinoma in a dog with a maldigestion syndrome. *Journal of the American Veterinary Medical Association* 187 (4): 420–421.

Chang, S.C., Liao, J.W., Lin, Y.C. et al. (2007). Pancreatic acinar cell carcinoma with intracranial metastasis in a dog. *The Journal of Veterinary Medical Science* 69 (1): 91–93. https://doi.org/10.1292/jvms.69.91.

Cony, F.G., Slaviero M., Santos I.R. et al. (2023). Pathological and immunohistochemical characterization of pancreatic carcinoma in cats. *Journal of Comparative Pathology* 201:123–129. https://doi: 10.1016/j.jcpa.2023.01.008.Cordner, A.P., Sharkey, L.C., Armstrong, P.J. et al. (2015). Cytologic findings and diagnostic yield in 92 dogs undergoing fine-needle aspiration of the pancreas. *Journal of Veterinary Diagnostic Investigation* 27 (2): 236–240. https://doi.org/10.1177/1040638715574862.

Cronin, K.A., Scott, S., Firth, A.U. et al. (2022). Annual report to the nation on the status of cancer, part 1: national cancer statistics. *Cancer* 128 (24): 4251–4284. https://doi.org/10.1002/cncr.34479.

Crozier, C., Wood, G.A., Foster, R.A. et al. (2016). KRAS mutations in canine and feline pancreatic acinar cell carcinoma. *Journal of Comparative Pathology* 155 (1): 24–28. https://doi.org/10.1016/j.jcpa.2016.05.007.

Dennis, M.M., O'brien, T.D., Wayne, T. et al. (2008). Hyalinizing pancreatic adenocarcinoma in six dogs. *Veterinary Pathology* 45 (4): 475–483. https://doi.org/10.1354/vp.45-4-475.

Dunn, A., Rao, S., Husbands, B. et al. (2024). Computed tomographic features of exocrine pancreatic carcinomas in dogs and cats. *Veterinary Radiology & Ultrasound* 65 (4): 400–407. https://doi.org/10.1111/vru.13370.

Gear, R.N., Bacon, N.J., Langley-Hobbs, S. et al. (2006). Panniculitis, polyarthritis and osteomyelitis associated with pancreatic neoplasia in two dogs. *Journal of Small Animal Practice* 47 (7): 400–404. https://doi.org/10.1111/j.1748-5827.2006.00162.x.

Healy, D.M., Cassidy, J.P., and Martin, S.A. (2022). A true congenital pancreatic cyst in a dog. *BMC Veterinary Research* 18 (1): 304. https://doi.org/10.1186/s12917-022-03215-6.

Hecht, S., Penninck, D.G., and Keating, J.H. (2007). Imaging findings in pancreatic neoplasia and nodular hyperplasia in 19 cats. *Veterinary Radiology & Ultrasound* 48 (1): 45–50. https://doi.org/10.1111/j.1740-8261.2007.00203.x.

Hines, B.L., Salisbury, S.K., Jakovljevic, S. et al. (1996). Pancreatic pseudocyst associated with chronic-active necrotizing pancreatitis in a cat. *Journal of the American Animal Hospital Association* 32 (2): 147–152. https://doi.org/10.5326/15473317-32-2-147.

Linderman, M.J., Brodsky, E.M., De Lorimier, L.P. et al. (2013). Feline exocrine pancreatic carcinoma: a retrospective study of 34 cases. *Veterinary and Comparative Oncology* 11 (3): 208–218. https://doi.org/10.1111/j.1476-5829.2012.00320.x

Monteiro, C.B. and O'brien, R.T. (2004). A retrospective study on the sonographic findings of abdominal carcinomatosis in 14 cats. *Veterinary Radiology & Ultrasound* 45 (6): 559–564. https://doi.org/10.1111/j.1740-8261.2004.04096.x.

Pinard, C.J., Hocker, S.E., and Weishaar, K.M. (2021). Clinical outcome in 23 dogs with exocrine pancreatic carcinoma. *Veterinary and Comparative Oncology* 19 (1): 109–114. https://doi.org/10.1111/vco.12645.

Priester, W.A. (1974). Data from eleven United States and Canadian colleges of veterinary medicine on pancreatic carcinoma in domestic animals. *Cancer Research* 34 (6): 1372–1375.

Quigley, K.A., Jackson, M.L., and Haines, D.M. (2001) Hyperlipasemia in 6 dogs with pancreatic or hepatic neoplasia: evidence for tumor lipase production. *Veterinary Clinical Pathology* 30 (3): 114–120. https://doi.org/10.1111/j.1939-165x.2001.tb00418.x.

Rawla, P., Sunkara, T., and Gaduputi, V. (2019). Epidemiology of pancreatic cancer: global trends, etiology and risk factors. *World Journal of Clinical Oncology* 10 (1): 10–27. https://doi.org/10.14740/wjon1166.

Seaman, R.L. (2004). Exocrine pancreatic neoplasia in the cat: a case series. *Journal of the American Animal Hospital Association* 40 (3): 238–245. https://doi.org/10.5326/0400238.

Selmic, L.E. (2020). Exocrine pancreatic cancer. In: *Withrow & MacEwen's Small Animal Clinical Oncology* (ed. D.M. Vail, D.H. Thamm, and J.M. Liptak), 451–452. St. Louis, Missouri: Elsevier.

Tasker, S., Griffon, D.J., Nuttall, T.J. et al. (1999). Resolution of paraneoplastic alopecia following surgical removal of a pancreatic carcinoma in a cat. *Journal of Small Animal Practice* 40 (1): 16–19. https://doi.org/10.1111/j.1748-5827.1999.tb03248.x.

Torner, K., Staudacher, M., Tress, U. et al. (2020). Histopathology and feline pancreatic lipase immunoreactivity in inflammatory, hyperplastic and neoplastic pancreatic diseases in cats. *Journal of Comparative Pathology* 174: 63–72. https://doi.org/10.1016/j.jcpa.2019.10.195.

Van Wettere, A.J. and Brown, D.L. (2022). Hepatobiliary system and exocrine pancreas. In: *Pathologic Basis of Veterinary Disease* (ed. J.F. Zachary), 486–546. St. Louis, Missouri: Elsevier.

Vanderperren, K., Haers, H., Van Der Vekens, E. et al. (2014). Description of the use of contrast-enhanced ultrasonography in four dogs with pancreatic tumours. *Journal of Small Animal Practice* 55 (3): 164–169. https://doi.org/10.1111/jsap.12153.

Vanenkevort, B.A., O'brien, R.T., and Young, K.M. (1999). Pancreatic pseudocysts in 4 dogs and 2 cats: ultrasonographic and clinicopathologic findings. *Journal of Veterinary Internal Medicine* 13 (4): 309–313.

Nutritional Management of Exocrine Pancreatic Disorders

CHAPTER 32

Cecilia Villaverde

Expert Pet Nutrition, Fermoy, County Cork, Ireland

KEY POINTS

- Patients with acute pancreatitis should be fed as soon as possible to minimize risk of malnutrition and other complications of fasting.
- Fat moderation in pancreatitis is a controversial topic, and each case must be assessed individually to decide on the best nutritional profile for both short- and long-term management.
- Patients with exocrine pancreatic insufficiency (EPI) can be managed with a variety of diets, and choice should be tailored to the individual, with therapeutic gastrointestinal diets being good choices in many cases if maintenance diets are not effective in controlling clinicals signs and promoting an ideal body condition. Low-fat diets are not recommended as first choice in patients with poor body condition.
- Cobalamin status should be assessed in all patients with EPI and supplemented if low. Diet should also be assessed to ensure it is replete in this nutrient.

INTRODUCTION

The two main exocrine pancreatic disorders include pancreatitis and exocrine pancreatic insufficiency (EPI). Both conditions can have serious implications in the nutritional status of the patient; EPI in particular can result in overt malnutrition. As such, providing a complete diet in sufficient amounts to meet energy needs is a priority in these cases. There is a lack of information on what are the best nutritional strategies to provide adequate nutrition and help control clinical signs, and some aspects are still controversial.

The goals of nutritional management in exocrine pancreatic disorders include preventing malnutrition and decreasing the rate of complications by providing energy and nutrients to ensure organ function and promote the integrity of the gastrointestinal tract.

EXOCRINE PANCREATIC INSUFFICIENCY

EFFECT ON NUTRITIONAL STATUS

This condition is a maldigestion and malabsorption syndrome resulting from low secretion of digestive enzymes by the acinar cells of the pancreas. The main treatment consists of exogenous enzyme replacement therapy, with nutritional therapy playing an important supportive role.

EPI patients cannot adequately digest macronutrients, which results in general malnutrition signs associated with low energy uptake (weight loss, thin) and catabolism and others such as diarrhea and polyphagia. Preliminary data (Oliveira et al. 2011) in six dogs with well-controlled EPI

Disorders of the Liver, Exocrine Pancreas, and Gastrointestinal Tract in Dogs and Cats, First Edition. Edited by Harry Cridge et al. Published 2026 by John Wiley & Sons, Inc. Companion Website: www.wiley.com/go/cridge/disorders

treated with exogenous enzymes, showed a decreased digestibility of macronutrients (and, therefore, energy) compared to healthy dogs. The intestinal environment is negatively affected by maldigestion, including worse gut permeability (Oliveira et al. 2022) and dysbiosis.

Fat malabsorption can cause steatorrhea and decrease the nutritional status of fat-soluble vitamins in the body. Some studies have noted a decrease in vitamin A and E even when adequately treated with enzyme replacement therapy.

The nutritional status of cobalamin (vitamin B12) can often be negatively affected in dogs (Soetart et al. 2019) and cats (Thompson et al. 2009) with EPI. Cobalamin requires binding to intrinsic factor, which is secreted mainly by the pancreas (also secreted by parietal cells in dogs) and the complex is absorbed via receptor in the ileum. Hypocobalaminemia (Figure 32.1) is frequently associated with intestinal disease including EPI.

The role of EPI on the status of other nutrients is unknown. One study found low blood taurine in 2 out of 18 dogs with this disease (Tayler et al. 2020). Another one noted low serum concentration of copper and zinc in dogs with experimental EPI versus healthy controls.

NUTRITIONAL STRATEGIES FOR MANAGEMENT

The main nutritional goals in patients with EPI are to provide energy and nutrients, in the form of a complete diet, to:

- Maintain weight (gain in the case of puppies/kittens) and an ideal body condition score (BCS)
- Avoid nutrient deficiencies for correct organ function
- Minimize diarrhea

Dietary Fat

Exogenous lipase activity is not comparable in treated patients versus those without EPI. In humans, exogenous lipase is destroyed at a much higher rate than trypsin and amylase. This explains why some treated patients can still show steatorrhea. For this reason, feeding a low-fat diet has been a common recommendation in EPI.

Studies have not been conclusive. One uncontrolled study in dogs with EPI (Simpson et al. 1994) noted clinical improvement when giving a low-fat diet and enzyme supplementation, but dogs were later changed to other diets without worsening of signs. Another study (Westermarck et al. 1995) switched treated, stable dogs with EPI fed a variety of diets to a low-fat diet (15 g fat/1000 kcal of metabolizable energy). While there was no statistical difference between groups before and after diet change, the authors report that there was a high individual variation in the response to diet. Another study with stable treated dogs with EPI compared three different diets in a cross-over, randomized

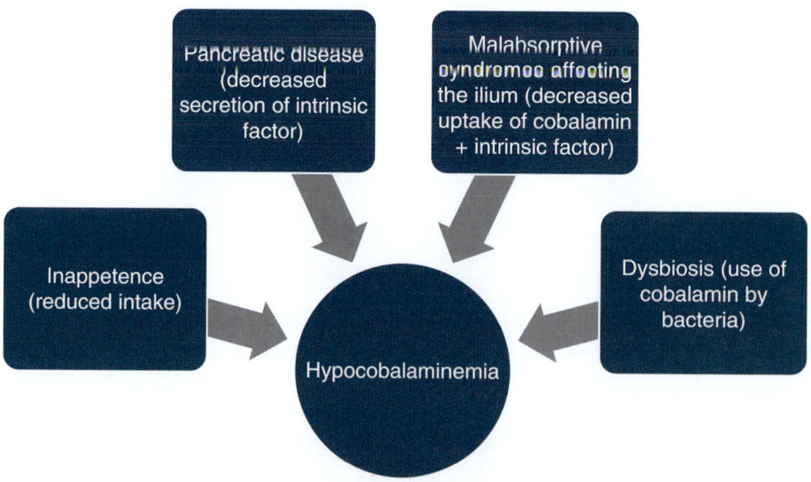

FIGURE 32.1 Causes of hypocobalaminemia in intestinal and pancreatic disease

design (Westermarck and Wiberg 2006). The fat content of the three diets was 57.6 g/1000 kcal (high-fat diet), 35 g/1000 kcal (highly digestible diet), and 30 g/1000 kcal (lower fat and high-fiber diet). Diets varied in several aspects, including fat but also fiber, protein, carbohydrate, and energy density, with the lower fat diet also being higher in fiber and lower in energy. Similarly to the previous study, the response to different strategies was highly variable, and in 8 out of 21 dogs, the original diet was the best fit. A case series (Biourge and Fontaine 2004) of three dogs with EPI and cutaneous adverse food reaction did well on a hydrolyzed high-fat diet (48 g/1000 kcal). A retrospective study (Batchelor et al. 2007) did not identify a benefit or a downside of changing to a low-fat diet in dogs with EPI. There are no studies in cats regarding the effect of dietary fat on clinical response. A retrospective paper (Xenoulis et al. 2016) did not find an association between diet change and clinical improvement.

In dogs with experimental EPI, a higher fat diet with 50 g/1000 kcal (vs. a low-fat diet providing 21 g/1000 kcal) can protect exogenous lipase during gastrointestinal transit and result in higher fat absorption. Moreover, lower fat diets tend to have a reduced energy density, and some patients might struggle to meet their energy needs with them. Given these results, low-fat diets should not be routinely recommended.

Modifying dietary fat has also been considered, particularly the use of diets enriched in medium chain triglycerides (MCTs). Compared to longer chain triglycerides, MCTs are believed to be absorbed mainly via portal circulation rather than the lymphatic system. For this reason, they could be a good source of energy in malabsorptive syndromes, although there is a dearth of data in veterinary medicine. One study (Rutz et al. 2004) in dogs with well-controlled EPI compared diets differing in their MCT content in a cross-over design for 12 weeks each. There were no differences in fecal characteristics, appetite and other subjective aspects, but blood concentration of vitamins E and A and cholesterol was higher with the high MCT diet. The clinical significance of these changes is unknown, and more research is needed to determine the usefulness of MCTs for EPI. There is no data in cats, and MCTs are reported to decrease palatability in this species.

Dietary Fiber and Digestibility

Different types and amounts of fiber have desirable effects on intestinal tract motility, fecal consistency, and microbiome composition, and this nutrient has received attention in the management of intestinal diseases. Patients with EPI can have dysbiosis, and prebiotic fiber theoretically could play a role in management. Unfortunately, the use of fiber-enriched diets or fiber supplementation has not been well studied in canine or feline EPI, including its role in managing dysbiosis.

High-fiber diets should be avoided in thin patients, as they tend to be bulky (low in energy density) and some dogs or cats with EPI might not eat enough to maintain their weight. Moreover, high dietary fiber levels can affect enzyme access to the substrate in the small intestine; therefore, using a low-fiber, highly digestible diet could be a benefit in this regard, potentially allowing for lower enzyme dosages. High dietary fiber also decreases overall digestibility. A low-fiber, highly digestible diet can be beneficial in EPI management. In one abstract (Oliveira et al. 2022), using a highly digestible diet resulted in improvements in protein and carbohydrate digestibility.

Cobalamin

Low cobalamin status is associated with worse prognosis in dogs (Batchelor et al. 2007; Soetart et al. 2019). Retrospective data in cats suggests that cobalamin supplementation can improve response to treatment (Xenoulis et al. 2016). It is important to ensure that any diet choice is not deficient in this vitamin. One abstract (Oliveira et al. 2022) using a highly digestible diet enriched in cobalamin (1.5 mg/kg) resulted in a higher blood cobalamin versus a control diet (0.17 mg/kg) in dogs with EPI.

FEEDING PLAN

All patients with EPI require a nutritional assessment (Freeman et al. 2011) to identify any nutritional risk factors, evaluate the adequacy of the current diet, and to assess current energy intake; the latter is particularly important in those individuals with an abnormal BCS.

1. Diet choice

Research suggests the best diet choice will vary depending on the patient, and there is not one diet type that will suit all EPI patients equally well. A nutritional assessment will help individualize the choice for each case, but there will be a component of trial and error.

In all cases, the diet must be complete and balanced for the species and life stage and be consistent day-to-day to ensure maximal efficacy of the exogenous enzymes. If a homemade diet is chosen over a commercial product, it should be balanced by a specialist to ensure it is complete, as generic books and online recipes can have nutritional adequacy issues.

Unless there is a comorbidity that requires it, diet change can be delayed until the patient has been on exogenous enzyme therapy for a few weeks and it might not even be required if good clinical control is achieved with the original diet. This is usually also more cost-effective than a veterinary therapeutic diet, which is desirable given the economic burden of EPI treatment.

If response is not ideal, there are several diet options that can be tried depending on the patient's situation:

- Highly digestible (also known as "gastrointestinal" or "low-residue") diets are a common choice. Some dogs have responded well to this approach (Westermarck and Wiberg 2006; Oliveira et al. 2022), and they can be helpful if the stool quality has not normalized on medical treatment, which can indicate abnormal digestion. These diets are often also adequate for growth, so they are a great choice for puppies and kittens. Within the veterinary gastrointestinal diets, there is variety in palatability, macronutrient profile, and energy density, which permit customization. For example, high-calorie gastrointestinal diets can be used in thin pets struggling to gain weight. In addition, gastrointestinal diets, while low in fiber, do contain small amounts of fiber, including prebiotics.
- Convalescence high-calorie diets can be used in pets with reduced BCS, if a gastrointestinal diet is not calorie dense enough.
- While high-fiber diets (defined as >40 g total dietary fiber/1000 kcal in dogs and >25 in cats, [Cridge et al. 2024]) should be avoided, fiber supplementation can be considered to improve stool quality, for example, with psyllium husk powder (in the author's experience, a good start is 1 tsp per day divided over the meals, and this can be titrated up every 3–4 days).
- In cats, EPI presents with comorbidities in about 60% of the cases (Thompson et al. 2009; Xenoulis et al. 2016), which will affect diet choice. Comorbidities can also happen in dogs. For nutrient-sensitive diseases, a diet adequate for the specific condition should be chosen. If multiple options are available, then the choice can be customized depending on energy density, fiber level, etc.
- Cobalamin should be supplemented if hypocobalaminemia is detected with a complete diet. Studies in dogs (Chang et al. 2022) and cats (Chang et al. 2024) with EPI show that oral supplementation can be efficacious in normalizing serum cobalamin.
- It is unknown at this time if supplementation of fat-soluble vitamins would be beneficial. Some of these vitamins (A and D) can have toxic effects at high dosages. As such, supplementation is not always safe and thus not generally recommended, and feeding a complete diet plus enzyme replacement therapy seems to be sufficient in most cases. Subcutaneous vitamin K can be initiated if there is evidence of coagulopathy (Cridge et al. 2024).

2. Daily allowance

The daily allowance depends on the energy needs. All patients should receive their maintenance energy requirements (MER), which can be calculated in two ways: calculating the current calorie intake or with formulas (Figure 32.2). The MER (kcal/day) can be divided by the energy content of the diet (kcal per kg, cup, can, etc.) to get the daily allowance. Alternatively, label recommendations can also be used (these are based on formulas as well). However, formulas and label recommendations have a high error, and are only a starting point; therefore, the daily allowance will require adjustment, initially every two weeks and once stable, monthly, to achieve weight and BCS goals.

In underweight patients, assessing current intake via a complete diet history to set up a baseline is invaluable. The daily allowance can be then set up to provide 10% more calories

Daily allowance calculation:

1. Calculate resting energy requirements (RER, kcal per day):

$$RER = 70 \times weight\ (kg)^{0.75}$$

2. Calculate maintenance energy requirements (MER) by multiplying RER by factor (F), depending on species and life stage:

$$MER = RER \times F$$

F for dogs		F for cats	
Intact adult	1.8	Intact adult	1.4
Neutered adult	1.6	Neutered adult	1.2
Puppy <4 months	3	Kitten	2.5
Puppy ≥4 months	2	—	—

3. Divide MER (kcal/day) by energy content of the diet of choice (kcal/g, kcal/cup, kcal/can...)

$$Daily\ allowance = \frac{MER\ patient}{Energy\ content\ diet}$$

FIGURE 32.2 Calculation of MER in dogs and cats. *Source*: Adapted from Gross et al. (2010)

than baseline to help achieve weight gain and an ideal BCS. These patients might suffer from low digestibility, so their energy needs might be notably higher than those estimated by formulas obtained from healthy pets and lead to underfeeding.

3. Feeding method
Patients with EPI need to be meal-fed, at least two meals daily: they need to receive exogenous enzyme supplementation with each meal; thus, free feeding is not a good option in these cases. These patients should not have access to unmonitored food sources, which can be an issue in multi-human households or in outdoor pets. Treats should not be fed between main meals.

PANCREATITIS

Nutritional management of pancreatitis is considered an important part of the supportive treatment in veterinary medicine; however, the evidence of specific nutritional modifications for both dogs and cats is scarce, and most recommendations are mainly based on clinical experience (Jensen and Chan 2014; Forman et al. 2021; Cridge et al. 2024; Lim et al. 2024). As such, pancreatitis management is clinician-dependent, and there will be some trial and error involved to find the best diet per case. Comorbidities are common, especially in cats, which will also affect the feeding plan.

NUTRITIONAL STRATEGIES

Early Feeding

Historical recommendations for pancreatitis included withholding food and water orally, especially in acute presenting cases associated with vomiting. The rationale was to "rest the pancreas" by minimizing pancreatic stimulation and attempt to reduce premature activation of the zymogens within the pancreatic tissue. Feeding does stimulate pancreatic secretions to make sure digestive enzymes are present in the small intestine to digest the food. Some nutrients stimulate more pancreatic secretion via cholecystokinin (CCK) than others, fat being the most potent followed by protein.

However, studies in dogs with experimental pancreatitis saw that early intrajejunal feeding did not increase pancreatic secretions into the gut, even while increasing the concentration of CCK in blood. Therefore, the inflamed pancreas might not respond to feeding the same way as a healthy one. Another reason for fasting includes minimizing aspiration pneumonia in patients that are actively vomiting. Finally, some cases can present with severe abdominal pain, which can reduce tolerance to oral feeding.

The current consensus is to encourage early enteral feeding, following data in human medicine, where early nutritional intervention is associated with better outcomes and helps prevent malnutrition, reduce inflammation, and decrease the rate of complications such as multiple organ failure in severe cases. Fasting can also have an important negative effect on intestinal barrier integrity. Thus, international guidelines for people recommend early nutritional support in this situation, if feasible.

In veterinary medicine, early enteral nutrition has been compared to fasting or parenteral nutrition in dogs with pancreatitis, although the studies have a small sample size. One pilot clinical study (Mansfield et al. 2011) with dogs diagnosed with severe acute pancreatitis fed them via esophagostomy feeding tube with a low-fat diet (5 dogs) or via parenteral nutrition (5 dogs), within 24 hours of admission. The enteral group had a lower incidence of intestinal complications, and they did not detect postprandial pain. Other researchers (Harris et al. 2017) looked at retrospective data (34 cases), comparing enteral feeding within 48 hours of admission versus delayed feeding in dogs with acute pancreatitis. Patients fed early met their energy requirements sooner and showed a faster return to voluntary food intake, in addition to having fewer intolerance issues. Dogs with experimental pancreatitis fed intrajejunally versus parenterally (Qin et al. 2003) had a better intestinal barrier function and lower bacterial translocation.

There are even less studies in cats. A retrospective paper (Klaus et al. 2009) looked at 55 cases with suspected pancreatitis fed via nasogastric feeding tube within two days of admission. This was well tolerated, with a low incidence of complications. Prolonged inappetence in cats can be associated with hepatic lipidosis, so nutritional support should be instituted as soon as possible if they are inappetent.

For milder pancreatitis cases, usually outpatients, fasting is not a consideration, as they do not usually present with anorexia, protracted vomiting, or severe abdominal pain.

Energy Provision

Patients with severe pancreatitis that require hospitalization might not meet their energy and nutrient needs via voluntary oral intake, and they will require assisted feeding or nutritional support. Appetite stimulants can be attempted but might not be enough in completely anorexic patients.

The goal during hospitalization, whatever the disease and the BCS of the patient, is to avoid weight loss and maintain a stable weight, since decreased food intake and loss of weight is associated with worse outcomes.

Dietary Fat: Dogs

Fat restriction is a common recommendation in canine pancreatitis. The rationale behind this recommendation is the relatively high potency of fat to stimulate pancreatic secretions and slow down gastric emptying via CCK compared to the other macronutrients. Some old studies with experimental high-fat diets (around 90 g /1000 kcal) worsened or caused pancreatitis in dogs, but other dietary characteristics might be involved. Anecdotally, the switch to high-fat diets in dogs, like urinary diets or ketogenic diets, can be associated with pancreatitis development in some dogs. Feeding table foods (which can be high fat) has also been associated to a higher risk of acute pancreatitis in dogs (Lem et al. 2008) and hyperlipidemia can be present in a small subset of canine pancreatitis patients, be it cause or consequence (Xenoulis et al. 2020).

However, the clinical evidence supporting this recommendation is scarce. One study (James et al. 2009) in 10 healthy dogs fed diets differing in fat (18 vs. 45 g/1000 kcal, with or without enzyme supplementation) for one week did not identify any differences in serum pancreatic lipase immunoreactivity, serum trypsin like immunoreactivity or gastrin. Another one (Zhang et al. 2023), also in healthy dogs fed high-fat diets (59 g/1000 kcal) from different sources (saturated, unsaturated, or MCTs) versus a low-fat control diet (3.5 g/1000 kcal), saw no changes in serum pancreatic lipase immunoreactivity, gastrin, or DGGR lipase up to 180 minutes after a meal. That said, the response could be different in dogs with pancreatitis. Unfortunately, there is almost no data on the effect of dietary fat on clinical outcomes. A retrospective study (Harris et al. 2017) in dogs with acute pancreatitis fed enterally did not really see a different outcome in dogs fed low-fat diets versus others, except for a trend to a better gastrointestinal tolerance; however, the sample size was small.

There is no consensus on what level of dietary fat is "low-fat". According to some authors (Cridge et al. 2024), low-fat canine diets provide 17–29 g/1000 kcal, moderate 30–50 g/1000 kcal, and high >50 g/1000 kcal. They also define ultra-low fat as <17 g/1000 kcal, which requires homemade diets, as currently no commercial diets are as low as that. While different authors might have different cutoffs, having a common reference would be helpful to communicate diet recommendations. Unfortunately, fat information on the label is provided as percentage as fed (g of fat per 100 g of food) and, in some areas of the world, it is provided as a minimum guarantee rather than the average value. As fed values are not comparable as they are affected by moisture content and energy density, converting as fed values to g/1000 kcal is important to evaluate and compare dietary fat (or other nutrients) content (Figure 32.3).

Dietary Fat: Cats

There is no evidence that modifying dietary fat can cause or worsen pancreatitis in cats, or that it can be used for treatment. The ACVIM consensus statement mentions avoidance of high-fat diets in some cases (Forman et al. 2021), on a case-by-case basis situation. For cats (Cridge et al. 2024), a low-fat diet has been proposed to be <40 g/1000 kcal, moderate 40–60 g/1000 kcal, and high >60 g/1000 kcal.

FEEDING PLAN

A nutritional assessment will help identify any nutritional risk factors, evaluate the adequacy of the current diet, and assess current energy intake.

Step 1: Obtain percentage as fed fat information from label or website → % fat as fed = grams fat/100 g food

Example: 7% fat

Step 2: Obtain kcal per kg of metabolizable energy of the food

a) Check label (mandatory in some countries)
b) Contact manufacturer
c) Can estimate with formulas (NRC 2006)

Example: 1200 kcal/kg

Step 3:

$$\frac{X\,g\,fat}{100\,g\,food} \times \frac{1000\,g\,food}{Y\,kcal} \times 1000 = z\,g\,fat/1000\,kcal$$

$$\frac{7\,g\,fat}{100\,g\,food} \times \frac{1000\,g\,food}{1200\,kcal} \times 1000 = 58.3\,g\,fat/1000\,kcal$$

For veterinary therapeutic diets, manufacturers can have the nutrient information already on a calorie basis (per 100 or 1000 kcal or per 1000 kJ):

- To convert g/100 kcal to g/1000 kcal → multiply by 10
- To convert g/1000 kJ to g/1000 kcal → multiply by 4.18

FIGURE 32.3 How to convert as fed information to calorie basis?

1. Diet choice

Dogs:

Cridge et al. (2024) recommend feeding a diet 50% lower in fat versus the diet at diagnostics in dogs with acute pancreatitis. For patients fed very high-fat diets, a gastrointestinal low-fat diet might not be needed, but those are excellent choices in many cases. For those fed via feeding tube, there are liquid low-fat diets available, and low-fat gastrointestinal diets can be made into slurries. An ultra-low-fat homemade diet might be needed if the diet at diagnostics is already moderate in fat or the commercial options do not control hyperlipidemia if present.

Low-fat diets can have some drawbacks related to palatability and energy density. However, in the author's opinion, the low-fat, low-fiber gastrointestinal diets have a decent energy density, and it is possible in many cases to meet energy needs, as long as the diet is liked by the patient.

This recommendation is not universal, and some authors recommend only low-fat diets if there is hyperlipidemia (Jensen and Chan 2014).

In acute cases, patients can be returned to their original diet (or to a maintenance diet with average fat content) once recovered, but chronic recurrent cases might require fat moderation long term. In such cases, care should be taken to advise caregivers not only on the main diet but also on treats (particularly for dogs), including commercial products, table foods, and supplements, as some might be an important source of fat. Fruits and vegetables are usually low in fat, but commercial treats can vary widely. Overall, unbalanced items should not provide more than 10% of the daily calories.

Cats:

Gastrointestinal diets are an excellent choice if pancreatitis is the only disease present, as they are highly digestible and can help facilitate nutrient digestion and absorption. If there is concurrent chronic enteropathy, feeding hydrolyzed diets can be helpful for diet-responsive disease (Kathrani 2021) and is a common recommendation. They are also highly digestible, and peptides are less of a stimulant of CCK secretion versus intact protein. Gastrointestinal and hydrolyzed protein diets vary in their fat content, so fat reduction (compared with diet at diagnostics) might be possible if desired, for example, in refractory cases or those associated with hyperlipidemia.

In both species, concurrent diseases will affect diet choice. Some veterinary therapeutic diets for specific diseases in dogs can be quite high in fat, especially if protein moderation is also present, and it is recommended to compare the fat content of the available choices or consult with a veterinary nutrition specialist for a homemade diet formulation.

2. Daily allowance

Outpatients should receive their MER, which can be calculated in two ways: calculating the current calorie intake or with formulas (Figure 32.2). The MER (kcal/day) can be divided by the energy content of the diet (kcal per kg, cup, can, etc.) to get the daily allowance. Alternatively, label recommendations can also be used (these are based on formulas as well). However, formulas and label recommendations have a high error, and are only a starting point; therefore, the daily allowance will require adjustment, initially every two weeks and once stable, monthly, to achieve weight and BCS goals.

In hospitalized patients, the initial goal is to feed the RER to prevent overfeeding (Figure 32.2) with adjustments to promote weight stability initially and weight gain after stabilization in underweight patients.

A weight loss plan using a therapeutic weight loss diet moderate in fat is indicated in overweight patients once they have recovered from their pancreatitis episode.

3. Feeding method

Feeding should be initiated as soon as possible. In the hospital, water (as is or as ice cubes) can be offered first to assess tolerance before offering a gastrointestinal (low-fat in the case of dogs) diet. Multiple meals per day might be better tolerated, especially if there is abdominal pain, and can result in faster gastric emptying in comparison to one or two big meals.

In both dogs and cats, assisted feeding is recommended with anorexia of three days, or earlier if preceded by days of hyporexia or the risk of feline hepatic lipidosis is high

(Jensen and Chan 2014). Enteral feeding is preferred to parenteral. Nasogastric (or nasoesophageal), esophagostomy and gastrostomy tubes can all be used. While jejunostomy tubes were the main recommendation for acute pancreatitis to by-pass the pancreas, they are complicated to place and maintain, and studies support that pre-gastric feeding is safe and effective.

Nasogastric/nasoesophageal tubes are less invasive than others and do not require anesthesia, which makes them excellent choice in cases where they are not stable enough to have a different tube placed. They do require the use of liquid veterinary diets (and, for dogs, low in fat) and can only be used for a few days. Liquid diets formulated for humans are not the best choice, especially for cats, and should only be used if there are no other choices and only short term. For longer nutritional support or to use slurries, esophagostomy or gastrostomy tubes are better choices.

Parenteral nutrition can be considered in the small number of patients when enteral nutrition is not possible (e.g., a tube cannot be placed, or the vomiting is intractable) or when they cannot protect their airway. There is no need to moderate the fat in this situation, except if there is hyperlipidemia.

REFERENCES

Batchelor, D.J., Noble, P.J.M., Taylor, R.H. et al. (2007). Prognostic factors in canine exocrine pancreatic insufficiency: prolonged survival is likely if clinical remission is achieved. *Journal of Veterinary Internal Medicine*, 21 (1). https://doi.org/10.1892/0891-6640(2007)21[54:PFICEP]2.0.CO;2.

Biourge, V.C. and Fontaine, J. (2004). Exocrine pancreatic insufficiency and adverse reaction to food in dogs: a positive response to a high-fat, soy isolate hydrolysate-based diet. *Journal of Nutrition*. https://doi.org/10.1093/jn/134.8.2166s.

Chang, C., Lidbury, J., Suchodolski, J.S. et al. (2024). Effect of oral or subcutaneous administration of cyanocobalamin in hypocobalaminemic cats with chronic gastrointestinal disease or exocrine pancreatic insufficiency. *Journal of Veterinary Internal Medicine* 38 (5): 2464–2479. https://doi.org/10.1111/jvim.17195.

Chang, C.H., Lidbury, J.A., Suchodolski, J.S. et al. (2022). Effect of oral or injectable supplementation with cobalamin in dogs with hypocobalaminemia caused by chronic enteropathy or exocrine pancreatic insufficiency. *Journal of Veterinary Internal Medicine* 36 (5). https://doi.org/10.1111/jvim.16528.

Cridge, H., Parker, V.J., and Kathrani, A. (2024). Nutritional management of pancreatitis and concurrent disease in dogs and cats. *Journal of the American Veterinary Medical Association* 262 (6): 834–840.

Forman, M.A., Steiner, J.M., Armstrong, P.J. et al. (2021). ACVIM consensus statement on pancreatitis in cats. *Journal of Veterinary Internal Medicine* 35 (2). https://doi.org/10.1111/jvim.16053.

Freeman, L., Becvarova, I., Cave, N. et al. (2011). WSAVA nutritional assessment guidelines. *Journal of Small Animal Practice* 52 (7): 385–396. https://doi.org/10.1111/j.1748-5827.2011.01079.x.

Gross, K.L., Yamka, R.M., Khoo, C. et al. (2010) Macronutrients, In: *Small Animal Clinical Nutrition*, 5e (ed. M.S. Hand, C.D. Thatcher, R.L. Remillard et al.), 49–105. Topeka, KS: Mark Morris Institute.

Harris, J.P., Parnell, N.K., Griffith, E.H. et al. (2017). Retrospective evaluation of the impact of early enteral nutrition on clinical outcomes in dogs with pancreatitis: 34 cases (2010–2013). *Journal of Veterinary Emergency and Critical Care* 27 (4). https://doi.org/10.1111/vec.12612.

James, F.E., Mansfield, C.S., Steiner, J.M. et al. (2009). Pancreatic response in healthy dogs fed diets of various fat compositions. *American Journal of Veterinary Research* 70 (5). https://doi.org/10.2460/ajvr.70.5.614.

Jensen, K.B. and Chan, D.L. (2014). Nutritional management of acute pancreatitis in dogs and cats. *Journal of Veterinary Emergency and Critical Care*. https://doi.org/10.1111/vec.12180.

Kathrani, A. (2021). Dietary and nutritional approaches to the management of chronic enteropathy in dogs and cats. *Veterinary Clinics of North America - Small Animal Practice*. https://doi.org/10.1016/j.cvsm.2020.09.005.

Klaus, J.A., Rudloff, E., and Kirby, R. (2009). Nasogastric tube feeding in cats with suspected acute pancreatitis: 55 cases (2001–2006). *Journal of Veterinary Emergency and Critical Care* 19 (4). https://doi.org/10.1111/j.1476-4431.2009.00438.x.

Lem, K.Y., Fosgate, G.T., Norby, B. et al. (2008). Associations between dietary factors and pancreatitis in dogs. *Journal of the American Veterinary Medical Association* 233 (9). https://doi.org/10.2460/javma.233.9.1425.

Lim, S.Y., Cridge, H., Twedt, D.C. et al. (2024). Management of acute-onset pancreatitis in dogs: a narrative review. *Journal of the American Veterinary Medical Association* 262 (9): 1231–1240.

Mansfield, C.S., James, F.E., Steiner, J.M. et al. (2011). A pilot study to assess tolerability of early enteral nutrition via esophagostomy tube feeding in dogs with severe acute pancreatitis. *Journal of Veterinary Internal Medicine* 25 (3). https://doi.org/10.1111/j.1939-1676.2011.0703.x.

NRC (National Research Council) (2006). *Nutrient Requirements of Dogs and Cats*. Washington, DC: The National Academies Press.

Oliveira, V.V., Henríquez, L.B.F., Rentas, M.F. et al. (2011). Comparison of macronutrient digestibility of client-owned dogs with exocrine pancreatic insufficiency given pancreatic enzymes and healthy dogs. In: *25th Congress of the European College of Veterinary and Comparative Nutrition*, 136–136.

Oliveira, V.V., Teixeira, F.A., Ishii, P.E. et al. (2022) High digestible diet with higher cobalamin and prebiotic content improves serum cobalamin and digestibility of dogs with exocrine pancreatic insufficiency but did not improve dysbiosis and gut permeability. In: *26th Congress of the European Society of Veterinary and Comparative Nutrition*, 94.

Qin, H.L., Su, Z.D., Hu, L.G. et al. (2003). Parenteral versus early intrajejunal nutrition: effect on pancreatitic natural course, entero-hormones release and its efficacy on dogs with acute pancreatitis. *World Journal of Gastroenterology* 9 (10). https://doi.org/10.3748/wjg.v9.i10.2270.

Rutz, G.M., Steiner, J.M., Bauer, J.E. et al. (2004). Effects of exchange of dietary medium chain triglycerides for long-chain triglycerides on serum biochemical variables and subjectively assessed well-being of dogs with exocrine pancreatic insufficiency. *American Journal of Veterinary Research* 65 (9). https://doi.org/10.2460/ajvr.2004.65.1293.

Simpson, J.W., Maskell, I.E., Quigg, J. et al. (1994). Long term management of canine exocrine pancreatic insufficiency. *Journal of Small Animal Practice* 35 (3). https://doi.org/10.1111/j.1748-5827.1994.tb03915.x.

Soetart, N., Rochel, D., Drut, A. et al. (2019). Serum cobalamin and folate as prognostic factors in canine exocrine pancreatic insufficiency: an observational cohort study of 299 dogs. *Veterinary Journal* 243. https://doi.org/10.1016/j.tvjl.2018.11.003.

Tayler, S., Seo, J., Connolly, D.J. et al. (2020). Blood taurine concentrations in dogs with exocrine pancreatic insufficiency. *American Journal of Veterinary Research* 81 (12). https://doi.org/10.2460/ajvr.81.12.958.

Thompson, K.A., Parnell, N.K., Hohenhaus, A.E. et al. (2009). Feline exocrine pancreatic insufficiency: 16 cases (1992–2007). *Journal of Feline Medicine and Surgery* 11 (12). https://doi.org/10.1016/j.jfms.2009.04.004.

Westermarck, E., Junttila, J.T., and Wiberg, M.E. (1995). Role of low dietary fat in the treatment of dogs with exocrine pancreatic insufficiency *American Journal of Veterinary Research* 56 (5). https://doi.org/10.2460/ajvr.1995.56.05.600.

Westermarck, E. and Wiberg, M.E. (2006). Effects of diet on clinical signs of exocrine pancreatic insufficiency in dogs. *Journal of the American Veterinary Medical Association* 228 (2). https://doi.org/10.2460/javma.228.2.225.

Xenoulis, P.G., Zoran, D.L., Fosgate, G.T. et al. (2016). Feline exocrine pancreatic insufficiency: a retrospective study of 150 cases. *Journal of Veterinary Internal Medicine* 30 (6). https://doi.org/10.1111/jvim.14560.

Xenoulis, P.G., Cammarata, P.J., Walzem, R.L. et al. (2020). Serum triglyceride and cholesterol concentrations and lipoprotein profiles in dogs with naturally occurring pancreatitis and healthy control dogs. *Journal of Veterinary Internal Medicine* 34 (2). https://doi.org/10.1111/jvim.15715.

Zhang, Y., Kirk, C.A., Tolbert, M.K. et al. (2023). Impact of fatty acid composition on markers of exocrine pancreatic stimulation in dogs. *PLoS One* 18 (8 August). https://doi.org/10.1371/journal.pone.0290555.

Laboratory Assessment of the Gastrointestinal Tract

CHAPTER 33

Romy M. Heilmann

Department of Small Animal Medicine, College of Veterinary Medicine, University of Leipzig, Leipzig, Saxony, Germany

KEY POINTS

- Obtaining a minimum laboratory database (MLDB) provides an important initial assessment of dogs and cats presenting with gastrointestinal (GI) signs, and it should be tailored to the individual patient.
- Diagnosing chronic GI diseases in dogs and cats often requires an integrated approach, including the patient's medical and dietary history, clinical signs, physical examination findings, diagnostic imaging, and sequential diagnostic interventions.
- Expanding the MLDB for dogs and cats suspected of GI disease with laboratory tests of GI function and/or inflammation will allow for evaluation of GI health, exclusion of pertinent differential or concurrent diagnoses, and establishment of a systematic approach.
- Several functional and inflammatory laboratory biomarkers are available for use with specimens from dogs and/or cats and can provide clinically useful diagnostic and/or prognostic information, particularly when evaluated in combination.
- Additional biomarkers that are currently not readily available (e.g., genomic markers) and algorithms that incorporate information from several biomarkers (e.g., biomarker panels) are likely a path to individualized patient management in the future.

INTRODUCTION

Clinical presentations of gastrointestinal (GI) diseases are one of the most common reasons for dogs and cats to be presented to the veterinarian. The optimal approach to these patients, both diagnostically and therapeutically, varies between both species and depends upon the severity and chronicity of the clinical problem. Common clinical signs in dogs and cats with GI diseases are reduced appetite (hyporexia) or anorexia, vomiting, and/or diarrhea. Weight loss is more likely associated with a chronic disease process, and tenesmus, steatorrhea, salivation, and regurgitation can also be displayed. The clinical picture in dogs can additionally include abdominal pain and borborygmus, which are infrequently detected in cats.

Acute GI presentations (e.g., acute gastritis associated with dietary indiscretion) can be self-limiting or resolve with supportive care of the patient without a need for further diagnostics, particularly if the clinical signs are mild and the patient is treated on an outpatient basis. However, dogs and cats presenting with either more severe acute GI signs (e.g., evidence of systemic consequences), an acute episode of an apparently more chronic recurrent disease process, and patients with chronic persistent clinical signs generally require more intensive treatment (e.g., inpatient stabilization and monitoring) and further diagnostic evaluation. The latter will aid in determining the overall condition of the patient and diagnosing the underlying disease.

Disorders of the Liver, Exocrine Pancreas, and Gastrointestinal Tract in Dogs and Cats, First Edition. Edited by Harry Cridge et al. Published 2026 by John Wiley & Sons, Inc. Companion Website: www.wiley.com/go/cridge/disorders

Suspicion of a chronic GI disease process such as chronic enteropathy (i.e., clinical signs persist or intermittently present for at least three weeks) warrants a stepwise diagnostic evaluation that includes laboratory tests, diagnostic imaging, and – in some dogs and cats – more invasive diagnostics such as endoscopy and biopsy for histopathologic evaluation (Jergens and Heilmann 2022; Marsilio 2021).

ROUTINE CLINICOPATHOLOGIC PARAMETERS

A minimum laboratory database (MLDB) in dogs and cats with GI signs (Figure 33.1) should include routine hematology (with differential blood cell counts if indicated), serum biochemistry profile with electrolytes, and urinalysis with urine sediment examination (and, if needed, bacterial culture and antimicrobial susceptibility testing).

Complete blood count (CBC) analysis often reveals nonspecific findings (e.g., mild non-regenerative, normocytic normochromic anemia reflecting anemia of inflammation or anemia of chronic disease). With severe acute disease, there can be evidence of hemoconcentration (i.e., an increased or falsely normal erythrocyte count), which can be verified by the hydration status of the patient and other biochemical parameters (e.g., high-normal serum albumin concentration or hyperalbuminemia). Non-regenerative microcytic anemia (and erythrocyte hypochromia) suggests iron deficiency anemia (IDA), and more subtle changes such as a decreased reticulocyte hemoglobin concentration reflect a state of iron-limited erythropoiesis (IDE) which can precede IDA. Together with, at most, moderate thrombocytosis and an increased blood urea nitrogen (BUN) level, IDA or IDE raises the suspicion for chronic (occult) GI hemorrhage.

Mild leukocytosis with neutrophilia is a characteristic finding of an inflammatory and/or stress leukogram in both dogs and cats. Leukopenia, and particularly neutropenia, can develop with viral infections of rapidly regenerating tissues (e.g., parvovirus enteritis). Lymphopenia is common in cats with parvovirus infection, resulting in panleukopenia. Lymphopenia can also be part of a stress leukogram or result from protein-losing enteropathy (PLE) in dogs. Lymphocytosis is frequently detected with infectious diseases (e.g., viral or vector-borne disease) but can also reflect hypoadrenocorticism or a malignant disease process (e.g., lymphoma). The blood neutrophil-to-lymphocyte ratio (NLR) can help detect dogs with (particularly eunatremic-eukalemic) hypoadrenocorticism

Minimum laboratory database (MLDB)

- ☑ Hematology (CBC ± differential blood cell counts)
  serum biochemistry panel with electrolytes (± SBA)
  urinalysis (± quantitative urine culture, UPC)
  retrovirus status [cats]
- ☑ Fecal examination (consistency score; parasitology: direct examination, flotation, *Giardia* spp. ELISA; ± other tests depending on risk factors/geographic location)
- ☑ Pancreatic disease markers (cPLI/fPLI, cTLI/fTLI) and B vitamin status (serum cobalamin, folate)
- ☑ Endocrine tests (resting cortisol ± ACTH stimulation test [dogs], tT4 ± fT4 [cats])

FIGURE 33.1 Minimum laboratory database (MLDB) in dogs and cats presenting with clinical signs of gastrointestinal disease. The laboratory diagnostics recommended for an initial assessment of patients with acute presentations are indicated in blue color. Particularly for chronic presentations, but in some instances also acute presentations (e.g., hemorrhagic diarrhea), the MLDB should be expanded (laboratory tests indicated in green color) depending upon findings on prior tests and pertinent differential diagnoses. ACTH, adrenocorticotropic hormone; CBC, complete blood count; cPLI, canine pancreatic lipase; cTLI, canine trypsin-like immunoreactivity; ELISA, enzyme-linked immunosorbent assay; fPLI, feline pancreatic lipase; fTLI, feline trypsin-like immunoreactivity; fT4, free thyroxin; SBA, serum bile acids; tT4, total thyroxin; UPC, urine protein/creatinine ratio and is a surrogate marker of disease severity in dogs with chronic intestinal inflammation (chronic inflammatory enteropathy, CIE) (Zeugswetter and Schwendenwein 2014). The blood NLR can help subclassify affected dogs based on their response to treatment – i.e., requiring anti-inflammatory or immunosuppressive treatment with immunosuppressant-responsive enteropathy (IRE) versus showing good clinical response to a therapeutic elimination diet with food-responsive enteropathy (FRE) – and evidence of PLE (Becher et al. 2021). In cats, a potential diagnostic or prognostic value of the blood NLR with GI diseases remains to be shown. Peripheral eosinophilia can occur in dogs and cats with enteric fungal or endoparasite infections, alimentary lymphoma, or mast cell tumor, and cats with eosinophilic gastroenteritis. Thrombocytosis and a reduced variation in platelet size have been linked to severe chronic GI disease in dogs (Mehain et al. 2019; Pierini et al. 2021). A normal CBC does not rule out a diagnosis of a relevant gastroenteropathy.

Serum biochemistry allows for the detection of consequences from acute or chronic GI disease and the exclusion of other differential diagnoses or concurrent conditions, such as hepatobiliary or renal disease, which can produce overlapping GI signs. Occasionally, mild to moderate increases in serum liver enzyme activities – particularly alkaline phosphatase and alanine aminotransferase activity – can occur with chronic intestinal disease and in the absence of a primary hepatic condition (reactive hepatopathy). Because similar increases in serum liver enzyme activities can reflect concurrent hepatopathy (e.g., chronic hepatitis in dogs, hepatic lipidosis in cats), cholangiohepatopathy (e.g., lymphocytic cholangitis in cats), or vascular disease (e.g., portosystemic shunt), functional liver substrates (serum albumin, BUN, cholesterol, bile acids, bilirubin, glucose, and potentially ammonia concentrations) should be evaluated and serum liver enzyme activities should be rechecked (keeping their shorter half-life in cats in mind).

Hypoalbuminemia or panhypoproteinemia can develop in dogs with severe hemorrhagic diarrhea and chronic diseases with intestinal protein loss (i.e., PLE secondary to CIE or primary intestinal lymphangiectasia, intestinal lymphoma, and parasite or fungal infection); hypoalbuminemia has prognostic value in canine CIE (Gianella et al. 2017a; Nakashima et al. 2015). In cats, hypoalbuminemia is a rare finding with GI disease, but severe infiltrative conditions (e.g., large-cell intestinal lymphoma or fungal enteritides such as histoplasmosis) can result in GI protein loss with hypoalbuminemia and carry a worse prognosis. Hyperglobulinemia can be detected with CIE, fungal enteritides, granulomatous feline infectious peritonitis (FIP), or alimentary neoplasia (e.g., lymphoma). However, extra-GI primary (e.g., lymphocytic cholangitis in cats) or secondary inflammatory (e.g., vector-borne diseases) and neoplastic diseases (e.g., plasmacytoma) are important differentials.

Total and ionized hypocalcemia, hypomagnesemia, and hypocholesterolemia can be detected in dogs with PLE, and increased BUN concentrations (presumably resulting from occult GI bleeding) are prognostic with this disease entity (Nakashima et al. 2015; Kathrani et al. 2019). Detecting hypoalbuminemia with concurrent hypercholesterolemia raises suspicion for protein-losing nephropathy (PLN). Hypocalcemia development in cats with CIE or intestinal lymphoma reflects more severe histologic lesions. Hypercalcemia can be a paraneoplastic sign (e.g., with T-cell lymphoma leading to a worse prognosis in dogs), result from granulomatous disease (e.g., schistosomiasis) or certain treatments (e.g., lactulose in cats), or present as a concurrent idiopathic condition in cats. However, extra-GI etiologies causing hypercalcemia (i.e., hypoadrenocorticism, renal disease, hyperparathyroidism, and neoplastic conditions) can also result in GI signs. Hypophosphatemia affects every other cat with chronic enteropathy, and BUN concentrations are generally higher in cats with intestinal lymphoma than with CIE (Gianella et al. 2017b; Reed et al. 2007).

Serum or plasma electrolyte (sodium, potassium, and chloride) concentrations should always be determined in dogs and cats with either acute or chronic GI presentations. Significant electrolyte shifts (e.g., marked hypokalemia, hyponatremia) can occur with vomiting and/or diarrhea, posing a risk of systemic consequences and requiring correction as part of the patient's initial treatment plan. Electrolyte abnormalities in canine CIE include hypokalemia (19% of dogs; no differentiation of IRE from FRE), hyponatremia (14%; predominantly with IRE and linked to diarrhea severity), and hypo- (5%) or hyperchloremia (11%) (Heilmann et al. 2022). Cats with CIE can also develop hyponatremia and hypo- or hyperkalemia, particularly with marked intestinal fibrosis and worse disease outcomes (Baker et al. 2024). Documenting acid–base disturbances requires a *blood gas analysis*, which most commonly detects metabolic acidosis in dogs and cats with acute or chronic GI presentations.

Urinalysis with a urine protein-to-creatinine (UPC) ratio can help exclude renal losses of protein (PLN) if the UPC is <0.5 (dogs) or <0.4 (cats). An active urine sediment and/or increased UPC warrants a quantitative urine culture with antimicrobial susceptibility testing and, if negative, measurement of systemic blood pressure and evaluation for chronic renal diseases (including secondary renal tubule dysfunction) or lower urinary tract pathologies.

In cats, the MLDB should include determining the *retrovirus* (feline leukemia virus and feline immunodeficiency virus) *status*, if unknown, and total thyroxine (tT4) concentration – combined with a free T4 if inconclusive – to screen for hyperthyroidism in cats ≥7 years of age and/or if an enlarged thyroid gland was palpated during the physical examination.

FECAL EXAMINATION

Fecal consistency, as an indicator of GI disease, can vary and should be evaluated using a standardized fecal scoring system (https://www.purinainstitute.com/sites/default/files/2024-02/fecal-chart.pdf; https://www.waltham.com/s3media/2020-05/waltham-scoring.pdf). Using defined criteria to assign a fecal score allows veterinary staff, as well as the owner, to evaluate the extent of abnormal fecal consistency and monitor for changes after initiating treatment. For correct assessment, the fecal consistency score is to be assessed on a fecal sample immediately after defecation.

A routine *fecal parasitological examination* using samples collected on three consecutive days helps evaluate the patient with acute or chronic GI signs for helminth infections (nematodes and/or cestodes via analysis of a fecal smear, sedimentation and/or flotation techniques, or coproantigen immunoassays) or the presence of protozoa (e.g., *Giardia* spp., *Tritrichomonas blagburni* [cats], *Cryptosporidium* spp. by immunoassays or molecular diagnostics). It is important to emphasize that *Giardia* spp. shedding also occurs in healthy dogs and cats and is more likely in clinically less severely affected dogs with CIE (Perrucci et al. 2020), questioning the role of *Giardia* spp. as a primary pathogen in immunocompetent dogs and cats. In addition, it is currently common practice to perform empirical deworming in some dogs and cats with particularly chronic diarrhea prior to more invasive diagnostics (e.g., GI endoscopy), even if fecal parasitology is negative.

Giardia spp. trophozoites can be visualized microscopically (100× magnification) in a fresh fecal smear or wet mount by the characteristic smooth "falling leaf" motility pattern. Adding methylene blue or Lugol's solution to the fecal wet mount can improve the detection of *Giardia* spp. trophozoites. Because *Giardia* spp. cysts have an increased resistance to environmental conditions, they can be microscopically detected in fecal material after enrichment via $ZnSO_4$ or sugar centrifugal flotation. Detection of *Giardia* spp. cysts using a direct immunofluorescence assay (IFA) is currently the reference (gold standard) diagnostic test, which can be combined with the evaluation of pathogen morphology. However, this diagnostic is time-consuming and costly for routine use. Fecal *Giardia* spp. antigen ELISAs offer a sensitive alternative diagnostic test but should only be used in dogs and cats with clinical signs of GI disease and with three fecal samples collected within five days. A patient-side *Giardia* spp. ELISA (SNAP *Giardia* test) is also available and compares well with IFA results and has low false-positive and false-negative rates. A PCR-based *Giardia* spp. assay is highly specific but less sensitive than antigen immunoassays and thus not recommended for routine diagnostics. The current recommendation for the routine laboratory diagnosis of *Giardia* spp. is to use a combination of centrifugal flotation and *Giardia* spp. antigen ELISA.

Infections with *T. blagburni* (formerly known as *T. foetus*) should be considered as a differential diagnosis in predominantly young cats (<2 years of age) with a history of chronic persistent, or recurrent (often malodorous) large-bowel diarrhea. Trophozoites of *T. blagburni* can be detected during direct microscopic examination of a fresh fecal smear or wet mount with saline solution (100× magnification) by their characteristic jerky and rapid pattern of anterior motion. However, this test is insensitive to detect *T. blagburni*, and the motile flagellates can be misidentified as either *Giardia* spp. trophozoites or apathogenic *Pentatrichomonas hominis*. Cultural enrichment and detection of *T. blagburni* using a fresh fecal sample (e.g., with the InPouch^{TM} TF) is moderately sensitive and specific. However, the final results can take up to 12 days. Diagnosis of *T. blagburni* by PCR-based testing of a fecal sample (collected immediately after natural defecation or via rectal loop technique) has the highest sensitivity and specificity.

Cryptosporidium spp. (*C. parvum* and *C. felis*) oocysts can be detected by traditional Ziehl-Neelsen staining of a fecal smear, but this test has a low sensitivity and is inferior to immunoassays with a moderate sensitivity for *Cryptosporidium* spp. PCR-based amplification of the organism offers a molecular diagnostic tool with improved sensitivity and specificity. However, the reference gold standard method for the noninvasive detection of *Cryptosporidium* spp. in dogs and cats remains the direct IFA on a fecal sample after centrifugal flotation.

Diagnosis of canine schistosomiasis, caused by the trematode *Heterobilharzia americana*, in endemic areas (states lining the Gulf Coast and southern Atlantic coast), is by fecal PCR for *H. americana* DNA or detection of *H. americana* eggs on fecal sedimentation.

Canine parvovirus (CPV) and feline parvovirus (FPV) infections can be diagnosed based on a positive fecal parvovirus antigen ELISA result. Such an ELISA is available as a point-of-care test (Parvo SNAP) and can rapidly detect CPV (antigenic variants CPV-2a, CPV-2b, and CPV-2c) and FPV with high specificity and moderate sensitivity. However, false-positive test results are possible within two weeks of vaccination using a modified-live vaccine against CPV or FPV (Patterson et al. 2007). A false-negative result with a strong suspicion of parvovirus enteritis in a dog (CPV infection) or panleukopenic cat (FPV or CPV infection) should be followed by a fecal CPV-/FPV-PCR analysis. PCR-based tests have the highest sensitivity and specificity for the detection of CPV/FPV and can differentiate infection from vaccine strain for CPV (currently not FPV) but are less practical than the point-of-care ELISA. Molecular assays can serve to evaluate other or additional causes of viral enteritides in dogs (e.g., canine circovirus, canine distemper virus, or canine enteric coronavirus) and are available as PCR-based diagnostic panels.

Fecal bacteriological examination should be carefully considered, particularly in dogs and cats with chronic GI signs, as its diagnostic value is limited to specific situations, such as the presence of risk factors (e.g., feeding a raw meat-based diet) or the implication of zoonotic concerns. Pathogens that are most commonly cultured from feces in dogs and cats are *Salmonella* spp., *Clostridium perfringens, Campylobacter* spp., and *Clostridium difficile*. However, these bacteria can also be isolated from healthy non-diarrheic animals and be transiently shed, making the clinical interpretation of a positive culture result challenging. Adding to the complexity, isolating these bacteria can reveal a cause of diarrhea or a consequence of intestinal bacterial dysbiosis resulting from underlying GI disease, and clinically affected dogs and cats often have acute uncomplicated (occasionally hemorrhagic) diarrhea that is self-limiting or resolves with supportive treatment. Adequate handling of fresh fecal specimens for bacterial culture is also imperative, and samples should either be processed within two hours of collection (for on-site analysis) or placed in a transport medium and shipped at 4–10 °C (for analysis off-site).

Salmonella spp. can be shed in healthy dogs and cats, especially those fed a raw meat-based diet. All *Salmonella* spp. strains express virulence genes, but isolating *Salmonella* spp. from feces in a diarrheic dog or cat is not proof of *Salmonella* spp.-induced enteritis. Given the zoonotic relevance of salmonellosis, this important differential is to be considered when isolating *Salmonella* spp. by culture or PCR amplification in a dog or cat with compatible clinical signs and potential risk factors (e.g., feeding of a raw meat-based diet, prior antimicrobial administration, environmental and housing conditions). *C. perfringens* is a commensal organism with a high prevalence in healthy dogs and cats. However, increased levels of *C. perfringens* enterotoxin (CPE) – presumably resulting from a disrupted intestinal microenvironment – have been linked to acute (hemorrhagic) diarrhea in dogs and cats. Fecal real-time PCR for enterotoxigenic (CPE-producing) *C. perfringens* and CPE immunodetection by coproantigen ELISA can secure the diagnosis. The pore-forming NetE and NetF toxins have been linked to severe acute *C. perfringens*-associated diarrhea in dogs (not yet reported in cats) and can be identified by quantitative analysis of the toxin genes (Sindern et al. 2019). *Campylobacter* spp. (*C. upsaliensis* and *C. helveticus*, but also *C. jejuni*) can be isolated via culture or quantitative PCR. *Campylobacter* spp. are also shed in healthy dogs and cats but more likely to be causative of diarrhea in young animals with certain risk factors (e.g., housing in a shelter, feeding of a raw meat-based diet). Diagnosis of *C. difficile* infection, which infrequently occurs in dogs and is rare in cats, is based on real-time PCR analysis of the organism and ELISA-based detection of toxin A (TcdA) and toxin B (TcdB).

Escherichia coli is a commensal bacterium in dogs and cats but acts as a pathogen when expressing certain virulence factors and facing an immunocompromised host. Different *E. coli* pathotypes exist, of which adherent and invasive *E. coli* (AIEC) strains can cause granulomatous colitis (GC; previously referred to as histiocytic ulcerative colitis) as a unique form of CIE in dogs (predisposed breeds are Boxers, French bulldogs, and Mastiffs) and cats. A diagnosis of GC is based on characteristic microscopic lesions in mucosal biopsy specimens of the colon (i.e., ulceration, accumulation of periodic-acid Schiff stain-positive macrophages, and reduction of goblet cell numbers) and AIEC localization within macrophages (by fluorescence in situ hybridization), isolation of AIEC by culture, and antimicrobial susceptibility testing (due to high rates of antimicrobial resistance in AIEC strains) (Craven et al. 2010). A causal role of invasive *E. coli* in the pathogenesis of GC supports the achievement of GC remission by eradicating these bacteria via enrofloxacin administration (Mansfield et al. 2009). Isolating *E. coli* from fecal specimens of dogs or cats with chronic diarrhea cannot establish a diagnosis of GC or *E. coli*-induced enterocolitis.

An infection with *Histoplasma capsulatum*, a fungal organism endemic to the southern USA, localized to the GI tract or presenting disseminated histoplasmosis, can be diagnosed by cytology (rectal scrape or fine-needle aspirate from a lymph node) or histopathology (intestinal tissue biopsies). An immunoassay can noninvasively detect and quantify *H. capsulatum* antigen in serum and/or urine samples. This test can help diagnose affected dogs and cats and monitor the response to treatment. *Pythium insidiosum* infection, a rare differential diagnosis in dogs and cats from the coastal areas along the Gulf of Mexico, is diagnosed by histopathology (hematoxylin/eosin and Gomori methenamine silver stain), *P. insidiosum*-immunohistochemistry, and culture- or PCR-based isolation. Immunoassays detecting *P. insidiosum* antigens or antibodies can help diagnose and monitor the disease.

FURTHER CLINICOPATHOLOGIC EVALUATION

Despite the importance of routine clinicopathologic tests, additional evaluation of biomarkers for exocrine pancreatic or endocrine diseases should be considered in dogs and cats, particularly with chronic or recurrent episodes of GI signs.

Serum canine or feline *specific pancreatic lipase* concentration (cPLI/fPLI, measured as Spec cPL/fPL or validated 1,2-o-dilauryl-rac-glycero-3-glutaric acid-[6'-methylresorufin] ester [DGGR] lipase assay) evaluates the possibility of pancreatitis as either primary etiology or concurrent condition (e.g., with chronic GI and/or hepatobiliary inflammation as feline triaditis). This test result is interpreted in light of the clinical signs and diagnostic imaging findings (i.e., abdominal ultrasonography). A semiquantitative point-of-care test (SNAP cPL/fPL) is available, and a positive result should be verified, and a baseline for monitoring obtained by a quantitative cPLI/fPLI test. Whereas increased serum cPLI concentrations are a negative prognostic factor in dogs with CIE, increased serum fPLI concentrations do not appear to affect outcomes in cats with CIE. Currently used cPLI/fPLI assays have been optimized for diagnosing pancreatitis in dogs/cats and are not useful to exclude or diagnose exocrine pancreatic insufficiency (EPI).

Decreased fasting serum canine or feline trypsin-like immunoreactivity (cTLI/fTLI) concentrations – reflecting the amount of functional exocrine pancreatic tissue – can identify dogs or cats with EPI, which produces a different clinical picture of maldigestion in dogs than in cats (see Chapters 29 and 30). Equivocal serum cTLI concentrations can be detected in dogs with chronic GI disease and dogs/cats developing EPI; they should be retested 3–4 weeks later. Oral enzyme replacement therapy in patients with EPI does not affect serum cTLI/fTLI concentrations.

A *resting serum cortisol* concentration may be considered to rule out a diagnosis of hypoadrenocorticism in dogs, which in its eunatremic-eukalemic form can be a cause of waxing and waning GI signs (not reported and probably very rare in cats) (Hauck et al. 2020). A normal or increased resting serum cortisol concentration rules out a diagnosis of hypoadrenocorticism, whereas a low concentration (≤ 2 μg/dL or ≤ 55 nmol/L) is followed by an ACTH stimulation test to rule out or confirm (eunatremic-eukalemic or hyponatremic and/or hyperkalemic) hypoadrenocorticism.

Given the rarity of hypoadrenocorticism in cats, routine measurement of serum cortisol (unstimulated or as an ACTH stimulation test) is not warranted in cats with clinical signs of GI disease.

A *bile acid stimulation* test can further evaluate dogs and cats suspected to have a diagnosis of a (cholangio)hepatopathy, but this test does not offer additional information in patients with hepatic or posthepatic hyperbilirubinemia. Severely increased *serum gastrin* concentrations can help identify rare cases of gastrinoma in dogs naïve to any gastric acid suppressant medication.

Coagulation testing may be considered in patients with severe acute GI disease and suspicion of acquired coagulopathy as a systemic consequence (e.g., disseminated intravascular coagulopathy), ideally including a full coagulation panel with clotting times (PT, aPTT), fibrinogen, antithrombin, and fibrin(ogen) degradation products or D-dimer concentrations. Coagulopathic findings are also common in dogs with CIE, particularly those dogs with PLE, but clotting times are insensitive to detect the hypercoagulability affecting 63–100% of dogs with CIE (Nagahara et al. 2021; Wennogle et al. 2021). Hypoantithrombinemia, hyperfibrinogenemia, and a global assessment of the coagulation status via thromboelastography (TEG) or rotational thromboelastometry (ROTEM) can help detect a CIE/PLE-associated hypercoagulable/hypofibrinolytic state, which may predispose affected dogs to thromboembolic complications. Plasma fibrinogen measurement can serve as a surrogate conventional coagulation parameter for the maximum amplitude or clot firmness (reflecting the maximum strength of a clot) when TEG or ROTEM is unavailable.

Serum *vitamin D* concentrations – measured as 25-hydroxyvitamin D (25-OH-D) – can help detect hypovitaminosis D, which is a common finding in dogs and cats with chronic GI inflammation or small-cell intestinal lymphoma and is linked to negative outcomes in dogs (Allenspach et al. 2017). More evidence is needed to determine the utility of routine serum 25-OH-D measurement in cats with chronic GI disease. Dysmetabolism of other fat-soluble vitamins (e.g., vitamin E or A) also occurs in chronic GI disease, but diagnostic testing is mostly reserved for specific questions (e.g., long-term feeding of a home-prepared diet).

Fluid analysis from an ultrasonography-guided diagnostic abdominocentesis in patients with ultrasonographic evidence of peritoneal effusion should include a macroscopic assessment, routine laboratory (specific gravity, protein concentration, and total and nucleated cell counts), cytological (direct smear and/or cytocentrifuge preparation) and, if indicated, microbiological examination (bacterial culture and antimicrobial susceptibility testing). These findings may dictate additional testing (e.g., PCR for FIP virus with a sterile exudate).

ADDITIONAL BIOMARKERS TO EVALUATE CHRONIC GI DISEASE

The further diagnostic investigation of dogs and cats with chronic GI signs usually follows a staged approach, where noninvasive tests precede more invasive diagnostics. Given the differential diagnoses to be considered, this process can demand a significant amount of time and resources, making client education an important cornerstone to optimize compliance during the diagnostic evaluation.

Chronic enteropathy in dogs and cats encompasses a spectrum of disease entities, including the CIE subcategories of FRE, steroid- or immunosuppressant-responsive enteropathy (IRE, with a subgroup showing evidence of secondary PLE), and an evolving group responding to treatments that primarily aim to modulate the intestinal microbiome composition and function, as well as alimentary lymphoma (particularly low-grade intestinal T-cell lymphoma [LGITL] in cats). The CIE subcategories are histologically indistinguishable and classified retrospectively based on the individual response to sequential treatment trials (see Chapter 41). Differentiating IRE from LGITL in cats can be challenging, whereas the diagnosis is typically more straightforward with large-cell intestinal lymphoma, which carries a worse prognosis. In contrast to dogs, PLE from primary intestinal lymphangiectasia is not reported in cats.

Several laboratory markers have been evaluated for their clinical utility in the diagnosis and management of canine and feline CIE. These include functional (cobalamin ± methylmalonic acid, folate, α_1-proteinase inhibitor), biochemical (serum C-reactive protein [CRP], fecal calprotectin), and microbiome biomarkers (fecal dysbiosis index [fDI]). Metabolomic, genetic, and cellular biomarkers are an important area of research but are currently not employed in clinical practice.

Detecting *food-specific serum IgG* and *IgE titers* reflects exposure to certain dietary ingredients (cross-reactions can occur) but does not confirm antigenic effects and a diagnosis of food allergy, food intolerance or FRE in dogs or cats.

Serum *cobalamin* (*vitamin B_{12}*) and *folate* (*vitamin B_9*) concentrations are not specific for CIE but have therapeutic relevance. Cobalamin from food is released in the stomach, complexed with intrinsic factor (originating primarily [dogs] or exclusively [cats] from the exocrine pancreas), and absorbed via cobalamin-intrinsic factor receptors in the distal small intestine. Hypocobalaminemia can occur with EPI (>80% in dogs and cats), CIE (19–61% in dogs and 13–17% in cats), and neoplastic infiltration of the intestinal wall (42–78% in cats with intestinal lymphoma) (Kather et al. 2020). Suboptimal serum cobalamin status (<400 ng/L) can result from small intestinal malabsorption, secondary small intestinal dysbiosis (increased cobalamin utilization by intestinal microbiota), increased demand by the host (essential for tissue regeneration), and/or alterations in cobalamin transport proteins (sequestration). Hypocobalaminemia is a negative prognostic factor in dogs with CIE, but normocobalaminemia does not preclude a diagnosis of relevant GI or exocrine pancreatic disease. Increases in the metabolite methylmalonic acid (MMA) can signal a lack of intracellular cobalamin availability, provided that renal insufficiency is excluded (Berghoff et al. 2013), but MMA testing on serum or urine is currently not (yet) routinely performed in dogs and cats. A transient hypocobalaminemic state is recognized in cats with newly diagnosed hyperthyroidism (up to 41%) and, with the absence of any concurrent GI or exocrine pancreatic disease, resolves with treatment of the underlying hyperthyroidism (Geesaman et al. 2016). Hypercobalaminemia (without prior supplementation) is detected in some dogs and cats with chronic GI inflammation or neoplasia. Hypocobalaminemia with concurrent hyperfolatemia can indicate secondary small intestinal dysbiosis (e.g., with CIE or LGITL) because some intestinal bacteria can produce folic acid, but folate also accumulates with cobalamin deficiency because of the interdependency of their intracellular pathways. Concurrent hypofolatemia more likely reflects diffuse GI disease, as folic acid is absorbed by carrier-mediated endocytosis in the proximal small intestine. Hypofolatemia is detected in up to 47% of dogs and 40% of cats with chronic GI disease, but normofolatemia does not exclude the diagnosis.

Increased fecal concentrations of *alpha$_1$-proteinase inhibitor* (α_1PI), a proteolysis-resistant protein, are reflective of protein loss into the GI lumen. Increased 3-day mean and/or 3-day maximum fecal concentrations are a good diagnostic test for PLE (primary intestinal lymphangiectasia or secondary to CIE) in dogs ≥1 year of age; they are also a marker for characteristic intestinal microscopic lesions of PLE in dogs (lacteal dilation, crypt lesions/abscesses) irrespective of the serum albumin concentration (Heilmann et al. 2016). Fecal α_1PI testing is also useful to detect GI protein loss in dogs prior to the onset of hypoalbuminemia/panhypoproteinemia and/or clinical disease and to differentiate GI protein loss from other causes of hypoalbuminemia (PLN, hepatic disease). The serum-to-fecal α_1PI ratio has improved diagnostic accuracy for PLE in hypoalbuminemic dogs (serum α_1PI can be depleted with chronic GI loss of α_1PI), provided that corticosteroids were not administered at the time of testing. Fecal α_1PI concentrations (determined using samples collected on three consecutive days) are increased in cats with marked chronic GI disease (severe IRE, GI lymphoma), but the feline α_1PI test is currently not routinely available.

Serum CRP, a positive type II acute-phase protein and nonspecific marker of inflammation, can increase with systemic infections, inflammation, or neoplasia. Serum CRP has utility as a surrogate biomarker for monitoring dogs with CIE after treatment initiation, but its high biological variability requires large increases or decreases (≥2.7-fold) to be assessed as clinically relevant. Increased serum CRP concentrations can further aid in distinguishing dogs with CIE that are categorized as IRE from those with FRE. Several assay formats with similar cut-offs are used to quantify serum CRP in dogs, but a high-sensitivity CRP test is currently not routinely available. CRP assays do not work with serum samples from cats. Serum *amyloid A* and *α_1-acid glycoprotein* are the major acute-phase proteins in cats but have not been studied as biomarkers of GI disease.

Calprotectin, a protein complex accumulating at sites of inflammation, is increased in the intestinal mucosa and fecal samples from dogs and cats with chronic GI inflammation (Heilmann et al. 2018). Fecal calprotectin levels are a surrogate marker of disease severity in dogs with CIE and can help predict the response to treatment in the IRE subgroup. Fecal calprotectin remains to be systematically studied in dogs with GI neoplasia, and the test cannot differentiate cats with CIE from those with LGITL (Riggers et al. 2023).

The fDI can aid in evaluating intestinal microbiome alterations (normobiosis vs. dysbiosis) as an individualized approach to managing dogs and cats with GI disease. The fDI evaluates eight bacterial groups known to have shifted abundances with CIE in dogs (*Blautia, Clostridium* [Peptacetobacter] *hiranonis, E. coli, Faecalibacterium, Fusobacterium, Streptococcus, Turicibacter*, and total bacteria) (AlShawaqfeh et al. 2017) and cats (*Bacteroides, Bifidobacterium, C. hiranonis, E. coli, Faecalibacterium, Streptococcus, Turicibacter*, and total bacteria) (Sung et al. 2022). Serum and fecal metabolome signatures in dogs and cats with CIE indicate associated functional alterations (e.g., bile acid dysmetabolism, eicosanoid imbalances, oxidative stress).

Other systemic and/or locally produced biomarkers of GI *inflammation* (3-bromotyrosine, N-methylhistamine, S100A12 protein, and several cytokines, chemokines, decoy receptors, autoantibodies, and other signaling molecules) or GI *function* (zonulin, citrulline, and other permeability or absorptive function markers) have been evaluated in dogs and/or cats with chronic GI disease but are currently not routinely available and/or lack reported diagnostic accuracy data. Laboratory techniques to assess GI *absorptive function* (^{51}Cr-EDTA or iohexol absorption), GI *permeability* (urine sucrose levels, serum, or urine lactulose/rhamnose or xylose/methyl-glucose ratio), or *gastric emptying* (^{13}C-octanoic acid breath test) are no longer performed in dogs and cats; more practical modalities have largely replaced these tests.

CONCLUDING REMARKS

A MLDB serves as an important initial assessment of the patient, recognizing that these tests are not specific for diagnosing most underlying GI etiologies in dogs and cats. In addition to these clinicopathologic parameters, a fecal examination and diagnostic imaging are essential to assess the overall health status of a dog or cat with acute or chronic GI signs, rule in or exclude various GI and extra-GI etiologies and clarify whether more invasive diagnostics or surgical intervention is required. Immunological or molecular-based diagnostic tests can help diagnose specific disease processes and determine the ideal treatment plan. The diagnosis of CIE remains a diagnosis of exclusion, requiring other GI and extra-GI causes to be ruled out, but patient and environmental factors will be important determinants of the best individual diagnostic strategy.

REFERENCES

Allenspach, K., Rizzo, J., Jergens, A.E. et al. (2017). Hypovitaminosis D is associated with negative outcome in dogs with protein losing enteropathy: a retrospective study of 43 cases. *BMC Veterinary Research* 13 (1): 96.

AlShawaqfeh, M.K., Wajid, B., Minamoto, Y. et al. (2017). A dysbiosis index to assess microbial changes in fecal samples of dogs with chronic inflammatory enteropathy. *FEMS Microbiology Ecology* 93 (11). https://doi.org/10.1093/femsec/fix136.

Baker, I., Heilmann, R., Knoll, R. et al. (2024). Serum electrolyte abnormalities in cats with chronic inflammatory enteropathy. *Journal of Veterinary Internal Medicine* 38 (6): 3038–3049.

Becher, A., Suchodolski, J.S., Steiner, J.M. et al. (2021). Blood neutrophil-to-lymphocyte ratio (NLR) as a diagnostic marker in dogs with chronic enteropathy. *Journal of Veterinary Diagnostic Investigation* 33 (3): 516–527.

Berghoff, N., Parnell, N.K., Hill, S.L. et al. (2013). Serum cobalamin and methylmalonic acid concentrations in dogs with chronic gastrointestinal disease. *American Journal of Veterinary Research* 74 (1): 84–89.

Craven, M., Dogan, B., Schukken, A. et al. (2010). Antimicrobial resistance impacts clinical outcome of granulomatous colitis in boxer dogs. *Journal of Veterinary Internal Medicine* 24 (4): 819–824.

Geesaman, B.M., Whitehouse, W.H., and Viviano, K.R. (2016). Serum cobalamin and methylmalonic acid concentrations in hyperthyroid cats before and after radioiodine treatment. *Journal of Veterinary Internal Medicine* 30 (2): 560–565.

Gianella, P., Lotti, U., Bellino, C. et al. (2017a). Klinischpathologische und prognostische Faktoren bei kurz- und langfristig überlebenden Hunden mit Eiweissverlustsyndrom. *Schweizer Archiv für Tierheilkunde* 159 (3): 163–169.

Gianella, P., Pietra, M., Crisi, P.E. et al. (2017b). Evaluation of clinicopathological features in cats with chronic gastrointestinal signs. *Polish Journal of Veterinary Sciences* 20 (2): 403–410.

Hauck, C., Schmitz, S.S., Burgener, I.A. et al. (2020). Prevalence and characterization of hypoadrenocorticism in dogs with signs of chronic gastrointestinal disease: a multicenter study. *Journal of Veterinary Internal Medicine* 34 (4): 1399–1405.

Heilmann, R.M., Becher, A., and Dengler, F. (2022). Electrolyte imbalances in dogs with chronic inflammatory enteropathies. *Topics in Companion Animal Medicine* 46: 100597.

Heilmann, R.M., Berghoff, N., Mansell, J. et al. (2018). Association of fecal calprotectin concentrations with disease severity, response to treatment, and other biomarkers in dogs with chronic inflammatory enteropathies. *Journal of Veterinary Internal Medicine* 32 (2): 679–692.

Heilmann, R.M., Parnell, N.K., Grützner, N. et al. (2016). Serum and fecal canine α_1-proteinase inhibitor concentrations reflect the severity of intestinal crypt abscesses and/or lacteal dilation in dogs. *Veterinary Journal* 207: 131–139.

Jergens, A.E. and Heilmann, R.M. (2022). Canine chronic enteropathy–Current state-of-the-art and emerging concepts. *Frontiers in Veterinary Science* 9: 923013.

Kather, S., Grützner, N., Kook, P.H. et al. (2020). Review of cobalamin status and disorders of cobalamin metabolism in dogs. *Journal of Veterinary Internal Medicine* 34 (1): 13–28.

Kathrani, A., Sánchez-Vizcaíno, F., and Hall, E.J. (2019). Association of chronic enteropathy activity index, blood urea concentration, and risk of death in dogs with protein-losing enteropathy. *Journal of Veterinary Internal Medicine* 33 (2): 536–543.

Mansfield, C.S., James, F.E., Craven, M. et al. (2009). Remission of histiocytic ulcerative colitis in Boxer dogs correlates with eradication of invasive intramucosal *Escherichia coli*. *Journal of Veterinary Internal Medicine* 23 (5): 964–969.

Marsilio, S. (2021). Feline chronic enteropathy. *The Journal of Small Animal Practice* 62 (6): 409–419.

Mehain, S.O., Haines, J.M., and Lee, P.M. (2019). Platelet indices as biomarkers for characterization and determination of severity in canine chronic enteropathy. *Veterinary Journal* 248: 37–41.

Nagahara, T., Ohno, K., Nagao, I. et al. (2021). Changes in the coagulation parameters in dogs with protein-losing enteropathy between before and after treatment. *Journal of Veterinary Medical Science* 83 (8): 1295–1302.

Nakashima, K., Hiyoshi, S., Ohno, K. et al. (2015). Prognostic factors in dogs with protein-losing enteropathy. *Veterinary Journal* 205 (1): 28–32.

Patterson, E.V., Reese, M.J., Tucker, S.J. et al. (2007). Effect of vaccination on parvovirus antigen testing in kittens. *Journal of the American Veterinary Medical Association* 230 (3): 359–363.

Perrucci, S., Berrilli, F., Procopio, C. et al. (2020). *Giardia duodenalis* infection in dogs affected by primary chronic enteropathy. *Open Veterinary Journal* 10 (1): 74–79.

Pierini, A., Esposito, G., Gori, E. et al. (2021). Platelet abnormalities and platelet-to-lymphocyte ratios in canine immunosuppressant-responsive and non-responsive enteropathy: a retrospective study in 41 dogs. *Journal of Veterinary Medical Science* 83 (2): 248–253.

Reed, N., Gunn-Moore, D., and Simpson, K. (2007). Cobalamin, folate and inorganic phosphate abnormalities in ill cats. *Journal of Feline Medicine and Surgery* 9 (4): 278–288.

Riggers, D.S., Xenoulis, P.G., Karra, D.A. et al. (2023). Fecal calprotectin concentrations in cats with chronic enteropathies. *Veterinary Sciences* 10 (7): 419.

Sindern, N., Suchodolski, J.S., Leutenegger, C.M. et al. (2019). Prevalence of *Clostridium perfringens* netE and netF toxin genes in the feces of dogs with acute hemorrhagic diarrhea syndrome. *Journal of Veterinary Internal Medicine* 33 (1): 100–105.

Sung, C.-H., Marsilio, S., Chow, B. et al. (2022). Dysbiosis index to evaluate the fecal microbiota in healthy cats and cats with chronic enteropathies. *Journal of Feline Medicine and Surgery* 24 (6): e1–e12.

Wennogle, S.A., Olver, C.S., and Shropshire, S.B. (2021). Coagulation status, fibrinolysis, and platelet dynamics in dogs with chronic inflammatory enteropathy. *Journal of Veterinary Internal Medicine* 35 (2): 892–901.

Zeugswetter, F.K. and Schwendenwein, I. (2014). Diagnostic efficacy of the leukogram and the chemiluminometric ACTH measurement to diagnose canine hypoadrenocorticism. *Tierarztliche Praxis. Ausgabe K, Kleintiere/Heimtiere* 42 (4): 223–230.

Diagnostic Imaging of the Gastrointestinal Tract

CHAPTER 34

Eimear Shorten[1] *and Séamus Hoey*[2]

[1] *Department of Equine Studies, Anaesthesia and Diagnostic Imaging, School of Veterinary Medicine, University College Dublin, Dublin, Belfield, Ireland*
[2] *School of Veterinary Medicine, University College Dublin, Ireland, Vet CT, Cambridge, UK, School of Veterinary Medicine, University of Wisconsin-Madison, USA*

KEY POINTS

- The gastrointestinal tract show similar layering ultrasonographically: hypoechoic mucosa, hyperechoic submucosa, hypoechoic muscularis and hyperechoic serosa/subserosa.
- Gastric dilatation-volvulus can be identified on right lateral view showing compartmentalization, with a tubular pylorus dorsally and a dilated fundus ventrally.
- Mechanical ileus (obstruction) of small intestines can be identified radiographically with two populations of intestine, one distended loop measuring greater than twice the height of L5 in the dog, and greater than 12mm in the cat. The distended loop measures more than twice the diameter of the smaller more normal loops.
- Functional ileus of small intestines, such as gastroenteritis, can be seen where all loops of intestine are distended, but no loop is twice the diameter of another loop.

GASTROINTESTINAL WALLS

The wall of the gastrointestinal tract, including the esophagus, stomach, small intestine, and large intestine, consists of four layers: mucosa, submucosa, muscularis, and adventitia or serosa. Radiographically, these layers are not distinct and can border efface with luminal content, making the normal wall appear thickened. Ultrasonographically, the wall layers can be identified as a hyperechoic lumen-mucosal interface, hypoechoic mucosa, hyperechoic submucosa, hypoechoic muscularis, and hyperechoic serosa.

THE ESOPHAGUS

The esophagus is the first component of the gastrointestinal tract and is a hollow tubular organ extending between the pharynx and gastric cardia, with a sphincter at each end. Radiography is frequently used to assess the esophagus. In the absence of pathology, the esophagus is not usually visible, but it may be outlined if incidental luminal gas or fluid is present. Static positive contrast esophagography (using barium or iodinated contrast) provides a more detailed structural evaluation of the esophagus, while contrast videofluoroscopy is required to assess esophageal motility and dynamic disorders. In patients with esophageal pathology, thoracic radiographs should also be evaluated for concurrent aspiration pneumonia.

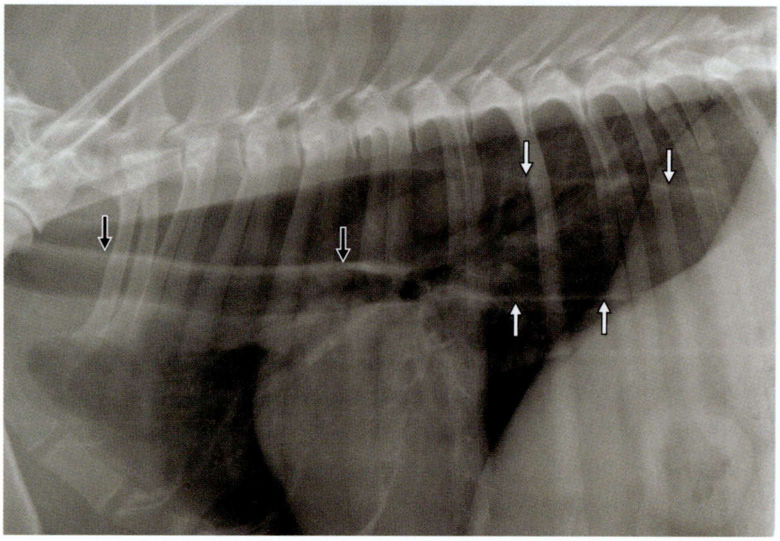

FIGURE 34.1 Left lateral radiograph of a dog with megaesophagus secondary to myasthenia gravis. The esophageal wall is visible as thin linear opacities (white arrows), and a tracheal stripe sign (black arrows) is present due to summation of the tracheal and esophageal walls, both outlined by gas in their respective lumens. Courtesy of University College Dublin

ESOPHAGEAL DILATION

Megaesophagus can be congenital or acquired and refers to segmental or generalized dilation of the esophagus, often accompanied by reduced muscle tone and hypomotility. Survey radiography of the neck and thorax is usually diagnostic for megaesophagus, identifying dilation of the esophagus with gas, ingesta, fluid, or mixed content. Depending on the severity of the dilation, there may be an associated mass effect, with ventral displacement of the cardiac silhouette and right-ventral displacement of the trachea. The presence of luminal gas produces a tracheal stripe sign with delineation of the normally indistinct dorsal tracheal wall as a uniform soft tissue band (Figure 34.1). Similarly, luminal gas may outline the esophageal wall as thin, linear soft tissue opacities extending in a craniocaudal direction. Esophageal dilation is not always pathological, and mild to moderate gas content may be observed on survey radiographs due to sedation, general anesthesia, or aerophagia. Conscious radiographs may be indicated to confirm the transient nature of the dilation in these cases.

Esophagitis is not readily identified on diagnostic imaging studies, but focal or generalized dilation or fluid accumulation may be present in some cases. Positive contrast esophagography provides a superior assessment of the esophageal wall and may reveal focal or generalized wall thickening, prominent mucosal striations, or mucosal irregularity in severe cases (Han et al. 2003).

Esophageal diverticula are rare outpouchings of the esophageal wall that may be congenital or acquired, forming secondary to esophageal or periesophageal disease and a focal weakening of the esophageal wall. Survey or contrast radiographs may show a dilated cavity associated with the esophagus (Park et al. 2012).

Redundant esophagus may be observed in brachycephalic dogs, characterized by a U-shaped deviation or dilation of the esophagus at the thoracic inlet (Eivers et al. 2019; Reeve et al. 2017).

Esophageal dysmotility can occur in association with structural or functional esophageal disorders, and contrast videofluoroscopy is an effective imaging technique that allows real-time, dynamic assessment of motility. Common features of dysmotility include prolonged esophageal transit time, abnormal propagation of peristaltic waves, and gastroesophageal reflux (Eivers et al. 2019; Reeve et al. 2017; Bexfield et al. 2006).

ESOPHAGEAL FOREIGN BODIES

Esophageal foreign bodies are more frequently diagnosed in dogs than in cats and can cause partial or complete esophageal obstruction. Bones, rawhides, dental chews, sticks, and fishhooks are common foreign bodies in dogs, while sewing needles and bones are common in cats (Figure 34.2).

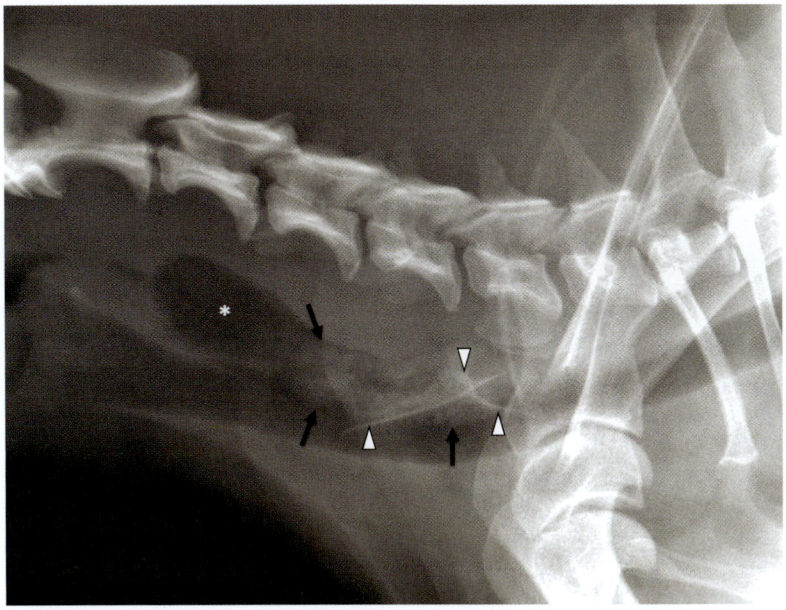

FIGURE 34.2 Lateral cervical radiograph of a dog showing a sharp marginated mineral foreign body (white arrowheads), lodged just cranial to the thoracic inlet with a surrounding heterogeneous soft tissue opacity (black arrows). There is moderate gas dilation of the esophagus cranial to the material (asterisk). Courtesy of University College Dublin

Common sites of lodgment include the cervical esophagus just caudal to the pharynx, the thoracic inlet, the heart base, and the esophageal hiatus. In dogs, obstructions most often occur in the caudal thorax, whereas in cats, they are more commonly found at the cervical esophagus and thoracic inlet (Abd Elkader et al. 2020; Gianella et al. 2009; Leib and Sartor 2008; Thompson et al. 2012). Survey radiographs of the neck and thorax are highly sensitive for detecting esophageal foreign bodies (Gianella et al. 2009; Leib and Sartor 2008; Thompson et al. 2012).

Opaque foreign bodies can be identified on survey images, while contrast administration may be required to identify lucent foreign bodies. CT offers higher resolution than radiography for detecting lucent foreign bodies, with the added benefit of providing a detailed assessment of the surrounding mediastinum. Additional radiographic signs include gas dilation cranial to the obstruction, adjacent soft tissue opacity, tracheal distortion/displacement, and mediastinal or pleural effusion (Houlton et al. 1985). Esophageal perforation can occur as a complication of foreign bodies or as a result of acute penetrating injury. Radiographic and CT indicators of perforation may include cervical emphysema, pneumomediastinum, pneumothorax, pleural effusion, and mediastinal widening suggesting mediastinitis (Gianella et al. 2009; Doran et al. 2008).

ESOPHAGEAL NARROWING

Esophageal strictures typically develop as a result of injury or inflammation of the esophageal mucosa. Strictures are characterized by varying degrees of luminal narrowing, which may be progressive. Other causes of esophageal narrowing include vascular ring anomalies, esophageal or extraluminal masses, and congenital esophageal stenosis. Survey radiographs are often unremarkable in patients with esophageal strictures, although focal or generalized dilation may be present depending on the location and severity of the stricture (Figure 34.3). Contrast esophagography provides information on the location, severity, number, and length of strictures. In particular, videofluoroscopy offers optimal assessment of the maximal dimension of the lesion and its effect on the passage of ingesta. Contrast studies typically reveal persistent luminal narrowing, and contrast retention may be evident proximal to the stricture (German et al. 2005).

Persistent right aortic arch (PRAA) is the most common vascular ring anomaly in dogs and cats. It occurs when the aorta arises anomalously from the right fourth aortic arch, leading to entrapment of the esophagus at the heart base. The right-sided aorta, together with the pulmonary artery and ligamentum

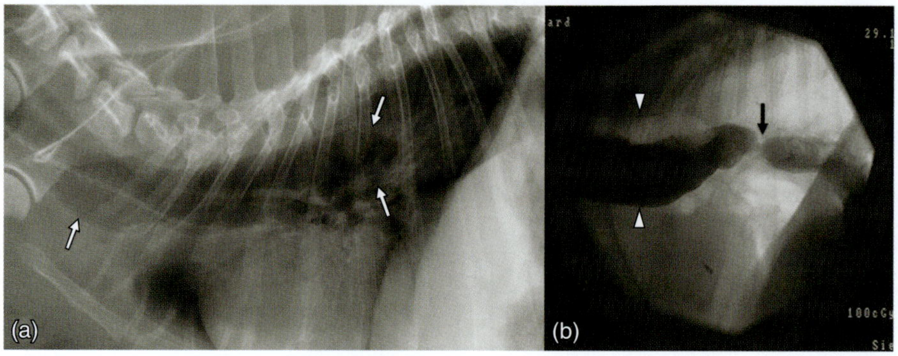

FIGURE 34.3 Lateral thoracic projections of dogs with strictures at the distal thoracic esophagus. (a) A survey radiograph reveals moderate gas dilation of the thoracic esophagus (white arrows) without clear visualization of the stricture. (b) A fluoroscopic still frame demonstrates focal narrowing of the distal esophagus (black arrow), with associated dilation of the cranial esophagus, containing barium-mixed ingesta and gas (white arrowheads). Courtesy of University College Dublin

arteriosum, surrounds the esophagus, causing a narrowing of the lumen. Common radiographic features include esophageal dilation cranial to the obstruction, ventral displacement of the trachea, focal narrowing of the trachea, and characteristic focal leftward deviation of the trachea at the cranial border of the heart (Buchanan 2004). Contrast studies confirm the site and severity of the obstruction, showing abrupt luminal narrowing at the heart base. CT provides superior assessment of the vascular anatomy and aids differentiation between the different types of vascular ring anomaly (Shua-Haim et al. 2023).

ESOPHAGEAL MASSES

Esophageal neoplasia is rare in dogs and cats. Malignant neoplasms are more common than benign ones and include squamous cell carcinoma, leiomyosarcoma, fibrosarcoma, and osteosarcoma. Common radiographic findings include the presence of a soft tissue mass, displacement of mediastinal structures, and variable esophageal dilation cranial to the mass (Farese et al. 2008). Contrast esophagography or videofluoroscopy can further characterize the mass by identifying its position relative to the lumen and aiding differentiation between mural and intraluminal masses. Circumferential mural masses may present with focal narrowing and mucosal irregularity, while filling defects suggest an intraluminal mass. CT with contrast provides a more detailed evaluation of the position, origin, and vascularity of the mass, as well as its relationship to surrounding structures, and has added benefits in assessing for local invasion and metastatic disease.

In endemic regions, sarcomas can develop as a consequence of *Spirocerca lupi* infection. Chronic inflammation and persistent esophageal nodules caused by the parasite can undergo malignant transformation, most commonly leading to fibrosarcoma or osteosarcoma. These esophageal nodules or masses typically occur in the caudal thorax, and additional radiographic features include thoracic aortic mineralization and spondylitis at the mid- to caudal thoracic vertebrae (Dvir et al. 2001; Ranen et al. 2004).

HIATAL DISORDERS

Hiatal disorders include sliding hiatal hernias, paraesophageal hernias, and gastroesophageal intussusception. Sliding hiatal hernias are the most common type of hiatal hernia, often observed in brachycephalic dogs, characterized by recurrent cranial displacement of the lower esophageal sphincter through the esophageal hiatus. Radiographically, sliding hiatal hernias may present as a soft tissue or mixed opacity between the aorta and caudal vena cava, silhouetting with the diaphragm. Given the transient nature of the herniation, videofluoroscopy is superior to radiography for detection. Gastroesophageal intussusception is an uncommon condition characterized by invagination of the stomach, with or without other abdominal organs, into the caudal esophageal lumen, usually requiring urgent surgical intervention. Radiographic features include a sharply defined soft tissue or mixed opacity mass within the caudal thoracic esophagus, often accompanied by esophageal dilation and displacement of adjacent structures.

THE STOMACH

The stomach is a hollow muscular organ located in the cranial abdomen between the esophagus and the small intestinal tract. The stomach is divided into distinct regions: the cardia, fundus, body, and pylorus. The body is the large central portion of the stomach, positioned between the dome-shaped saccular fundus at the left dorsal aspect and the more tubular right ventral pylorus.

Survey radiography and ultrasonography are commonly used to assess gastric disorders. Ultrasonography facilitates dynamic assessment of contractility and gastric emptying, as well as evaluation of the gastrointestinal wall. For this reason, it is often favored over the more time-consuming contrast radiography. The radiographic appearance of the stomach depends on its luminal contents. Radiographically, the presence of intraluminal gas or ingesta outlines the size and position of the stomach, while assessment is limited when the lumen is empty or fluid filled. In addition to ventrodorsal or dorsoventral projections, it is advisable to perform both left and right lateral projections. Gas moves to fill the nondependent portion of the stomach, and this gravitational variation in gas distribution can be used to improve evaluation. Ultrasonographically, the normal gastric thickness ranges up to 5 mm in dogs and cats (Table 34.1) (Penninck et al. 1989; Newell et al. 1999). Gas-related artifacts can limit visibility, while luminal fluid provides an optimal acoustic window. Adjusting patient positioning during the examination helps redistribute gas and fluid, allowing for a more comprehensive assessment of all gastric regions.

GASTRIC DILATATION-VOLVULUS

Gastric dilatation-volvulus (GDV) is an acute life-threatening condition that is more common in large-breed, deep-chested dogs. Variable degrees of dilation and torsion can occur, typically rotating 180° to 360° in a clockwise direction, leading to left craniodorsal displacement of the pylorus. Following patient stabilization, radiographs may confirm the diagnosis and aid differentiation between GDV and gastric dilation (GD) without volvulus. Right lateral projections are widely considered to be the most useful to diagnose GDV, although acquisition of both laterals is advisable. Typical features of 180° rotation include GD, compartmentalization, and displacement of the fundus and pylorus (Figure 34.4) (Fischetti et al. 2004; Mur et al. 2025). Compartmentalization refers to the presence of a soft tissue band between the craniodorsally displaced tubular pylorus and the gastric body or fundus, often seen in right lateral projections. Due to the gastrosplenic ligament attachment, varying degrees of splenic displacement may also be observed. It is important to note that radiographs have low sensitivity for detecting 360° GDV, as the more anatomically normal pyloric position can lead to misdiagnosis as simple GD (Mur et al. 2025). This limitation has significant implications when determining the need for surgical intervention. Gastric pneumatosis is infrequently identified as linear or curvilinear accumulations of gas within the gastric wall, and this finding can be indicative of gastric wall necrosis (Fischetti et al. 2004). The presence of free peritoneal gas on radiographs raises concern for gastric rupture or necrosis, necessitating immediate surgical intervention (Fischetti et al. 2004;

Table 34.1 Published Upper Values of Normal Wall Thickness of the Stomach, Small Intestine, Colon in the Dog and Cat

	Dog			Cat
Gastric Fundus	5 mm			5 mm
Weight	0–20 kg	20–29.9 kg	Over 30 kg	All
Duodenum	5.1 mm	5.3 mm	6.0 mm	2.2 mm
Weight	0–20 kg	20–39.9 kg	Over 40 kg	All
Jejunum	4.1 mm	4.4 mm	4.7 mm	2.2 mm
Ileum	3.8 mm			2.8 mm
Weight	0–15 kg	15–30 kg	>30 kg	All
Colon	1.8 mm	1.9 mm	2 mm	1.7 mm

Source: Penninck et al. (1989); Newell et al. (1999); Delaney et al. (2003); Di Donato et al. (2014).

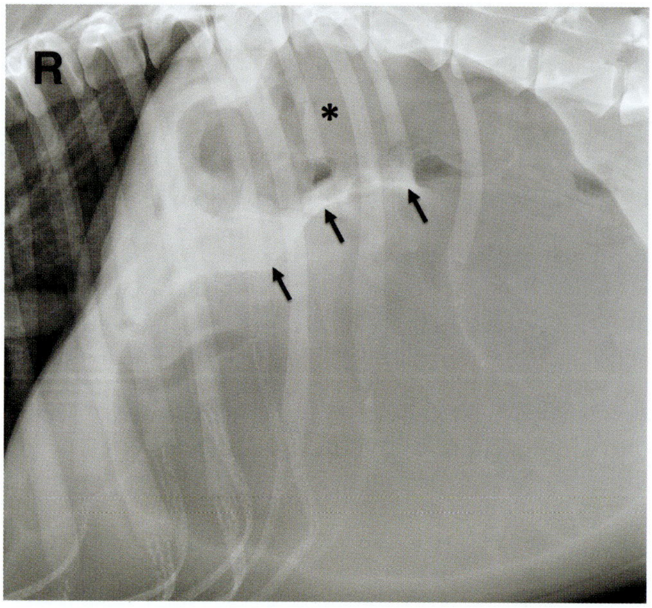

FIGURE 34.4 Right lateral radiograph of a dog with gastric dilatation-volvulus (GDV). The stomach is markedly dilated, with dorsal displacement of the pylorus (asterisk) and compartmentalization, seen as a soft tissue band (arrows) separating the dorsally displaced pylorus from the gastric body and fundus. Courtesy of University College Dublin

Probst et al. 1984). GDV is rare in cats and may be spontaneous or associated with diaphragmatic hernia (Leary and Sinnott-Stutzman 2018; Formaggini et al. 2008). Radiographs typically show gas distension and mispositioning of the stomach with or without compartmentalization.

PYLORIC OUTFLOW OBSTRUCTION

Pyloric obstruction occurs due to a mechanical or functional impairment in the normal passage of gastric contents through the pyloric canal. Chronic partial obstruction can be caused by hypertrophic pyloric stenosis, hypertrophic pyloric gastropathy, masses, inflammation, or fibrosis, whereas acute obstruction is more commonly caused by the presence of foreign material. Functional delays in gastric emptying typically occur in association with gastric motility disorders. Survey radiographs may be normal or show varying degrees of gastric distention, depending on the cause, severity, and duration of the obstruction. A gravel sign suggests chronic partial obstruction, whereby liquid and more soluble material can pass, and larger granular opacities are retained in the pyloric antrum, proximal to the site of obstruction. Often, radiography does not identify the cause of the obstruction, and ultrasonography offers significant advantages in evaluating the morphology of the pylorus. Hypertrophic gastropathy is characterized ultrasonographically by uniform hypoechoic thickening of the muscularis layer (Biller et al. 1994). Similarly, congenital hypertrophic pyloric stenosis may present as circumferential thickening of the pyloric wall, primarily affecting the muscularis layer. Gastric hyperplastic polyps are sessile or pedunculated mucosal nodules that may protrude into the pyloric lumen and contribute to outflow obstruction depending on their size and location (Diana et al. 2009). Likewise, neoplastic or inflammatory processes involving the pylorus can cause varying degrees of outflow obstruction.

GASTRIC FOREIGN BODIES

Opaque foreign bodies are readily visible on survey radiographs with variable characteristics depending on the shape and composition of the material. In contrast, lucent or less opaque foreign bodies are more challenging to detect and often require ultrasonography, CT, or contrast radiography for accurate identification. Visibility improves when the foreign body is surrounded by gas, so performing multiple projections is advisable to enhance visibility and increase the likelihood of detection. If there is associated outflow obstruction, concurrent GD may be evident. The ultrasonographic appearance and visibility of foreign bodies depend on the composition, position, and surrounding gastric contents. Intraluminal fluid provides an ideal acoustic window for foreign body detection, while excessive gas may obscure deeper structures due to reverberation artifacts. Strategic patient positioning can help to optimize visibility (Tidwell and Penninck 1992). Foreign bodies often produce a linear or curvilinear echogenic acoustic interface with variable distal acoustic shadowing, depending on the properties of the material (Tidwell and Penninck 1992; Hoffmann 2003; Boysen et al. 2003). Appreciation of the shape of the object is influenced by how much it transmits or attenuates the ultrasound beam (Tidwell and Penninck 1992).

Gastroduodenal linear foreign bodies often become anchored at the pylorus, and survey radiographs taken in left lateral recumbency may delineate the foreign material within the pyloric antrum. Additional findings include small intestinal plication with small, fragmented luminal gas accumulations, and bunching or gathering of the small intestines in the mid- to ventral abdomen (Root and Lord 1971). Ultrasonographically, the anchored portion of a linear foreign body may be appreciated as strongly shadowing material within the pylorus (Hoffmann 2003). Sharp foreign bodies can perforate the gastric wall, making it important to assess for local changes such as gastric wall thickening and signs of peritonitis. Ingested wooden foreign bodies can perforate the gastrointestinal tract, leading to extensive inflammatory changes in the thorax and abdomen (Boysen et al. 2003; Hunt et al. 2004; Costas and Cervera 2024; Penninck and Mitchell 2003). Wooden foreign bodies are inconsistently visualized radiographically, and CT may be particularly useful in such cases for identifying the foreign body while providing a comprehensive assessment of the affected structures and body cavities (Costas and Cervera 2024).

GASTRIC NEOPLASIA

Gastric neoplasia is rare in dogs and cats. Benign differentials include leiomyoma and adenoma, while malignant differentials include adenocarcinoma, lymphoma, leiomyosarcoma, histiocytic sarcoma, fibrosarcoma, mast cell tumor, and gastrointestinal stromal tumor (GIST). Adenocarcinoma is the most common malignant gastric neoplasm in dogs, with frequent metastasis to regional lymph nodes, liver, and lungs. In cats, lymphoma is the most common type, presenting either in isolation or as a component of systemic disease.

Radiographic detection of gastric neoplasia depends on the size and position of the lesion, and visualization is only possible if the mass is imaged tangentially and highlighted by luminal gas. In such cases, a soft tissue opacity may be evident, protruding into the lumen. Care must be taken not to misinterpret gastric contents in contact with the wall as pathological wall thickening. Ultrasonography and CT have higher sensitivity and provide the added advantage of assessing regional lymph nodes and adjacent abdominal structures. Common ultrasonographic findings include gastric wall thickening, loss of wall layering, and reduced or altered wall echogenicity (Figure 34.5) (Penninck et al. 1994; Kaser-Hotz et al. 1996; Lamb and Grierson 1999;

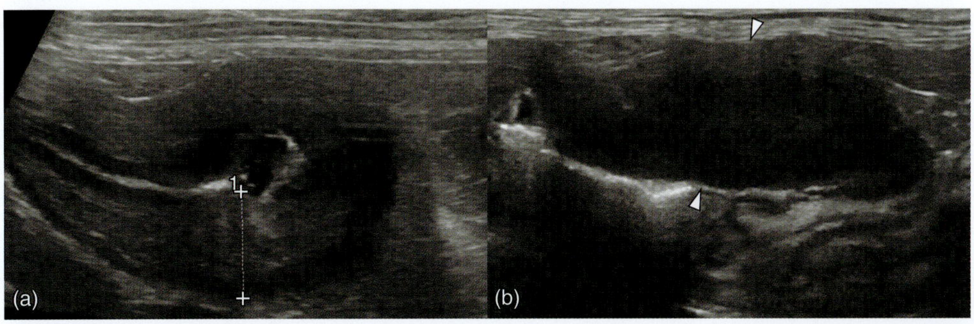

FIGURE 34.5 (a) Ultrasonographic image of a dog with gastritis, showing diffuse gastric wall thickening with preserved wall layering (calipers). (b) Ultrasonographic image of a cat with lymphoma, demonstrating marked gastric wall thickening, hypoechogenicity, and loss of normal wall layering (arrowheads). Courtesy of University College Dublin

Hobbs et al. 2015). Lymphoma often causes generalized transmural thickening, although asymmetric or focal mass lesions may also occur (Penninck et al. 1994). Additional features of gastric carcinoma include extension of the lesion through the serosal layer and "pseudolayering," which refers to the appearance of hypoechoic inner and outer layers separated by a more echogenic central layer (Lamb and Grierson 1999; Penninck et al. 1998). Gastric leiomyoma and leiomyosarcoma often present as distinct focal masses arising from the gastric wall (Lamb and Grierson 1999; Penninck et al. 1998). CT is valuable for determining the precise origin of gastric masses and offers superior assessment of local invasion and metastatic disease (Tanaka et al. 2019; Zuercher et al. 2021). There is considerable overlap in the imaging characteristics of gastric tumors, and definitive diagnosis requires sampling for cytological or histological evaluation. It is worth noting that gastric wall thickness in a contracted stomach must be interpreted with caution, as physiologic thickening can mimic a mass lesion (Lamb and Forster-van Hijfte 1994).

GASTRITIS

Inflammatory diseases of the stomach typically cause diffuse wall thickening with preserved wall layering on ultrasound (Figure 34.5) (Manczur and Vörös 2000). However, considerable overlap exists between the imaging features of inflammatory and neoplastic diseases, making it essential to integrate clinical history and physical examination findings for accurate diagnosis. Granulomatous conditions, such as eosinophilic gastritis, feline gastrointestinal sclerosing fibroplasia, and pythiosis, can present with more severe changes, including loss of normal wall layering and mass lesions (Graham et al. 2000; McConnell et al. 2007; Weissman et al. 2013). Similarly, acute pancreatitis can disrupt normal gastric wall layering. Cytological or histological analysis may be necessary to reach a definitive diagnosis. *Emphysematous gastritis* is a serious condition characterized by the presence of gas within the gastric wall, typically due to infection. Survey radiographs may reveal gastric wall thickening and intramural gas, while ultrasonographic features include diffuse gastric wall thickening, loss of normal wall layering, and intramural gas-associated artifacts (Thierry et al. 2019). *Uremic gastropathy* occurs in patients with chronic uremia. Radiography may reveal subtle thin curvilinear mineral opacities within the gastric wall, and ultrasonographic findings include gastric wall thickening, loss of wall layering, and a highly echogenic, minimally shadowing line at the gastric mucosa representing mucosal mineralization (Grooters et al. 1994). Presumed gastric wall edema appears ultrasonographically as altered gastric wall layering and thickening, often involving the submucosal layer (Murakami et al. 2019). On CT, it presents as wall thickening with a three-layered pattern and a non-enhancing middle layer (Murakami et al. 2022).

GASTRIC ULCERATION

The stomach is the most common site of gastrointestinal ulceration, with several causes, including inflammatory gastrointestinal disease, neoplasia, and the use of anti-inflammatory or corticosteroid medications (Fitzgerald et al. 2017). Gastric ulceration can be recognized ultrasonographically as a mucosal defect containing hyperechoic microbubbles due to gas extending from the lumen into the ulcer. This may be accompanied by local wall thickening, luminal fluid accumulation, and reduced gastric motility. Non-perforated ulcers pose a diagnostic challenge with ultrasonography and CT displaying superior sensitivity compared to radiography, while CT has the highest sensitivity for detecting perforated ulcers (Pennick et al. 1997; Murakami et al. 2022). Additional findings in patients with gastrointestinal perforation include hyperechoic mesenteric fat, peritoneal effusion, and pneumoperitoneum (Boysen et al. 2003).

SMALL INTESTINE

The small intestine is composed of the duodenum, jejunum, and ileum. The duodenum has descending, transverse, and ascending portions. Although radiography is frequently the initial imaging modality in the investigation of small intestinal disease, it has limitations in the assessment of many disease processes, in particular, mural changes or functional abnormalities. Radiography allows evaluation of intestinal diameter, wall opacity, and luminal contents and is particularly useful for detecting luminal dilation and obstruction. In dogs, normal small intestinal loops should measure less than 1.6 times the height of the midbody of L5 in diameter, and in cats they should measure less than 12 mm in diameter.

The small intestinal walls, like other areas of the gastrointestinal tract, are composed of multiple layers, which are best appreciated on ultrasonography and can be partially seen on post-contrast computed tomographic images, namely the mucosa, submucosa, muscularis, and serosa. These layers are important in the assessment of disease. Ultrasonography can be useful in the assessment of small intestinal wall thickness, with published values available in the dog and cat (Table 34.1).

Arterial phase CT images show mucosal enhancement; however, the poorer spatial resolution of CT compared to ultrasonography makes differentiation of the small intestinal wall layers difficult. In intestinal loops with no luminal gas or content, delineation of the mucosal margins is often not possible. CT has been shown to be superior to ultrasonography in the assessment of the abdomen of dogs larger than 25 kg. CT also allows for assessment of the adjacent lymph nodes and can evaluate the lung for staging purposes.

SMALL INTESTINAL ILEUS

The absence of normal movement of the intestinal contents is termed ileus. This can be divided into functional or mechanical ileus.

MECHANICAL ILEUS: OBSTRUCTION

Small intestinal mechanical obstruction is most commonly caused by intraluminal obstructions such as foreign bodies; however, other causes such as luminal neoplasia can be identified. Less common causes include extraluminal mass effect secondary to neoplasia or intraluminal stenosis.

The most common radiographic feature of small intestinal mechanical obstruction is variable degrees of intestinal dilation, with segments often measuring more than 1.6 times the midbody height of L5 in the dog and >12 mm in the cat. Two distinct populations of small intestine are often identified, where one loop is twice the diameter of another. At a ratio of 1.73 times the midbody height of L5, the reported probability of obstruction is 50%. As the size of the larger loop increases, the likelihood of obstruction is greater. However, one study reported that 29% of cases of mechanical obstruction in dogs did not show evidence of small intestinal dilation (Figure 34.6).

Luminal foreign bodies vary in opacity, depending on their composition. Mineral foreign bodies such as bones, or gas-filled balls may be readily identified, but others, which are soft tissue

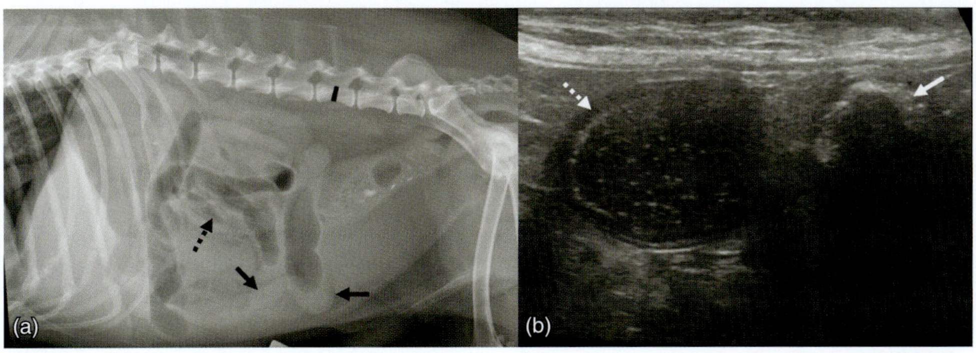

FIGURE 34.6 A composite right lateral abdominal view (a) and ultrasonographic image of the jejunum (b) of a dog with a mechanical small intestinal obstruction. There are two populations of small intestine, with one loop of intestine dilated with a mixture of gas and soft tissue opaque material. This loop is greater than 1.6 times the mid-body height of L5 vertebral body (black line). There are other smaller loops of intestine measuring less than half the diameter of the larger loops (dashed black arrow). Ultrasonographically, there is a large well-defined hyperechoic structure within a jejunal loop, with distal acoustic shadowing (white arrow). The adjacent small intestinal loop is distended with heterogeneous fluid material (white dashed arrow). Courtesy of University College Dublin

opaque, are difficult to discern from the intestinal wall and normal intestinal content. Some foreign bodies, such as fruit seeds or corn cobs, may trap gas or have characteristic shapes.

When small intestinal mechanical obstruction is suspected, it may be important to determine if an intestinal loop is small intestinal or colonic, especially when segments measure larger than normal (>1.6 times the midbody height of L5) (Finck et al. 2014; Graham et al. 1998). To make this distinction, gas can be introduced into the descending colon/rectum via a flexible tube, at volumes of 1–3 mL/kg in dogs and 20–30 mL in cats. By filling the colon with gas, the enlarged loop can be identified as either colonic or small intestinal.

Ultrasonography is excellent at diagnosing small intestinal diameter enlargement and identifying intraluminal foreign bodies. Foreign bodies are usually identified as well-defined, hyperechoic structures with a hyperechoic margin and strong distal acoustic shadowing (Tidwell and Penninck 1992). Ultrasonography has been reported to show higher sensitivity than radiography for identifying obstructive gastrointestinal lesions. One study found that ultrasonography identified intestinal obstruction in 96% of cases, while radiography diagnosed only 52% of cases (Sharma et al. 2011).

Computed tomography can be used to detect mechanical obstruction and has been shown to have a higher sensitivity and specificity compared to abdominal radiographs when assessed by a board-certified radiologist. Similarly, CT has been reported to have comparable sensitivity and higher specificity compared to ultrasonography in the diagnosis of mechanical obstruction. Radiologists have also correctly identified the small intestinal foreign body location in 96% of patients.

FUNCTIONAL ILEUS

In cases of functional ileus, there is a decrease or absence of normal peristaltic waves leading to dilation of the small intestinal loops. This may be due to inflammation, electrolyte imbalances, trauma, or drug administration. Radiographically, functional ileus presents as small intestinal dilation, often measuring >1.6 × mid-body height of L5 in the dog or 12 mm in the cat. In contrast to mechanical obstruction, functional ileus typically shows one population of small intestine, with all loops of similar size and no segment measuring twice the diameter of another. Ultrasonographic findings may include generalized fluid dilation of the small intestines with normal wall layering. In normal jejunal segments, content should move only in an oral-to-aboral direction, whereas bidirectional movement is suggestive of ileus.

LINEAR FOREIGN BODIES

Linear foreign bodies can be challenging to identify radiographically, especially in dogs. Linear foreign bodies such as string, twine, or fishing line can become tethered to a focal point proximally, such as the base of the tongue or within the stomach. The linear material then extends aborally (distally) with the normal peristaltic waves. When the linear material becomes taut, the peristaltic waves cause bunching or "plication" of the small intestines (Felts et al. 1984). Radiographically, this appears as an accumulation of intestinal loops in one region of the peritoneal cavity, forming a stacked appearance between adjacent loops. Gas bubbles within the intestinal lumen can be organized into "comma-shapes" due to the bunching (Figure 34.7). Linear foreign bodies may cause secondary obstruction, and concurrent radiographic features of obstruction may be evident (Root and Lord 1971). Ultrasonography typically reveals a hyperechoic linear structure within the small intestinal lumen surrounded by undulating walls. With chronicity, linear foreign bodies may have a "cheese-wire" effect, where repeated peristaltic movements against taut linear material cause wall perforation. Leakage of small intestinal contents may lead to adjacent peritoneal effusion and peritonitis, and additional radiographic features include a loss of peritoneal serosal detail and pneumoperitoneum (Boysen et al. 2003).

SMALL INTESTINAL NEOPLASIA

Small intestinal neoplastic infiltration causes thickening of the small intestinal wall, which can be circumferential or eccentric in nature. In severe cases, the lesion may be associated with secondary stenosis or obstruction.

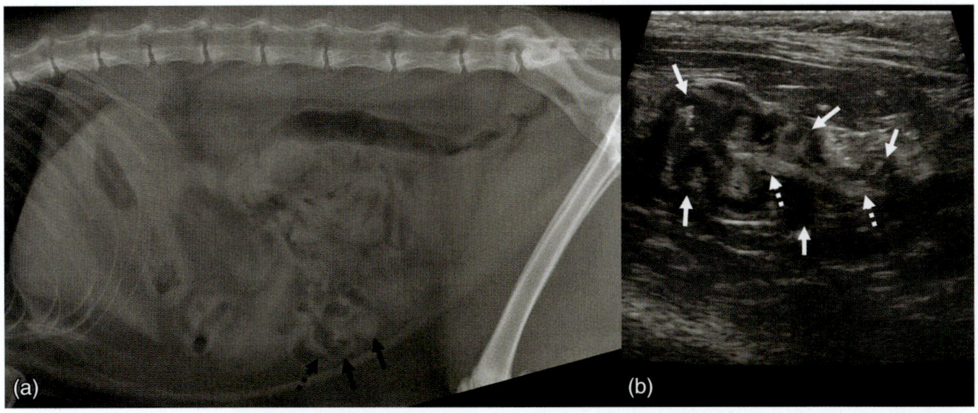

FIGURE 34.7 A right lateral radiograph (a) and corresponding ultrasonographic image (b) of the abdomen of a cat with a jejunal linear foreign body. There is corrugation and bunching of several small intestinal loops within the caudoventral abdomen (black arrows) with some comma-shaped gas bubbles (dashed black arrow). Ultrasonographic image shows a linear hyperechoic structure within the jejunal lumen (dashed white arrows) with corrugated small intestinal loops around the foreign body (white arrows). Courtesy of University College Dublin

Small intestinal neoplasia is best appreciated on ultrasonographic images and typically presents as wall thickening, loss of normal wall layering, and homogeneous or heterogeneous hypoechogenicity of the intestinal wall. Normal small intestinal wall thickness has been previously published (Table 34.1).

The most common neoplasms are adenocarcinoma and lymphoma in dogs, and lymphoma and adenocarcinoma in cats. Other differentials include leiomyosarcomas and GISTs. Both lymphoma and adenocarcinoma are associated with thickening of the wall. Lymphoma typically causes more circumferential wall thickening and affects a longer section of small intestine, whereas carcinoma more often presents as eccentric thickening, affecting a more focal section of small intestine (Penninck et al. 1994). Adenocarcinoma is more likely to extend into the lumen of the intestine; however, there is overlap in the imaging findings, and tissue sampling is necessary to confirm the diagnosis. With intestinal neoplasia, the adjacent lymph nodes are frequently moderately enlarged and rounded, and there may be adjacent malignant effusion. In cats, the ileum is a common site of neoplasia, although it is important to recognize that the feline ileal wall is generally thicker than the remainder of the small intestine.

CT can be used to investigate the small intestines for signs of malignancy and may identify wall thickening, evidence of small intestinal mechanical obstruction, adjacent lymph node enlargement, or peritoneal malignant effusion.

SMALL INTESTINAL INFLAMMATION

Small intestinal inflammation, or enteritis, may be infectious or noninfectious. Infectious enteritis can be bacterial, viral, or fungal in nature. Noninfectious enteritis includes inflammatory bowel disease (IBD), also called chronic enteropathy; a complex condition involving inflammatory cell infiltration in the small intestines, such as lymphocytic-plasmacytic enteritis or eosinophilic enteritis. Radiographs are often unremarkable, but increased luminal gas or evidence of functional ileus may be observed. On ultrasonographic images, there may be mild thickening of the small intestinal wall, although normal wall layering is usually maintained. The different forms of enteritis and intestinal wall infiltration are usually indistinguishable. In fungal enteritis, such as blastomycosis or histoplasmosis, the organisms can cause thickening of the intestinal wall and loss of wall layering, similar to neoplasia.

LYMPHANGIECTASIA

Lymphangiectasia refers to dilation, obstruction, or dysfunction of the small intestinal lymphatic vessels and lacteals. Lymphangiectasia can be seen in various conditions, including chronic enteropathies and intestinal neoplasia, such as lymphoma. It has been within the small

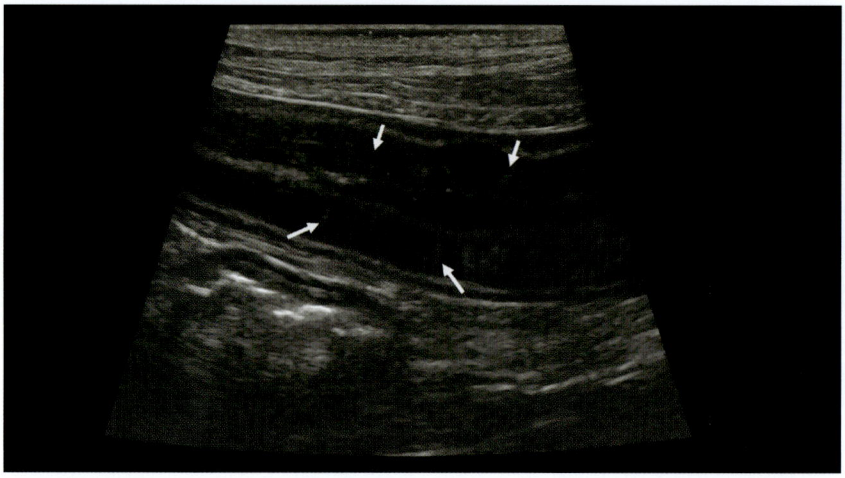

FIGURE 34.8 An ultrasonographic image of a dog with lymphocytic-plasmacytic enteritis. The image shows the jejunum in long axis, showing mild thickening of the jejunal wall, with intact wall layers but with multiple linear hyperechoic lines perpendicular to the lumen (arrows). Courtesy of University College Dublin

intestines and is reported to be seen in 46% of dogs with cases of protein-losing enteropathy. Ultrasonography may identify multiple parallel hyperechoic striations within the intestinal mucosa, oriented perpendicular to the lumen. Importantly, lacteal dilation can occur after a recent meal in normal patients, so this finding should be interpreted in conjunction with the clinical history (Figure 34.8).

INTUSSUSCEPTION

Intussusception is most commonly seen in young animals and can be due to inflammation (viral, parasitic, or bacterial), foreign bodies, neoplasia, or metabolic abnormalities causing asynchrony of the peristaltic waves. Intussusception occurs when a small intestinal segment invaginates into the lumen of an adjacent segment, often due to the asynchrony of the peristaltic waves. The invaginated portion is called the intussusceptum, with the outer portion called the intussuscipiens. Often mesenteric fat and vessels are also displaced into the intussusception. There may be secondary mechanical obstruction or adjacent peritoneal effusion. Chronic intussusception may cause swelling of the intestinal loops and compression of the vessels trapped within the intussusceptum. The vessel occlusion can lead to vascular compromise and ischemia of the wall. Radiographs may show enlargement of the intestinal loop and associated mass effect. A meniscal sign may be evident, characterized by a rounded soft tissue opacity with a gas interface. Poor peritoneal serosal detail secondary to peritoneal effusion can be seen. However, radiographs may be normal in some cases. Ultrasonographic findings are more conclusive. The characteristic appearance is "a loop within a loop" of intestine, appearing as alternating hyperechoic and hypoechoic concentric rings surrounding a hyperechoic center. Doppler can be used to interrogate the vessels within the intussuscipiens, with the identification of Doppler signal associated with improved reducibility in surgery. CT can identify the alternating hypoattenuating and hyperattenuating rings of the intussusception. It is also valuable for determining the location of the intussusception, as well as assessing the mesenteric vessels involved, adjacent lymph nodes, and the presence of peritoneal effusion.

MESENTERIC VOLVULUS

Mesenteric volvulus is rare in dogs and very rare in cats. There is rotation of the intestine around the mesenteric axis, resulting in occlusion of the cranial mesenteric artery. With the arterial supply affected, the duodenum, jejunum, ileum, cecum, and colon become ischemic, with subsequent wall necrosis and rupture (Junius et al. 2004; Spevakow et al. 2010). Radiography shows markedly gas-distended small intestines, which are stacked in loops (one population of intestine) (Figure 34.9).

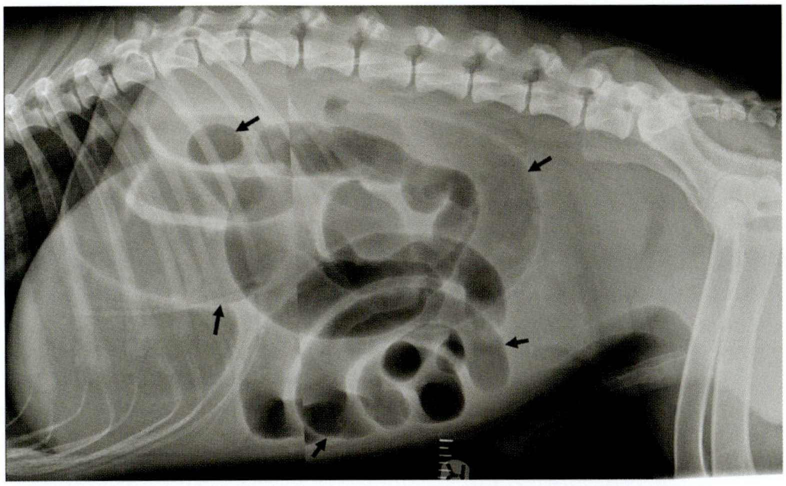

FIGURE 34.9 A composite right lateral radiograph of a dog with mesenteric torsion. Marked gas dilation and stacking of the intestinal loops (arrows). Courtesy of University College Dublin

With rupture, pneumoperitoneum may be identified. Ultrasonography may be limited due to the small intestinal gas causing reverberation artifact, preventing imaging of the deeper abdomen. Peritoneal effusion and pneumoperitoneum may be detected ultrasonographically. On CT, marked gas distension of the small intestines and stacking can be identified, and twisting of the mesenteric vessels can be recognized as a "whirl sign."

CECUM

The cecum is a blind-ended dilation of the proximal colon, which communicates with the ascending colon at the ileocolic junction in the dog and cat. The normal cecum can contain a mild amount of gas and be corkscrew- or comma-shaped, usually located within the right dorsal abdomen. In the cecum there are similar wall layers to the rest of the gastrointestinal tract, with one study in the cat describing the combined mucosa and submucosa as a "follicular layer," due to multiple lymphoid follicles bridging between the layers. The normal follicular layer has a reported maximal thickness of 2 mm in cats (Hahn et al. 2017).

TYPHLITIS

Typhlitis is rare in dogs and cats. It can occur in association with viral (such as feline infectious peritonitis), parasitic (such as *Trichuris* or *Giardia*), or bacterial (such as *Campylobacter*) infections. Radiographically there may be no changes identified. Ultrasonographically there may be thickening of the cecal wall, alteration to the cecal wall layering, adjacent hypoechoic free fluid, and local lymphadenopathy.

COLON AND RECTUM

The colon is divided into three portions: the ascending, transverse, and descending colon, terminating with the rectum. The colon and rectum have similar wall layers to the small intestine; however, the colon and rectum have relatively thin walls, and generally the wall layers are indistinct (Table 34.1).

INTUSSUSCEPTION

Multiple variations of large intestinal intussusceptions can occur, including ileocolic (the ileum invaginates into the colon), cecocolic (the cecum invaginates within the colon), and colocolic (a colonic segment invaginates into an adjacent segment) types. Cecocolic intussusception is also called cecal inversion. The ileocolic junction is the most commonly affected region. The radiographic appearance is similar to that of small intestinal intussusceptions, with a large tubular soft tissue opacity in the mid-abdomen. There may be a crescent-shaped gas opacity with a smooth margin at the interface between the intussusceptum and intussuscipiens. Similar to small intestinal intussusceptions, ultrasonography will reveal "a loop within a loop" with alternating hyperechoic and hypoechoic rings and a central hyperechoic region. The mesenteric fat and vessels within the intussuscipiens can be assessed and evaluated for Doppler signal, with the absence of signal raising concern for ischemia.

COLORECTAL NEOPLASIA

Colonic neoplasia is rare in cats and dogs. The most common colorectal neoplasia in dogs was reported to be adenoma or polyp in 71% of cases, with 29% reported as carcinoma in situ or carcinoma. In cats the most common colorectal neoplasia was adenocarcinoma and lymphoma. This study found no changes in abdominal radiography, while ultrasonography revealed colonic wall thickening, a mass at the colorectal junction, and adjacent lymphadenopathy. Abdominal ultrasonography generally shows eccentric or concentric thickening of the colonic wall and an absence of wall layering.

Colorectal polyps are rare in dogs, with one study reporting that West Highland White terriers are overrepresented (Méric et al. 2023). Polyps have been divided into three forms: nonneoplastic hyperplastic polyps, benign neoplasia, and malignant neoplasia. The size of the masses may be such that they cause colorectal stenosis or obstruction and associated clinical constipation or obstipation. More commonly, patients present with hematochezia, diarrhea and tenesmus.

COLONIC TORSION

Colonic torsion is a rare condition in small animals in which the colon twists around its longitudinal axis. Plain radiographs may show segmental distention of the colon, displacement of the descending colon to the right, focal narrowing of the colonic lumen, and displacement of the cecum to the left, usually with normal small intestinal loops (Gremillion et al. 2018). Barium enemas can be administered and may demonstrate a narrowing of the colon with helical striations, called a "torsion sign." Ultrasonography may not be useful due to the gas-filled colonic segment causing reverberation artifact.

MEGACOLON

Megacolon is an irreversible dilation of the colon, often associated with a loss of colonic motility and mechanical function. It is more commonly seen in cats than in dogs. Megacolon can be idiopathic, caused by chronic constipation or obstipation, or due to neurologic disorders such as spinal cord injuries or dysautonomia. Radiographically, megacolon presents as a distended colon, measuring greater than 1.48 times the length of the body of L5 in the cat, and may be suspected if the colonic diameter is greater than the length of L7 in the dog. Ultrasonography is not useful in the diagnosis of megacolon.

ATRESIA ANI

Atresia ani is a rare congenital abnormality whereby there is an absence of the anal opening or terminal rectum, and the distal colon or rectum does not communicate with the anus. There may be a blind pouch formed by the rectum, cranial to the anus, or there may be a persistent communication between the rectum and vagina (rectovaginal fistula). If the condition is not identified quickly, the colonic contents may build up with a resultant megacolon secondary to prolonged distension (Vianna and Tobias 2005). Radiography may identify a digesta-filled distended colon. In females a dilated colon may not occur due to the rectovaginal fistula allowing the passage of materials from the rectum into the vagina. Positive contrast radiography, such as a barium enema, may be useful to show a blind-ended anal region that does not communicate with the distal colon. Ultrasonography is not useful because of the intrapelvic location of the lesion. CT may be useful in identifying the colon, rectum, and anus, and negative or positive contrast enemas may be useful to assess a connection.

PERIANAL REGION

The anal sacs are paired structures located between the internal and external sphincter muscles. The sacs store secretions from the anal glands within the sac, with a duct that connects to the skin surface at the left and right lateral aspects of the anus. Perianal glands are small glands located in the dermis around the anus and adjacent skin.

ANAL SAC INFLAMMATION

Anal sac impactions and inflammation (sacculitis) may occur in the dog and cat, with some suggesting that loose stools or constipation may be a cause. With sacculitis, there may be subsequent abscessation (Corbee et al. 2021). This is generally identified clinically without the use of diagnostic imaging. In complex sacculitis and abscessation, CT may be useful to characterize the extent of the abscessation for surgical planning.

PERIANAL NEOPLASIA

The most common perianal neoplasms are apocrine gland anal sac adenocarcinoma (AGASACA) and perianal adenomas and carcinomas (Adamovich-Rippe et al. 2017). These neoplasms can present as large, irregular perianal masses. CT is useful for assessing the size, shape, and extent of the masses, as well as evaluating the adjacent lymph nodes. A recent CT study suggested that perianal adenomas and adenocarcinomas are more likely to be bilateral in location compared to AGASACAs, which are more likely unilateral (Figure 34.10) (Jeong et al. 2025). Tissue sampling is necessary to achieve a definitive diagnosis. Thoracic radiography may be useful for staging purposes, and abdominal assessment is indicated to identify metastatic disease. Similarly, ultrasonography may not be useful in characterizing the lesion but facilitates staging of the neoplasia.

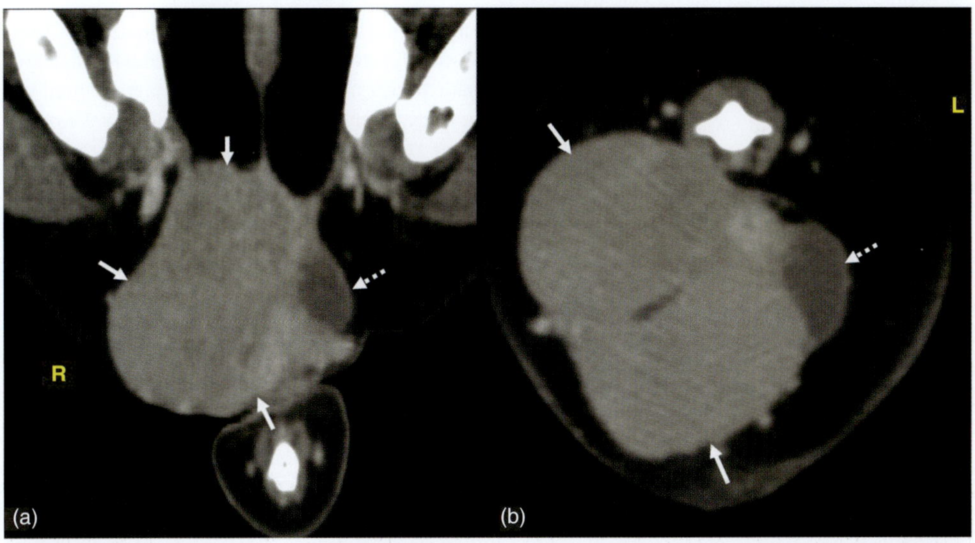

FIGURE 34.10 Computed tomographic dorsal (a) and transverse (b) multiplanar reconstruction post-contrast images of the perineal region of a dog. A large strongly contrast-enhancing rounded mass (arrows) is within the perineal tissues to the right of the rectum and anus. The anus and left anal sac (dashed arrows) are displaced to the left by the mass. Courtesy of University College Dublin

REFERENCES

Abd Elkader, N.A., Emam, I.A., Farghali, H.A. et al. (2020). Oesophageal foreign bodies in cats: clinical and anatomic findings. *PLoS One* 15 (6): e0233983. https://doi.org/10.1371/journal.pone.0233983.

Adamovich-Rippe, K.N., Mayhew, P.D., Marks, S.L. et al. (2017). Colonoscopic and histologic features of rectal masses in dogs: 82 cases (1995–2012). *Journal of the American Veterinary Medical Association* 250 (4): 424–430. https://doi.org/10.2460/javma.250.4.424.

Bexfield, N.H., Watson, P.J., and Herrtage, M.E. (2006). Esophageal dysmotility in young dogs. *Journal of Veterinary Internal Medicine* 20 (6): 1314–1318. https://doi.org/10.1892/0891-6640(2006)20[1314:edivd]2.0.co;2.

Biller, D.S., Partington, B.P., Miyabayashi, T. et al. (1994). Ultrasonographic appearance of chronic hypertrophic pyloric gastropathy in the dog. *Veterinary Radiology & Ultrasound* 35 (1): 30–33. https://doi.org/10.1111/j.1740-8261.1994.tb00174.x.

Boysen, S.R., Tidwell, A.S., and Penninck, D.G. (2003). Ultrasonographic findings in dogs and cats with gastrointestinal perforation. *Veterinary Radiology & Ultrasound* 44 (5): 556–564. https://doi.org/10.1111/j.1740-8261.2003.tb00507.x.

Buchanan, J.W. (2004). Tracheal signs and associated vascular anomalies in dogs with persistent right aortic arch. *Journal of Veterinary Internal Medicine* 18 (4): 510–514. https://doi.org/10.1892/0891-6640(2004)18<510:tsaava>2.0.co;2.

Corbee, R.J., Woldring, H.H., van den Eijnde, L.M. et al. (2021). A cross-sectional study on canine and feline anal sac disease. *Animals (Basel)* 12 (1): 95. https://doi.org/10.3390/ani12010095.

Costas, A. and Cervera, V. (2024). CT findings in seven dogs with perforating wooden skewer foreign bodies from the gastrointestinal tract. *Open Veterinary Journal* 14 (4): 1002–1011. https://doi.org/10.5455/OVJ.2024.v14.i4.7.

Delaney, F., O'Brien, R.T., and Waller, K. (2003). Ultrasound evaluation of small bowel thickness compared to weight in normal dogs. *Veterinary Radiology & Ultrasound* 44 (5): 577–580. https://doi.org/10.1111/j.1740-8261.2003.tb00510.x.

Di Donato, P., Penninck, D., Pietra, M. et al. (2014). Ultrasonographic measurement of the relative thickness of intestinal wall layers in clinically healthy cats. *Journal of Feline Medicine and Surgery* 16 (4): 333–339. https://doi.org/10.1177/1098612x13509080.

Diana, A., Penninck, D.G., and Keating, J.H. (2009). Ultrasonographic appearance of canine gastric polyps. *Veterinary Radiology & Ultrasound* 50 (2): 201–204. https://doi.org/10.1111/j.1740-8261.2009.01517.x.

Doran, I.P., Wright, C.A., and Moore, A.H. (2008). Acute oropharyngeal and esophageal stick injury in forty-one dogs. *Veterinary Surgery* 37 (8): 781–785. https://doi.org/10.1111/j.1532-950X.2008.00448.x.

Dvir, E., Kirberger, R.M., and Malleczek, D. (2001). Radiographic and computed tomographic changes and clinical presentation of spirocercosis in the dog. *Veterinary Radiology & Ultrasound* 42 (2): 119–129. https://doi.org/10.1111/j.1740-8261.2001.tb00914.x.

Eivers, C., Chicon Rueda, R., Liuti, T. et al. (2019). Retrospective analysis of esophageal imaging features in brachycephalic versus non-brachycephalic dogs based on videofluoroscopic swallowing studies. *Journal of Veterinary Medical Science* 33 (4): 1740–1746. https://doi.org/10.1111/jvim.15547.

Farese, J.P., Bacon, N.J., Ehrhart, N.P. et al. (2008). Oesophageal leiomyosarcoma in dogs: surgical management and clinical outcome of four cases. *Veterinary and Comparative Oncology* 6 (1): 31–38. https://doi.org/10.1111/j.1476-5829.2007.00134.x.

Felts, J.F., Fox, P.R., and Burk, R.L. (1984). Thread and sewing needles as gastrointestinal foreign bodies in the cat: a review of 64 cases. *Journal of the American Veterinary Medical Association* 184 (1): 56–59.

Finck, C., D'Anjou, M.A., Alexander, K. et al. (2014). Radiographic diagnosis of mechanical obstruction in dogs based on relative small intestinal external diameters. *Veterinary Radiology & Ultrasound* 55 (5): 472–479. https://doi.org/10.1111/vru.12153.

Fischetti, A.J., Saunders, H.M., and Drobatz, K.J. (2004). Pneumatosis in canine gastric dilatation-volvulus syndrome. *Veterinary Radiology & Ultrasound* 45 (3): 205–209. https://doi.org/10.1111/j.1740-8261.2004.04034.x.

Fitzgerald, E., Barfield, D., Lee, K.C. et al. (2017). Clinical findings and results of diagnostic imaging in 82 dogs with gastrointestinal ulceration. *Journal of Small Animal Practice* 58 (4): 211–218. https://doi.org/10.1111/jsap.12631.

Formaggini, L., Schmidt, K., and De Lorenzi, D. (2008). Gastric dilatation-volvulus associated with diaphragmatic hernia in three cats: clinical presentation, surgical treatment and presumptive aetiology. *Journal of Feline Medicine and Surgery* 10 (2): 198–201. https://doi.org/10.1016/j.jfms.2007.09.010.

German, A.J., Cannon, M.J., Dye, C. et al. (2005). Oesophageal strictures in cats associated with doxycycline therapy. *Journal of Feline Medicine and Surgery* 7 (1): 33–41. https://doi.org/10.1016/j.jfms.2004.04.001.

Gianella, P., Pfammatter, N.S., and Burgener, I.A. (2009). Oesophageal and gastric endoscopic foreign body removal: complications and follow-up of 102 dogs. *Journal of Small Animal Practice* 50 (12): 649–654. https://doi.org/10.1111/j.1748-5827.2009.00845.x.

Graham, J.P., Lord, P.F., and Harrison, J.M. (1998). Quantitative estimation of intestinal dilation as a predictor of obstruction in the dog. *Journal of Small Animal Practice* 39 (11): 521–524. https://doi.org/10.1111/j.1748-5827.1998.tb03698.x.

Graham, J.P., Newell, S.M., Roberts, G.D. et al. (2000). Ultrasonographic features of canine gastrointestinal pythiosis. *Veterinary Radiology & Ultrasound* 41 (3): 273–277. https://doi.org/10.1111/j.1740-8261.2000.tb01490.x.

Gremillion, C.L., Savage, M., and Cohen, E.B. (2018). Radiographic findings and clinical factors in dogs with surgically confirmed or presumed colonic torsion. *Veterinary Radiology & Ultrasound* 59 (3): 272–278. https://doi.org/10.1111/vru.12595.

Grooters, A.M., Miyabayashi, T., Biller, D.S. et al. (1994). Sonographic appearance of uremic gastropathy in four dogs. *Veterinary Radiology & Ultrasound* 35 (1): 35–40. https://doi.org/10.1111/j.1740-8261.1994.tb00175.x.

Hahn, H., Freiche, V., Baril, A. et al. (2017). Ultrasonographic, endoscopic and histological appearance of the caecum in clinically healthy cats. *Journal of Feline Medicine and Surgery* 19 (2): 85–93. https://doi.org/10.1177/1098612x15602740.

Han, E., Broussard, J., and Baer, K.E. (2003). Feline esophagitis secondary to gastroesophageal reflux disease: clinical signs and radiographic, endoscopic, and histopathological findings. *Journal of the American Animal Hospital Association* 39 (2): 161–167. https://doi.org/10.5326/0390161.

Hobbs, J., Sutherland-Smith, J., Penninck, D. et al. (2015). Ultrasonographic features of canine gastrointestinal stromal tumors compared to other gastrointestinal spindle cell tumors. *Veterinary Radiology & Ultrasound* 56 (4): 432–438. https://doi.org/10.1111/vru.12253.

Hoffmann, K.L. (2003). Sonographic signs of gastroduodenal linear foreign body in 3 dogs. *Veterinary Radiology & Ultrasound* 44 (4): 466–469. https://doi.org/10.1111/j.1740-8261.2003.tb00486.x.

Houlton, J.E.F., Herrtage, M.E., Taylor, P.M. et al. (1985). Thoracic oesophageal foreign bodies in the dog: a review of ninety cases. *Journal of Small Animal Practice* 26 (9): 521–536. https://doi.org/10.1111/j.1748-5827.1985.tb02230.x.

Hunt, G.B., Worth, A., and Marchevsky, A. (2004). Migration of wooden skewer foreign bodies from the gastrointestinal tract in eight dogs. *Journal of Small Animal Practice* 45 (7): 362–367. https://doi.org/10.1111/j.1748-5827.2004.tb00249.x.

Jeong, J., Goh, J., Nam, C. et al. (2025). Comparison of computed tomography findings between perianal tumors originating from the anal sacs and perianal glands in dogs. *Veterinary Radiology & Ultrasound* 66 (1): e13453. https://doi.org/10.1111/vru.13453.

Junius, G., Appeldoorn, A.M., and Schrauwen, E. (2004). Mesenteric volvulus in the dog: a retrospective study of 12 cases. *Journal of Small Animal Practice* 45 (2): 104–107. https://doi.org/10.1111/j.1748-5827.2004.tb00211.x.

Kaser-Hotz, B., Hauser, B., and Arnold, P. (1996). Ultrasonographic findings in canine gastric neoplasia in 13 patients. *Veterinary Radiology & Ultrasound* 37 (1): 51–56. https://doi.org/10.1111/j.1740-8261.1996.tb00812.x.

Lamb, C.R. and Forster-van Hijfte, M. (1994). Ultrasound corner beware the gastric pseudomass. *Veterinary Radiology & Ultrasound* 35 (5): 398–399. https://doi.org/10.1111/j.1740-8261.1994.tb02060.x.

Lamb, C.R. and Grierson, J. (1999). Ultrasonographic appearance of primary gastric neoplasia in 21 dogs. *Journal of Small Animal Practice* 40 (5): 211–215. https://doi.org/10.1111/j.1748-5827.1999.tb03062.x.

Leary, M.L. and Sinnott-Stutzman, V. (2018). Spontaneous gastric dilatation-volvulus in two cats. *Journal of Veterinary Emergency and Critical Care (San Antonio)* 28 (4): 346–355. https://doi.org/10.1111/vec.12734.

Leib, M.S. and Sartor, L.L. (2008). Esophageal foreign body obstruction caused by a dental chew treat in 31 dogs (2000-2006). *Journal of the American Veterinary Medical Association* 232 (7): 1021–1025. https://doi.org/10.2460/javma.232.7.1021.

Manczur, F. and Vörös, K. (2000). Gastrointestinal ultrasonography of the dog: a review of 265 cases (1996-1998). *Acta Veterinaria Hungarica* 48 (1): 9–21. https://doi.org/10.1556/AVet.48.2000.1.2.

McConnell, J.F., Sparkes, A.H., Blunden, A.S. et al. (2007). Eosinophilic fibrosing gastritis and toxoplasmosis in a cat. *Journal of Feline Medicine and Surgery* 9 (1): 82–88. https://doi.org/10.1016/j.jfms.2006.11.005.

Méric, T., Issard, J., Maufras, T. et al. (2023). Recurrence and survival in dogs with excised colorectal polyps: a retrospective study of 58 cases. *Journal of Veterinary Internal Medicine* 37 (6): 2375–2384. https://doi.org/10.1111/jvim.16876.

Mur, P.E., Appleby, R., Phillips, K.L. et al. (2025). Radiographic findings in dogs with 360 degrees gastric dilatation and volvulus. *Veterinary Radiology & Ultrasound* 66 (1): e13445. https://doi.org/10.1111/vru.13445.

Murakami, M., Heng, H.G., and Sola, M. (2022). CT features of confirmed and presumed gastric wall edema in dogs. *Veterinary Radiology & Ultrasound* 63 (6): 711–718. https://doi.org/10.1111/vru.13123.

Murakami, M., Heng, H.G., Lim, C.K. et al. (2019). Ultrasonographic features of presumed gastric wall edema in 14 dogs with pancreatitis. *Journal of Veterinary Internal Medicine* 33 (3): 1260–1265. https://doi.org/10.1111/jvim.15507.

Newell, S.M., Graham, J.P., Roberts, G.D. et al. (1999). Sonography of the normal feline gastrointestinal tract. *Veterinary Radiology & Ultrasound* 40 (1): 40–43. https://doi.org/10.1111/j.1740-8261.1999.tb01837.x.

Park, H.A., Kim, J.W., and Park, H.M. (2012). Characteristics of esophageal diverticula using computed tomography and three-dimensional reconstruction in a Maltese dog. *Journal of Veterinary Medical Science* 74 (9): 1233–1236. https://doi.org/10.1292/jvms.11-0546.

Penninck, D. and Mitchell, S.L. (2003). Ultrasonographic detection of ingested and perforating wooden foreign bodies in four dogs. *Journal of the American Veterinary Medical Association* 223 (2): 206–209, 196. https://doi.org/10.2460/javma.2003.223.206.

Penninck, D., Matz, M., and Tidwell, A. (1997). Ultrasonography of gastric ulceration in the dog. *Veterinary Radiology & Ultrasound* 38 (4): 308–312. https://doi.org/10.1111/j.1740-8261.1997.tb00860.x.

Penninck, D.G., Moore, A.S., and Gliatto, J. (1998). Ultrasonography of canine gastric epithelial neoplasia. *Veterinary Radiology & Ultrasound* 39 (4): 342–348. https://doi.org/10.1111/j.1740-8261.1998.tb01618.x.

Penninck, D.G., Moore, A.S., Tidwell, A.S. et al. (1994). Ultrasonography of alimentary lymphosarcoma in the cat. *Veterinary Radiology & Ultrasound* 35 (4): 299–306. https://doi.org/10.1111/j.1740-8261.1994.tb02045.x.

Penninck, D.G., Nyland, T.G., Fisher, P.E. et al. (1989). Ultrasonography of the normal canine gastrointestinal tract. *Veterinary Radiology* 30 (6): 272–276. https://doi.org/10.1111/j.1740-8261.1989.tb01799.x.

Probst, C.W., Bright, R.M., Ackerman, N. et al. (1984). Spontaneous pneumoperitoneum subsequent to gastric volvulus in two dogs. *Veterinary Radiology* 25 (1): 37–42. https://doi.org/10.1111/j.1740-8261.1984.tb00743.x.

Ranen, E., Lavy, E., Aizenberg, I. et al. (2004). Spirocercosis-associated esophageal sarcomas in dogs. A retrospective study of 17 cases (1997-2003). *Veterinary Parasitology* 119 (2-3): 209–221. https://doi.org/10.1016/j.vetpar.2003.10.023.

Reeve, E.J., Sutton, D., Friend, E.J. et al. (2017). Documenting the prevalence of hiatal hernia and oesophageal abnormalities in brachycephalic dogs using fluoroscopy. *Journal of Small Animal Practice* 58 (12): 703–708. https://doi.org/10.1111/jsap.12734.

Root, C.R. and Lord, P.F. (1971). Linear radiolucent gastrointestinal foreign bodies in cats and dogs: their radiographic appearance. *Veterinary Radiology* 12(1):45–52. https://doi.org/10.1111/j.1740-8261.1971.tb00401.x.

Segarra, A., Herrtage, M.E., and Salgüero, R. (2022). Diagnostic imaging appearance of canine gastric leiomyomas: four cases. *Veterinary Record Case Reports* 10 (3): e357. https://doi.org/10.1002/vrc2.357.

Sharma, A., Thompson, M.S., Scrivani, P.V. et al. (2011). Comparison of radiography and ultrasonography for diagnosing small-intestinal mechanical obstruction in vomiting dogs. *Veterinary Radiology & Ultrasound* 52 (3): 248–255. https://doi.org/10.1111/j.1740-8261.2010.01791.x.

Shua-Haim, T., Vilaplana Grosso, F.R., Suarez Fuentes, D. et al. (2023). Computed tomographic features of double aortic arch in six dogs. *Veterinary Radiology & Ultrasound* 64 (4): 669–676. https://doi.org/10.1111/vru.13257.

Spevakow, A.B., Nibblett, B.M., Carr, A.P. et al. (2010). Chronic mesenteric volvulus in a dog. *The Canadian Veterinary Journal* 51 (1): 85–88. https://doi.org/10.4141/cjas71-011.

Tanaka, T., Akiyoshi, H., Mie, K. et al. (2019). Contrast-enhanced computed tomography may be helpful for characterizing and staging canine gastric tumors. *Veterinary Radiology & Ultrasound* 60 (1): 7–18. https://doi.org/10.1111/vru.12677.

Thierry, F., Ferreira, M.F., Paterson, G.K. et al. (2019). Canine and feline emphysematous gastritis may be differentiated from gastric emphysema based on clinical and imaging characteristics: five cases. *Veterinary Radiology & Ultrasound* 60 (2): 136–144. https://doi.org/10.1111/vru.12691.

Thompson, H.C., Cortes, Y., Gannon, K. et al. (2012). Esophageal foreign bodies in dogs: 34 cases (2004-2009). *Journal of Veterinary Emergency and Critical Care (San Antonio)* 22 (2): 253–261. https://doi.org/10.1111/j.1476-4431.2011.00700.x.

Tidwell, A.S. and Penninck, D.G. (1992). Ultrasonography of gastrointestinal foreign bodies. *Veterinary Radiology & Ultrasound* 33 (3): 160–169. https://doi.org/10.1111/j.1740-8261.1992.tb01439.x.

Vianna, M.L. and Tobias, K.M. (2005). Atresia ani in the dog: a retrospective study. *Journal of the American Animal Hospital Association* 41 (5): 317–322. https://doi.org/10.5326/0410317.

Weissman, A., Penninck, D., Webster, C. et al. (2013). Ultrasonographic and clinicopathological features of feline gastrointestinal eosinophilic sclerosing fibroplasia in four cats. *Journal of Feline Medicine and Surgery* 15 (2): 148–154. https://doi.org/10.1177/1098612x12464224.

Zuercher, M., Vilaplana Grosso, F., and Lejeune, A. (2021). Comparison of the clinical, ultrasound, and CT findings in 13 dogs with gastric neoplasia. *Veterinary Radiology & Ultrasound* 62 (5): 525–532. https://doi.org/10.1111/vru.12980.

Gastrointestinal Endoscopy

CHAPTER 35

Edward Hall

Bristol Veterinary School, University of Bristol, Langford, Bristol, UK

KEY POINTS

- Flexible endoscopy permits examination of the upper and lower GI tract but not the mid small intestine, and is safer than surgical biopsy.
- The ideal endoscope should be 1–1.4 m long, with a tip diameter of 7–9 mm, and four-way tip deflection.
- Multiple biopsies should always be collected (except from the esophagus) even if the organ appears grossly normal.
- Success depends on understanding the endoscope controls and normal anatomy, and on practice.

INTRODUCTION

Endoscopy, derived from Greek meaning "to view within", was developed as a minimally invasive method for observing lesions within the gastrointestinal (GI) tract. However, technological advances since the first flexible endoscopes were invented over 60 years ago now provide the ability to steer (including retroflexion), enhanced imaging (e.g., video, HD quality, magnification, narrowband) with digital recording, and the ability to collect biopsies and other specimens, and to perform therapeutic procedures such as removing foreign bodies (FBs), dilating strictures, placing gastrostomy feeding tubes, and resecting mucosal masses.

EQUIPMENT

RIGID ENDOSCOPES

Hollow rigid endoscopes have limited utility in investigating GI diseases; such colonoscopes can be used to examine the left colon although the field of view is very limited; they can also be used to protect the proximal esophagus when retrieving sharp FBs. However, rigid proctoscopes can provide a better view of the rectum than a flexible endoscope, because adequate insufflation is difficult because adequate insufflation is difficult as air leaks from the anus.

FLEXIBLE ENDOSCOPES

Endoscope

Flexible endoscopes can be used for both upper and lower GI endoscopy. Video endoscopes are preferred over fiberoptic as they are easier to steer and give an image of better quality, which can be recorded digitally.

With the right equipment and the necessary expertise, all parts of the GI tract can be examined. However, standard veterinary gastroscopes are typically too short to examine the majority of the jejunum even when accessing it via both the duodenum and ileum. Dedicated enteroscopes which are long enough are rarely available and are difficult to advance without special oversleeves and/or balloon attachments (Albors et al. 2011). The jejunum can be more easily visualized by video capsule endoscopy.

Disorders of the Liver, Exocrine Pancreas, and Gastrointestinal Tract in Dogs and Cats, First Edition. Edited by Harry Cridge et al. Published 2026 by John Wiley & Sons, Inc. Companion Website: www.wiley.com/go/cridge/disorders

Endoscopes for dogs and cats have an insertion tube (the part inserted into the patient) that range from 1.0 to 1.4 m in length. A longer length enables pyloric intubation in large and giant breeds of dog but makes steering more unwieldy in cats and small dogs due to the length of insertion tube draped outside the patient. Gastroscopes designed for humans can be used but are only 1 m long and cannot reach the duodenum in giant breed dogs. However, human colonoscopes ranging from 1.4 to 1.7 m can be used in giant breeds as their larger tip diameter does not preclude pyloric intubation in these dogs.

The diameter of the insertion tube tip is also critical in determining the size of patient that can be examined. The smallest diameter tip, but with the largest biopsy/working channel possible, is ideal, as the bigger the biopsy is, the more reliable the histological diagnosis. However, these features are inversely proportional: a larger channel increases the tip diameter; a narrow insertion tube has a smaller channel. For most dogs and all cats, the insertion tube tip diameter should be less than 1 cm or pyloric and ileal intubation may be impossible, and the biopsy channel should be no less than 2 mm diameter or intestinal biopsies will fragment. Referral centers often have a range of endoscopes, with a dedicated feline/small dog video endoscope (or a human transnasal gastroscope) only 1 m long, with a tip diameter of 5.5 and a 2.0 mm working/biopsy channel as well as standard gastroscopes. As most primary care practices only possess one gastroscope, a 1.4 m insertion tube with a tip diameter of 8–9 mm and a biopsy channel of 2.7 mm is the best compromise.

Gastroscopes must have four-way tip deflection capability at the terminal bending section: 90 degrees left-right and down with 180–210 degrees up. The ability to retroflex the tip in one direction is essential to be able to visualize and biopsy the cardia and can aid orientation within the stomach. A retroflexed view of the rectum during lower GI endoscopy can also be obtained in large dogs.

Endoscopy Tower

The tower holds the equipment necessary to perform endoscopy. The light source houses not only a xenon arc or an LED lamp but also an air pump for the air–water channel. Towers for video endoscopes also hold a video processor to allow display of the live image on a monitor. Essential ancillary equipment includes a suction pump to allow removal of liquid and deflation of a viscus. Some types of image recording equipment are ideal, but not essential. Optional equipment includes a peristaltic flushing pump, a CO_2 insufflator, and electrosurgical devices.

Endoscopic Instruments

A range of instruments is available: biopsy forceps for collecting biopsies; balloons, snares, and injector needles for performing therapeutic procedures; and grasping and basket forceps, and a Roth net for retrieving FBs.

Biopsy forceps are essential to maximize the yield from diagnostic endoscopy. Historically, forceps were reusable but were expensive if they broke prematurely. Single-use, disposable forceps are now a more affordable option. The design of the biopsy cups is varied, but ellipsoid-shape, fenestrated, alligator edge, and "swing-jaw" are considered the best for obtaining good quality tissue samples (Danesh et al. 1985; Goutal-Landry et al. 2013). The presence of a spike may enable biopsies from tough tissues such as the esophagus and some tumors. However, the main factors affecting sample quality are the size of the cups, which is dictated by the size of the biopsy channel and the pressure exerted by the endoscopist. Swing-jaw forceps hinge the cups into the tissue allowing pressure to be exerted more perpendicular to the surface.

VIDEO CAPSULE ENDOSCOPY

Capsules containing a battery-powered light source and 360-degree camera coverage are swallowed by the patient to enable observation of the whole GI tract. However, they are only able to visualize the mucosa and cannot collect biopsies (Mabry et al. 2019). Therefore, their use is mainly limited to look for sources of bleeding beyond the reach of conventional endoscopes where a focal bleeding lesion is suspected but is too small to be found with ultrasonography, such as vascular ectasia, or when a practice does not possess a flexible endoscope, or where extremes of environmental temperature may damage a flexible endoscope. They can be used in patients where anesthesia is unsafe or refused by the owner, but the study is more likely to be incomplete in patients less than ~8 kg (St-Jean et al. 2025).

Images are either transmitted by telemetry to sensors on the body surface or recorded onto a flash drive within the capsule. In the former, images are recorded in real time, but in the latter, the capsule must be retrieved after defecation and images downloaded for analysis with the risk that the capsule may be lost. Retention in the stomach can be a problem unless the video capsule is delivered via an endoscopic device directly into the duodenum.

ENDOSCOPIC PROCEDURE

Endoscopy is rarely indicated in acute GI diseases except for FB retrieval. It is a relatively safe method for obtaining biopsies in chronic enteropathies compared to open surgery, but perforation is a potential risk, particularly with lower GI endoscopy, as the colonic wall is thinner than the small intestinal wall (Irom et al. 2014). Bacteremia may develop due to endoscopic mucosal trauma, but clinically significant infections have not been reported (Gaspardo et al. 2020).

PATIENT PREPARATION

No special measures are needed to prepare patients for upper GI endoscopy. Withholding food for 12 hours is recommended, as the healthy stomach should then be empty, and finding retained food provides some basic functional information about gastric emptying. Water does not need to be withheld; any liquid in the GI tract can be aspirated via the endoscope.

Conversely, lower GI endoscopy requires significant patient preparation to remove all solid fecal material. Solid food is withheld for 24–48 hours, and fecal material is cleared either by repeated, high, warm water enemas, or by lavage with an oral cleanser. Polyethylene glycol (PEG 3350) solutions made isotonic with electrolytes are most effective, but large volumes (~25 ml/kg given three times two hours apart) are needed. However, they are not palatable to most patients, even when mixed with a meat broth, and have to be given by stomach tube in dogs or via a nasogastric tube in cats. Gavage carries a risk of inhalation which can be fatal (Leib et al. 2004). However, low-volume solutions containing sodium or magnesium salts can cause vomiting and abdominal discomfort and are not such effective cleansers (Daugherty et al. 2008). Gavage with PEG solutions produces optimal cleansing but can be technically challenging and potentially dangerous, but more aesthetic than repeated enemas.

SEDATION AND ANESTHESIA

Premedication with sedatives is recommended as it reduces swallowing of frothy saliva by anxious animals, which can reduce visibility. Oral administration of a 1:5 mixture of acetyl cysteine and simethicone given at the time of premedication has been suggested as a way to abolish froth.

General anesthesia with endotracheal intubation is necessary for GI endoscopy but there is no need for a special protocol as the safest one is the one that is most familiar. The author uses sedation with dexmedetomidine and butorphanol, induction with propofol or alfaxalone, and maintenance with isoflurane or sevoflurane. There is limited evidence that butorphanol makes pyloric intubation slightly easier than methadone (McFadzean et al. 2017). However, there are geographic variations in drug availability, and use of the local standard anesthetic protocol is recommended.

For upper GI endoscopy, it is mandatory to place a gag to prevent potential damage to the endoscope. Spring-loaded gags should be avoided in cats as opening the mouth too wide can occlude the maxillary artery leading to brain and retinal ischemia and post-anesthetic blindness (Martin-Flores et al. 2014). For lower GI endoscopy, an assistant can hold the anus shut to allow insufflation of the left colon and prevent the endoscope tip falling out of the rectum. Whether the assistant is used to advance and withdraw the endoscope depends on the personal preference of the endoscopist.

PATIENT POSITIONING

For both upper and lower GI diagnostic endoscopy, the patient is placed in left lateral recumbency. With insufflation, air will rise to fill the antrum and right colon, allowing visualization and intubation of the pylorus and ileo-colic valve, respectively. Air is usually used for all insufflation, but warm saline in the intestine is preferred by some endoscopists, claiming it improves visualization (Galiazzo et al. 2020).

Right lateral recumbency is only used when placing percutaneous endoscopic gastrostomy (PEG) tubes, sometimes when trying to retrieve a gastric FB initially near the cardia, or when resecting a mass in the left colon.

ENDOSCOPIC TECHNIQUE

The endoscope can be steered by manipulating the steering wheels, torquing the insertion tube on its long axis and by inserting/withdrawing it. Written descriptions of how to steer are of little value, and proficiency only comes from repeated practice and understanding the principle that the center of the image on the monitor is the direction in which the endoscope tip will move when advanced. Thus, to steer, one should adjust the image position to where one wants to go rather than thinking about which way one should turn the steering wheels. To pass through a sphincter, it is necessary to continually readjust the image position so that the sphincter is in the center of the screen because advancement of the endoscope can distort the viscus and move the sphincter away from this position.

Insufflation is necessary to be able to visualize the GI mucosa, because red-out (loss of vision) occurs if the endoscope tip is too close to the mucosa. However, overinflation of the stomach should be avoided as it makes pyloric intubation more difficult and can compromise the patient's cardiorespiratory function by compressing the caudal vena cava and splinting the diaphragm.

BIOPSY TECHNIQUE

To maximize the diagnostic yield from GI endoscopy, biopsies should always be obtained unless a FB is the cause of GI signs. This rule applies even if the mucosa looks grossly normal, as discordance between one's subjective interpretation of the gross appearance and the histopathology is recognized. Furthermore, the development of HD quality imaging and the ability to see individual intestinal villi has required reappraisal of the assessment of the significance of the irregularity of the small intestinal mucosa. The only region where biopsies are not routinely collected is the esophagus. The normal esophageal mucosa is too tough to be able to obtain diagnostic biopsies routinely and a diagnosis of esophagitis is usually based on the gross appearance. Esophageal biopsies are only attempted if dysplasia or neoplasia is suspected, but then the tissue will be more amenable to biopsy.

RECORDING

The procedure can be recorded digitally on a DVD recorder, a USB stick, or with dedicated software, and this is recommended both for medico-legal purposes and for patient follow-up. Simple recording forms for upper and lower GI endoscopy are available from the WSAVA website (GI Endoscopy Report Forms).

UPPER GI ENDOSCOPY

In most cases, the upper GI endoscopy procedure involves esophago-gastro-duodenoscopy, with proximal jejunoscopy potentially achieved in cats and small dogs depending on the length of the insertion tube. Examination of the whole upper GI tract and biopsy (except in the esophagus) is indicated in patients with vomiting and diarrhea, but there can sometimes be specific indications for focusing on just one region.

ESOPHAGOSCOPY

Indications

Examination of the esophagus is indicated in patients with signs of regurgitation or reflux (gulping, lip-smacking) or when there is radiographic evidence of an esophageal lesion. However, caution is required if megaesophagus (ME) is suspected, as there is a risk of inhalation on anesthesia induction because retained fluid may be inhaled before endotracheal intubation can be achieved; the head should be held up until after intubation.

Method

After passing the endoscope tip through the upper esophageal sphincter, often achieved blindly as the sphincter is normally closed, insufflation of the esophagus enables visualization. Having examined the body of the esophagus, time is spent observing the lower esophageal sphincter (LES) for signs of a sliding hiatal hernia. Biopsies of the esophagus are not routinely collected.

Normal Findings

The esophagus should contain no solid material nor large volumes of liquid, although a small amount of saliva or refluxed bile is not abnormal. A healthy mucosa is normally pale pink, but areas of pigmentation are seen in those dog breeds with pigmented tongues. Indentation by the trachea to the level of the heart base and the heart and great vessels of the thorax pulsating against the wall should be visible. Distal circumferential folds and submucosal vessels are only seen in cats. The LES is usually closed but, if open, a sharp demarcation between the oesophageal and darker gastric mucosa should be seen.

Abnormal Findings

Esophagoscopy can reveal a number of pathologies affecting the lumen and mucosa listed in Table 35.1.

Table 35.1 Endoscopic Diagnoses of Esophageal Diseases

Diagnosis	Findings
Megaesophagus	• Massive dilation • Thin wall and prominent submucosal vessels • ± Retained food and liquid
Esophagitis	• Reddening or ulceration of the mucosa • Location near the lower esophageal sphincter (LES) suggests spontaneous reflux esophagitis
Hiatal hernia	• Cranial bulging of the LES • “Crease” around the LES • Esophagitis
Gastro-esophageal intussusception	• Protrusion of rugal folds through the LES
Diverticulum	• Outpocketing of esophageal wall • Debris accumulated in the diverticulum • Diverticulum wall may have abnormal mucosal appearance
Neoplasia	• Rounded mass in distal esophagus of dogs due to a leiomyoma/sarcoma • Ulcerated mass in older cats due to squamous cell carcinoma
Granuloma (*Spirocerca lupi*)	• Masses with the mucosa • Motile worms may be seen
Foreign body[a]	• Bones, chews, fishhooks most common in dogs • Needle and thread more common in cats
Stricture[a]	• Narrowing of the esophageal lumen • Esophagitis proximally

[a]Findings that can be treated endoscopically.

Endoscopic assessment of ME is not recommended once a radiographic diagnosis has been made, not only because of the high risk of inhalation, but also because the normal esophagus is flaccid under anesthesia and its dilation by excessive insufflation can mimic ME. The presence of food and/or large volumes of liquid are very suggestive of ME, but if the esophagus is empty, a thin mucosa, as evidenced by prominent submucosal vessels, also supports the diagnosis as in this German shepherd (Video 35.1) with the LES being closed.

The presence of a sliding hiatal hernia may be suggested by evidence of distal esophagitis and a characteristic "crease" around the LES (Figures 35.1a, b). The hernia may bulge cranially with inspiration but often will not manifest once the patent is intubated, as herniation is normally provoked by increase negative intrathoracic pressure associated with upper airway obstruction in brachycephalic dogs and patients with laryngeal paralysis, and this is abolished by intubation. Herniation can be elicited either by abdominal compression often leading to opening of the LES and consequent reflux (Video 35.2) or by occluding the endotracheal tube for three spontaneous breaths whilst observing the LES endoscopically (Broux et al. 2018).

Esophagitis is diagnosed by the gross appearance of reddened mucosa (Figure 35.1c) and/or ulceration with bleeding in severe cases (Figure 35.1d), without the need for biopsy. Obstruction of the esophagus by strictures and FBs (Figure 35.1e) are easily recognized and can be managed endoscopically. Extra-luminal causes of a narrowed esophagus, such as vascular ring anomalies or mediastinal masses, may be observed, but ultimately the diagnosis will depend on other imaging modalities.

Neoplasia of the esophagus is rare with leiomyoma/sarcoma in dogs (Figure 35.1f) and squamous cell carcinoma in cats being the most common; adenocarcinomas are extremely rare. A diverticulum is also rare, whilst granulomas caused by the parasite *Spirocerca lupi* are only seen in dogs in regions such as Mediterranean countries, southern Africa, and southern USA.

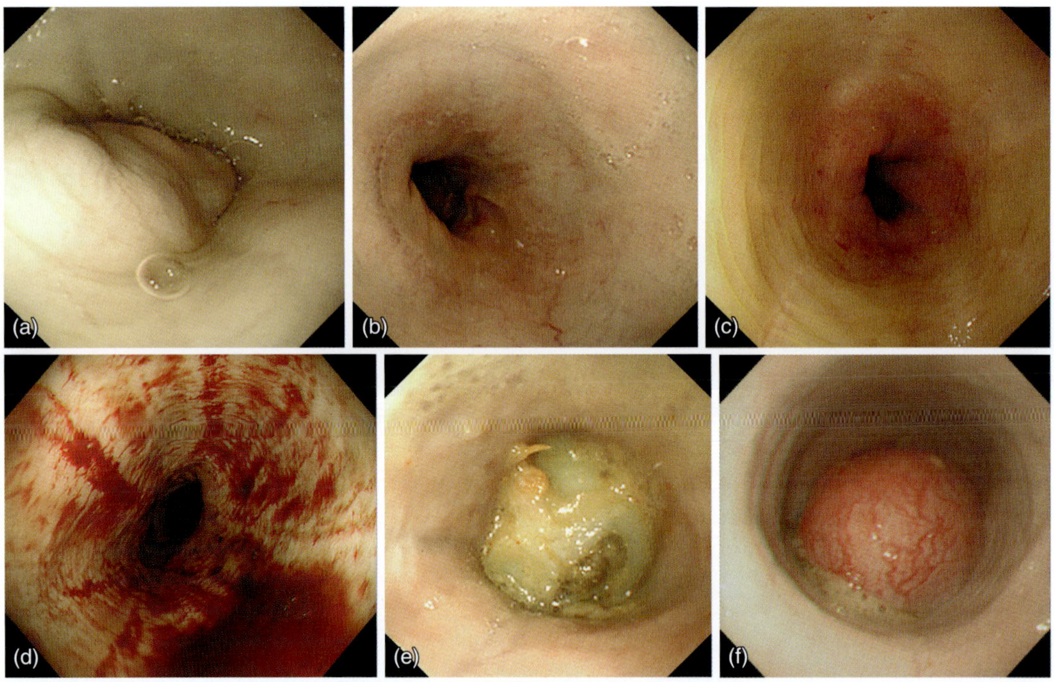

FIGURE 35.1 Endoscopic images of esophageal lesions. (a) Bulging of a hiatal hernia in a French bulldog with chronic diarrhea during temporary occlusion of the endotracheal tube. However, there is no evidence of esophagitis. (b) Spontaneous opening of the lower esophageal sphincter and associated reflux esophagitis due to a hiatal hernia in a Boston terrier. (c) Reflux esophagitis in a cat with a suspected hiatal hernia. Note the normal, circumferential, mucosal folds seen in cats. (d) Severe esophagitis in a cat following ingestion of a caustic liquid. (e) Bone esophageal foreign body. (f) Leiomyoma in the distal esophagus of a dog

GASTROSCOPY

Indications

Specific endoscopic examination of the stomach is indicated in animals with chronic vomiting, significant hematemesis, and for gastric FB removal. However, the stomach is also examined and biopsied when investigating intestinal disease, as there may be gastritis as part of a chronic inflammatory enteropathy.

Method

The entrance of the gastroscope to the stomach through the LES is at an oblique angle but once through, the tip is pointing at the rugal folds on greater curvature at the junction of the fundus and body. Insufflation and then deflection of the tip allow a view along the body, following roughly parallel rugal folds toward the antrum, where the folds flatten out (Figure 35.2a). At this point, it is usual to advance into the antrum to achieve pyloric intubation unless a diagnosis, such as a gastric FB, has been made. After examination and biopsy of the small intestine, the gastroscope is withdrawn to enable complete examination and biopsy of the stomach.

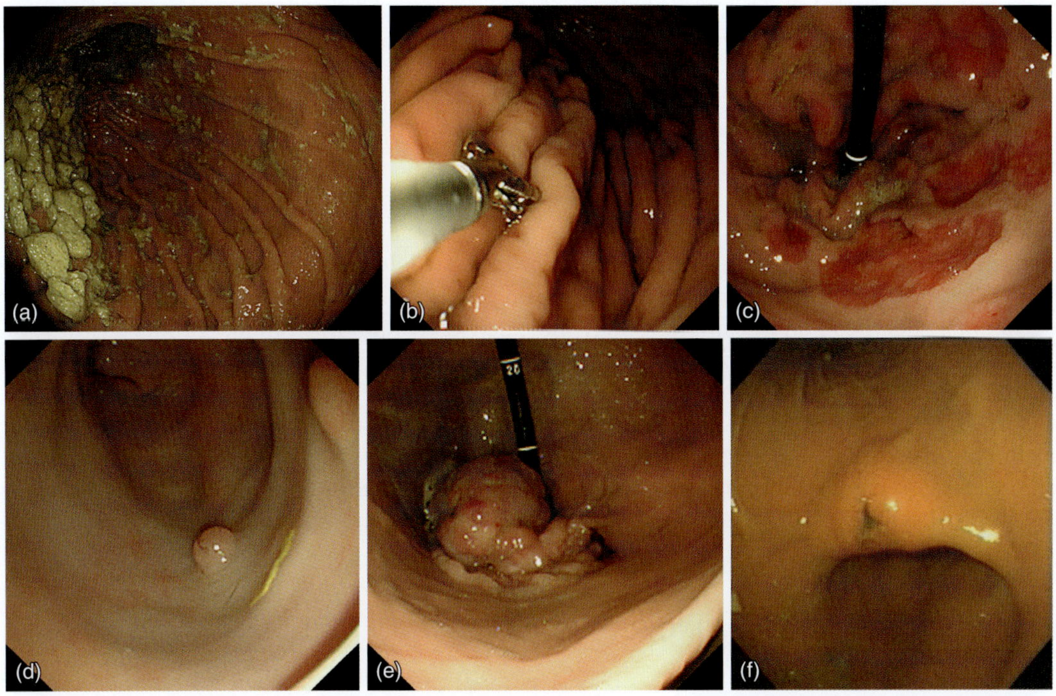

FIGURE 35.2 Endoscopic images of gastric lesions. (a) Gastroscopic image showing retained food in the stomach of a dog with intestinal malabsorption causing delayed gastric emptying. Note the normal parallel rugal folds running along the greater curvature toward the antrum. (b) Endoscopic biopsy of the stomach of dog with moderate lymphoplasmacytic gastritis. Although the rugal folds run parallel as normal, there is a subtle irregularity in the mucosal surface, although biopsies were needed to confirm the diagnosis. (c) Retroflexed gastroscopic view of the cardia, showing severe ulceration associated with eosinophilic gastritis. (d) Gastroscopic view of a small benign polyp in the antrum of an old dog with chronic diarrhea. Such lesions are of no clinical significance. (e) Retroflexed gastroscopic view of the cardia and fundus of a dog showing a large irregular mass shown by excisional biopsy to be a leiomyosarcoma. (f) Gastroscopic view of an ulcerated mass on the angle of the lesser curvature in an 8-year-old Rough collie. The signalment, its gross appearance, and site were very suggestive of a gastric carcinoma. Although it appeared to be a circumscribed lesion, CT imaging revealed diffuse spread throughout the lesser curvature of the stomach and to gastric lymph nodes

Retroflexion of the endoscope allows observation of the angle of the lesser curvature, with the endoscope entering through the LES and the fundus and cardia visible above it, and the antrum and pylorus below. As mentioned previously, some insufflation is necessary but overinflation should be avoided. However, toward the end of the procedure full insufflation to flatten rugal folds should be performed to ensure no lesions between rugae have been missed Biopsies are always taken as there may be microscopic pathology: 10–15 samples are either collected randomly from various regions or more systematically (Candido et al. 2022). Specific lesions should be biopsied, and samples submitted separately.

Normal Findings

The stomach should be empty after withholding food for 8–12 hours although a small amount of fluid or bile may be present. The rugal folds should flatten on insufflation and re-form on deflation. The normal mucosa is dark pink, glistening, and smooth. Dark spots indicating lymphoid follicles, usually associated with *Helicobacter* infection, may be seen but may not be clinically significant.

Diagnostic Findings

The presence of food in the stomach after adequate patient preparation indicates delayed gastric emptying (Figure 35.2a). This may be caused by an outflow obstruction, gastric inflammation, ulceration, or neoplasia but can also be due to intestinal malabsorption inhibiting gastric emptying.

Nonerosive gastritis may cause subtle irregularities in the mucosal surface and excessive mucus but is sometimes only detected by biopsy (Figure 35.2b). The presence of large numbers of lymphoid follicles may be indicative of follicular gastritis although the role of *Helicobacter* remains controversial.

Finding fresh or changed blood in the gastric lumen should prompt full examination of the stomach to look for a sharp or abrasive FB and for ulcers (Figure 35.2c), assuming coagulopathies and swallowed blood have been ruled out. After ruling out non-GI causes of ulceration, such as mast cell tumors, superficial and deep ulcers may indicate NSAID administration, chronic gastritis, or neoplasia. Fibrosis associated with chronic gastritis or carcinoma may make the stomach wall rigid and prevent adequate insufflation.

In old dogs, benign antral polyps are common and are rarely clinically significant (Figure 35.2d). Smooth muscle tumors may be pedunculated but can be sessile and can ulcerate (Figure 35.2e). Gastric carcinomas in dogs typically arise along the angle of the lesser curvature and are ulcerated as shown in Figure 35.2f and Video 35.3, whereas smooth muscle tumors are found in other areas. Gastric lymphoma must be confirmed by biopsy.

DUODENOSCOPY (AND JEJUNOSCOPY)

Indications

Making a diagnosis in cases of chronic diarrhea has historically relied on histological examination of surgical biopsies. However, as endoscopic biopsy is relatively safe, milder cases often undergo the procedure now, although the vast majority of canine patients have inflammatory disease (Volkmann et al. 2017). Yet biopsies do not necessarily indicate the cause of any inflammation, and clinicians now rely on the response to treatment trials (Dupouy-Manescau et al. 2024). As food-responsive enteropathy appears to represent approximately two-thirds of all chronic enteropathies in dogs, it makes sense to perform adequate diet trials before performing endoscopy in most cases. Intestinal biopsies first are indicated in patients with anorexia, profound weight loss, significant GI bleeding, protein-losing enteropathy, or imaging abnormalities within reach of the endoscope. Biopsies are also needed when investigating chronic vomiting, as this may be the only sign of intestinal disease, especially in cats. Also in older cats, biopsies are required to distinguish small cell lymphoma from lymphoplasmacytic enteritis, although it can be argued that biopsies make no difference to the treatment or outcome.

Method

After a quick inspection of the stomach to enable orientation and prevent misinterpretation of any artefacts seen after duodenal intubation, pyloric intubation should be performed. Overinflation of the stomach should be avoided as it displaces the pylorus by bending the stomach into a U-shape and also stimulates peristalsis. It should be possible to reach the distal duodenal flexure in most patients and the proximal jejunum in cats and small dogs.

Normal Findings

Depending on the image quality of the endoscopy system, the normal mucosa may appear smooth or villous. The major duodenal papilla is visible in dogs and cats, and a minor papilla is seen in some dogs (Figure 35.3a). Peyer's patches are whitish depressions on the antimesenteric duodenal wall seen only in dogs. Roundworms are incidental findings.

Diagnostic Findings

The most common finding is irregularity of the mucosa, sometimes with ulceration and spontaneous bleeding (Figures 35.3b, c). Fat-filled lacteals are consistent with lymphangiectasia (Figure 35.3d), Biopsies are required to distinguish inflammation from lymphoma (Figures 35.3e, f). Solid neoplasms are rare, but occasionally *Uncinaria* hookworms, appearing as small white worms embedded in the intestinal mucosa are seen (Video 35.4), although infection should have been diagnosed by fecal examination.

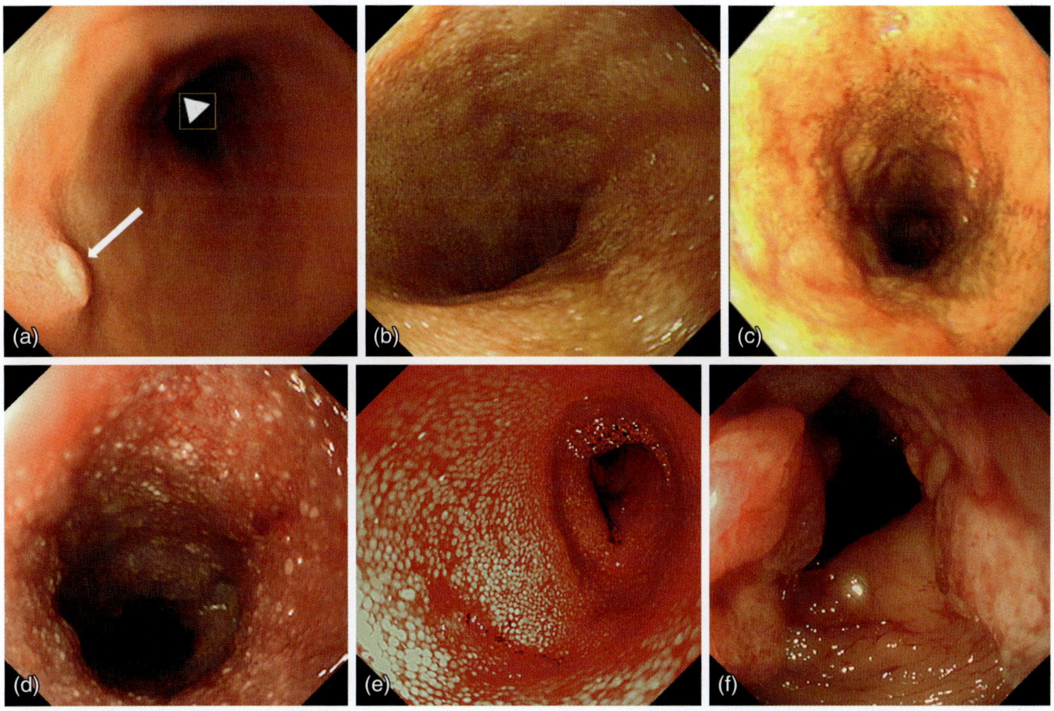

FIGURE 35.3 Endoscopic images of duodenal lesions. (a) Grossly normal duodenal mucosa with major (arrow) and minor (arrowhead) duodenal papillae visible. Despite the gross appearance, biopsies confirmed moderate lymphoplasmacytic enteritis. (b) Irregular duodenal mucosa in a German shepherd due to lymphoplasmacytic enteritis confirmed by biopsy. (c). Irregular duodenal mucosa in a Labrador due to eosinophilic enteritis confirmed by biopsy. (d) Duodenum of a Border collie with a protein-losing enteropathy. The white spots are fat-filled lacteals consistent with a diagnosis of lymphangiectasia. (e) Small cell lymphoma in an old cat. The blood is from biopsy sites but helps highlight the irregularity of the mucosa. (f) Large cell lymphoma in the duodenum of an English pointer

LOWER GI ENDOSCOPY

Examination of the whole large intestine may be a stand-alone procedure, but in chronic enteropathies, it often follows upper GI endoscopy, especially if ileal biopsies are desired. The combined examinations are termed "top-and-tail" procedures.

RECTO-COLONOSCOPY

Indications

Examination of just the large intestine is indicated if there is significant hematochezia, and a focal lesion is suspected. Stand-alone cases of chronic colitis are unusual, and top-and-tail procedures are generally indicated in chronic diarrhea. The exception is when granulomatous (histiocytic ulcerative) colitis of young Boxers and French bulldogs is suspected. Severe ulceration and bleeding restricted to the colon is seen (Video 35.5). However, colonic biopsies are required for both histological confirmation and culture/sensitivity before antimicrobial treatment (Video 35.5).

Method

Patient preparation with oral lavage and/or enemas is crucial in achieving a successful procedure, which requires the ileo-ceco-colic region to be reached. Steering around flexures is by tip deflection and torquing the insertion tube, although, as the tip passes, it may cause artefactual damage to the outer radius, which must then be recognized as artefact as the endoscope is withdrawn. Significant complications are rare (Leib et al. 2004).

Normal Findings

A healthy colonic mucosa is smooth and glistening with a small amount of mucus. Lymphoid follicles are seen in the canine rectum and submucosal vessels should be visible in the colon as the wall is thinner than in the small intestine (Figures 35.4a, b). Any residual liquid must be aspirated but can cause suction marks (red spots) in the mucosa (Figure 35.4c).

Diagnostic Findings

Obscuration of submucosal vessels suggests mucosal thickening, and diffusely irregular and/or ulcerated mucosa likely indicate colitis (Figure 35.4d), although biopsies are necessary to rule out the rarer colo-rectal lymphoma. Focal bleeding lesions are most often found in the left descending colon and rectum, with polyps and adenocarcinomas often within reach of digital rectal examination (Figure 35.4e). Cecal inversion (ceco-colic intussusception) and angiodysplasia are rare causes of focal bleeding. Finding *Trichuris* whipworms, usually in the cecum, is a failure to adequately investigate before endoscopy.

ILEOSCOPY

Indications

There is evidence in dogs with chronic enteropathies that ileal biopsies are more likely to yield a diagnosis (Casamian-Sorrosal et al. 2010; Caulfield et al. 2021). In cats, ileal biopsies are more sensitive for finding lymphoma than upper GI biopsies (Scott et al. 2011). Therefore, ileoscopy as part of a top-and-tail procedure is optimal in chronic enteropathies. However, ileal intubation is technically difficult and potentially risks perforation, especially in cats (Woolhead et al. 2020).

Method

In some patients it may be possible to simply steer the endoscope through the button-like ileo-colic valve. When this fails, biopsy forceps passed through the valve can act as a guide for the endoscope to follow. A couple of blind biopsies may be obtained if intubation fails (Figure 35.4f).

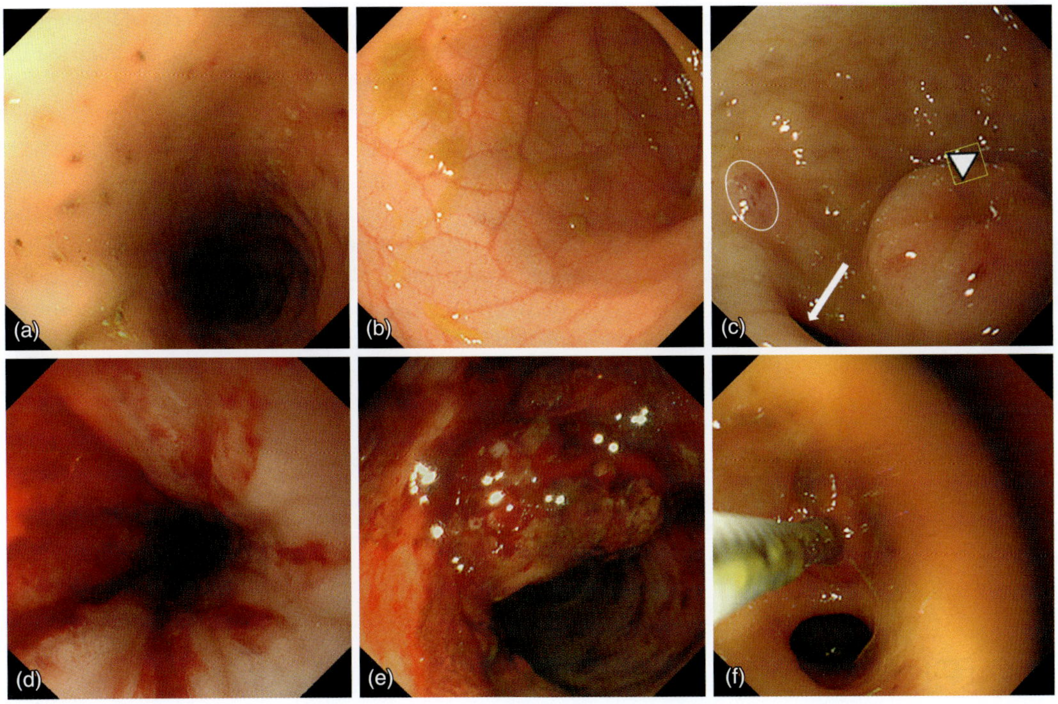

FIGURE 35.4 Endoscopic images of the canine large intestine. (a) Endoscopic image of normal rectal mucosa. The dark spots are lymphoid follicles. (b) Endoscopic image of normal colonic mucosa. Submucosal vessels are visible, which is considered normal. (c) Endoscopic image of the ileo-ceco-colic region. The ceco-colic orifice (arrow) and button-like ileocolic valve (arrowhead). There is evidence of some trauma whilst trying to intubate the ileum and a suction mark (circle). (d) Thickened and ulcerated mucosa with spontaneous hemorrhage in a dog with lymphoplasmacytic colitis. (e) Ulcerated mass in the distal left colon in a dog with dyschezia and hematochezia and confirmed as an adenocarcinoma by biopsy. (f) Passage of endoscopic forceps through the ileo-colic valve of a dog to obtain blind biopsies. The ceco-colic opening is seen below the ileo-colic valve

Normal Findings

The ileal mucosa appears grossly similar to the upper jejunum, except that lymphoid follicles may be obvious. The mucosa is thinner and bleeds more after biopsy.

Diagnostic Findings

Mucosal irregularity and ulceration are suggestive of inflammatory disease.

THERAPEUTIC ENDOSCOPIC TECHNIQUES

FB RETRIEVAL

This is the most common therapeutic endoscopic technique (Binvel et al. 2018; Dollo et al. 2020; Gianella et al. 2009; Smit et al. 2018). A range of grasping instruments that can be inserted down the working channel is available. However, for FBs wedged in the esophagus, using long rigid forceps under guidance from a flexible endoscope is often more successful. Gastric FBs may fall toward the cardia and become difficult to grasp with the patient in left lateral recumbency. Rolling the patient to the right lateral can aid retrieval. Sharp FBs such as cocktail, kebab sticks, and fishhooks can be difficult to find if they have been swallowed with food or fishing bait. One can wait for the food to empty but there is a risk of perforation. Using a peristaltic flushing pump allows visualization by washing the food away. Techniques for retrieving golf balls using a plastic bottle liner and ferrous FBs with a magnet have been published (Skinner et al. 2024; Le Boedec et al. 2024). However, larger gastric FBs may not be retrievable endoscopically even though the patient managed to swallow them.

ESOPHAGEAL STRICTURE DILATION

Strictures can be dilated by balloons or bougies, ranging from 2 to 4 cm diameter depending on the patient's size, ideally used under endoscopic guidance (Bissett et al. 2009; Da Riz et al. 2021; Sami et al. 2018). The procedure may need to be repeated many times, although four quadrant injections of triamcinolone into the stricture before it is dilated may reduce the risk of recurrence (Fraune et al. 2009; Ricart et al. 2022).

ENDOSCOPIC MUCOSAL RESECTION

Polypoid masses can be removed endoscopically using hot biopsy forceps or snares with diathermy. Sessile masses can also be removed with snares and electrosurgery, having first raised the mass up by injecting sterile saline into the submucosa with an endoscopic injector needle (Coleman et al. 2014). Insufflation with CO_2 is recommended because of the risk of explosion of intestinal gases when using electrosurgery.

PEG FEEDING TUBES

Although largely superseded by esophagostomy tubes as the main route for assisted enteral feeding, PEG tubes allow feeding directly into the stomach when a diseased esophagus needs to be bypassed. The endoscope is used to insufflate the stomach to identify the site of the percutaneous needle entry and to grasp the wire or thread fed into the stomach via the needle and pull it out through the mouth (McCrackin et al. 1993).

REFERENCES

Albors, O.L., Rojo, D., Sarriá, R. et al. (2011). Morphometry of the canine intestine with reference to the use of double balloon endoscopy. *Veterinary Journal* 190: 113–118. https://doi.org/10.1016/j.tvjl.2010.08.017

Binvel, M., Poujol, L., Peyron, C. et al. (2018). Endoscopic and surgical removal of oesophageal and gastric fish-hook foreign bodies in 33 animals. *Journal of Small Animal Practice* 59: 45–49. https://doi.org/10.1111/jsap.12794

Bissett, S.A., Davis, J., Subler, K. et al. (2009). Risk factors and outcome of bougienage for treatment of benign esophageal strictures in dogs and cats: 28 cases (1995–2004). *Journal of the American Veterinary Medical Association* 235: 844–850. https://doi.org/10.2460/javma.235.7.844

Broux, O., Clercx, C., Etienne, A.L. et al. (2018). Effects of manipulations to detect sliding hiatal hernia in dogs with brachycephalic airway obstructive syndrome. *Veterinary Surgery* 47: 243–251. https://doi.org/10.1111/vsu.12735

Candido, M.V., Syrjä, P., Kilpinen, S. et al. (2022). Can chromoendoscopy improve the early diagnosis of gastric carcinoma in dogs? *Animals* 12: 19. https://doi.org/10.3390/ani12172253

Casamian-Sorrosal, D., Willard, M.D., Murray, J.K. et al. (2010). Comparison of histopathologic findings in biopsies from the duodenum and ileum of dogs with enteropathy. *Journal of Veterinary Internal Medicine* 24: 80–83. https://doi.org/10.1111/j.1939-1676.2009.0427.x

Caulfield, S., Priestnall, S.L., and Kathrani, A. (2021). Concordance of the histopathologic diagnosis of concurrent duodenal and ileal biopsy specimens in dogs. *Animals* 11: 13. https://doi.org/10.3390/ani11102938

Coleman, K.A., Berent, A.C., and Weisse, C.W. (2014). Endoscopic mucosal resection and snare polypectomy for treatment of a colorectal polypoid adenoma in a dog. *Javma-Journal of the American Veterinary Medical Association* 244: 1435–1440. https://doi.org/10.2460/javma.244.12.1435

Da Riz, F., Béguin, J., Manassero, M. et al. (2021). Outcome of dogs and cats with benign oesophageal strictures after balloon dilatation or stenting: 27 cases (2002-2019). *Journal of Small Animal Practice* 62: 886–894. https://doi.org/10.1111/jsap.13392

Danesh, B.J.Z., Burke, M., Newman, J. et al. (1985). Comparison of weight, depth, and diagnostic adequacy of specimens obtained with 16 different biopsy forceps designed for upper gastrointestinal endoscopy. *Gut* 26: 227–231.

Daugherty, M.A., Leib, M.S., Rossmeisl, J.H. et al. (2008). Safety and efficacy of oral low-volume sodium phosphate bowel preparation for colonoscopy in dogs.

Journal of Veterinary Internal Medicine 22: 31–36. https://doi.org/10.1111/j.1939-1676.2007.0025.x

Dollo, V., Chambers, G., and Carothers, M. (2020). Endoscopic retrieval of gastric and oesophageal foreign bodies in 52 cats. *Journal of Small Animal Practice* 61: 51–56. https://doi.org/10.1111/jsap.13074

Dupouy-Manescau, N., Méric, T., Sénécat, O. et al. (2024). Updating the classification of chronic inflammatory enteropathies in dogs. *Animals* 14: 17. https://doi.org/10.3390/ani14050681

Fraune, C., Gaschen, F., and Ryan, K. (2009). Intralesional corticosteroid injection in addition to endoscopic balloon dilation in a dog with benign oesophageal strictures. *Journal of Small Animal Practice* 50: 550–553. https://doi.org/10.1111/j.1748-5827.2009.00785.x

Galiazzo, G., Costantino, F., Foglia, A. et al. (2020). Water immersion vs. air insufflation in canine duodenal endoscopy: is the future underwater? *Polish Journal of Veterinary Sciences* 23: 581–588. https://doi.org/10.24425/pjvs.2020.135804

Gaspardo, A., Sabetti, M.C., Zanoni, R.G. et al. (2020). Incidence of bacteremia consequent to different endoscopic procedures in dogs: a preliminary study. *Animals* 10: 9: https://doi.org/10.3390/ani10122265

GI Endoscopy Report Forms. https://wsava.org/global-guidelines/gastrointestinal-guidelines

Gianella, P., Pfammatter, N.S., and Burgener, I.A. (2009). Oesophageal and gastric endoscopic foreign body removal: complications and follow-up of 102 dogs. *Journal of Small Animal Practice* 50: 649–654. https://doi.org/10.1111/j.1748-5827.2009.00845.x

Goutal-Landry, C.M., Mansell, J., Ryan, K.A. et al. (2013). Effect of endoscopic forceps on quality of duodenal mucosal biopsy in healthy dogs. *Journal of Veterinary Internal Medicine* 27: 456–461. https://doi.org/10.1111/jvim.12085

Irom, S., Sherding, R., Johnson, S. et al. (2014). Gastrointestinal perforation associated with endoscopy in cats and dogs. *Journal of the American Animal Hospital Association* 50: 322–329. https://doi.org/10.5326/jaaha-ms-5727

Le Boedec, K., Flageollet, J., and Touzet, C. (2024). Endoscopic removal of gastric foreign bodies with a bottle liner in 12 dogs (2020-2023). *Journal of the American Animal Hospital Association* 60: 60–67. https://doi.org/10.5326/jaaha-ms-7394

Leib, M.S., Baechtel, M.S., and Monroe, W.E. (2004). Complications associated with 355 flexible colonoscopic procedures in dogs. *Journal of Veterinary Internal Medicine* 18: 642–646.

Mabry, K., Hill, T., Marks, S.L. et al. (2019). Use of video capsule endoscopy to identify gastrointestinal lesions in dogs with microcytosis or gastrointestinal hemorrhage. *Journal of Veterinary Internal Medicine* 33: 1964–1969. https://doi.org/10.1111/jvim.15584

Martin-Flores, M., Scrivani, P.V., Loew, E. et al. (2014). Maximal and submaximal mouth opening with mouth gags in cats: implications for maxillary artery blood flow. *Veterinary Journal* 200: 60–64. https://doi.org/10.1016/j.tvjl.2014.02.001

McCrackin, M.A., Denovo, R.C., Bright, R.M. et al. (1993). Endoscopic placement of a percutaneous gastroduodenostomy feeding tube in dogs. *Journal of the American Veterinary Medical Association* 203: 792–797.

McFadzean, W.J.M., Hall, E.J., and van Oostrom, H. (2017). Effect of premedication with butorphanol or methadone on ease of endoscopic duodenal intubation in dogs. *Veterinary Anaesthesia and Analgesia* 44: 1296–1302. https://doi.org/10.1016/j.vaa.2017.05.004

Ricart, M.C., Rodriguez, S., and Dova, G. (2022). Intralesional steroid injection after endoluminal esophageal stricture dilatation in a cat. *Open Veterinary Journal* 12: 192–196. https://doi.org/10.5455/OVJ.2022.v12.i2.6

Sami, S.S. Haboubi, H.N., Ang, Y. et al. (2018). UK guidelines on oesophageal dilatation in clinical practice. *Gut* 67: 1000–1023. https://doi.org/10.1136/gutjnl-2017-315414

Scott, K.D., Zoran, D.L., Mansell, J. et al. (2011). Utility of endoscopic biopsies of the duodenum and ileum for diagnosis of inflammatory bowel disease and small cell lymphoma in cats. *Journal of Veterinary Internal Medicine* 25: 1253–1257. https://doi.org/10.1111/j.1939-1676.2011.00831.x

Skinner, S.M., Gilor, C., Berg, A.S. et al. (2024). Magnet-assisted endoscopic removal of ferromagnetic metallic gastric foreign bodies in 4 dogs. *Journal of Veterinary Internal Medicine* 38: 2348–2352. https://doi.org/10.1111/jvim.17105

Smit, I., Crnogaj, M., Brkljačić, M. et al. (2018). Endoscopic removal of esophageal and gastric foreign bodies in dogs: the prevalence, risk factors and efficacy of removal. *Veterinarski Arhiv* 88: 481–496. https://doi.org/10.24099/vet.arhiv.0039

St-Jean, C., Collier, A., Zur Linden, A. et al. (2025). Feasibility and complications of videocapsule endoscopy in dogs weighing 7 kg or less. *Journal of Veterinary Internal Medicine* 39: 7. https://doi.org/10.1111/jvim.17286

Volkmann, M. Steiner, J.M., Fosgate, G.T. et al. (2017). Chronic diarrhea in dogs - retrospective study in 136 cases. *Journal of Veterinary Internal Medicine* 31: 1043–1055. https://doi.org/10.1111/jvim.14739

Woolhead, V.L., Whittemore, J.C., and Stewart, S.A. (2020). Multicenter retrospective evaluation of ileocecocolic perforations associated with diagnostic lower gastrointestinal endoscopy in dogs and cats. *Journal of Veterinary Internal Medicine* 34: 684–690. https://doi.org/10.1111/jvim.15731

CHAPTER 36

Cytology and Histopathology of the Gastrointestinal Tract (Dogs and Cats)

Simon L. Priestnall and Alejandro Suárez-Bonnet

Department of Pathobiology and Population Sciences, Royal Veterinary College, London, United Kingdom

KEY POINTS

- Biopsy sample quality and quantity can greatly affect the ability to reach a histopathologic diagnosis.
- Microscopic standards for reporting endoscopic biopsies can ensure all morphological and inflammatory parameters are assessed in a uniform manner between pathologists.
- Routine hematoxylin and eosin staining is sufficient to achieve a diagnosis in the vast majority of samples with ancillary tests, such as special histochemical stains or immunohistochemistry, available to confirm or refine a diagnosis.

INTRODUCTION

The majority of the gastrointestinal (GI) tract is a mucosal surface and as such has a resident population of leukocytes, principally lymphocytes and plasma cells. Numbers and distribution of these cells vary with location, age (and possibly breed), immune status, concurrent medication, and even diet. When assessing inflammatory lesions in the GI tract, an awareness of what is considered "normal" is required. This has been helped by published standards for histopathologic scoring of inflammatory and morphological changes on endoscopically obtained GI biopsies in dogs and cats (Day et al. 2008).

Lesions affecting the GI tract typically have morphologic changes, e.g., villous necrosis or atrophy, erosion/ulceration, lacteal ectasia, or inflammatory changes, e.g., infiltrates of neutrophils, eosinophils, or both. This chapter will review disease processes affecting the various microscopic/histological components of the GI tract with examples.

SAMPLE QUALITY

Perhaps more than in any other organ or tissue, the quality and quantity of samples, particularly for histopathology, can significantly affect the ability to reach a successful diagnosis (Jergens et al. 2016). The majority of biopsies are taken endoscopically, which somewhat limits access and visibility, especially in the distal small intestine. Careful handling of samples to avoid crushing, which can cause artifacts, is essential, and indeed as little handling as possible is usually preferred, both during sample collection and laboratory processing. Many lesions are either focal, multifocal, or even segmental/regional, and so the greater number of samples, the greater chance of including a diagnostically useful region. Many changes are not visible grossly, e.g., inflammatory or neoplastic infiltrates in the propria mucosa, and thus even in a grossly "normal" GI tract, at least 10 biopsies of each region should be obtained if possible. Providing the pathologist with clinically relevant history and especially the endoscopic appearance of the GI tract is very important and can help significantly to form and frame a useful comment with the microscopic diagnosis.

Disorders of the Liver, Exocrine Pancreas, and Gastrointestinal Tract in Dogs and Cats, First Edition. Edited by Harry Cridge et al. Published 2026 by John Wiley & Sons, Inc. Companion Website: www.wiley.com/go/cridge/disorders

CYTOLOGY

Fine-needle aspiration (FNA) of the intestinal wall or GI masses under ultrasound guidance has been compared with histopathology (considered the gold standard), with 58% cases in agreement (Henry et al. 2004). This was higher for mass lesions or when sampling of enlarged mesenteric lymph nodes. Challenges to FNA techniques in the bowel are access (and risks of perforation), a thin bowel wall and the resident inflammatory cell population, which, without the context of architecture can be very hard to interpret, i.e., lymphocytes and plasma cells would be expected in the healthy mucosa but not only millimeters away in the submucosa. When comparing the diagnosis based on impression smears from GI masses with histology, there appears to be a much greater degree of agreement (94% in one study (Bonfanti et al. 2006)), presumably since the architectural position of the cells (and potentially improved cell morphological preservation) is maintained.

A study comparing diagnosis between endoscopically obtained cytology with histology samples found 81.4% agreement overall, but this increased to 98.6% when differentiating enteritis from GI lymphoma (Maeda et al. 2017).

MUCOSA

EPITHELIUM AND PROPRIA MUCOSA

Beyond the esophagus (which is lined by stratified squamous non-keratinizing epithelium), the remainder of the GI tract is lined by simple columnar epithelium up to the anus, where there is a transition back to stratified squamous epithelium. Villi are present throughout the small intestine, although they tend to become shorter and slightly broader more distally. Additionally, the proportion of mucus-secreting goblet cells relative to simple columnar epithelial cells is increased in the ileum versus the duodenum and then greatly increases further in the cecum and colon. In general, the epithelium has a large capacity for repair if damaged, and if the basement membrane is intact, e.g., erosion, then this can be complete. Damage to the basement membrane leads to ulceration, which is usually repaired by collagen (fibrosis/scarring), thus reducing functional capacity. Ulceration is most often seen in the stomach and proximal duodenum, e.g., due to NSAID overdose or foreign bodies. Histopathologically the lesions can vary in size and depth, although they usually have abundant fibrin, necrotic cellular debris, and neutrophilic inflammation within the region of ulcerated mucosa. The epithelium bordering ulcers can be highly thickened as repair and re-epithelialization are attempted. Ulceration is also a frequent presentation of gastric carcinoma, and care needs to be taken when examining gastric ulcers for evidence of neoplastic cells, which can be challenging at these highly reactive ulcer margins.

Viral infections, such as canine enteric coronavirus or rotavirus, can induce sometimes subtle changes in enterocytes, such as vacuolation and sloughing, although these are rarely sampled for histopathology, as lesions tend to be transient and purely functional, as the basement membrane is not damaged; thus, repair is by replacement of enterocytes from crypts. Bacterial infections, particularly Clostridial infections where toxins may be involved, tend to cause more damage, including to the basement membrane, and in these cases, there may be a thick layer of necrotic material, fibrin, and inflammatory cells overlying the mucosa in areas of ulceration (diphtheritic membrane).

Hyperplasia of both surface (and cryptal) epithelium is seen in polyps – these are nonneoplastic, reactive lesions that typically occur following focal injury or chronic irritation/inflammation. Most often encountered in the stomach, they can occur throughout the GI tract. Differentiation of polypoid lesions from epithelial tumors can be challenging when only endoscopically retrieved samples are available for histopathologic assessment. Polyps are typically composed of a hyperplastic epithelium overlying a core of fibrovascular connective tissue (propria mucosa), which is invariably infiltrated by increased lymphocytes and plasma cells. Polyps can often have an ulcerated surface and persistently bleed.

Chronic inflammatory lesions in the small intestine are often accompanied by villous atrophy. This is usually observed as reduced villous to crypt length, broadening of villi, and in more severe cases by fusion of adjacent villi. The cumulative effect is a reduced surface area for nutrient uptake and thus osmotic diarrhea. Increased deposition of collagen (fibrosis) is observed variably in the canine and feline GI tract, and although its origins are often obscure, it is believed to be due to the effects of chronic inflammation. More defined linear bands of collagen can occasionally be observed in the feline small intestinal mucosa and have been associated with a worse clinical outcome; the pathogenesis of their formation is unknown (Bandara et al. 2023).

CRYPTS AND GLANDS

The classic viral infection of dogs and cats primarily targeting crypts is that caused by either feline or canine parvovirus. These infections can even spare the villous/surface enterocytes but target the rapidly dividing cryptal epithelial cells. Cryptal necrosis and loss ultimately lead to loss of surface epithelium as it is not replaced (Figure 36.1). Occasionally small intranuclear inclusion bodies can be observed in cryptal epithelium early in the time course of infection. Parvoviruses also target the GI lymphoid tissue, e.g., Peyer's patches, causing lymphocytolysis (necrosis) and ultimately depletion.

Crypts can also become distended and filled with mucus and variable numbers of sloughed necrotic epithelial cells and neutrophils in various noninfectious inflammatory lesions such as chronic inflammatory enteropathies (e.g., dietary or antibiotic responsive) in both dogs and cats. These so-called "crypt abscesses" are a useful indicator that there may be an underlying inflammatory process, although a specific etiology is often elusive. An altered microbiome is one possibility, as is increased inflammation leading to physical distortion and altered drainage of crypts to the lumen.

In malignant epithelial neoplasms of the small and large intestine, the finding of small acini or nests of cells, resembling cryptal epithelium, deep to the mucosa is a hallmark finding in adenocarcinomas. These invasive nests of cells have breached the basement membrane and, in doing so, often induce a marked spindle-cell response (scirrhous response/desmoplasia). This latter desmoplasia can sometimes be so severe that it occupies a much greater percentage of a "mass" than the actual tumor cells and can result in narrowing of the lumen, especially in cats.

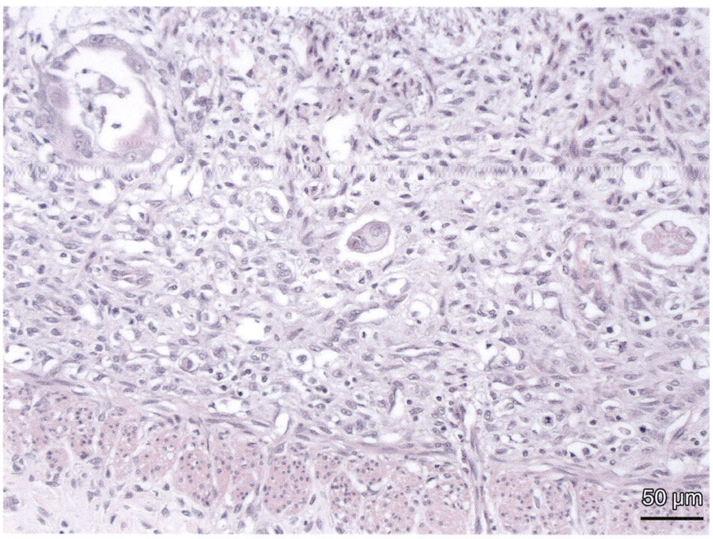

FIGURE 36.1 Parvoviral enteritis in a dog. The intestinal mucosa is effaced and necrotic with fusion and collapse of villi. Only occasional crypts remain supported by a fibrotic lamina propria that contains scant lymphocytes. Intestinal crypts are frequently lined by multinucleated and cytomegalic cells that are an attempt to restore the necrotic mucosa

In the stomach, carcinomas arising from the fundic glands can be very challenging to diagnose on endoscopically retrieved samples where invasion is almost impossible to assess. One exception is the so-called "signet cell" carcinoma, where large, round, discohesive glandular epithelial cells contain a large clear eccentric vacuole that peripheralizes the nucleus and can be recognized quite readily with adequate samples (Hardas et al. 2021).

LYMPHATIC VESSELS

Thin-walled lymphatic vessels can undergo only limited changes, which include dilation (ectasia) or rupture. Dilation (lymphangiectasia) can be primary in dogs with PLE or secondary to obstructed drainage, most often due to increased infiltrates of either inflammatory or, less often, neoplastic cells within the propria mucosa (Jablonski 2022). In dogs and cats, lymphangiectasia is a frequent feature of chronic enteropathies when large infiltrates of lymphocytes and plasma cells cause widespread dilation of the lymphatics within both the cores of villi and sometimes the deeper propria mucosa.

Rupture of lymphatic vessels leads to quite a marked inflammatory reaction, which usually involves an influx of macrophages (granulomatous) and is seen in cases where the lymphatic vessels are the primary target, e.g., lipogranulomatous lymphangitis. Inflammation specifically targets and usually obliterates the lymphatic vessel, both within the bowel wall and also within adjacent mesenteric lymphatic vessels.

BLOOD VESSELS

Specific targeting of either arteries (arteritis), veins (phlebitis), or both (vasculitis) is generally an unusual lesion in the GI tract of cats and dogs (compared with farmed species), with the one exception of feline infectious peritonitis. Mutated feline coronavirus (FCoV) characteristically causes inflammation around veins (periphlebitis), which can involve the wall of the vein itself, although it is not a true vasculitis (Tasker et al. 2023). The inflammation is typically very mixed, involving not only lymphocytes and plasma cells but also macrophages and neutrophils, which are unusual for a viral etiology, and fibrin (Figure 36.2). The histopathologic lesions in a cat with compatible

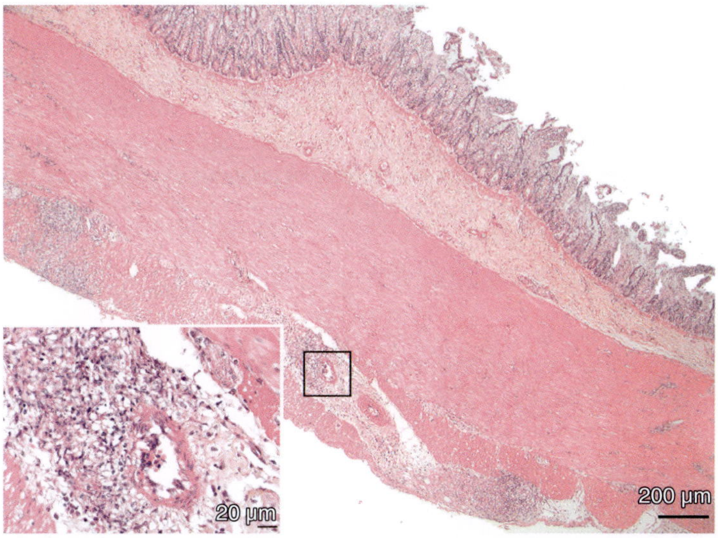

FIGURE 36.2 Feline infectious peritonitis (FIP). The walls of blood vessels within the tunica muscularis and serosa are expanded by dense inflammatory infiltrates. Inset: A higher magnification of the area within a box shows a necrotic blood vessel (artery) in which the wall is expanded by necrotic debris, lymphocytes, degenerate neutrophils, and macrophages that also expand the perivascular space

clinical/gross findings are almost pathognomonic, but immunohistochemical detection of FCoV within the regions of inflammation is the gold standard for diagnosis.

Vasculitis is also a feature of some bacterial, such as salmonellosis, and fungal (e.g., disseminated aspergillosis) infections. Targeting of blood vessels by vasculotropic pathogens results in focal thrombosis and ischemia, which can present as quite sharply defined regions of mucosal ulceration sometimes known as "button ulcers."

In processes in which segments of the intestine become mispositioned, e.g., volvulus, torsion, or intussusception, the primary lesion is vascular compromise due to compression. The pathogenesis of this usually begins with compression of the lymphatics since they have the thinnest walls; this leads to edema development and further compression of veins. Venous compression leads to congestion of the tissue and ultimately, unless corrected, the arterial flow is compromised, leading to tissue ischemia and/or infarction. This is often transmural, affecting all layers of the bowel from mucosa to serosa and may also involve mesentery. A devitalized bowel readily sloughs the mucosa, which can then lead to bacteremia/toxemia and/or potential rupture.

INFLAMMATORY CELLS

All levels of the GI tract have a resident population of inflammatory cells. These are predominantly lymphocytes (both T- and B-cells) and plasma cells with much fewer eosinophils. In the healthy cat or dog, the total number of cells varies along the GI tract, with the stomach containing the least and the ileum the most resident cells.

LYMPHOCYTES

The relative proportions of lymphocytes versus plasma cells can vary dramatically with an approximate ratio of 50 : 50 in the healthy animal and marked increases in plasma cells, particularly in cases of chronic inflammatory enteropathy due to either dietary or microbiome-responsive hypersensitivity. Lymphocytes are present both in the propria mucosa and within the surface enterocytes (intraepithelial). In general, these are a mixture of both CD3+ and CD8+ T-cells and B-cells. When lymphocytes are the predominant cell type, then consideration should always be given to GI lymphoma, which can be either T- or B-cell and large or small cell size (Marsilio et al. 2023). In cats small cell T-cell lymphoma is by far the most common subtype and in many cases exhibits very high levels of epitheliotropism (i.e., presence of lymphocytes within surface and cryptal enterocytes), which can be a helpful diagnostic feature. However, histopathologic diagnosis of early stage GI lymphoma can be very challenging and can often mean a tentative diagnosis based on H&E being supported by immunohistochemical labeling, e.g., CD3 (T-cell) and CD20 (B-cell) based on the predominant type (Figure 36.3). Even then an adequate number of well-oriented samples is essential for a reliable diagnosis. Alternatively, clonality testing (PCR for Antigen Receptor Rearrangements, PARR) of the infiltrate may be used to determine if the population is polyclonal (most likely inflammatory) or monoclonal (most likely neoplastic) (Waugh et al. 2016).

PLASMA CELLS

Plasma cell predominant inflammation in the small intestine (and often stomach and colon) is typical of a number of chronic enteropathies in both cats and dogs. Diet- and microbiome-responsive hypersensitivity can often manifest as plasmacytic (and/or eosinophilic) inflammation. Additional histopathologic characteristics include crypt abscesses, villous atrophy (shortening and fusion), and potentially proprial fibrosis in more chronic cases. In 2008, the first comprehensive grading system for both inflammatory and morphological changes observed in endoscopic GI tract biopsies was published by WSAVA. This series of "standards" provided a reference for pathologists when reporting severity of lesions. In subsequent years the standards have been updated and refined to include only those parameters where, when used in practice, pathologists broadly agreed and were correlated with measurable clinical disease severity or outcomes (Allenspach et al. 2019). Each measure,

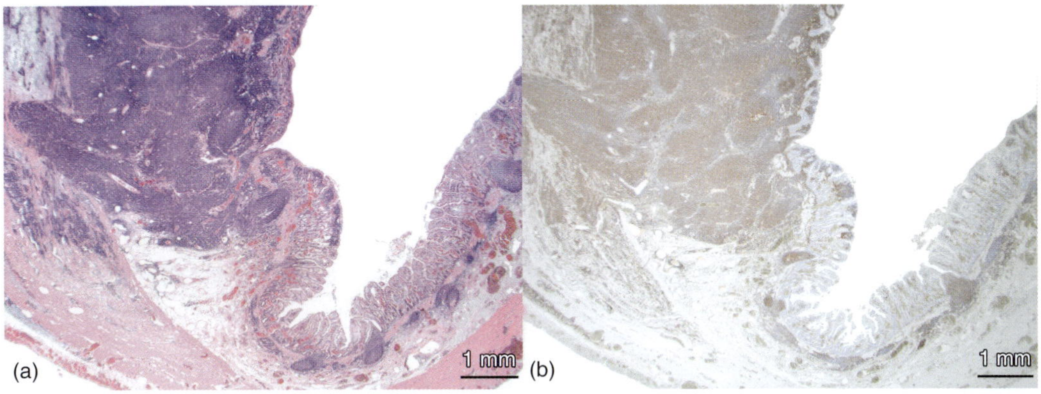

FIGURE 36.3 Intestinal lymphoma in a cat. (a) A lymphoma has expanded, effaced, and caused ulceration of a large segment of the jejunum. The lymphoma invades the submucosa and tunica muscularis. Adjacent villous profiles are blunted and the lamina propria expanded by oedema and increased numbers of lymphocytes. The lacteals within villi are dilated (lymphangiectasia). (b) A serial section immunolabelled with an anti-CD20 antibody identifies this neoplasm as a B-cell lymphoma

such as lamina propria lymphocytes and plasma cells, is scored from normal (zero) to three (marked infiltrate), and individual parameter scores are sometimes summed to give a total histopathologic score for a portion of the GI tract. Clearly with endoscopic biopsies these measures only apply to the mucosa and not deeper lesions. Provision of GI tract histopathological scores has now become a routine part of the histopathology report and can be used to assess or monitor lesion progression or response to treatment. However, thus far, evidence points to histopathological changes lagging behind clinical expression of GI disease and, in some cases, poorly correlating. As with any scoring system, there is scope for individual interpretation, but scores can be a useful research tool, e.g., for prospective studies comparing response to treatment between groups.

Plasma cell tumors are infrequently found in the GI tract, most often in the stomach, but can occur at any level. A hallmark histopathologic feature is the production of amyloid (AL) by the neoplastic plasma cells, which can become quite abundant in some lesions.

EOSINOPHILS

Low numbers of eosinophils are found at all levels of the GI tract but can increase in response to parasite infestations, e.g., roundworms (*Toxocara* spp.), hookworms (*Ancylostoma* spp.), and whipworms (*Trichuris* spp.), hypersensitivity, or in feline conditions such as feline eosinophilic sclerosing fibroplasia (Linton et al. 2015). Increased numbers of eosinophils can also be seen secondary to mast cell neoplasia, particularly in the stomach, and are attracted chemotactically in some T-cell lymphomas.

NEUTROPHILS

Neutrophils are considered abnormal at any level of the GI tract, although their presence is often possibly unspecific as to a cause. Clearly, infections, particularly bacterial will induce large numbers of neutrophils through the bowel wall, but also ulcerative or penetrating lesions involving bacteria secondarily.

MACROPHAGES/HISTIOCYTES

Macrophages/histiocytes are generally unusual in the GI tract of cats and dogs. In both species histiocytic/granulomatous (usually in conjunction with neutrophils, thus pyogranulomatous) inflammation is typical of fungal infections, especially *Histoplasma capsulatum*, which is found within the cytoplasm of macrophages. Other fungi, such as *Pythium insidiosum* and *Blastomyces dermatitidis*, can also cause lesions in the bowel of dogs (less often cats) and tend to be geographically restricted. Macrophages are also the predominant cell type with algal infections, e.g., *Prototheca* spp., which can be challenging to identify and often require the use of special histochemical stains such as Periodic Acid Schiff (PAS). The presence of abundant macrophages in the canine colon may suggest a specific condition such as granulomatous (histiocytic ulcerative) colitis in which the propria mucosa is filled and expanded by macrophages containing numerous PAS-positive granules, which are invariably enteroinvasive *Escherichia coli*. This same condition has also been described, rarely, in cats (Matsumoto et al. 2019).

TUNICA MUSCULARIS

The two muscle layers of the bowel are rarely the primary source of GI lesions, with one exception being intestinal leiomyositis, which is considered an autoimmune process involving lymphocytic destruction of the smooth muscle of the tunica muscularis (Zacuto et al. 2016). Typically, the effect of this, initially at least, is functional with lack of peristalsis, and thus it often presents as a pseudo-obstruction. Smooth muscle tumors can arise either from the thin layer of muscularis mucosa or, more often, the actual tunica. Leiomyomas are relatively frequent masses at all levels for the bowel and generally cause problems through physical obstruction. Leiomyosarcomas are less common, infiltrative/poorly demarcated, and potentially more likely to cause ulceration of the overlying mucosa. Smooth muscle tumors can be challenging to differentiate from tumors arising from components of the enteric nervous system, the interstitial cells of Cajal, which act as "pacemakers" for peristalsis and are found in both the submucosal and myenteric nerve plexi (see nervous tissue). Gastrointestinal stromal tumors (GISTs) most often arise from these cells and can be challenging to differentiate from smooth muscle tumors, and this is best done using immunohistochemistry (Figure 36.4).

SEROSA

The serosa is a thin layer of fibrovascular connective tissue that is covered by a single layer of mesothelium. Mesothelial cells are highly reactive and have phagocytic and proliferative abilities. Hypertrophy of mesothelial cells is frequently seen with any type of peritoneal effusion, e.g., ascites.

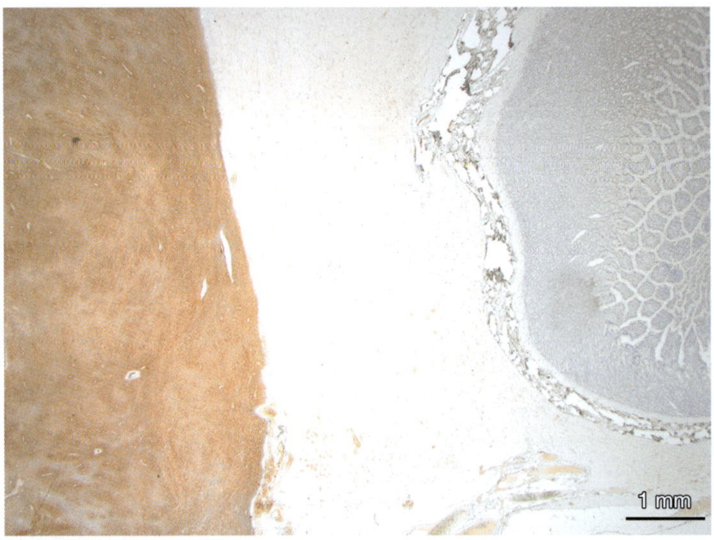

FIGURE 36.4 Gastrointestinal stromal tumor (GIST) in a dog. A section immunolabeled with an anti-CD117 (C-Kit) antibody strongly labels all the neoplastic cells of the GIST that expands and effaces the tunica muscularis of the jejunum

Mesothelial proliferation can occur with inflammatory processes, including those originating in the abdominal cavity (peritonitis/serositis), e.g., due to leakage of bile or with viral infections such as FIP or can occur locally due to perforating lesions of the GI wall. Neoplasia of the mesothelium, mesotheliomas, are less frequent in dogs and cats than in humans but are equally challenging to diagnose and manage. Pleomorphic and atypical mesothelial cells readily exfoliate into peritoneal fluid, but cytologically differentiating reactive versus neoplastic mesothelial cells is very difficult and, in many cases, impossible and requires histological evidence of invasion beyond the serosal layer.

NERVOUS SYSTEM

The autonomic nervous system innervates the bowel via the submucosal and myenteric plexi and controls peristalsis. There are relatively few changes that specifically target the enteric nerve plexi, but degeneration of nerve cell bodies is encountered in dysautonomia (Key-Gaskell-like syndrome) in cats, particularly affecting the colon. The characteristic lesion in this unusual condition is central chromatolysis, or dissolution of the Nissl substance of myenteric and submucosal plexi, leading eventually to neuronal loss, which is usually the only finding. In advanced cases plexi are identified with difficulty as small foci of residual glial cells.

REFERENCES

Allenspach, K.A., Mochel, J.P., Du, Y. et al. (2019). Correlating gastrointestinal histopathologic changes to clinical disease activity in dogs with idiopathic inflammatory bowel disease. *Veterinary Pathology* 56 (3): 435–443.

Bandara, Y., Priestnall, S.L., Chang, Y.M. et al. (2023). Characterization of intestinal fibrosis in cats with chronic inflammatory enteropathy. *Journal of Veterinary Internal Medicine* 37 (3): 936–947. https://doi.org/10.1111/jvim.16688. Epub 2023 Apr 13. PMID: 37052621; PMCID: PMC10229354.

Bonfanti, U., Bertazzolo, W., Bottero, E. et al. (2006). Diagnostic value of cytologic examination of gastrointestinal tract tumors in dogs and cats: 83 cases (2001–2004). *Journal of The American Veterinary Medical Association* 229 (7): 1130–1133.

Day, M.J., Bilzer, T., Mansell, J. et al. (2008). Histopathological standards for the diagnosis of gastrointestinal inflammation in endoscopic biopsy samples from the dog and cat: a report from the world small animal veterinary association gastrointestinal standardization group. *Journal of Comparative Pathology* 138 (1): S1–S43.

Hardas, A., Suarez-Bonnet, A., Beck, S. et al. (2021). Canine gastric carcinomas: a histopathological and immunohistochemical study and similarities with the human counterpart. *Animals (Basel)* 11 (5): 1409.

Henry, P.M.N., Boag, A.M., Dandrieux, J.R.S. et al. (2024). Diagnostic yield of percutaneous, ultrasound-guided, fine needle aspirates of the gastrointestinal wall: a retrospective analysis of 152 samples. *Journal of Small Animal Practice* 65 (10): 749–758.

Jablonski, S.A. (2022). Pathophysiology, diagnosis, and management of canine intestinal lymphangiectasia: a comparative review. *Animals (Basel)* 12 (20): 2791.

Jergens, A.E., Willard, M.D., and Allenspach, K. (2016). Maximizing the diagnostic utility of endoscopic biopsy in dogs and cats with gastrointestinal disease. *The Veterinary Journal* 214: 50–60.

Linton, M., Nimmo, J.S., Norris, J.M. et al. (2015). Feline gastrointestinal eosinophilic sclerosing fibroplasia: 13 cases and review of an emerging clinical entity. *Journal of Feline Medicine and Surgery* 17 (5): 392–404.

Maeda, S., Tsuboi, M., Sakai, K. et al. (2017). Endoscopic cytology for the diagnosis of chronic enteritis and intestinal lymphoma in dogs. *Veterinary Pathology* 54 (4): 595–604.

Marsilio, S., Freiche, V., Johnson, E. et al. (2023). ACVIM consensus statement guidelines on diagnosing and distinguishing low-grade neoplastic from inflammatory lymphocytic chronic enteropathies in cats. *Journal of Veterinary Internal Medicine* 37 (3): 794–816.

Matsumoto, I., Nakashima, K., Morita, H. et al. (2019). *Escherichia coli*-induced granulomatous colitis in a cat. *Journal of Feline Medicine and Surgery Open Reports* 5 (1): 2055116919836537.

Tasker, S., Addie, D.D., Egberink, H. et al. (2023). Feline infectious peritonitis: European advisory board on cat diseases guidelines. *Viruses* 15 (9): 1847.

Waugh, E.M., Gallagher, A., Haining, H. et al. (2016). Optimisation and validation of a PCR for antigen receptor rearrangement (PARR) assay to detect clonality in canine lymphoid malignancies. *Veterinary Immunology and Immunopathology* 182: 115–124.

Zacuto, A.C., Pesavento, P.A., Hill, S. et al. (2016). Intestinal leiomyositis: a cause of chronic intestinal pseudo-obstruction in 6 dogs. *Journal of Veterinary Internal Medicine* 30 (1): 132–140.

CHAPTER 37

Diseases of the Oral Cavity, Oropharynx, and Salivary Glands

Sarah Tayler

Department of Clinical Sciences & Services, Royal Veterinary College, Hatfield Hertfordshire, UK

KEY POINTS

- Oral cavity, oropharynx, and salivary gland disorders may present with very varied clinical signs, and therefore thorough examination of the oral cavity and associated structures should be performed in all patients. Sedation or anesthesia will often be required to allow full assessment and probing of these structures.
- Dental radiographs should be regarded as standard of care when investigating patients with dental disease and should form part of the standard dental assessment.
- Oral mass lesions may be inflammatory or neoplastic in origin, with biopsies required for definitive diagnosis in most cases. For neoplastic causes such as squamous cell carcinoma, electrochemotherapy represents an appealing alternative to previous treatment options (surgery and radiotherapy), particularly in cases in which surgical resection may not be possible and may result in good median survival times.

INTRODUCTION

The oral cavity, oropharynx, and salivary glands are essential structures involved in the prehension of food, digestion, and formation of a food bolus for swallowing. Clinical signs associated with disease largely depend upon the structure affected; however, any patient with hyporexia/anorexia should be evaluated for the presence of disease affecting the oral cavity, oropharynx, and salivary glands that may be impairing their ability to eat.

DISEASES OF THE ORAL CAVITY

Diseases associated with the oral cavity generally result in clinical signs of dysphagia, pain when eating, ptyalism, and halitosis. Structures within the oral cavity that may be implicated in disease include the teeth, periodontium, tongue, maxilla, mandible, and hard and soft palate. Examination of the oral cavity in the conscious patient can be challenging, and a thorough examination involving full dental examination and probing will usually require the patient to be sedated or anesthetized. Often, lesions affecting the oral cavity must be severe to result in inappetence in both dogs and cats, with many patients maintaining their appetite despite the presence of marked abnormalities.

Disorders of the Liver, Exocrine Pancreas, and Gastrointestinal Tract in Dogs and Cats, First Edition. Edited by Harry Cridge et al. Published 2026 by John Wiley & Sons, Inc. Companion Website: www.wiley.com/go/cridge/disorders

DISEASES OF THE TEETH AND PERIODONTIUM

The normal dental formula for an adult dog is 2x (I3/I3, C1/C1, P4/P4, M2/M3), totaling 42 teeth, and for an adult cat is 2x (I3/I3, C1/C1, P3/P2, M1/M1), totaling 30 teeth. Puppies and kittens have fewer teeth than adults, with the dental formula for puppies being 2x (I3/I3, C1/C1, P3/P3), totaling 28 teeth, and for kittens being 2x (I3/I3, C1/C1, P3/P2), totaling 26 teeth.

Full dental assessment requires general anesthesia for thorough visual inspection, probing of the teeth, and intraoral radiographs. Dental charts can be useful aids for thoroughly assessing all aspects of the teeth when performing dental assessments.

Periodontal disease is one of the most common disorders affecting both dogs and cats presenting to primary care practices (O'Neill et al. 2014a; O'Neill et al. 2014b). The periodontium is comprised of the gingiva, periodontal ligament, alveolar bone, and cementum. Inflammation of the periodontium occurs secondary to dental plaque on the surface of the teeth, which then induces a local inflammatory response. Gingivitis is the mildest form of periodontal disease, and with appropriate treatment may be reversible, in comparison to periodontitis, which results in loss of attachment of the tooth from its surrounding structures and often will require dental extractions for resolution.

Patients with periodontal disease will most commonly have minimal to no clinical signs present and will have presented for unrelated problems or routine appointments such as annual vaccinations. There must be very severe periodontal disease present to result in clinical signs such as hyporexia or dysphagia. Consequences of severe periodontal disease include tooth root abscessation and the formation of oronasal fistulae. These patients may present with more marked clinical signs such as pyrexia, reluctance to eat and a mass lesion for tooth root abscessation, and purulent nasal discharge and sneezing for oronasal fistulae.

Approach to patients with gingivitis and/or periodontitis should include full dental examination, probing, and charting under general anesthesia. Dental radiographs may also be obtained to further assess for evidence and severity of periodontal disease (e.g., alveolar bone loss). Treatment consists of manually scaling dental plaque where present and polishing of the teeth. Dental extractions are often required in more advanced cases of periodontitis.

Prevention of periodontitis is key, and owners should be educated on the importance of regular dental brushing at puppy and kitten initial consultations. Most dogs will accept regular dental brushing if introduced at a young age, and many cats also will if instigated from kittenhood. Brushing of the teeth is the only proven method for control of plaque and prevention of periodontal disease. Early recognition and treatment of periodontal disease is key, and dental examinations should be carried out at annual check-ups so that recommendations and treatment can be made promptly to stop disease progression.

Feline Resorptive Lesions

Feline odontoclastic resorptive lesions (FORLs) are painful lesions thought to be associated with dysregulated odontoclastic resorption of the tooth. FORLs are thought to affect over 60% of cats over the age of six years old, with an increased incidence with age. Various factors, including diet, microbiome, and viral agents, have been investigated as underlying factors that may be implicated in the development of FORLs; however, their pathogenesis is still poorly understood.

Patients with FORLs may present with pain when eating or reluctance to eat; however, many FORLs will be identified at routine annual appointments or during routine dental assessments. Full assessment must be performed under general anesthesia along with intraoral dental radiographs. The American Veterinary Dental College (AVDC) suggests a staging system for classifying the location and severity of tooth resorption based on appearance and radiographic changes (Table 37.1).

Treatment of FORLs is through removal of the affected teeth in their entirety. Dental radiographs may be utilized postoperatively to ensure that the extraction of each root is complete. These can be challenging, lengthy procedures if there are multiple teeth affected, and for this reason it may be beneficial to separate the assessment, radiographs, and scaling and polishing of the remaining teeth from the dental extractions into two general anesthetics.

Table 37.1 The American Veterinary Dental College Classification System for Tooth Resorption

Stage of tooth resorption	Type of tooth resorption (based on radiographic appearance)
Stage 1: mild dental hard tissue loss (cementum or cementum and enamel)	Type 1: a focal or multifocal radiolucency is present in the tooth with otherwise normal radiopacity and normal periodontal ligament space
Stage 2: moderate dental hard tissue loss (cementum or cementum and enamel with loss of dentin that does not extend to the pulp cavity)	Type 2: there is narrowing or disappearance of the periodontal ligament space in at least some areas and decreased radiopacity of part of the tooth
Stage 3: deep dental hard tissue loss (cementum or cementum and enamel with loss of dentin that extends to the pulp cavity); most of the tooth retains its integrity	Type 3: features of both type 1 and type 2 are present in the same tooth. A tooth with this appearance has areas of normal and narrow or lost periodontal ligament space, and there is focal or multifocal radiolucency in the tooth and decreased radiopacity in other areas of the tooth
Stage 4: extensive dental hard tissue loss (cementum or cementum and enamel with loss of dentin that extends to the pulp cavity); most of the tooth has lost its integrity	
Stage 5: remnants of dental hard tissue are visible only as irregular radiopacities, and gingival covering is complete	

Feline Chronic Gingivostomatitis

Feline chronic gingivostomatitis (FCGS) is a severe, painful condition resulting in severe inflammation of the caudal oral cavity, involving the palatoglossal folds (Lee et al. 2020). It is thought to be caused by an abnormal immune response to antigenic stimuli in the oral cavity. Various factors have been implicated in the etiopathogenesis, including dental disease and chronic viral infections (feline calicivirus [FCV], and feline herpesvirus [FHV-1], feline immunodeficiency virus [FIV] and feline leukemia virus [FeLV]) (Lee et al. 2020). Of these viral diseases, FCV appears to have the most convincing evidence base for its involvement in the development of FCGS (Thomas et al. 2017).

Clinical signs include hyporexia, pain when eating, dysphagia, and ptyalism. The hallmark finding on physical examination is severe inflammation of the mucosa of the caudal oral cavity, which may be ulcerated or proliferative in nature. In the majority of cases there will be significant gingivitis and periodontitis present, possibly along with FORLs. If viral infections are implicated, then other clinical signs associated with the underlying viral pathogen (e.g., ocular and nasal discharge) may be present. Diagnosis is largely based on clinical examination; however, pharyngeal swabs for viral disease testing may also be useful.

Treatment may be attempted medically, including the use of corticosteroids, modified cyclosporine, mesenchymal stem cell therapy, and recombinant feline interferon omega. However, medical management as sole therapy is unlikely to result in acceptable long-term control of the disease. Analgesia is key and often multimodal analgesia will be required, e.g., nonsteroidal anti-inflammatory drugs, transmucosal buprenorphine, gabapentin, and amantadine. The most effective treatment option in many cases is full (or nearly full mouth) extractions; often the canines and incisors can be preserved if they are otherwise healthy. Full mouth extractions are thought to minimize the antigenic stimulation that leads to the abnormal immune response seen in FCGS. Surgical management may be combined with medical management in cases that do not fully resolve with full mouth extractions. Prognosis is highly dependent upon response to treatment, and many cats may only exhibit a partial response to surgical and medical management, necessitating long-term management with analgesic agents.

Canine Chronic Ulcerative Stomatitis

Canine chronic ulcerative stomatitis (CCUS) (previously termed chronic ulcerative paradental stomatitis [CUPS] or 'kissing lesions') is an inflammatory condition thought to have an immune-mediated etiopathogenesis. The terminology CCUS is preferred over CUPS, as the lesions observed are not exclusively paradental and may affect other parts of the oral cavity, including the tongue, lips, palatine folds, and palate. Approximately 40% of lesions seen in CCUS will in fact affect areas of the mouth without teeth present.

Patients with CCUS may present with halitosis, hypersalivation, pain when eating, and dysphagia. Physical examination will reveal ulcerative lesions affecting the oral mucosa or any of the aforementioned locations. These lesions can sometimes become purulent and markedly necrotic, with a foul smell. Breeds observed to be predisposed to CCUS include Cavalier King Charles Spaniels, Maltese Terriers, Labrador Retrievers, and Greyhounds. Diagnosis is through biopsy of the lesions and ruling out other immune-mediated or neoplastic conditions that could present with similar appearing lesions.

Treatment often involves a combination of dental care and immunosuppressive therapy. In cases where the lesions are in contact with areas of dental plaque/tartar, scaling and polishing or removal of the affected teeth may be required. Immunosuppressive treatment with cyclosporine or prednisolone should be considered. Use of antimicrobial mouthwashes can also be of use. Broad-spectrum antibiotics (e.g., amoxycillin–clavulanate) may be required in cases with clear secondary bacterial involvement; however, are unlikely to be effective as sole therapy.

Feline Eosinophilic Granuloma Complex

Feline eosinophilic granuloma complex (FEGC) may present with a very diverse range of clinical signs and lesions affecting the oral cavity. The etiology of FEGC is poorly understood; however, it is thought to represent a hypersensitivity response to environmental allergens such as ectoparasites (fleas), pollen, dust mites, and food allergens. Cats with FEGC may present with a wide variety of lesions that may affect almost any location within the oral cavity or the lips. Lesions may range from raised, plaque-like lesions to large masses that may be easily confused for neoplasia on oral examination.

Diagnosis of FEGC may be made through a combination of thorough oral examination, fine needle aspirates and/or biopsies, and histopathology of the lesions. Bacterial involvement is common; however, it is unclear if this is primary and involved in the development of FEGC or simply represents secondary infection. Therefore, the use of broad-spectrum antibiotics may be considered, with one study demonstrating a moderate to marked response to amoxycillin–clavulanate in cats with eosinophilic plaques and lip ulcers (Wildermuth et al. 2012). Immunosuppressive therapy is, however, the mainstay of treatment. Use of immunosuppressive doses of glucocorticoids (e.g., 2–3 mg/kg prednisolone PO SID) generally results in rapid and complete resolution of lesions. Modified cyclosporine may be used alongside prednisolone or considered as an alternative sole therapy in cases in which corticosteroids are poorly tolerated or contraindicated. Modified cyclosporine not only works to suppress the immune system through inhibition of IL-2 production, induction of apoptosis in feline peripheral blood mononuclear cells, and blocking recruitment and activation of eosinophils (Cridge et al. 2020). Careful history taking to identify and eliminate any potential contributing factors is also important to consider, e.g., ectoparasite control.

Malignant Neoplasms Affecting the Oral Cavity

Mass lesions affecting the structures of the oral cavity may be benign in nature, such as inflammatory lesions (e.g., eosinophilic granuloma complex) and benign neoplasms (e.g., peripheral odontogenic fibroma, acanthomatous ameloblastoma, etc.), or may be malignant neoplasms such as squamous cell carcinoma, malignant melanoma, and fibrosarcoma. Squamous cell carcinoma (SCC) is the most frequently reported oral neoplasm in the cat, with malignant melanoma the most frequently reported in the dog. SCC and fibrosarcoma are the second and third most frequently reported canine oral neoplasms.

Squamous cell carcinoma may affect many of the structures of the oral cavity, including the rostral mandible (canine) and oropharynx, tongue, and tonsils (feline). In cats there has been a reported predilection for SCC development in cats that use flea collars and those that eat canned foods, particularly canned tuna. There has also been a possible association with exposure to tobacco smoke. Lesions can be ulcerative or proliferative and often result in regional bone lysis. The bone lysis observed can be debilitating and result in marked pain when eating.

Malignant melanoma affecting the oral cavity is a highly malignant neoplasm, and the majority of dogs (~80%) will have evidence of regional (local lymph node) or distant (most commonly pulmonary) metastases at the time of diagnosis or go on to develop metastatic disease at a later date. Metastases to the central nervous system have also been frequently reported (Razmara et al. 2022).

Fibrosarcoma is most commonly observed in large-breed dogs such as Labrador Retrievers and Golden Retrievers. They tend to be locally invasive with a lower rate of regional and distant metastases in comparison to malignant melanoma. Histopathology can often reveal relatively benign/low-grade tumors; however, biologically the tumor behaves in a much more aggressive fashion.

For all oral mass lesions, definitive diagnosis requires a large incisional biopsy for histopathology. There is, however, a good level of agreement documented between fine needle aspiration, fine needle insertion (without aspiration), and impression smears with histopathology in dogs and cats with oral tumors; therefore, this may be considered as a noninvasive first step (Bonfanti et al. 2015). In malignant melanoma, histopathologic diagnosis can be challenging in amelanotic cases (which represent up to 38% of all cases), and immunohistochemistry may be required to aid diagnosis. Advanced imaging and sampling of local lymph nodes may be warranted to assess for the extent of local invasion of the tumor and assess for local or distant metastases. Sentinel lymph node mapping may be useful for assessing for local lymph node metastases, given the unpredictable nature of lymphatic drainage documented in patients with oral tumors. This involves injection of contrast around the primary tumor (or surgical site if an excisional biopsy has already been performed) and assessment of the drainage pattern via computed tomography to help guide sampling.

Treatment of oral neoplasia will depend largely on tumor location. If amenable to surgical resection, then this will generally be the preferred primary approach. Depending upon the location, radical surgical approaches such as partial or total mandibulectomy/maxillectomy may need to be considered. Dogs appear to be highly adaptable and tolerant of this procedure; however, cats are thought to be less tolerant of mandibulectomy/maxillectomy. Despite this, there are multiple successful reports of mandibulectomy in cats in the veterinary literature, therefore, this may still be considered an appropriate treatment option (Northrup et al. 2006). Feeding tubes are highly likely to be required in feline patients postoperatively and may need to be considered in canine patients.

Radiotherapy may then be recommended as an adjunctive treatment following surgical removal depending upon the margins achieved with surgical removal. Radiotherapy could be considered as sole therapy in cases in which surgery is not considered an option; however, it would not be expected to result in similar survival times to surgical management. Complications from radiotherapy include glossitis, mucositis, and oronasal fistula formation. Feeding tube placement may also be required temporarily in patients that develop side effects.

Chemotherapy tends to be ineffective as a sole therapy for oral neoplasia. It may be recommended in cases with incomplete margins following surgical excision or with evidence of local or distant metastatic disease. Toceranib has been documented to result in increased median survival times in cats with oral squamous cell carcinoma and appears to be well tolerated (Wiles et al. 2017). Cats with squamous cell carcinoma that is locally invading osseous structures may also benefit from the administration of bisphosphonates such as zoledronate to assist with bone-related pain. A vaccine has been developed for use in malignant melanoma in dogs, which appears safe to use; however, with varying reports of efficacy.

Electrochemotherapy involves the use of electrical pulses in order to transiently increase the permeability of cell membranes and allow for the uptake of drugs that the cell would otherwise be impermeable to. It has been well documented in the treatment of squamous cell carcinoma affecting the nasal planum in cats; however, it has also been reported to be of use in oral tumors in both dogs and cats. In a study of dogs with non-tonsillar squamous cell carcinoma treated with electrochemotherapy combined with intravenous bleomycin, there was a response rate of 90.9%, with 8 of the 11 dogs achieving complete remission and an overall recurrence rate of 27.3% (Simčič et al. 2020). Electrochemotherapy is therefore a very appealing novel treatment option for patients with oral neoplasia and may even be considered the first-line treatment option for selected cases in the future.

Benign Neoplasms Affecting the Oral Cavity

Peripheral odontogenic fibromas (POF), otherwise known as fibromatous epulis of periodontal ligament origin (FEPLO), are benign neoplastic or neoplastic-like masses arising from the periodontal ligament. Their classification as neoplastic lesions is at present uncertain, with no general consensus amongst pathologists. They tend to be expansile, noninvasive lesions that may displace teeth and can be single or multiple. Boxer dogs appear predisposed to POF/FEPLO formation, and there are only rare case reports of them affecting cats. Treatment is through surgical excision of the lesion/lesions.

Acanthomatous ameloblastoma is a relatively common odontogenic tumor seen in dogs, most commonly affecting the rostral mandible of large-breed dogs such as Golden Retrievers. They exhibit variable behavior, with some being very slow growing with minimal local tissue invasion compared to others, which grow rapidly and cause severe bone lysis. Recurrence is common after surgical removal if margins are not achieved; therefore, rostral mandibulectomy will often be required to obtain complete remission of disease.

DISEASES OF THE TONGUE

The tongue is composed of skeletal muscle, and its primary function is for drinking and to aid in the formation of a food bolus in preparation for swallowing. Its motor innervation is from the hypoglossal nerve (CN XII), and its sensory innervation comes from the lingual branch of the trigeminal (CN V) for the rostral two-thirds, and the glossopharyngeal (CN IX) for the most caudal one-third. Disease affecting these cranial nerves may present as an inability to move the tongue or atrophy of the tongue, which may be most noticeable if unilateral.

Neoplastic Conditions of the Tongue

Neoplasia is the most commonly reported abnormality associated with the tongue in dogs, with the majority (64%) being malignant in origin and including malignant melanoma, squamous cell carcinoma, and fibrosarcoma (Dennis et al. 2006). Squamous cell carcinoma is the most common malignant neoplasia affecting the tongue and/or oral cavity in cats (Figure 37.1).

The behavior and management of these neoplasms is similar to neoplasms of the oral cavity. The mainstay of treatment for the majority of neoplastic conditions of the tongue is surgical removal of the tumor. Major, subtotal, and partial glossectomy have all been described as potential surgical

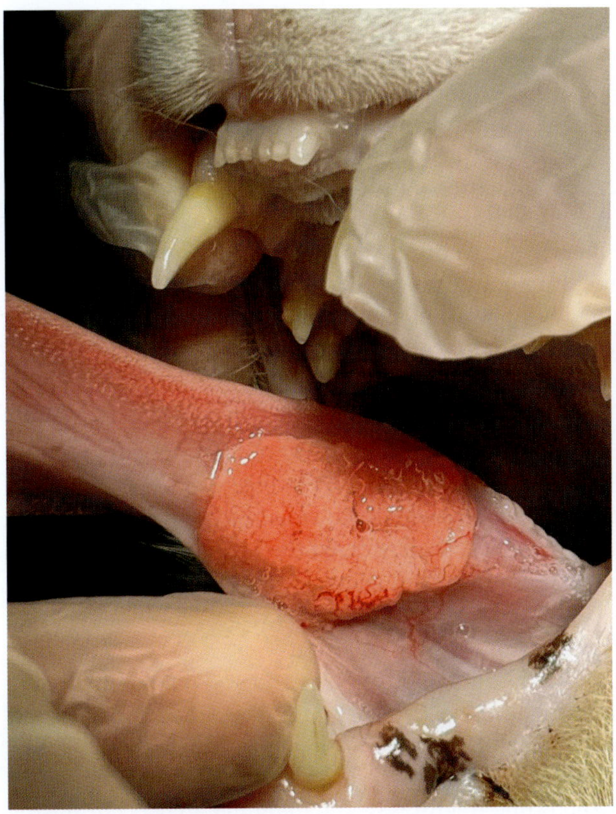

FIGURE 37.1 A lingual squamous cell carcinoma present in a cat. Picture courtesy of Dr. Andy Yale

techniques; however, dogs are observed to be more tolerant of aggressive surgical procedures. Feeding tube placement may be required at the time of surgery to allow for enteral nutrition while the patient adapts post-surgery. Electrochemotherapy may also be considered for these cases, especially where surgical removal is not possible.

DISEASES OF THE MAXILLA AND MANDIBLE

The maxilla and mandible are joined by the temporomandibular joint (TMJ) and together function to facilitate prehension and mastication of food. Conditions affecting the maxilla and mandible will tend to present with pain or inability to open the mouth (trismus). Occasionally, pathology affecting structures in close proximity to the TMJ may present with similar clinical signs, for example, in patients with otitis media or retrobulbar disease. It is important to consider these differentials when assessing patients for diseases associated with the jaw.

Craniomandibular Osteopathy

Craniomandibular or temporomandibular osteopathy (CMO) is a progressive condition in which there is new bone formation along the mandible and TMJ; however, in rare cases, other bones may be affected too, e.g., cervical vertebrae, radius, and ulna. Certain breeds appear to be predisposed to CMO, with West Highland White Terriers and Scottish Terriers the most frequently reported breeds. Patients present at a young age with progressive, firm swelling of the jaw and difficulty or reluctance to eat. Diagnostic imaging is required for diagnosis, with computed tomography potentially revealing osteoproliferation not only of the jaw but also of the cranium and the tympanic bulla too (Perez Lopez et al. 2024).

Generally, disease progression stops beyond 12 months of age. Treatment is focused on provision of pain relief (e.g., use of nonsteroidal anti-inflammatory drugs) and nutritional support. Prognosis depends on the extent of the disease, with the prognosis considered poorer if there are significant changes involving the TMJ. In cases that can be nursed through the clinical phase, there may be some regression of the osteoproliferative changes following closure of the growth plates.

Fibrous Osteodystrophy

Fibrous osteodystrophy, also known as "rubber jaw," is a consequence of hyperparathyroidism, which may be primary in origin but more commonly is seen in secondary cases due to renal disease or secondary nutritional hyperparathyroidism. The excess parathyroid hormone causes increased resorption of bone, which may be more pronounced in the jaw. The bone is replaced by fibrous tissue, causing swelling/thickening of the jawbone, increased tooth mobility, and widening of the gaps between the teeth. Diagnostic imaging with radiographs or computed tomography may reveal osteopenia of the jawbones and, to a lesser extent, other bones included in the study. Diagnosis and treatment rely upon correct identification of the underlying cause of hyperparathyroidism. In most cases the prognosis is considered very poor, especially those with advanced renal failure. Patients with secondary nutritional hyperparathyroidism may improve with feeding of a complete and balanced diet.

Neoplasia of the Maxilla and Mandible

In addition to the previously described neoplasms that affect the oral cavity, osteosarcoma has also been reported to affect the maxilla and mandible. These masses tend to behave in a more benign manner than osteosarcoma of the appendicular skeleton, with a slower speed of progression and lower risk of metastasis. Surgical excision with margins is considered the best first-line treatment option and may be combined with radiation therapy and/or adjuvant chemotherapy.

Idiopathic Osteonecrosis of the Jaw

Idiopathic osteonecrosis of the jaw is a reported consequence in patients undergoing treatment with bisphosphonates and has also been reported as a complication following radiation therapy of the jaw area. It has been most consistently reported in cats undergoing long-term treatment with alendronate for idiopathic hypercalcemia. In many cases, osteonecrosis of the jaw may only be recognized at the point of dental treatment, at which time fractures of the mandible may occur during tooth extraction. Other bones may be affected (e.g., proximal tibia). Fractures will generally require surgical correction; however, due to the underlying pathology, these can be complicated procedures with an increased risk of failure, with approximately 35% requiring at least one revision surgery (Hatunen et al. 2024). It is recommended that any cat receiving bisphosphonates undergoing dental treatment should have dental radiographs prior to extractions, and ideally consideration should be given to performing dental treatment prior to bisphosphonate administration.

DISEASES OF THE HARD AND SOFT PALATE

The hard and soft palate separate the oral cavity from the nasal cavity and nasopharynx. The hard palate is comprised of the maxillary and palatine bones with overlying mucosa, which folds palatal rugae. The soft palate is made up of muscular tissue covered with mucosa and tends to be longer in dogs than cats. In cats there is a sensory vomeronasal organ (Jacobson's organ) located just behind the incisors on the hard palate that is a normal anatomical finding.

Cleft Palate

A cleft palate is an abnormal communication between the oral and nasal cavities. Most commonly this is a congenital defect; however, an acquired cleft palate may develop secondary to trauma affecting the head. In puppies with a congenital cleft palate, breeders may notice difficulties when suckling, milk coming from the nose, failure to gain weight, gagging, coughing, and sneezing. Brachycephalic and Mastiff-type breeds appear to be predisposed to cleft palates along with other orofacial clefts (e.g., cleft lip).

The extent of the cleft palate can be highly variable, with defects ranging from being slit-like in some cases to very wide clefts in others. The location of the cleft is also variable, with some being situated more rostrally over the hard palate, while others may affect larger portions of both the hard and soft palate. The more caudal lesions are thought to be associated with more severe clinical signs.

Diagnosis of a cleft palate is generally straightforward through thorough examination of the oral cavity. Definitive treatment is through surgical correction of the defect; however, surgery ideally should be delayed until four months of age. Surgery has been described in puppies as young as 8–10 weeks. Orogastric feeding may be required in young puppies that are unable to suckle prior to weaning. Use of a temporary palatal prosthesis has been described in three dogs, which allowed for successful bottle feeding and then corrective surgery at the age of 5–6 months (Conze et al. 2018). Conservative management may also be attempted in the long term, with reports of good quality of life and only minor complications associated with the presence of the defect (e.g., material lodging in the cleft) (Monck et al. 2025).

Hypoplasia of the Soft Palate

Hypoplasia of the soft palate may be unilateral or bilateral and is a congenital defect resulting in lack of growth of the caudal aspect of the soft palate. Patients may present with similar clinical signs to a cleft palate; however, there is also an association between palatine hypoplasia and middle ear disease (White et al. 2009). Treatment is through surgical correction of the defect by a three-layer appositional repair or a nasopharyngeal mucosal flap.

Elongated Soft Palate

Elongation of the soft palate is part of the brachycephalic obstructive airway syndrome (BOAS), along with other abnormalities such as stenotic nares, everted laryngeal saccules, and a hypoplastic trachea. Patients will generally present with stertor with or without respiratory compromise (particularly when stressed or in hot weather), snoring, and regurgitation secondary to increased intrathoracic pressure and/or a concurrent hiatal hernia, which is also common in brachycephalic breeds. Assessment of the palate length requires airway examination under general anesthesia. Treatment is through partial staphylectomy, alongside correction of any other anatomical abnormalities (e.g., resection rhinoplasty for stenotic nares). In patients presenting with regurgitation, BOAS surgery can often significantly improve clinical signs, even with concurrent hiatal hernia. The prognosis for an elongated soft palate is generally considered good; however, complications, including airway obstruction, can be seen in the immediate postoperative period, which might warrant temporary tracheostomy placement.

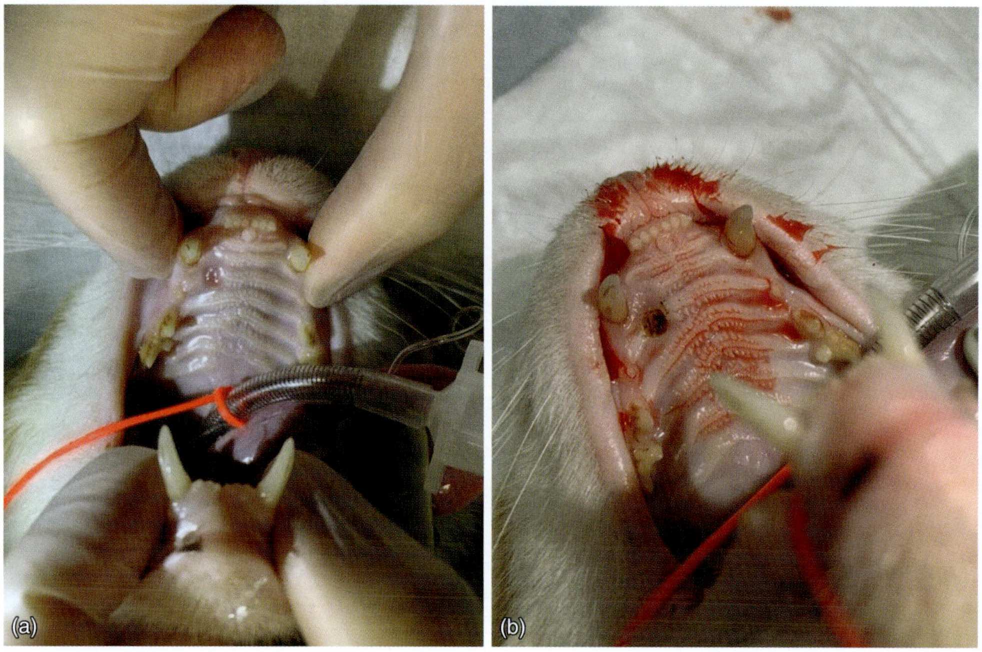

FIGURE 37.2 A palatine (Menrath's) ulcer in a cat presenting with hemoptysis and anemia; pre-cauterization (left) of the palatine artery and post-cauterization (right). Pictures courtesy of Dr. Frederick Allan

Palatine (Menrath's) Ulcer

"Menrath's ulcers" are ulcerations located on the hard palate over the palatine artery (Figure 37.2). They are exclusively reported in cats and are thought to be associated with conditions that lead to overgrooming, such as allergic skin disease and ectoparasites (e.g., fleas). Presenting complaints include melena and hemoptysis. All anemic cats with concerns for blood loss should be evaluated for the presence of a palatine ulcer through thorough oral examination. In many cases, owners will not have reported any hemoptysis or melena prior to presentation or will require prompting to recognize the presence of melena. Treatment is through surgical ligation and/or cauterization of the palatine artery. Any predisposing skin disease (e.g., fleas) should be addressed and treated as necessary, and a buster collar may be required to prevent further overgrooming and damage to the surgical site in the postoperative period. Blood transfusions are often required for stabilization prior to surgery. The prognosis with surgical management is excellent.

Palatitis/Ulcerations

Ulcerations or inflammation of the hard and soft palate may be observed as part of more widespread ulceration of the oral cavity (e.g., immune-mediated disease) or can occasionally be seen in patients with gastroesophageal reflux, in particular brachycephalic dogs. In these cases, a fluoroscopic swallow study may be useful to diagnose gastroesophageal reflux and assess for the presence of a hiatal hernia. Management should be aimed at controlling the gastroesophageal reflux with proton pump inhibitors (e.g., omeprazole), sucralfate, and dietary changes (e.g., low-fat diet), and correcting the underlying BOAS if this is thought to have played a role.

Canine Oral Eosinophilic Granuloma

Oral eosinophilic granuloma is far less frequently encountered in dogs compared to cats and may present in a different way to FEGCs. Cavalier King Charles Spaniels appear predisposed to oral eosinophilic disease. Lesions may present as mass-like lesions in the oral cavity or more diffuse plaque-like lesions of the palate (Figure 37.3). Patients may present for dysphagia, gagging/retching, or if severe lesions are present, inspiratory dyspnea and stertor may be noted.

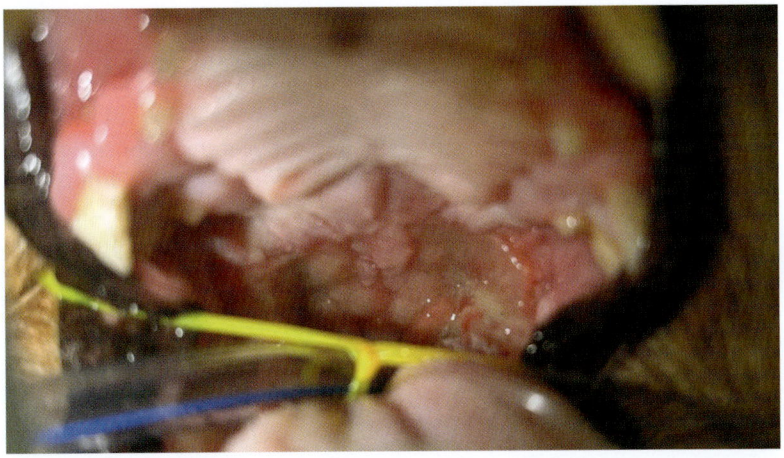

FIGURE 37.3 Plaque like lesions on the hard palate of a cavalier King Charles spaniel with oral eosinophilic granuloma. Picture courtesy or Dr. Sarah Tayler

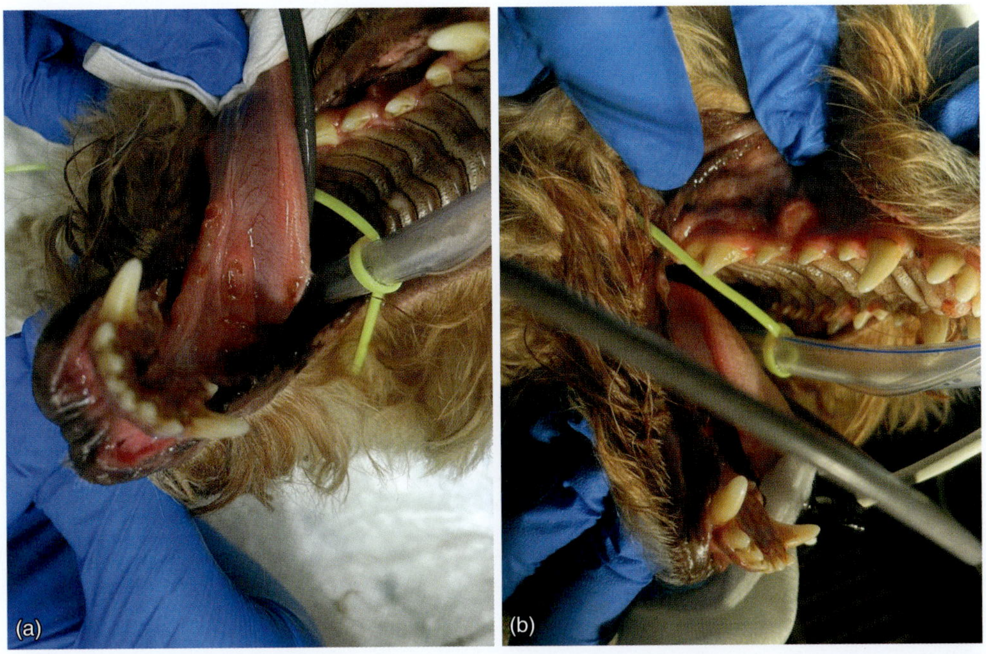

FIGURE 37.4 Gingival and sublingual ulcerations in a crossbreed dog presenting with halitosis, inappetence and reluctance to drink. Histopathology revealed an autoimmune subepidermal blistering disease, and the patient demonstrated a markedly positive response to immunosuppressive therapy. Pictures courtesy of Dr. Ed Shelton

Diagnosis can be made through incisional biopsy of the lesions under general anesthesia. Treatment comprises immunosuppression with glucocorticoids and/or a second-line immunosuppressive agent. Cyclosporine is considered the second agent of choice due to its recognized and well-documented efficacy in eosinophilic disease in cats. Response to treatment should be rapid; however, relapses may be observed with tapering of medications.

MISCELLANEOUS ORAL CAVITY DISORDERS

The oral cavity may be involved in the development of immune-mediated disease, with varying presentations and locations of lesions (Figure 37.4). Ulcerations, bullae, and erosions may be present on the gingiva, tongue, and/or palate. Biopsies with histopathology are required for definitive diagnosis and to rule out other causes (e.g., infectious, neoplastic), however, the response to immunosuppressive treatment with glucocorticoids will often further support a diagnosis of immune-mediated disease.

Ingestion of caustic substances may also cause lesions of the oral cavity, particularly the tongue and palate. These lesions may be linear in appearance, consistent with the passage of the caustic substance over the surface of the tongue/palate. If caustic injury is suspected, then management should be focused around providing analgesia, nutritional support, limiting secondary bacterial infection (e.g., use of chlorhexidine mouthwash), and assessing the patient for involvement beyond the oral cavity (e.g., esophagitis). Thermal injury or electrical burns may also cause similar lesions and require similar management.

Rarely, severe uremia may result in the development of oral ulceration, particularly affecting the lateral aspects of the tongue and buccal mucosa. This can sometimes progress to necrosis of the tip of the tongue, which may result in sloughing of the necrotic portion. Treatment is aimed at addressing and correcting the underlying cause of uremia and providing analgesia and nutritional support for any oral cavity ulcerations and/or tongue necrosis.

Viral papillomas present as cauliflower-like small mass lesions of the lips, gingiva, and tongue. Often many lesions may be present in the same animal. They are most common in young dogs. Generally, they are asymptomatic and will regress with age. Occasionally they may be observed in patients on immunosuppressive treatment and will regress when the immunosuppressive therapy is withdrawn.

Gingival hyperplasia is a recognized complication with long-term usage of certain drugs. It has mainly been associated with chronic cyclosporine and chronic amlodipine administration. Affected cases are generally asymptomatic; however, the hyperplastic gingiva may catch when eating and be prone to bleeding. Discontinuation of the inciting drug should result in resolution of the condition.

DISEASES OF THE OROPHARYNX

Structures within the oropharynx include the caudal aspect of the soft palate, the caudal portion of the tongue, tonsils, and the pharyngeal walls. The oropharynx functions to help with formation of the food bolus, and storage of the bolus prior to swallowing. Patients with oropharyngeal disease will often present with a combination of gagging/retching and difficulty eating.

The swallowing process involves three phases:

1. Oral phase: this is initially a voluntary phase and involves the prehension of food, chewing, and mixing of food with saliva in the oral cavity. The tongue then moves the food to the oropharynx.
2. Pharyngeal phase: this is an involuntary phase in which the soft palate is lifted to prevent food from entering the nasopharynx, and the epiglottis moves to cover the larynx and prevent aspiration. There is coordinated contraction of the pharyngeal muscles with synchronous relaxation of the cricopharyngeus muscle of the upper esophageal sphincter, which allows the food bolus to pass into the cranial portion of the esophagus.
3. Esophageal phase: in this involuntary phase, esophageal peristalsis moves the food bolus from the cranial esophagus to the lower esophageal sphincter, which relaxes to allow food to pass into the stomach.

DISEASES OF THE TONSILS

The palatine tonsils are paired lymphoid organs situated at the caudal aspect of the oral cavity in the tonsillar crypts. Lingual, paraepiglottic, and pharyngeal tonsils are also present in both dogs and cats; however, they are often not able to be visualized macroscopically. The tonsils play a key role in coordinating the immune response to antigens that enter the oral cavity.

Tonsillar Neoplasia

Tonsillar carcinoma (squamous cell carcinoma) is the most frequently diagnosed neoplasm of the tonsils in both dogs and cats. Patients will often present with gagging/retching and pain when attempting to eat or swallow. Metastasis to local lymph nodes is relatively common, and occasionally patients may present for large cervical mass lesions associated with metastatic lymph nodes as opposed to the primary mass itself. It is therefore important to perform thorough visual examination of the tonsils in any patient presenting with enlargement of the lymph nodes in the region of the tonsils, e.g., retropharyngeal lymphadenopathy. Other neoplasms reported to affect the tonsils are lymphoma and melanoma.

Treatment for tonsillar neoplasia depends upon tumor type. For tonsillar carcinoma treatment modality will likely depend on the presence of regional metastases and the size of the mass lesion present. Overall prognosis is considered relatively poor, with a reported median survival time regardless of treatment option of 126 days (Treggiari et al. 2023).

CRICOPHARYNGEAL ACHALASIA AND CRICOPHARYNGEAL ASYNCHRONY

The cricopharyngeus muscle, which largely forms the upper esophageal sphincter, is a band of muscle located between the pharynx and esophagus that aids in passage of the food bolus from the oral cavity into the proximal esophagus. It is usually closed to prevent air from entering the esophagus and will only open in response to the presence of a food bolus in the oropharynx. It also prevents retrograde movement of esophageal contents into the oropharynx. It is innervated by the glossopharyngeal nerve (CN IX) and the pharyngeal branch of the vagus nerve (CN X).

Cricopharyngeal dysphagia may be characterized by cricopharyngeal achalasia, in which there is an inability of the cricopharyngeus to relax and allow the bolus to pass into the esophagus, or cricopharyngeal asynchrony, in which there is uncoordinated relaxation of the cricopharyngeus in response to the presence of the bolus. Cricopharyngeal achalasia is more common than asynchrony; however, in some cases, there may be a combination of both achalasia and asynchrony present in cases of cricopharyngeal dysphagia.

Dogs with cricopharyngeal achalasia typically present earlier in life (often soon after weaning) with dysphagia and regurgitation. They will make repeated attempts to swallow their food, which may be variably successful or result in dropping of the food out of their mouth. They often particularly struggle when drinking and when eating food of liquid consistency. They may also present for coughing and respiratory compromise if aspiration pneumonia is present. Breeds predisposed to cricopharyngeal achalasia include the Cocker Spaniel and Cockerpoo, with Labradoodles also anecdotally reported to be overrepresented.

Diagnosis is made through fluoroscopic swallow study. Barium may be used as a contrast medium; however, it can be persistent and irritant if aspirated. Water-based contrast media (e.g., iohexol) may be used in cases in which there is a high concern for aspiration, as this may be less damaging if aspirated. In situations in which fluoroscopy is unavailable, plain radiographs may reveal a prominent "bar" in the proximal esophagus consistent with a hypertrophied cricopharyngeus muscle. Thoracic radiographs may also be useful in evaluating the patient for the presence of aspiration pneumonia.

Supportive treatment involves addressing aspiration pneumonia if clinically relevant and optimizing feeding techniques. Many patients will tolerate wet food made into "meatballs" or dry kibble better than liquid preparations. Thickening substances can be added to water to aid in drinking. However, if left untreated, the majority of patients will succumb to repeated bouts of aspiration pneumonia early in life.

Medical treatment can be trialed with botulinum toxin injections into the cricopharyngeus muscle. This can cause relaxation of the muscle and improve signs for approximately 2–4 months, however, is not a permanent solution. Therefore, in the majority of cases surgery is the recommended treatment option. A cricopharyngeal myotomy or myectomy involves either 'releasing' or excising the abnormal cricopharyngeal muscle. Postoperative complications include treatment failure and aspiration pneumonia. Outcome is largely dependent on recovery in the postoperative period – if surgery is successful with improvement of the clinical signs, then long-term outcome can be favorable.

MISCELLANEOUS CONDITIONS OF THE OROPHARYNX

Foreign bodies may become lodged in the oropharynx, requiring removal. Stick or bone foreign bodies in dogs may become lodged across the hard palate, requiring removal under sedation or general anesthesia. Cats may ingest blades of grass that become stuck in the oropharynx and/or nasopharynx behind the soft palate. Retroflex nasopharyngoscopy may be useful in these cases for direct visualization and retrieval of the foreign body. If endoscopy is unavailable, the patient may be anesthetized and positioned in dorsal recumbency. The soft palate can then be pulled forward using a spay hook or Allis tissue forceps, and the area examined for the presence of a foreign body. The spay hook may also be used to sweep behind the palate from side to side, which may sometimes capture a grass blade if present and allow for its removal. A retroesophageal approach to the nasopharynx has also been described, whereby the tip of the endoscope is protected by a flared red rubber catheter and inserted into the cervical esophagus through the same technique used for esophagostomy tube placement (Derré et al. 2021). This allows superior visualization and access to the nasopharynx compared to retroflex nasopharyngoscopy and may be beneficial for foreign bodies that are hard to retrieve through the standard retroflex approach.

Jugular foramen syndrome is a condition in which the cranial nerves crossing the jugular foramen (glossopharyngeal [CN IX], vagus [CN X], and accessory [CN XI]) are compromised due to a lesion at the jugular foramen. Most commonly this is due to a neoplastic lesion, with meningioma the most frequently reported cause in dogs. Patients with jugular foramen syndrome may present with clinical signs relatable to oropharyngeal disease, such as gagging, retching, and coughing, due to the structures innervated by these cranial nerves. Therefore, it is important to consider this as a differential diagnosis in patients presenting for oropharyngeal disease and consider full neurological examination in these patients. Not all patients will have neurological deficits present on examination, however, and therefore advanced imaging such as CT scan or MRI may be required to further interrogate the jugular foramen.

Pharyngeal weakness may result in an inability for the patient to move the bolus from the pharynx through the upper esophageal sphincter and into the cranial esophagus. This may result in signs of dysphagia and regurgitation of food and/or water. Diagnosis may be made through a fluoroscopic swallow study, with specific focus on the pharyngeal phase of swallowing. Differentials are similar to those for megaesophagus or esophageal dysmotility, and include polyneuropathies/polymyopathies, endocrine disease (hypothyroidism and hypoadrenocorticism), and myasthenia gravis. A thorough neurological examination should therefore be performed in all cases. Treatment should be targeted at the underlying condition if identified. In the absence of an underlying condition, treatment should be focused upon optimization of feeding through identifying different textures of food that are better tolerated and the use of water thickening agents if liquids are poorly tolerated.

DISEASES OF THE SALIVARY GLANDS

The salivary glands are paired glands that secrete saliva, which aids in commencing digestion of food and lubricating the bolus prior to swallowing. The major salivary glands present in dogs and cats are the mandibular, parotid, sublingual, and zygomatic glands. Minor salivary glands are present throughout the oral cavity (e.g., buccal), with cats having a prominent molar salivary gland that may be mistaken for a mass lesion. The production of saliva is largely controlled by the parasympathetic nervous system in response to visual, olfactory, taste, and tactile stimuli from within the oral cavity. Saliva consists of mucus for lubrication of the bolus, ions (mainly potassium and bicarbonate), and enzymes such as ptyalin, which are involved in the digestion of starches.

Disorders affecting the salivary glands may present with ptyalism, swelling of the salivary glands, or pain when opening the mouth/eating. Thorough palpation of the salivary glands should be performed should a salivary gland disorder be suspected. Due to the location of the zygomatic salivary glands and their close proximity to the orbit, these patients may actually present for suspected retrobulbar disease, e.g., exophthalmos and pain on ocular retropulsion (Cannon et al. 2011).

Investigations into salivary gland disease will often require advanced imaging such as computed tomography of the head in order to determine the true nature and extent of the disease process and rule out other conditions that may present in a similar way. Ultrasound-guided or palpation-guided aspirates of the salivary glands may be useful for cytological analysis.

SIALADENITIS

Sialadenitis may affect any of the salivary glands, however, has been most frequently described to affect the zygomatic salivary gland, resulting in signs associated with retrobulbar disease. These patients may also be pyrexic and inappetent. Often these patients are noted to have undergone some form of general anesthesia or have had prior gastrointestinal signs (e.g., intestinal foreign body surgery). Cytological examination may reveal neutrophilic inflammation, and samples could be obtained for culture and sensitivity in case of a bacterial origin. Treatment involves anti-inflammatory medication such as NSAIDs and broad-spectrum antibiotics if an underlying bacterial cause is confirmed during investigations.

PHENOBARBITAL RESPONSIVE SIALADENOSIS

The etiology of phenobarbital-responsive sialadenosis is poorly understood; however, it is thought to potentially represent a form of limbic epilepsy. This condition has been exclusively reported in canine patients. Dogs may present with profuse hypersalivation, vomiting/regurgitation, gagging, gulping, and reluctance to eat and/or open the mouth. Physical examination may reveal markedly symmetrically enlarged, firm, painful salivary glands.

Diagnosis is based upon exclusion of other conditions such as sialadenitis and neoplasia that may result in salivary gland enlargement. Advanced imaging (computed tomography) and fine needle aspiration of the enlarged salivary glands are often warranted. Sialadenosis is nonneoplastic and non-inflammatory in origin, therefore, cytology or histopathology would be expected to be relatively normal in these cases.

Treatment is with phenobarbital, at a starting dose of 2 mg/kg PO q8h (or intravenously if oral medications are unable to be tolerated). The response to treatment is generally rapid and complete and can be used to support a diagnosis. Generally, long-term treatment with phenobarbital is required. If no response to treatment is observed, alternative differentials should be considered.

SIALOCOELE (SALIVARY MUCOCOELE)

Sialocoeles are caused by accumulation of mucinous salivary material within a subcutaneous or submucosal fibrous capsule. Any of the salivary glands may be implicated in their development; however, they are most commonly reported to form in the sublingual gland in dogs. Sublingual gland sialocoeles are also termed ranulae, which refers to the fluid-filled structure identified underneath the tongue in these cases. In the majority of cases no underlying cause resulting in their development is identified; however, trauma, neoplasia, sialadenitis, foreign bodies, and sialolithiasis may rarely result in sialocoele formation. There has also been a potential link between hypercortisolism (endogenous or exogenous) and sialocoele formation reported in dogs (Bae et al. 2023). Sialocoele formation is reported in cats, albeit more rarely than in the dogs.

Animals with sialocoeles will generally present with signs relatable to a mass lesion associated with the affected salivary gland – this may be intraoral if, for example, the sublingual gland is affected (ranula) or subcutaneously if, for example, the parotid gland is affected. The mass lesion will feel fluid-filled and should be non-painful. Osseous metaplasia of sialocoeles has been reported in a small number of dogs in which case the mass may be firm on palpation (Olimpo et al. 2023). Diagnosis may be made through aspiration of viscous, mucoid fluid from the mass lesion. Computed tomography may aid in diagnosis and may also be useful to rule out secondary causes of sialocoele formation (e.g., foreign body or sialolithiasis).

Treatment of sialocoeles generally involves surgical excision of the sialocoele and affected gland and duct (sialoadenectomy). Recurrence of the sialocoele is a recognized complication of surgery that owners should be warned of. Radiation therapy has also been described to result in either a complete or partial response to treatment in 54–45% of patients, respectively (Poirier et al. 2018). Prognosis with successful treatment is considered excellent.

NEOPLASIA OF THE SALIVARY GLANDS

The most common neoplasia reported to affect the salivary glands in both dogs and cats is adenocarcinoma. Commonly owners will present patients for a palpable mass lesion in the region of the affected gland, however, other complaints may be dysphagia, halitosis, and exophthalmos. Siamese cats may be overrepresented in the development of salivary gland neoplasia. Diagnosis is through fine needle aspiration and biopsies. Metastasis to local lymph nodes occurs in approximately 30% of patients, therefore, sentinel lymph node mapping and sampling of the appropriate nodes may be performed prior to treatment.

Treatment requires surgical removal of the affected gland and local lymph nodes if metastatic disease is confirmed or suspected. Prognosis can be considered good with successful surgical removal of the gland; however, the presence of regional lymph node metastases is associated with a poorer prognosis and significantly decreased median survival times.

REFERENCES

Bae, J.Y., Kim, J.I., Kim, J.Y. et al. (2023). Sialocele and its association with hypercortisolism and long-term glucocorticoid treatment in dogs: retrospective case–control study. *Animals* 14 (1): 120.

Bonfanti, U., Bertazzolo, W., Gracis, M. et al. (2015). Diagnostic value of cytological analysis of tumours and tumour-like lesions of the oral cavity in dogs and cats: a prospective study on 114 cases. *The Veterinary Journal* 205 (2): 322–327.

Cannon, M.S., Paglia, D., Zwingenberger, A.L. et al. (2011). Clinical and diagnostic imaging findings in dogs with zygomatic sialadenitis: 11 cases (1990–2009). *Journal of the American Veterinary Medical Association* 239 (9):1211–1218. https://doi.org/10.2460/javma.239.9.1211.

Conze, T., Ritz, I., Hospes, R. et al. (2018). Management of cleft palate in puppies using a temporary prosthesis: a report of three cases. *Veterinary Sciences* 5 (3): 61.

Cridge, H., Kordon, A., Pinchuk, L.M. et al. (2020). Effects of cyclosporine on feline lymphocytes activated in vitro. *Veterinary Immunology and Immunopathology* 219: 109962.

Dennis, M.M., Ehrhart, N., Duncan, C.G. et al. (2006). Frequency of and risk factors associated with lingual lesions in dogs: 1,196 cases (1995–2004). *Journal of the American Veterinary Medical Association* 228 (10): 1533–1537.

Derré, M.G., Snead, E.C., Beaufrère, H.H. et al. (2021). Investigation of a retroesophagoscopic approach to nasopharyngoscopy as an alternative to the conventional retroflexed endoscopic approach for selected indications in feline cadavers and client-owned cats. *American Journal of Veterinary Research* 82 (9): 752–759.

Hatunen, S.L., Anderson, J.G., Bell, C.M. et al. (2024). A retrospective case series on bisphosphonate related osteonecrosis of the jaw in 20 cats. *Frontiers in Veterinary Science* 11: 1436988.

Lee, D.B., Verstraete, F.J., and Arzi, B. (2020). An update on feline chronic gingivostomatitis. *Veterinary Clinics: Small Animal Practice* 50 (5): 973–982.

Monck, S.L., Mathews, K.G., Lascelles, B.D.X. et al. (2025). Conservative management of canine cleft palate can be a viable treatment option: 65 cases (2006–2023). *Journal of the American Veterinary Medical Association* 263 (1): 1–10.

Northrup, N.C., Selting, K.A., Rassnick, K.M. et al. (2006). Outcomes of cats with oral tumors treated with mandibulectomy: 42 cases. *Journal of the American Animal Hospital Association* 42 (5): 350–360.

O'Neill, D.G., Church, D.B., McGreevy, P.D. et al. (2014a). Prevalence of disorders recorded in cats attending primary-care veterinary practices in England. *The Veterinary Journal* 202 (2): 286–291.

O'Neill, D.G., Church, D.B., McGreevy, P.D. et al. (2014b). Prevalence of disorders recorded in dogs attending primary-care veterinary practices in England. *PloS One* 9 (3): e90501.

Olimpo, M., Ferraris, E.I., Parisi, L. et al. (2023). Diagnostic findings and surgical management of three dogs affected by osseous metaplasia secondary to a salivary mucocele. *Animals* 13 (9): 1550.

Perez Lopez, L.A., Almansa Ruiz, J.C., Steenkamp, G. et al. (2024). Computed tomographic characteristics of craniomandibular osteopathy in 20 dogs. *Frontiers in Veterinary Science* 11: 1436356.

Poirier, V.J., Mayer Stankeová, S., Buchholz, J. et al. (2018). Efficacy of radiation therapy for the treatment of sialocele in dogs. *Journal of Veterinary Internal Medicine* 32 (1): 107–110.

Razmara, A.M., Wittenburg, L.A., Al-Nadaf, S. et al. (2022). Prevalence and clinicopathologic features of canine metastatic melanoma involving the central nervous system: a retrospective analysis and comparative review. *Frontiers in Oncology* 12: 868004. https://doi.org/10.3389/fonc.2022.868004.

Simčič, P., Lowe, R., Granziera, V. et al. (2020). Electrochemotherapy in treatment of canine oral non-tonsillar squamous cell carcinoma. A case series report. *Veterinary and Comparative Oncology* 18 (3): 428–432.

Thomas, S., Lappin, D.F., Spears, J. et al. (2017). Prevalence of feline calicivirus in cats with odontoclastic resorptive lesions and chronic gingivostomatitis. *Research in Veterinary Science* 111: 124–126.

Treggiari, E., Pellin, M.A., Romanelli, G. et al. (2023). Tonsillar carcinoma in dogs: Treatment outcome and potential prognostic factors in 123 cases. *Journal of Veterinary Internal Medicine* 37 (1): 247–257. https://doi.org/10.1111/jvim.16623.

White, R.N., Hawkins, H.L., Alemi, V.P. et al. (2009). Soft palate hypoplasia and concurrent middle ear pathology in six dogs. *Journal of Small Animal Practice* 50 (7): 364–372.

Wildermuth, B.E., Griffin, C.E., and Rosenkrantz, W.S. (2012). Response of feline eosinophilic plaques and lip ulcers to amoxicillin trihydrate–clavulanate potassium therapy: a randomized, double-blind placebo-controlled prospective study. *Veterinary Dermatology* 23 (2): 110–e25.

Wiles, V., Hohenhaus, A., Lamb, K. et al. (2017). Retrospective evaluation of toceranib phosphate (Palladia) in cats with oral squamous cell carcinoma. *Journal of Feline Medicine and Surgery* 19 (2): 185–193.

CHAPTER 38 Aerodigestive Disorders

Beatrice Ruggerone and Fabio Procoli

Anicura Ospedale Veterinario I Portoni Rossi, Zola Predosa, BO, Italy

KEY POINTS

- **Update on the use of gastroprotectants in dogs:** The recent ACVIM consensus has reviewed the scientific evidence regarding the use of commonly prescribed drugs in veterinary medicine as gastroprotectants, demonstrating the actual efficacy of a limited group of molecules – particularly proton pump inhibitors – in very specific clinical conditions, such as reflux esophagitis and gastroduodenal ulcers.
- **Update on treatment of megaesophagus:** In addition to selecting the most appropriate food consistency for the individual patient and feeding in an upright position, recent scientific evidence supports the use of sildenafil in patients with megaesophagus. Its efficacy in reducing regurgitation episodes has been demonstrated, likely due to its action on the lower esophageal sphincter. In certain cases, the placement of a percutaneous endoscopic gastrostomy (PEG) tube and the management of aspiration pneumonia may also be necessary.
- **Update on treatment of aspiration pneumonia:** It is now well established that antibiotic therapy for aspiration pneumonia should be reserved for patients exhibiting systemic signs of infection – such as fever, marked neutrophilia or neutropenia, left shift, hyperbilirubinemia, or hypoglycemia – while conservative management (including nebulization, coupage, and prevention of further aspiration) may be sufficient in other cases. Furthermore, the duration of antibiotic treatment should be short (5–7 days) and guided by both clinical assessment and inflammatory markers, such as C-reactive protein.

INTRODUCTION

Aerodigestive disorders (ADs) refer to a wide range of diseases characterized by functional and/or mechanical defects pathologically linking the respiratory and the digestive tracts (Grobman and Reinero 2023).

ADs are a well-recognized entity in human medicine, to the extent that specific departments exist that are solely dedicated to the diagnosis and management of these diseases, which mostly affect the pediatric and geriatric population. Numerous specialty experts are involved in the evaluation of patients suffering from ADs, including otolaryngologists, gastroenterologists, pulmonologists, neurologists, and sleep medicine experts. On the contrary, ADs are poorly characterized and often overlooked in veterinary medicine, partly because of a lack of widely accessible expertise in addition to diagnostic limitations.

ADs typically result from defects in the swallowing reflex or in airway protection or from a combination of both, which can initiate or worsen respiratory and/or digestive diseases. Clinical signs of ADs can be subtle and insidious in onset and can span from chronic cough of different severity, with or without concurrent gastrointestinal signs, to severe aspiration pneumonia and associated respiratory distress.

Disorders of the Liver, Exocrine Pancreas, and Gastrointestinal Tract in Dogs and Cats, First Edition. Edited by Harry Cridge et al. Published 2026 by John Wiley & Sons, Inc. Companion Website: www.wiley.com/go/cridge/disorders

This chapter will review recognized ADs, classified based on their anatomical location, highlighting overall clinical presentation, and presenting available diagnostic and treatment strategies.

CLASSIFICATION

Aerodigestive defects can be classified based on the anatomical location and are listed in Table 38.1, together with the suggested diagnostic method and available treatments.

Table 38.1 Recognized Aerodigestive Diseases in Dogs and the Corresponding Diagnostic Methods and Treatment (When Known)

Upper airway disorders	Diagnostic method	Treatment
BOAS	Upper airway exam, endoscopy	Resection of laryngeal saccules, correction of soft palate and stenotic nares
Rhinitis	Endoscopy, histopathology	According to the etiology: antimicrobials, NSAIDs, corticosteroids, reflux treatment (small frequent meals with a low-fat diet, PPI, and/or prokinetics)
Nasal masses	CT, endoscopy, histopathology	Surgery/radiotherapy/chemotherapy
Nasopharyngeal foreign body	Endoscopy	Endoscopic removal
Laryngeal paresis and paralysis	Upper airway exam, endoscopy	Weight loss, reduction of exercise, NSAIDs, unilateral arytenoid lateralization
Laryngeal collapse	Upper airway exam, endoscopy	Resection of laryngeal saccules, correction of soft palate and stenotic nares
Pharyngeal collapse	Endoscopy, VFSS	Surgery
Sleep-disordered breathing	Radiography, VFSS, CT	
Lower airway and pulmonary parenchyma		
Large airway obstruction	Radiography, VFSS, CT, endoscopy	Endoscopy/Surgery (foreign body)
Tracheitis	Endoscopy, VFSS	According to the etiology: antimicrobials, reflux medical therapy
Chronic bronchitis	Radiography, CT, endoscopy, BAL	Weight loss, inhalatory/systemic steroids, cough suppressant
Bronchiectasis	Radiography, CT, endoscopy, BAL	Antimicrobials (in case of infection), mucoactive drugs
Diffuse aspiration bronchiolitis	CT, histopathology	Antimicrobials (in case of secondary infection)
Aspiration pneumonia	Radiology, CT, BAL	Antimicrobials (in case of infection), *coupage*, nebulization
Interstitial lung disease	Radiography, CT, BAL, histopathology	Antimicrobials (in case of infection), aerosol, steroids
Idiopathic cough	Radiography, CT, endoscopy, BAL	Aerosol, steroids, reflux medical therapy
Upper digestive tract and esophageal gastric junction		
Pharyngeal weakness	VFSS	Surgery, treatment of the primary cause if present

Upper airway disorders	Diagnostic method	Treatment
Pharyngeal mass	VFSS, CT, endoscopy, histopathology	Surgery/chemotherapy
Cricopharyngeal achalasia and dyssynchrony	VFSS	Surgical myotomy/myectomy, botulin injection
Esophageal dysmotility	VFSS	Treatment of the primary cause (see Algorithm 1), vertical feeding, PEG tube
Megaesophagus	Radiography	Treatment of the primary cause (see Algorithm 1), sildenafil, vertical feeding, PEG tube, PPI
Esophagitis	Endoscopy, histology, VFSS	Small, frequent low-fat meals, PPI
Lower esophageal sphincter achalasia-like syndrome	VFSS	Myotomy with partial fundoplication, Botox injection, balloon dilation
Gastroesophageal reflux	VFSS	Small, frequent low-fat meals, PPI, prokinetics
Sliding hiatal hernia	Radiography, VFSS, endoscopy	Medical management with small, frequent low-fat meals, PPI, prokinetics, surgery
Esophageal diverticula/strictures	Radiography, VFSS, CT angiography, endoscopy	Surgery if possible (e.g., persistent right aortic arch), balloon dilation

CT, computed tomography; VFSS, videofluoroscopic swallow study; BAL, bronchoalveolar lavage; PEG, percutaneous endoscopic gastrostomy; PPI, proton pump inhibitors.
Source: Adapted from Grobman and Reinero (2023).

SIGNALMENT, HISTORY, AND CLINICAL SIGNS

Although ADs can affect dogs of any breed and age, brachycephalic (from the Greek "short head") dogs are undoubtedly the most overrepresented, often presenting with earlier onset and more severe signs. Uncontrolled breed selection has significantly reduced the cranial space allocated to the upper airways and the initial portion of the digestive tract in these breeds, leading to the syndrome known as brachycephalic obstructive airway syndrome (BOAS) and dramatic health consequences.

It is important to be aware of certain breed predispositions to specific ADs: West Highland White Terriers, for example, are predisposed to pulmonary fibrosis possibly, secondary to recurrent microaspiration; the Bouvier des Flandres and Shar Peis are predisposed to esophageal motility disorders, while retrievers, German Shepherds, and Fox Terriers are predisposed to megaesophagus.

Clinical signs associated with ADs may primarily involve the respiratory system, the gastrointestinal system, or both simultaneously, according to the anatomical regions affected by functional and/or mechanical defects. The reoccurrence of aspiration pneumonia, the presence of coughing during swallowing of food or water, or the presence of regurgitation should prompt clinicians to suspect an underlying AD.

In cases of BOAS, the most common clinical signs include stertor, stridor, coughing, regurgitation, inspiratory dyspnea, poor exercise and heat tolerance, and syncope. Disorders affecting the nose and nasopharynx are characterized by sneezing, nasal discharge, stertor, gagging, and reverse sneezing. Laryngeal defects present with stridor, dysphonia, exercise and heat intolerance, and collapse.

Lower airway diseases, such as tracheitis and chronic bronchitis, are often associated with coughing. Patients with bronchiectasis are at a higher risk of developing bacterial pneumonia, which can lead to clinical and clinicopathological findings indicative of systemic inflammation (e.g., fever, lethargy, neutrophilic leukocytosis or neutropenia, and elevated serum C-reactive protein concentration).

If aspiration pneumonia develops, signs may be exclusively respiratory (e.g., cough, dyspnea) or systemic, depending on the development of bacterial pneumonia because of alveolar damage.

Cough, tachypnea, and exercise intolerance, with varying degrees of severity, are the main clinical signs in interstitial lung diseases. Functional or structural disorders of the pharynx may lead to dysphagia, a sign often poorly recognized by owners. Therefore, it is important to investigate for the presence of indirect signs associated with dysphagia (e.g., coughing during the intake of water or food, recurrent episodes of aspiration pneumonia, difficulty drinking).

Esophageal disorders (e.g., motility disorders, focal or generalized megaesophagus, esophagitis, lower esophageal sphincter achalasia-like syndrome) will typically present with regurgitation, often confused by owners with vomiting (from which it can be distinguished by the absence of a prodromal phase and abdominal muscle contractions). Since regurgitation is often associated with aspiration pneumonia, patients with esophageal disorders may present with coughing, as well as signs of malnutrition due to reduced food intake.

Dogs affected by sliding hiatal hernia are predisposed to developing gastroesophageal reflux and lower esophageal dysmotility, and will therefore frequently present with regurgitation, frequent swallowing, and odynophagia secondary to esophagitis.

Gastroesophageal reflux disease (GERD) can be asymptomatic or associated with signs such as regurgitation, odynophagia, hypersalivation, anorexia, bloating, or even respiratory signs, such as cough, sneezing, or nasal discharge secondary to inhalation of refluxate and resulting chronic rhinitis.

Among the multiple causes of laryngeal paralysis, polyneuropathies and polymyopathies are recognized, so affected animals may also exhibit peripheral neurological and neuromuscular signs (MacPhail, 2020). Myasthenia Gravis (MG), a known cause of megaesophagus, can present in a generalized form with weakness and exercise intolerance, in addition to regurgitation and dysphonia. A neurological examination is therefore recommended if these conditions are suspected.

DIAGNOSTIC MODALITIES

The diagnostic approach to ADs involves a combination of clinical evaluation, imaging techniques, and functional tests to assess the integrity and coordination of the aerodigestive system. Key diagnostic tools may include:

1. **Endoscopic examination**: flexible laryngoscopy or bronchoscopy to visualize the airways and detect structural abnormalities or signs of aspiration. This system enables direct visualization of the anatomical region of interest, facilitates the collection of cytological or histological samples or bronchoalveolar fluid and allows for therapeutic interventions.
2. **Videofluoroscopic swallow study (VFSS)**: to assess all phases of the swallowing reflex and detect the presence of gastro-esophageal or nasopharyngeal reflux or aspiration. This technique represents the gold standard to evaluate dogs with dysphagia. The patient is fed meal boluses of varying consistency containing radiopaque contrast medium to identify potential anatomical and functional defects. VFSS is also useful to determine the best food consistency in patients with esophageal dysmotility, and to evaluate the efficacy of medical treatment or the response to surgical intervention in patients with GERD.
3. **Imaging**: Radiographic studies, such as a barium swallow or computed tomography (CT), help to assess anatomical structures and detect any pathological changes. Nuclear scintigraphy can measure mucociliary clearance in dogs, reflux, and cumulative small volume aspiration.

UPPER AIRWAY DISORDERS

BOAS is a common cause of upper airway dyspnea. In the vast majority of affected patients, concomitant gastrointestinal tract conditions have been demonstrated, along with a reciprocal worsening of signs until surgical correction of airway abnormalities is performed. During the procedure, histological sampling of the gastrointestinal tract may be useful to confirm a concurrent inflammatory condition.

Upper airway abnormalities in brachycephalic dogs lead to increased resistance to airflow, resulting in airway collapse due to elevated negative pressure. Commonly observed associated conditions include hiatal hernia, esophageal reflux, and esophageal dysmotility. This explains why BOAS patients typically present with concurrent respiratory and gastrointestinal signs.

Surgical correction of anatomical defects is essential to improve prognosis and quality of life in these dogs. Surgical management of hiatal hernia and BOAS, together with medical treatment of gastroesophageal reflux, has led to an improvement in regurgitation in all the treated dogs, despite VFSS findings remaining unchanged before and after surgery (Mayhew et al. 2022).

In human medicine, the presence of extraesophageal reflux can act as an inflammatory stimulus for the upper airways, leading to chronic rhinitis and nasopharyngeal stenosis. In dogs, although this mechanism has not yet been confirmed and remains a hypothesis, clinical signs potentially associated with this condition include sneezing, reverse sneezing, nasal discharge, stertor, and gagging.

Preventing extraesophageal and gastroesophageal reflux should therefore be a therapeutic strategy to consider. The use of proton pump inhibitors, low-fat diets, and prokinetic agents to promote gastric emptying are possible therapeutic options.

LOWER AIRWAYS AND PULMONARY PARENCHYMA

Cough is the sign most commonly associated with lower airway diseases. Chronic tracheitis and bronchitis may result from repeated microaspirations of gastric contents, which exert a significant inflammatory stimulus. Bronchiectasis, an irreversible dilation of the bronchi, can similarly be a consequence of inflammatory stimuli caused by extraesophageal reflux.

The mucociliary damage caused by reflux increases the risk of secondary bacterial infections in these patients. Primary management focuses on controlling reflux and administering antibiotic therapy when secondary bacterial infections develop, particularly if they cause systemic effects consistent with SIRS or sepsis. Clinical signs may include fever, lethargy, neutrophilic leukocytosis, elevated inflammatory markers, hypoglycemia, and hyperbilirubinemia.

Aspiration pneumonia is the most recognized and readily diagnosable condition resulting from the inhalation of gastrointestinal contents following vomiting or regurgitation. The volume of aspirated material can vary, leading to variable outcomes ranging from asymptomatic cases to significant clinical signs such as dyspnea, fever, generalized weakness, or complications such as systemic inflammatory response syndrome (SIRS), or death due to respiratory arrest.

The resulting damage to local defenses predisposes the patient to bacterial pneumonia, requiring appropriate treatment. Radiographically, aspiration pneumonia is identified by an alveolar pattern, typically localized in the right cranial or middle lung lobes, and/or the left cranial lung lobe. A thoracic point-of-care ultrasound (T-POCUS) is a useful method to detect a variety of pulmonary disorders, including pneumonia, and has minimal impact on a dyspneic dog.

In patients with recurrent episodes of aspiration pneumonia, it is crucial to investigate underlying anatomical or functional abnormalities (e.g., airway defects) to prevent recurrences and refine the prognosis.

In addition to localization and anamnesis, the diagnosis of aspiration pneumonia should be confirmed by performing a bronchoalveolar lavage (BAL), which enables culture and sensitivity testing. In cases where confirmation via BAL is not possible but sepsis is suspected, broad-spectrum antibiotic therapy is recommended, along with nebulization and coupage to facilitate sputum expulsion, or oxygen therapy for patients with inadequate oxygenation.

In recent years, the clinical and laboratory monitoring of these patients has been emphasized to determine the appropriate duration of antibiotic therapy. Historically, prolonged antibiotic courses (4–6 weeks) were advised. However, a study by Rodrigues and colleagues (2022) suggests that most dogs with aspiration pneumonia can generally be stabilized with a short (5–7 day) course of antibiotic therapy. Additionally, monitoring of serum CRP concentrations has proven more reliable than repeated radiographic evaluation, as radiographic remission tends to lag behind clinical remission.

UPPER DIGESTIVE TRACT

Pharyngeal weakness or the presence of pharyngeal lesions (e.g., polyps, abscesses, neoplasms) are significant causes of dysphagia in both human and veterinary medicine. The primary condition is common in brachycephalic breeds but can also result from muscular, neurological, or systemic disorders (e.g., cranial nerve deficits, MG, hypothyroidism). Additionally, although not confirmed, extra-esophageal reflux may potentially lead to myositis, causing functional impairment of the pharynx.

Rubin and colleagues (2015) described 28 dogs with dynamic pharyngeal collapse and reported coughing and stertor as common signs. In 27 of 28 cases, a concurrent or previously diagnosed respiratory or cardiac disorder was detected (e.g., tracheal collapse, BOAS, pneumonia, pulmonary hypertension); even if it is unknown whether these diseases were attributed to the pharyngeal collapse, to the concurrent respiratory disease, or a combination of both, this finding is useful to confirm the association between respiratory and gastrointestinal tract disorders.

Achalasia and cricopharyngeal dyssynchrony result in a lack of coordination of the upper esophageal sphincter during the swallowing process, explaining their role in causing dysphagia. These conditions may be acquired (e.g., hypothyroidism, gastroesophageal reflux, MG) or congenital (e.g., focal neuropathy).

Esophageal hypomotility and megaesophagus cause regurgitation, characterized by the effortless expulsion of ingested material through the esophagus. Regurgitation is a risk factor for the development of aspiration and pneumonia, which are among the leading causes of death in these patients, alongside malnutrition, if not properly managed.

Congenital megaesophagus often manifests during weaning and the transition to solid food, leading to stunted growth in affected dogs (see Table 38.2). It appears to result from a defect in vagal afferent innervation. The acquired form is idiopathic in approximately 30% of cases or secondary to various pathological conditions that can influence prognosis. MG is diagnosed in 25–30% of dogs with secondary acquired megaesophagus and is a neuromuscular junction disorder. In affected dogs, the production of autoantibodies against acetylcholine (ACh) receptors reduces receptor uptake, impairing neuromuscular function. This condition may be focal, when involving only the esophagus, or generalized, leading to progressive weakness and exercise intolerance with variable severity and progression.

In a patient with megaesophagus, it is crucial to evaluate all the possible associated conditions, including MG, to guide specific treatment. For idiopathic acquired megaesophagus, the mortality rate is reported at 78%. However, in secondary forms, appropriate treatment of the underlying disease can result in remission of megaesophagus, as seen in 56% of MG cases (Gomes et al. 2020).

MG can be either idiopathic or secondary (see Figure 38.1); for example, in cases of thymoma, the similarity between neoplastic cells and acetylcholine receptors has been demonstrated.

Table 38.2 Main Predisposed Breeds to Megaesophagus

Congenital	Acquired
German Shepherd	Great Dane
Smooth Fox Terrier	German Shepherd
Miniature Schnauzer	Labrador Retriever
Samoyed	Irish Setter
Jack Russell Terrier	Shar Pei
Dachshund	Newfoundland
English Springer Spaniel	Akita Inu
—	Scottish Terrier
—	German Pointer
—	Pug

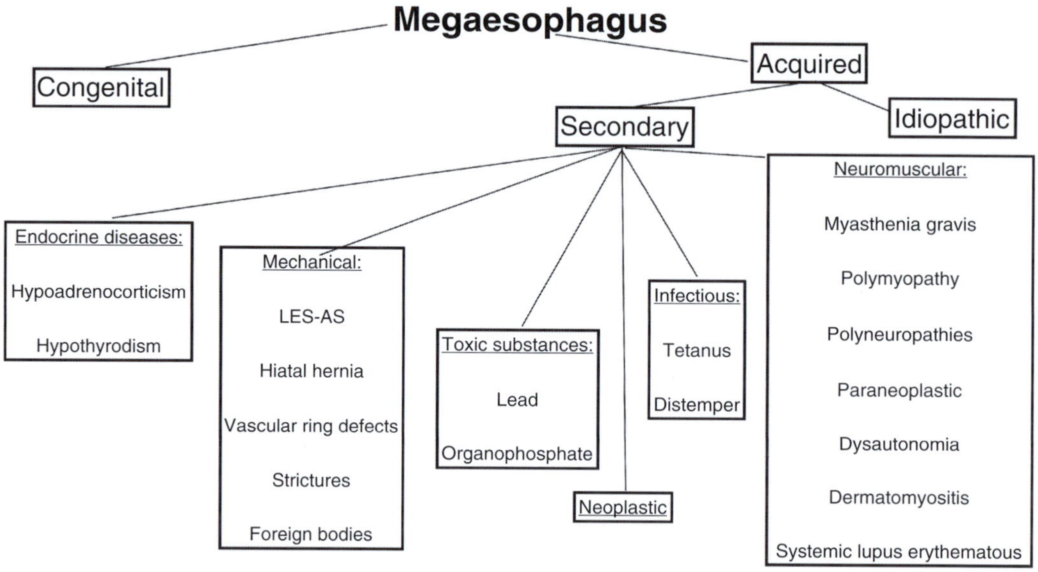

FIGURE 38.1 Suggested classification of megaesophagus in dogs. For the acquired secondary form, main etiologies are reported. LES-AS, lower esophageal sphincter achalasia-like syndrome

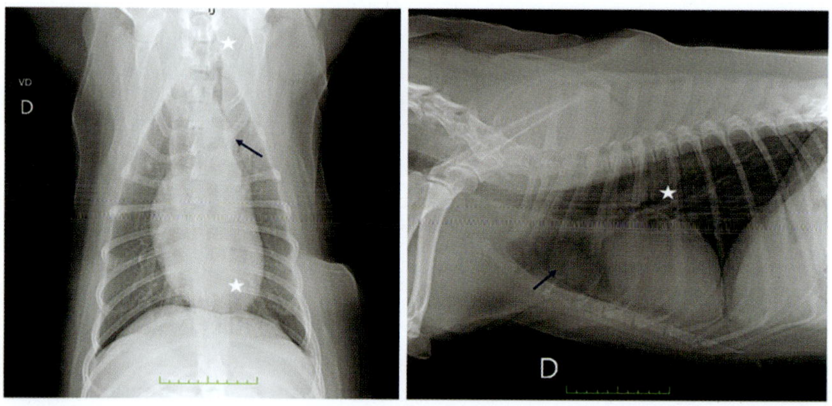

FIGURE 38.2 Thoracic radiographic study of a 6-year-old neutered female Golden Retriever presented for regurgitation. A diffuse megaesophagus (star) was detected, and a mediastinal mass (arrow) was histologically indicative of thymoma. Before surgery, MG was confirmed as the cause of megaesophagus through the detection of an increased level of anti-ACh receptor antibodies (0.7 nmol/L, reference interval <0.6); three days after thymoma removal, megaesophagus was no longer detected, and anti-ACh receptor antibodies were within normal reference intervals

This resemblance stimulates the immune system to produce autoantibodies. Thymoma removal can, therefore, promote the resolution of megaesophagus, as illustrated in the case presented in Figure 38.2.

Once primary causes of megaesophagus have been investigated, excluded, or treated, and if the condition persists, adjunctive treatments become necessary. This includes:

1. Feeding in an upright position, utilizing a Bailey chair, and keeping the patient in this position for at least 20 minutes after meals to facilitate bolus transit to the stomach.
2. Identifying the consistency best tolerated by the patient, such as using gelled water if liquids are not well tolerated or blending food to achieve the most suitable texture.
3. Utilizing a PEG tube to bypass oral feeding, combined with an esophagostomy tube to allow aspiration of persistent esophageal secretions (which could lead to aspiration).

4. Using sildenafil (1 mg/kg PO q8h), which reduces basal tone and increases electrically induced relaxation of LES in dogs with megaesophagus, thereby reducing the number of regurgitation episodes and increasing body weight.

5. Administering antibiotic therapy and performing nebulization and coupage in cases of aspiration (bacterial) pneumonia.

The study by Grobman and colleagues (2019) identified VFSS criteria to detect functional lower esophageal sphincter achalasia-like syndrome (LES-AS), which includes a baseline esophageal fluid line and "bird beak" frequently associated with esophageal motility disorders. Megaesophagus was present in almost 74% of dogs with LES-AS, and the association between these two conditions suggests that LES dysfunction may be a risk factor for the development of megaesophagus. Clinical signs can significantly improve with botulinum toxin injection into the LES associated with pneumatic dilatation, although the procedure must be repeated approximately every 40 days. Surgical myotomy with partial fundoplication is a more permanent therapeutic option.

The loss of integrity of the gastroesophageal barrier is responsible for gastroesophageal reflux (GER). The damage caused by acidic pH, pepsin, trypsin, and bile salts to the esophageal mucosa can lead to esophagitis. Episodes of GER are common during general anesthesia when LES pressure decreases, in cases of delayed gastric emptying (e.g., gastric atony, pyloric outflow obstructions), or with hiatal hernia.

The therapeutic management of GER depends on the underlying cause. For reflux secondary to a hiatal hernia, surgical intervention should be considered if medical management with small frequent meals with a low-fat diet, PPI, or prokinetics is ineffective. In patients with delayed gastric emptying, the use of antral prokinetics (e.g., metoclopramide, cisapride) combined with frequent meals of a low-fat diet is recommended. Metoclopramide increases the release of acetylcholine at the postsynaptic level and antagonizes the effect of dopamine on intestinal motility. It has been shown to enhance gastric contractions in fasted dogs but not in the postprandial phase, whereas it is effective in accelerating gastric emptying in fed cats. Given its short half-life, it should be administered intravenously (0.3 mg/kg/h CRI) or every six hours at a dose of 0.2–0.5 mg/kg IM/PO. Cisapride (dog: 0.1–0.5 mg/kg PO q8–12h; cat: 2.5–5 mg/cat PO q8–12h)—unavailable in some countries—has been shown to increase both the frequency and duration of pyloric contractions as well as enhance intestinal peristalsis. It is more effective than metoclopramide; however, a potential adverse effect associated with its use is diarrhea in both dogs and cats. Additionally, QT interval prolongation has been observed in humans and cats, particularly when higher doses are administered. For secondary esophagitis, the ACVIM consensus on the use of gastroprotectants (Marks et al. 2018) highlights the superiority of proton pump inhibitors (PPIs, such as omeprazole and esomeprazole) over other agents, recommending administration every 12 hours and gradual tapering if used for more than 14 days. In contrast, there is only weak evidence supporting the use of sucralfate for preventing reflux esophagitis, and combining sucralfate with PPIs is not recommended.

REFERENCES

Gomes, S.A., Van Ham, L., Van Ham, A. et al. (2020). Canine nonstructural megaesophagus as a clinical sign of potential neurological disease: 99 cases. *Journal of the American Animal Hospital Association* 56: 7–16. https://doi.org/10.5326/JAAHA-MS-6955.

Grobman, M. and Reinero, C. (2023). A One Health review of aerodigestive disease in dogs. *Journal of Veterinary Internal Medicine* 37: 817–834. https://doi.org/10.1111/jvim.16661.

Grobman, M.E., Schachtel, J., Gyawali, C.P. et al. (2019). Videofluoroscopic swallow study features of lower esophageal sphincter achalasia-like syndrome in dogs. *Journal of Veterinary Internal Medicine* 33: 1954–1963. https://doi.org/10.1111/jvim.15578.

MacPhail, M.C. (2020). Laryngeal disease in dogs and cats: an update. *Veterinary Clinics of North America: Small Animal Practice* 50: 295–310. https://doi.org/10.1016/j.cvsm.2019.11.001.

Marks, S.L., Kook, P.H., Papich, M.G. et al. (2018). ACVIM consensus statement: support for rational administration of gastrointestinal protectants to dogs and cats. *Journal of Veterinary Internal Medicine* 32: 1823–1840. https://doi.org/10.1111/jvim.15337.

Mayhew, P.D., Marks, S.L., Pollard, R. et al. (2022). Effect of conventional multilevel brachycephalic obstructive airway syndrome surgery on clinical and video fluoroscopic evidence of hiatal herniation and gastroesophageal reflux in dogs. *Veterinary Surgery* 52: 238–248. https://doi.org/10.1111/vsu.13906.

Rodrigues, N.F., Giraud, L., Bolen, G. et al. (2022). Antimicrobial discontinuation in dogs with acute aspiration pneumonia based on clinical improvement and normalization of C-reactive protein concentration. *Journal of Veterinary Internal Medicine* 36: 1082–1088. https://doi.org/10.1111/jvim.16405.

Rubin, J.A., Holt, D.E., Reetz, J.A. et al. (2015). Signalment, clinical presentation, concurrent disease, and diagnostic findings in 28 dogs with dynamic pharyngeal collapse (2008–2013). *Journal of Veterinary Internal Medicine* 29: 815–821. https://doi.org/10.1111/jvim.12598.

Disorders of the Esophagus – Megaesophagus

CHAPTER 39A

Jillian M. Haines

Department of Veterinary Clinical Sciences, College of Veterinary Medicine, Washington State University, Pullman, WA, USA

KEY POINTS

- Sildenafil is a promising treatment for management of clinical signs associated with megaesophagus in dogs. It can improve esophageal clearance, reduce frequency of regurgitation, and improve weight gain.
- Therapies targeting the lower esophageal sphincter such as direct injection of botulinum toxin, pneumatic dilation, or surgical myotomy can benefit patients with achalasia.

INTRODUCTION

Megaesophagus is a condition characterized by hypomotility and dilation of the esophagus. While recognized as a major cause of regurgitation in dogs, it remains rare in cats (Washabau 2003; Johnson et al. 2009). It is typically classified as congenital or acquired and can be idiopathic or secondary to a variety of disease conditions (Washabau 2003).

Congenital megaesophagus is thought to arise from dysfunctions in the esophageal afferent sensory pathways within the vagal nerve or anomalies in esophageal muscle properties (Holland et al. 1996; Tan and Diamant 1987). Acquired idiopathic megaesophagus likely results from a failure of vagal afferents to respond appropriately to esophageal distension or defective esophageal muscle function (Johnson et al. 2009). Other acquired forms arise secondary to a variety of systemic or localized diseases (Table 39a.1). Breed associations have been described in dogs and cats for congenital and acquired idiopathic megaesophagus, though any breed can be affected (Table 39a.2).

CLINICAL SIGNS AND PHYSICAL EXAM FINDINGS

Most commonly dogs or cats with megaesophagus will present with regurgitation, which must be differentiated from other signs such as vomiting, expectoration, or oropharyngeal dysphagia (Washabau 2003). Therefore, evaluation begins with a thorough history and physical examination, focusing on distinguishing vomiting from regurgitation or other signs. This can at times be challenging and video footage of the events may be useful. Weight loss or failure to gain weight may be present, but depending on chronicity, patients may have a normal body condition. Puppies may be underweight or smaller than littermates. Other signs that may be described include ptyalism, painful swallowing, halitosis, and dysphagia especially in situations of esophagitis, esophageal foreign material, stricture, or other obstructions. Distension of the ventral esophagus, particularly at the neck or thoracic inlet, may be observed. If present, animals with aspiration pneumonia may present with dyspnea, tachypnea, coughing, lethargy, fever, and/or nasal discharge. On physical exam, findings further suggestive of aspiration pneumonia may be seen such as respiratory distress and pulmonary crackles. Other physical exam findings depend on the presence of any underlying conditions or comorbidities, especially in cases of non-idiopathic acquired megaesophagus.

Disorders of the Liver, Exocrine Pancreas, and Gastrointestinal Tract in Dogs and Cats, First Edition. Edited by Harry Cridge et al. Published 2026 by John Wiley & Sons, Inc. Companion Website: www.wiley.com/go/cridge/disorders

Table 39a.1 Causes of Acquired Megaesophagus

Cause	Description	References
Congenital		
Congenital idiopathic megaesophagus	Most common in pediatric patients, especially those under 3 months of age	Washabau (2003), Boudrieau and Rogers (1985)
Vascular ring anomaly	Includes conditions like persistent right aortic arch, which may lead to esophageal compression	Buchanan (2004)
Acquired		
Myasthenia gravis	The most common cause of acquired secondary megaesophagus in both dogs and cats	Shelton (2002), Shelton et al. (2000), Haines (2019)
Idiopathic	Cause unknown	Washabau (2003)
Esophageal disease	Includes achalasia, esophagitis, foreign body obstruction, and esophageal strictures	Moses et al. (2000), Kempf et al. (2014), Gaynor et al. (1997), Sellon and Willard (2003)
Endocrine diseases	Includes hypoadrenocorticism and hypothyroidism	Haines (2019), Gaynor et al. (1997), Whitley (1995), Jaggy et al. (1994), David (2001), Ko et al. (2018), Bartges and Nielson (1992)
Gastrointestinal disease	Conditions like gastric dilatation–volvulus, hiatal hernia, pyloric dysfunction (cats), and gastroesophageal reflux disease	Gaynor et al. (1997), Keeley et al. (2008), Pearson et al. (1974), Han et al. (2003)
Toxicity	Toxins such as acrylamide, lead, thallium, organophosphates, and various venoms (e.g., Australian tiger snake, tick paralysis)	Gaynor et al. (1997), Satchell and McLeod (1981), Maddison and Allan (1990), Puschner et al. (2012), Harris et al. (1960), Satoh et al. (1967), Hopper et al. (2001), Atwell and Campbell (2001)
Dermatomyositis	Rare, associated with skin and muscle lesions	Hargis et al. (1984)
Geriatric onset laryngeal paralysis polyneuropathy	Seen in older dogs, particularly with underlying polyneuropathy	Bookbinder et al. (2016)
Infectious diseases	Includes canine distemper, *Spirocerca lupi* infection, and trypanosomiasis	Mosallanejad et al. (2010), van der Merwe et al. (2008), Boudrieau and Rogers (1985)
Immune-mediated diseases	e.g., systemic lupus erythematosus affecting neuromuscular function	Boudrieau and Rogers (1985)
Muscular disorders	e.g., glycogen storage disease II, muscular dystrophy, polymyopathy/polymyositis	Dillard et al. (2013), Walvoort (1985), Bedu et al. (2012)
Nasopharyngeal disease	Nasopharyngeal polyps and stenosis in cats	DeSandre-Robinson et al. (2011), Byron et al. (2010), Itoh et al. (2015)
Neuromuscular junction disorders	Botulism and tetanus	Uriarte et al. (2010), Dieringer and Wolf (1991)
Neoplastic/paraneoplastic diseases	Thymoma, brainstem tumors, leiomyomas, lymphoma	Gaynor et al. (1997), Atwater et al. (1994), Long et al. (2001), Kook et al. (2009)
Medications	Potassium bromide and vincristine	Chae et al. (2018), Rossmeisl Jr and Inzana (2009)
Peripheral neuropathy	Dysautonomia, ganglioradiculitis, giant axonal neuropathy, polyneuritis/polyneuropathy, and polyradiculoneuritis	Gaynor et al. (1997), Boudrieau and Rogers (1985), Harkin et al. (2002), Porter et al. (2002), Duncan et al. (1981), Shell et al. (1987)

Cause	Description	References
Select commercial diets	Unknown causative agents linked to food-associated megaesophagus/ polyneuropathy	Hurley et al. (2021)
Trauma	Brainstem trauma or bilateral vagal nerve damage	Gaynor et al. (1997)

Table 39a.2 Breed Associations for Congenital and Acquired Megaesophagus

Condition	Breed	References
Dogs		
Congenital Megaesophagus	Dachshund, Fox Terrier, German Shepherd Dog, Great Dane, Labrador Retriever, Miniature Schnauzer, Newfoundland, Shar Pei, Mixed breeds (especially Goldendoodle)	Haines (2019), Cox et al. (1980), Osborne et al. (1967), Schwartz et al. (1976), Knowles et al. (1990), Glidewell (1983)
Acquired Megaesophagus	Boxer, Chihuahua, Dachshund, German Shepherd Dog, Golden Retriever, Great Dane, Irish Setter, Labrador Retriever, Rottweiler, Mixed breeds	Haines (2019), Boudrieau and Rogers (1985), Gaynor et al. (1997)
Cats		
Congenital Megaesophagus	Domestic Shorthairs (British Shorthair, American Shorthair), Siamese	Forbes and Leishman (1985)

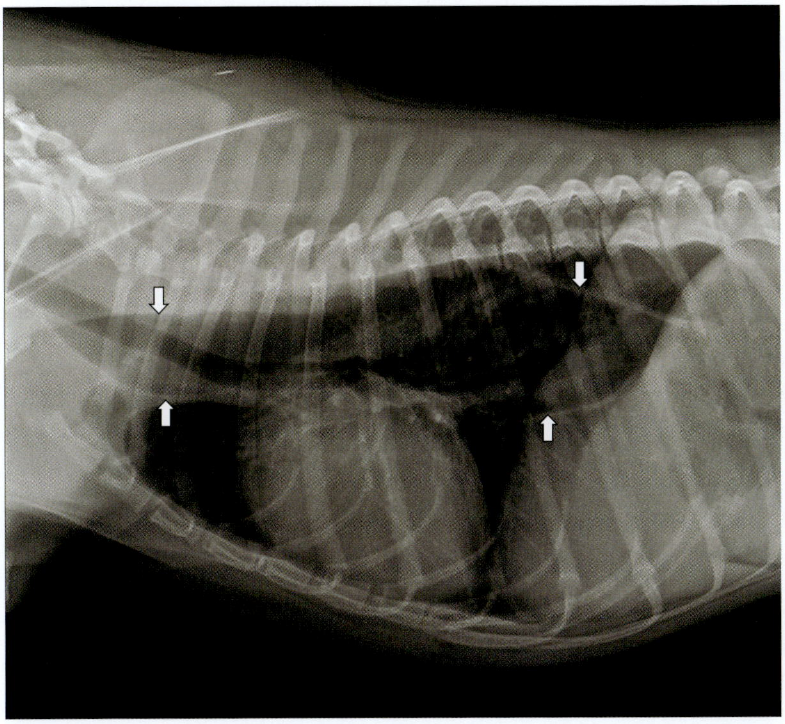

FIGURE 39a.1 Right lateral thoracic radiograph of a dog with diffuse megaesophagus (arrows)

DIAGNOSTIC TESTING

Thoracic radiographs are considered a key diagnostic tool for megaesophagus. Animals with megaesophagus may have diffuse or segmental gas, fluid, or ingesta dilation of the esophagus (Figure 39a.1). Differentiation of dilation secondary to aerophagia can be aided by evidence of gas accumulation elsewhere in the gastrointestinal tract. In some cases of congenital megaesophagus, dilation may be limited to the cranial esophagus if a vascular ring anomaly is present (Buchanan 2004). Aspiration pneumonia typically appears as an alveolar-interstitial pattern. Other abnormalities may be seen if an underlying condition is present such as hiatal hernia, neoplasia, or foreign material.

Contrast esophagrams and videofluoroscopy provide further insights into esophageal motility and structure, especially when survey radiographs are inconclusive (Haines et al. 2019). Videofluoroscopy is particularly useful for detecting swallowing abnormalities, identifying subtle motility issues, and making dietary management recommendations (Bonadio et al. 2009; Haines et al. 2019; Lyngby et al. 2022). Endoscopy, though less commonly utilized, may aid in identifying underlying issues like esophagitis, obstructions, or strictures (Sellon and Willard 2003). Laboratory testing, including complete blood count, biochemistry panel, acetylcholine receptor antibody titers, adrenocorticotropic hormone (ACTH) stimulation, and thyroid panels, aid in identifying underlying diseases contributing to acquired megaesophagus (Shelton 2002; Gaynor et al. 1997; Jaggy et al. 1994). Additional diagnostics, such as muscle biopsies or nerve conduction studies, may be warranted in cases of suspected neuromuscular disease (Cuddon 2002).

MANAGEMENT AND TREATMENT

Treatment of megaesophagus in dogs requires a multifaceted approach aimed at addressing the underlying cause when possible, minimizing regurgitation, ensuring adequate nutrition and hydration, and preventing secondary complications such as aspiration pneumonia and esophagitis. The management of acquired megaesophagus depends on the underlying etiology. In cases where an underlying cause can be identified, such as myasthenia gravis, hypothyroidism, or neuromuscular disorders, treatment of the primary condition may help mitigate the severity of megaesophagus, although resolution of the condition is not guaranteed (Washabau and Day 2013; Johnson et al. 2009; Shelton 2002).

Dietary management is the cornerstone of treatment for megaesophagus. Feeding strategies aim to optimize esophageal clearance to therefore minimize regurgitation risk. Upright feedings are an important part of dietary management as positioning the animal at a 45- to 90-degree angle during and after meals can aid in gravity-assisted esophageal clearance. Feeding devices such as the Bailey chair (Figure 39a.2), stepstool or ladder, feeding platform, or sling may be used (Haines et al. 2019). Meals should be calorically dense to reduce volume, and consistencies such as slurry, gruel, or soaked kibble are often tolerated better than dry kibble (Washabau 2003; Lyngby et al. 2022). There is no standard ideal diet consistency that works for all animals with megaesophagus, requiring that diet plans be individually tailored to each patient (Haines et al. 2019). Small, frequent meals may be necessary in animals with reduced gastric capacities or severe esophageal retention. Water can be problematic, as it may not stimulate lower esophageal sphincter (LES) relaxation in some dogs, potentially leading to prolonged esophageal retention and increased risk of regurgitation (Lyngby et al. 2022; Haines et al. 2019; Mehain et al. 2022). Therefore, it may be best to provide water as part of meals or in thickened forms (e.g., via gelatin cubes, ice cubes, starch-based thickeners), or via subcutaneous administration. For dogs with persistent clinical signs despite medical therapy, placement of a feeding tube, such as a percutaneous endoscopic gastrostomy (PEG) tube, may be considered to bypass the esophagus and provide nutritional support (Gaynor et al. 1997).

Prokinetic medications, such as metoclopramide and cisapride, are effective only on smooth muscle and will not improve motility of the striated muscle of the canine esophagus. They may, however, be effective on the smooth muscle portion of the distal feline esophagus. Cisapride is favored for use in cats due to their increased cholinergic innervation of the esophagus (Schuurkes et al. 1989). These medications can potentially increase LES tone, thus contributing to esophageal retention, making their use contraindicated in many patients (Kempf et al. 2014; Ullal et al. 2016). A response to prokinetic therapy could still be seen when esophageal reflux or delayed gastric emptying is contributing to regurgitation. The use of bethanechol, a cholinergic agent, has been described, but may also result in increases in LES pressures, and its use is not currently well supported in the veterinary literature (Diamant et al. 1974). In some cases, administration of phosphodiesterase inhibitors, such as sildenafil, may help reduce LES tone, improve esophageal clearance, reduce regurgitation

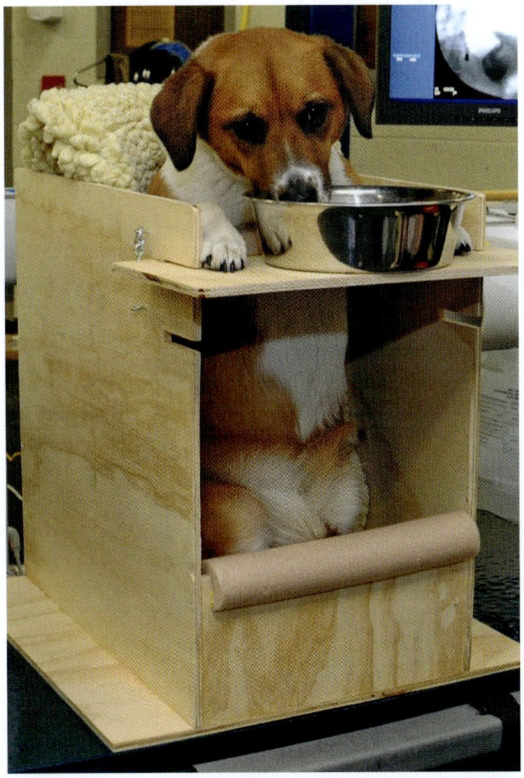

FIGURE 39a.2 Dog utilizing a Bailey chair during a videofluoroscopic imaging study

frequency, lead to increased weight gain, and reduce radiographic esophageal diameter in dogs with megaesophagus (Quintavalla et al. 2017; Mehain et al. 2022).

Other medical therapies focus on managing complications. Antibiotic therapy for aspiration pneumonia should ideally be guided by bacterial culture and susceptibility testing. Broad-spectrum antibiotics can be used empirically when indicated. Commonly used antibiotics include enrofloxacin (dogs) or pradofloxacin (cats), amoxicillin-clavulanic acid, and ampicillin-sulbactam (Levy 2011; Kogan et al. 2008). Proton pump inhibitors (omeprazole) are recommended for treatment of esophagitis and pain management may also be warranted.

Surgical intervention is generally reserved for cases where structural anomalies such as vascular ring anomalies are identified as the underlying cause. LES myotomy has shown potential in patients with achalasia-like syndromes but requires careful patient selection (Grobman et al. 2019). Botulinum toxin injections into the LES or pneumatic dilation of the LES may serve as a diagnostic and therapeutic trial before pursuing surgery (Grobman et al. 2019). Myotomy is generally avoided in patients without confirmed achalasia, as it may worsen clinical signs (Harvey et al. 1974).

Additional supportive care measures can be provided to further reduce aspiration of saliva or esophageal contents such as elevating the head during recumbency to reduce saliva pooling or the use of an esophagostomy tube to suction out material from the dilated esophagus (Manning et al. 2016). Integrative therapies, such as slippery elm or acupuncture, are sometimes used based on anecdotal reports, though evidence supporting their efficacy is limited (Setright 2017).

PROGNOSIS

The prognosis for megaesophagus varies with etiology, severity, and response to treatment. Congenital forms may improve as the animal matures, with some cases achieving resolution before one year of age (Lyngby et al. 2022; Cox et al. 1980). Prognosis for acquired forms depends on the underlying cause and response to therapy (Lainesse et al. 1996; Harjes et al. 2018; Itoh et al. 2015; Ko et al. 2018; Bartges and Nielson 1992). Idiopathic and acquired idiopathic forms often carry a guarded prognosis due to the risk of complications like aspiration pneumonia and malnutrition (McBrearty et al. 2011). Gastroesophageal intussusception is thought to occur at a greater frequency in animals with megaesophagus and carries a grave prognosis (Grimes et al. 2020; Van Geffen et al. 2006). Patient management requires significant owner education and commitment, as lifelong adjustments are frequently necessary to maintain quality of life. Despite these challenges, many animals can lead fulfilling lives with proper care (Haines 2019; Lyngby et al. 2022; Mehain et al. 2022).

REFERENCES

Atwater, S., Powers, B., Park, R. et al. (1994). Thymoma in dogs: 23 cases (1980–1991). *Journal of the American Veterinary Medical Association* 205: 1007–1013.

Atwell, R. and Campbell, F. (2001). Megaoesophagus in dogs with tick paralysis (*Ixodes holocyclus*). *Australian Veterinary Practitioner* 31: 75–79.

Bartges, J. and Nielson, D. (1992). Reversible megaesophagus associated with atypical primary hypoadrenocorticism in a dog. *Journal of the American Veterinary Medical Association* 201: 889–891.

Bedu, A.S., Labruyère, J.J., Thibaud, J.L. et al. (2012). Age-related thoracic radiographic changes in Golden and Labrador Retriever muscular dystrophy. *Veterinary Radiology & Ultrasound* 53: 492–500.

Bonadio, C., Pollard, R., Dayton, P.A. et al. (2009). Effects of body positioning on swallowing and esophageal transit in healthy dogs. *Journal of Veterinary Internal Medicine* 23: 801–805.

Bookbinder, L.C., Flanders, J., Bookbinder, P.F. et al. (2016). Idiopathic canine laryngeal paralysis as one sign of a diffuse polyneuropathy: an observational study of 90 cases (2007–2013). *Veterinary Surgery* 45: 254–260.

Boudrieau, R. and Rogers, W. (1985). Megaesophagus in the dog: a review of 50 cases. *The Journal of the American Animal Hospital Association* 21: 33–40.

Buchanan, J.W. (2004). Tracheal signs and associated vascular anomalies in dogs with persistent right aortic arch. *Journal of Veterinary Internal Medicine* 18: 510–514.

Byron, J.K., Shadwick, S.R., and Bennett, A.R. (2010). Megaesophagus in a 6-month-old cat secondary to a nasopharyngeal polyp. *Journal of Feline Medicine and Surgery* 12: 322–324.

Chae, M.-J., Kim, T.-W., Park, H.-M. et al. (2018). Acquired megaesophagus associated with accidental overdose of vincristine in a dog. *Pakistan Veterinary Journal* 39: 320–322.

Cox, V., Wallace, L., Anderson, V. et al. (1980). Hereditary esophageal dysfunction in the Miniature Schnauzer dog. *American Journal of Veterinary Research* 41: 326–330.

Cuddon, P.A. (2002). Acquired canine peripheral neuropathies. *Veterinary Clinics: Small Animal Practice* 32: 207–249.

David, L.P. (2001). Conditions associated with canine hypothyroidism. *Veterinary Clinics of North America: Small Animal Practice* 31: 935–950.

Desandre-Robinson, D.M., Madden, S.N., and Walker, J.T. (2011). Nasopharyngeal stenosis with concurrent hiatal hernia and megaesophagus in an 8-year-old cat. *Journal of Feline Medicine and Surgery* 13: 454–459.

Diamant, N., Szczepanski, M., and Mui, H. (1974). Idiopathic megaesophagus in the dog: reasons for spontaneous improvement and a possible method of medical therapy. *The Canadian Veterinary Journal* 15: 66.

Dieringer, T. and Wolf, A. (1991). Esophageal hiatal hernia and megaesophagus complicating tetanus in two dogs. *Journal of the American Veterinary Medical Association* 199: 87–89.

Dillard, K.J., Vainio-Siukola, K., Vidgren, G. et al. (2013). Glycogen storage disease II in Lapland dogs. *Federation of American Societies for Experimental Biology* 27 (S1): 874.10.

Duncan, I.D., Griffiths, I.R., Carmichael, S. et al. (1981). Inherited canine giant axonal neuropathy. *Muscle & Nerve* 4: 223–227.

Forbes, D.C. and Leishman, D.E. (1985). Megaesophagus in a cat. *The Canadian Veterinary Journal* 26: 354.

Gaynor, A.R., Shofer, F.S., and Washabau, R.J. (1997). Risk factors for acquired megaesophagus in dogs. *Journal of the American Veterinary Medical Association* 211: 1406–1412.

Glidewell, H. (1983). Clinical signs of idiopathic megaesophagus in great-dane puppies. *Veterinary Medicine and Small Animal Clinician* 78: 202–205.

Grimes, J.A., Fleming, J.T., Singh, A. et al. (2020). Characteristics and long-term outcomes of dogs with gastroesophageal intussusception. *Journal of the American Veterinary Medical Association* 256: 914–920.

Grobman, M., Hutcheson, K., Lever, T. et al. (2019). Mechanical dilation, botulinum toxin A injection, and surgical myotomy with fundoplication for treatment of lower esophageal sphincter achalasia-like syndrome in dogs. *Journal of Veterinary Internal Medicine* 33: 1423–1433.

Haines, J.M. (2019). Survey of owners on population characteristics, diagnosis, and environmental, health, and disease associations in dogs with megaesophagus. *Research in Veterinary Science* 123: 1–6.

Haines, J.M., Khoo, A., Brinkman, E. et al. (2019). Technique for evaluation of gravity-assisted esophageal transit characteristics in dogs with megaesophagus. *Journal of the American Animal Hospital Association* 55: 167–177.

Han, E., Broussard, J., and Baer, K.E. (2003). Feline esophagitis secondary to gastroesophageal reflux disease: clinical signs and radiographic, endoscopic, and histopathological findings. *Journal of the American Animal Hospital Association* 39: 161–167.

Hargis, A.M., Haupt, K.H., Hegreberg, G.A. et al. (1984). Familial canine dermatomyositis. Initial characterization of the cutaneous and muscular lesions. *American Journal of Pathology* 116: 234–44.

Harjes, L., Le Pommellet, H., Hostnik, E. et al. (2018). Resolution of esophageal dysmotility following treatment of nasal disease in a dog. *The Canadian Veterinary Journal* 59: 147.

Harkin, K.R., Andrews, G.A., & Nietfeld, J.C. (2002). Dysautonomia in dogs: 65 cases (1993–2000). *Journal of the American Veterinary Medical Association* 220: 633–639.

Harris, L.D., Ashworth, W., and Ingelfinger, F.J. (1960). Esophageal aperistalsis and achalasia produced in dogs by prolonged cholinesterase inhibition. *The Journal of Clinical Investigation* 39: 1744–1751.

Harvey, C.E., O'brien, J.A., Durie, V.R. et al. (1974). Megaesophagus in the dog: a clinical survey of 79 cases. *Journal of the American Veterinary Medical Association* 165: 443–6.

Holland, C., Satchell, P., and Farrow, B. (1996). Vagal esophagomotor nerve function and esophageal motor performance in dogs with congenital idiopathic megaesophagus. *American Journal of Veterinary Research* 57: 906–913.

Hopper, K., Beck, C., and Slocombe, R. (2001). Megaoesophagus in adult dogs secondary to Australian tiger snake envenomation. *Australian Veterinary Journal* 79: 672–675.

Hurley, K.J., Mansfield, C., Vanhoutan, I.M. et al. (2021). A comparative analysis of two unrelated outbreaks in Latvia and Australia of acquired idiopathic megaesophagus in dogs fed two brands of commercial dry dog foods: 398 cases (2014–2018). *Journal of the American Veterinary Medical Association* 259: 172–183.

Itoh, T., Nishi, A., Uchida, K. et al. (2015). Resolution of megaesophagus after excision of a nasopharyngeal polyp in an 8-month-old cat. *Japanese Journal of Veterinary Anesthesia & Surgery* 46: 77–79.

Jaggy, A., Oliver, J.E., Ferguson, D.C. et al. (1994). Neurological manifestations of hypothyroidism: a retrospective study of 29 dogs. *Journal of Veterinary Internal Medicine* 8: 328–336.

Johnson, B.M., Denovo, R.C., and Mears, E.A. (2009). Canine megaesophagus. In: *Kirk's Current Veterinary Therapy*, 14e (ed. J.D. Bonagura and D.C. Twedt), 486–492. Saunders.

Keeley, B., Puggioni, A., and Pratschke, K. (2008). Congenital oesophageal hiatal hernia in a pug. *Irish Veterinary Journal* 61: 389.

Kempf, J., Lewis, F., Reusch, C.E. et al. (2014). High-resolution manometric evaluation of the effects of cisapride and metoclopramide hydrochloride administered orally on lower esophageal sphincter pressure in awake dogs. *American Journal of Veterinary Research* 75: 361–366.

Knowles, K., O'brien, D., and Amann, J. (1990). Congenital idiopathic megaesophagus in a litter of Chinese shar peis: clinical, electrodiagnostic, and pathological findings. *Journal of the American Animal Hospital Association* 26: 313–318.

Ko, G.-B., Kim, J., Choi, H.-I. et al. (2018). Improvement of megaesophagus after treatment of concurrent hypothyroidism. *Journal of Veterinary Clinics* 35: 19–21.

Kogan, D.A., Johnson, L.R., Sturges, B.K. et al. (2008). Etiology and clinical outcome in dogs with aspiration pneumonia: 88 cases (2004–2006). *Journal of the American Veterinary Medical Association* 233: 1748–1755.

Kook, P., Wiederkehr, D., Makara, M. et al. (2009). Megaesophagus secondary to an esophageal leiomyoma and concurrent esophagitis. *Schweizer Archiv fur Tierheilkunde* 151: 497–501.

Lainesse, M., Taylor, S.M., Myers, S.L. et al. (1996). Focal myasthenia gravis as a paraneoplastic syndrome of canine thymoma: improvement following thymectomy. *Journal of the American Animal Hospital Association* 32: 111–117.

Levy, N.A. (2011). *Aspiration Pneumonia: Risk Factors and Diagnosis in Dogs and Cats.* MI.

Long, S.N., Johnston, P.E., and Anderson, T.J. (2001). Primary T-cell lymphoma of the central nervous system in a dog. *Journal of the American Veterinary Medical Association* 218: 719–722.

Lyngby, J.G., Haines, J.M., and Guess, S.C. (2022). Use of a videofluoroscopic feeding evaluation to guide management of dogs with congenital idiopathic megaoesophagus. *Veterinary Medicine and Science* 8: 1434–1442.

Maddison, J. and Allan, G. (1990). Megaesophagus attributable to lead toxicosis in a cat. *Journal of the American Veterinary Medical Association* 197: 1357.

Manning, K., Birkenheuer, A., Briley, J. et al. (2016). Intermittent at-home suctioning of esophageal content for prevention of recurrent aspiration pneumonia in 4 dogs with megaesophagus. *Journal of Veterinary Internal Medicine* 30: 1715–1719.

Mcbrearty, A.R., Ramsey, I.K., Courcier, E.A. et al. (2011). Clinical factors associated with death before discharge and overall survival time in dogs with generalized megaesophagus. *Journal of the American Veterinary Medical Association* 238: 1622–8.

Mehain, S.O., Haines, J.M., and Guess, S.C. (2022). A randomized crossover study of compounded liquid sildenafil for treatment of generalized megaesophagus in dogs. *American Journal of Veterinary Research* 83: 317–323.

Mosallanejad, B., Ghadiri, A., and Avizeh, R. (2010). The possible relationship of megaesophagus and canine distemper in two German shepherd dogs. *Iranian Journal of Veterinary Research* 11: 379–382.

Moses, L., Harpster, N., Beck, K., et al. (2000). Esophageal motility dysfunction in cats: a study of 44 cases. *Journal of the American Animal Hospital Association* 36; 309–312.

Osborne, C., Clifford, D., and Jessen, C. (1967). Hereditary esophageal achalasia in dogs. *Journal of the American Veterinary Medical Association* 151: 572–581.

Pearson, H., Gaskell, C., Gibbs, C. et al. (1974). Pyloric and oesophageal dysfunction in the cat. *Journal of Small Animal Practice* 15: 487–502.

Porter, B., Schatzberg, S., McDonough, S., et al. (2002). Ganglioradiculitis (sensory neuronopathy) in a dog: clinical, morphologic, and immunohistochemical findings. *Veterinary Pathology* 39: 598–602.

Puschner, B., Basso, M.M., and Graham, T.W. (2012). Thallium toxicosis in a dog consequent to ingestion of Mycoplasma agar plates. *Journal of Veterinary Diagnostic Investigation* 24: 227–230.

Quintavalla, F., Menozzi, A., Pozzoli, C. et al. (2017). Sildenafil improves clinical signs and radiographic features in dogs with congenital idiopathic megaoesophagus: a randomised controlled trial. *The Veterinary Record* 180: 404.

Rossmeisl Jr, J.H. and Inzana, K.D. (2009). Clinical signs, risk factors, and outcomes associated with bromide toxicosis (bromism) in dogs with idiopathic epilepsy. *Journal of the American Veterinary Medical Association* 234: 1425–1431.

Satchell, P. and Mcleod, J. (1981). Megaoesophagus due to acrylamide neuropathy. *Journal of Neurology, Neurosurgery & Psychiatry* 44: 906–913.

Satoh, H., Nishimura, A., Hirota, K. et al. (1967). An experimental development of esophageal achalasia: achalasia-like dogs after the administration of phthalimidomethyl o, o dimethylphosphorodithioate (pmp: cholinesterase inhibitor). *Gastroenterologia Japonica* 2: 214–214.

Schuurkes, J., Van Bergen, P., and Van Nueten, J. (1989). Cholinergic innervation of the feline esophagus. *British Journal of Pharmacology* 96: 50.

Schwartz, A., Ravin, C.E., Greenspan, R.H. et al. (1976). Congenital neuromuscular esophageal disease in a litter of newfoundland puppies 1. *Veterinary Radiology* 17: 101–105.

Sellon, R.K. and Willard, M.D. (2003). Esophagitis and esophageal strictures. *Veterinary Clinics: Small Animal Practice* 33: 945–967.

Setright, R. (2017). Prevention of symptoms of gastric irritation (GERD) using two herbal formulas: an observational study. *Journal of the Australian Traditional-Medicine Society* 23: 68.

Shell, L., Jortner, B., Leib, M. (1987). Spinal muscular atrophy in two Rottweiler littermates. *Journal of the American Veterinary Medical Association* 190: 878–880.

Shelton, G.D. (2002). Myasthenia gravis and disorders of neuromuscular transmission. *Veterinary Clinics of North America: Small Animal Practice* 32: 189–206.

Shelton, G.D., Ho, M., and Kass, P.H. (2000). Risk factors for acquired myasthenia gravis in cats: 105 cases (1986–1998). *Journal of the American Veterinary Medical Association* 216: 55–57.

Tan, B. and Diamant, N. (1987). Assessment of the neural defect in a dog with idiopathic megaesophagus. *Digestive Diseases and Sciences* 32: 76–85.

Ullal, T.V., Kass, P.H., Conklin, J.L. et al. (2016). High-resolution manometric evaluation of the effects of cisapride on the esophagus during administration of solid and liquid boluses in awake healthy dogs. *American Journal of Veterinary Research* 77: 818–827.

Uriarte, A., Thibaud, J.-L., and Blot, S. (2010). Botulism in 2 urban dogs. *The Canadian Veterinary Journal* 51: 1139.

Van Der Merwe, L.L., Kirberger, R.M., Clift, S. et al. (2008). *Spirocerca lupi* infection in the dog: a review. *The Veterinary Journal* 176: 294–309.

Van Geffen, C., Saunders, J., Vandevelde, B. et al. (2006). Idiopathic megaoesophagus and intermittent gastro-oesophageal intussusception in a cat. *Journal of Small Animal Practice* 47: 471–475.

Walvoort, H. (1985). Glycogen storage disease type II in the Lapland dog. *Veterinary Quarterly* 7: 187–190.

Washabau, R.J. (2003). Gastrointestinal motility disorders and gastrointestinal prokinetic therapy. *Veterinary Clinics of North America: Small Animal Practice* 33: 1007–1028.

Washabau, R.J. and Day, M.J. (2013). *Canine and Feline Gastroenterology*. St. Louis, MO: Elsevier Saunders.

Whitley, N. (1995). Megaoesophagus and glucocorticoid-deficient hypoadrenocorticism in a dog. *Journal of Small Animal Practice* 36: 132–135.

Disorders of the Esophagus (Excluding Megaesophagus)

CHAPTER 39B

Dan Batchelor

Department of Veterinary Clinical Sciences, School of Veterinary Science, University of Liverpool, Neston, UK

KEY POINTS

- Careful history taking is essential when investigating esophageal disorders – to distinguish between dysphagia and regurgitation, and between regurgitation and vomiting.
- Acid-suppressant drugs are overprescribed in veterinary practice but might be indicated in various esophageal disorders such as esophagitis. Proton-pump inhibitors (PPIs) are the drugs of choice to reach pH targets that have been established for treatment of acid-related disorders in humans and should usually be given twice daily rather than once daily. After prolonged administration, tapering of the dose is recommended, to avoid rebound acid hypersecretion. PPIs can have adverse effects – they alter the intestinal microbiome, and diarrhea is a common adverse effect in dogs. Oral H2-receptor antagonists are generally not recommended, either alone or in combination with PPIs.
- Some conditions, such as gastroesophageal reflux disease and sliding hiatal hernia, can be very difficult to diagnose. The clinician might ultimately only be able to make a tentative diagnosis based on the clinical presentation, exclusion of other causes for the clinical signs, or response to trial treatment.

NORMAL STRUCTURE AND FUNCTION

The major function of the esophagus is to move food from the oropharynx to the stomach. Anatomically, it begins at the upper esophageal sphincter (UES, composed of the cricopharyngeus and thyropharyngeus muscles), continues as the esophageal body, with cervical and thoracic portions, and a very short abdominal portion, and ends at the lower esophageal sphincter (LES).

The esophageal layers are mucosa, submucosa, muscularis, and adventitia. In dogs, the muscularis comprises two layers of striated muscle, with the LES having an outer layer of longitudinal striated muscle and an inner layer of circular smooth muscle. In cats, the muscularis caudal to the heart base, and the LES, are solely smooth muscle. The endoscopic appearance also varies between species: in dogs, longitudinal folds are present while in cats both longitudinal and transverse folds are present, giving the characteristic "herringbone" appearance distal to the heart base (Figure 39b.1). The esophageal mucosa has a stratified squamous epithelium that terminates at the stomach, with the sharp demarcation to columnar gastric mucosa clearly identifiable on endoscopy.

SWALLOWING

Swallowing is a sequence of coordinated events that transport food or liquid from mouth to stomach. In the oral phase, movements of the tongue, jaws, and hyoid muscles move the bolus to the pharynx. In the pharyngeal phase, there is synchronized contraction of pharyngeal muscles together with relaxation of the cricopharyngeus muscle to allow passage of the bolus into the esophagus. At the same time, breathing pauses, and closure of the glottis and elevation of the soft palate prevent food entering the

Disorders of the Liver, Exocrine Pancreas, and Gastrointestinal Tract in Dogs and Cats, First Edition. Edited by Harry Cridge et al. Published 2026 by John Wiley & Sons, Inc. Companion Website: www.wiley.com/go/cridge/disorders

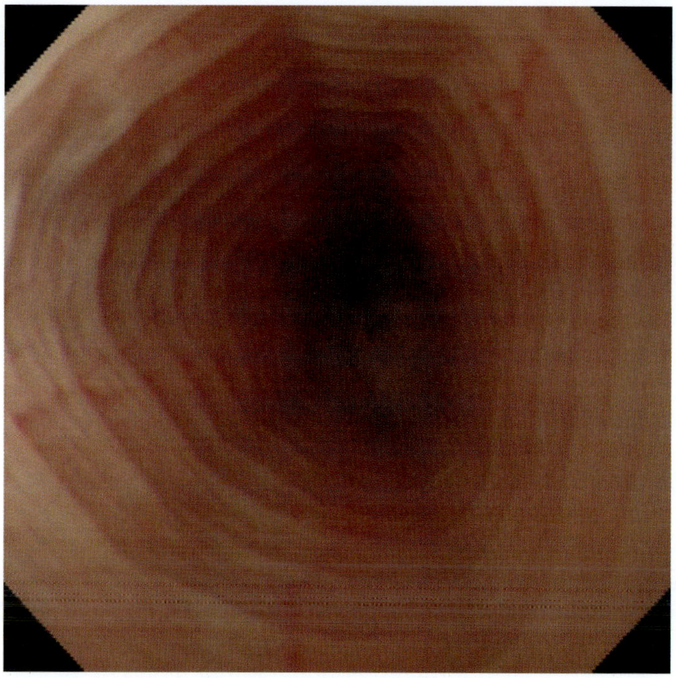

FIGURE 39b.1 Normal endoscopic appearance of the esophagus of a cat, showing the characteristic "herringbone" appearance

airway or nasopharynx. In the esophageal phase, an involuntary primary peristaltic wave moves the bolus along the esophagus. A secondary peristaltic wave is triggered by local distension of the esophagus if any material is left behind. The LES relaxes ahead of the peristaltic wave to allow food to enter the stomach, and then contracts again, acting to prevent reflux of stomach content back into the esophagus.

CRICOPHARYNGEAL MUSCLE DYSFUNCTION

Also known as cricopharyngeal dysphagia, cricopharyngeal muscle dysfunction refers to a group of disorders in which either the cricopharyngeus fails to relax (achalasia), or there is weak pharyngeal contraction leading to asynchrony between the contraction of the pharynx and relaxation of the UES. The etiology is unknown but hypothesized to be a focal neuropathy.

RECOGNITION AND DIAGNOSIS

Animals typically show signs from a young age, at the time of or soon after weaning. Careful information gathering during the clinical history, as well as direct observation of the animal eating, helps to identify a problem of dysphagia rather than regurgitation. Clinical signs are characterized by multiple ineffectual swallowing attempts, gagging, retching, discomfort, and salivation. Coughing or nasal discharge may be present if ingesta enters the airways or nasopharynx. Cricopharyngeal achalasia cannot be distinguished from cricopharyngeal weakness or asynchrony from clinical signs alone.

Once structural causes of dysphagia, such as foreign body or mass in the pharynx, have been excluded, definitive diagnosis of cricopharyngeal muscle dysfunction relies on videofluoroscopy.

TREATMENT

Treatment of cricopharyngeal achalasia is surgical, by performing myotomy or myectomy of the cricopharyngeus. Prognosis is guarded; dysphagia completely resolves immediately in some dogs after surgery, but others show no improvement or only partial resolution (Niles et al. 2001; Warnock et al. 2003). Bilateral myectomy can be considered for dogs that fail unilateral myectomy (Langlois et al. 2014).

Myectomy can also be beneficial in some cases of cricopharyngeal asynchrony, but if videofluoroscopy shows pharyngeal weakness, owners must be warned that surgery can exacerbate the problem if the weakness is not a consequence of the obstructing cricopharyngeus muscle. If doubt exists, one option is to treat the animal using injections of botulinum toxin into the cricopharyngeus as is done in people (Wei 2022). The temporary (3–4 months) effect can be used to screen for dogs that might benefit from myectomy.

ESOPHAGITIS

Esophagitis can result from ingestion of caustic substances, thermal injury (for example, the dog that snatches a dropped hot potato or sausage), lodged foreign bodies, or gastroesophageal reflux. General anesthesia is a common cause of gastroesophageal reflux (Wilson et al. 2005; Zacuto et al. 2012; Paran et al. 2023), most injectable anesthetic or sedative agents are associated with reduced LES pressure as are all inhalant anesthetics. Other causes of gastroesophageal reflux include upper airway obstruction (including brachycephalic airway obstruction syndrome [BOAS]), hiatal hernia, pyloric obstruction, gastric atony, and chronic vomiting. Some medications, such as doxycycline or clindamycin, are an irritant to the esophageal mucosa, especially in cats, so administration of 5 ml water by syringe is recommended after each oral dose of these drugs to a cat.

Esophagitis is affected by the frequency and composition of the reflux: gastric acid alone leads to mild esophagitis, but gastric acid combined with pepsin or trypsin, or bile salts with bicarbonate, can lead to severe esophagitis. Esophageal inflammation can itself lead to hypomotility, that is reversible after healing.

RECOGNITION AND DIAGNOSIS

Clinical signs of esophagitis can include pain on swallowing, extension of the head and neck while swallowing, lip-smacking, retching, regurgitation, discomfort, halitosis, and refusal to eat despite seeming hungry. If associated with anesthesia-induced reflux, clinical signs usually start 1–3 days after the anesthetic.

Diagnosis is best made on endoscopy, and this is normally enough for diagnosis: esophagitis is characterized by increased vascularity, a roughened, granular surface, and sometimes linear erythematous striations. If severe, ulceration may be present. Mild esophagitis can appear normal endoscopically. Biopsy can be performed, if desired, but it can be difficult to obtain good quality samples unless the esophagitis is severe.

TREATMENT

Management consists of gastric acid suppression and medication to increase LES pressure.

GASTRIC ACID SUPPRESSION

Proton-pump inhibitors (PPIs) (e.g., omeprazole, pantoprazole, esomeprazole, lansoprazole) are the drugs of choice and have been shown to be superior to H2-receptor antagonists for increasing gastric pH in animals (Tolbert et al. 2011; Grady et al. 2024). Inhibition of gastric acid secretion is about 30% of maximal on day 1 of treatment and reaches a maximum in 2–4 days. PPIs are most effective if taken either shortly before a meal, or with a meal.

PPIs are overprescribed in veterinary practice, and while esophagitis is a valid reason for their use, they should still be prescribed judiciously. Evidence for serious adverse effects in dogs or cats is lacking to date, but numerous adverse effects are associated with their use in humans, including kidney disease, pneumonia, dementia, cobalamin deficiency, and osteoporosis, in addition to several other conditions, though often based on low-quality evidence. Hypergastrinemia associated with chronic administration of PPIs has been linked to gastric tumors in rats, but this is not thought to be a concern in human medicine. PPIs can alter the intestinal microbiome and therefore may result in the consequential effects of that, and it is unknown whether use of probiotics will mitigate these effects. Diarrhea is a common adverse effect in dogs, but not in cats.

Twice-daily, rather than once-daily, administration of PPIs is recommended in both dogs and cats to reach pH targets that have been established for treatment of acid-related disorders in humans. Esomeprazole may be an exception, as a study in healthy beagles suggested that once-daily dosing may be adequate (Hwang et al. 2017). There is no conclusive evidence to show that one PPI is more effective than another. After prolonged administration (>4 weeks), tapering of the dose is recommended, to avoid rebound acid hypersecretion.

Oral H2-receptor antagonists are not recommended in the management of esophagitis, either alone or in combination with PPIs (Marks et al. 2018). They can in fact compromise the efficacy of PPIs.

OTHER ASPECTS OF TREATMENT

Cisapride and metoclopramide are frequently used in an attempt to increase LES pressure. In a placebo-controlled study using manometry, cisapride caused a significant increase in LES pressure whereas metoclopramide did not (Kempf et al. 2014).

Sucralfate is frequently used and anecdotally seems to be of benefit although it is doubtful that much orally administered sucralfate will bind to ulcerated esophageal mucosa. If anorexic, a gastrostomy tube allows provision of enteral nutrition, but continuing to feed the animal by mouth has been recommended to potentially reduce the risk of stricture formation. Depending on the underlying cause of the esophagitis, a low-fat diet could be considered to help hasten gastric emptying and therefore reduce gastroesophageal reflux.

Esophagitis normally heals well, especially if mild, but esophageal stricture can be a serious consequence of ulcerative esophagitis, especially if it affects >180 degrees of the circumference of the esophagus.

GASTROESOPHAGEAL REFLUX DISEASE (GERD)

GERD is a disorder of the LES, allowing gastric content to enter the esophagus aborally. Some degree of gastroesophageal reflux is normal in dogs and the point at which it becomes abnormal or excessive is unknown. A scintigraphic study of 12 healthy dogs fed a test meal containing radiolabelled technetium documented reflux of variable magnitude in all 12 (Grobman et al. 2020).

GERD is commonly diagnosed in people and while it may be more common in dogs than previously thought, especially given the increase in popularity of brachycephalic breeds, its significance is difficult to establish in animals. Diagnosis in people relies on the affected person reporting their symptoms to the doctor via a detailed questionnaire (ideally with ambulatory pH monitoring showing a temporal association between reflux and symptoms). Dogs and cats obviously cannot describe their symptoms, so we rely on owner perception of signs. However, clinical signs of GERD in animals are nonspecific, overlap with signs of other gastrointestinal diseases (e.g., chronic enteropathy), and may well be prone to overinterpretation by owners, or alternatively dismissed as "normal for the breed."

A clinical study of 7 healthy dogs and 22 dogs with clinical signs commonly attributed to gastroesophageal reflux used a wireless pH monitoring capsule in the distal esophagus to record reflux events, while owners simultaneously recorded observed clinical signs (Kook et al. 2014). Considerable variation was found in the number of refluxes as well as the amount of time esophageal pH was below 4, and differences were not detected between dogs with clinical signs and healthy dogs. When owner-reported clinical signs were correlated with reflux events detected by pH changes, the median percentage of clinical signs temporally associated with reflux was only 12.5%, and no dog had a convincingly positive relationship between clinical signs and reflux events.

In a separate study of 51 brachycephalic dogs, 84% showed reflux that was considered abnormal, but there was no association between the severity of reflux and severity of respiratory or gastrointestinal signs (Appelgrein et al. 2022).

In 11 French Bulldogs with sliding hiatal hernia, wireless pH monitoring capsules placed endoscopically in the esophagus were used to record up to 96 hours of data, while owners recorded clinical signs at the same time (Ullal et al. 2024). Median acid exposure time was 3.3%, and dogs showed 34–173 reflux events (median 70). Severity of clinical signs and severity of BOAS were not correlated with acid exposure time in this study. However, reflux did improve after BOAS surgery.

RECOGNITION AND DIAGNOSIS

Clinical signs are very similar to those for esophagitis (regurgitation, eructation, pain on swallowing with extension of the head and neck, and ptyalism). Mild cases may show very intermittent regurgitation or be asymptomatic. Regurgitation may occur in the early morning hours because of the transient relaxation of the LES during sleep.

Diagnosis can be difficult and ultimately may only be tentative based on clinical suspicion. In people, the most common form of GERD is the nonerosive form, in which symptoms are present but there are no visible lesions on endoscopy. If this is true for animals, then the diagnosis becomes one of exclusion and response to treatment.

Videofluoroscopy may show gastroesophageal reflux and possibly reduced distal oesophageal motility but can also be normal because gastroesophageal reflux is usually intermittent. Occasional gastroesophageal reflux on videofluoroscopy should not be overinterpreted, as it can be seen in normal animals. Endoscopy can be used to document concomitant esophagitis and gauge its severity. If endoscopy shows an open LES, this should not be overinterpreted, as it may simply be an effect of the anesthetic.

Definitive diagnosis relies on continuous ambulatory measurement of LES pressure and/or esophageal pH. Catheter-based systems are poorly tolerated but the catheter-free, wireless "Bravo" pH monitoring system has been used in dogs.

TREATMENT

Treatment of GERD is similar to that for esophagitis, by increasing LES tone (e.g., cisapride) and reducing gastric acid secretion (e.g., PPIs). Low-fat diets are usually recommended, as long as the animal is not severely underconditioned, to hasten gastric emptying. Underlying conditions should be corrected (e.g., BOAS, hiatal hernia). In humans, surgical management (fundoplication) is employed for management, but to date, trials are lacking in animals.

HIATAL HERNIA

A hiatal hernia refers to protrusion of abdominal contents such as the abdominal esophagus, the LES, parts of the stomach, or other abdominal organs through the esophageal hiatus of the diaphragm into the thorax. The esophagus can never tightly fill its hiatus because it must be able to expand to accommodate swallowed food boluses. Therefore, abnormalities of the phrenicoesophageal attachments can permit herniation. In a CT study, esophageal hiatus cross-sectional surface area in brachycephalic dogs was considerably larger than that in nonbrachycephalic dogs of similar body size (Conte et al. 2020), and this likely predisposes brachycephalics to both GERD and hiatal hernia.

The most common type is the sliding hiatal hernia in which the abdominal esophagus and/or parts of the stomach slide cranially into the mediastinum. This is usually congenital in origin and can be seen in Chinese Shar-peis and brachycephalic breeds, especially French Bulldogs, English Bulldogs, Pugs, and Boston terriers (Reeve et al. 2017). An acquired form may be seen after trauma, or in association with airway obstruction such as severe BOAS or laryngeal paralysis.

Paraesophageal hiatal hernia, in which the fundus of the stomach protrudes into the thorax next to the esophagus (with the LES remaining in the abdomen), is much less common.

RECOGNITION AND DIAGNOSIS

Diagnosis of sliding hiatal hernia is challenging because the herniation is typically intermittent. Clinical signs can include regurgitation, hypersalivation, or vomiting, with signs often triggered by exercise or excitement. Dogs with sliding hiatal hernia may present with a mixture of gastrointestinal and respiratory signs such as cough or exclusively respiratory signs (Grobman et al. 2019; Luciani et al. 2022). Concurrent BOAS may well be present. In fact, BOAS, GERD, and sliding hiatal hernia are now considered as "aerodigestive diseases."

Radiography of the thorax may show a soft tissue opacity in the region of the caudal esophagus, but it is frequently normal because the herniation is dynamic. Videofluoroscopy may demonstrate the herniation but again may be normal (false negative) in the case of a sliding hiatal hernia. Endoscopy allows concurrent esophagitis to be diagnosed. Hiatal hernia is not easy to confirm endoscopically but applying manual pressure to the abdomen or employing a maneuver in which the endotracheal tube is occluded for three breaths can allow more accurate diagnosis, as the associated increase in transdiaphragmatic pressure can provoke the herniation, so that the clinician can see the stomach protrude cranially (Broux et al. 2018 ; Vangrinsven et al. 2021).

TREATMENT

Treatment is usually attempted medically at first, along the same lines as for esophagitis or GERD, with gastric acid suppressants, and prokinetics (such as cisapride or metoclopramide), with or without sucralfate. Feeding a low-fat diet in small, frequent meals might help. Surgical correction of BOAS, if present, will likely be beneficial. If response is inadequate, surgical options, including a laparoscopic approach (Monnet 2021; Marvel and Monnet 2024), have been described. Early surgical intervention is recommended in Shar-peis with congenital hiatal hernias. In sliding hiatal hernia, clinical signs may persist even after successful surgery, because of ongoing gastroesophageal reflux (Mayhew et al. 2017; Mayhew et al. 2021).

STRICTURE

An esophageal stricture is an abnormal narrowing of the esophageal lumen, usually a consequence of severe esophagitis following gastroesophageal reflux under anesthesia, lodgment of a foreign body, or thermal or chemical injury from swallowed substances. In cats, doxycycline or clindamycin-associated esophagitis can be the cause. Damage to the deeper layers of the esophagus leads to a fibrotic reaction, and subsequent contraction causes luminal narrowing and stricture.

RECOGNITION AND DIAGNOSIS

Clinical signs include regurgitation that becomes progressively more severe, along with typical signs of esophageal disease (pain on swallowing, salivation, extension of the neck while swallowing, and sometimes refusal to eat, although most animals remain hungry). Weight loss may occur.

Diagnosis is based on the suggestive history. Up to 65% of cases have a history of recent anesthesia, with stricture formation usually occurring 1–2 weeks after the anesthetic.

A contrast radiograph using barium can be used to confirm the diagnosis, showing focal narrowing at the site of the stricture. Videofluoroscopy will also be diagnostic (Figure 39b.2). Endoscopy allows definitive diagnosis, as well as distinguishing benign from malignant strictures (Figure 39b.3).

TREATMENT

Management is usually by balloon dilation (Figure 39b.4). After initial dilation, the procedure is repeated every 4–7 days, as strictures tend to recur; typically, 2–4 procedures per animal are needed. Multiple dilations are sometimes needed. Intralesional injections of triamcinolone (2.5 mg of triamcinolone injected into each of the 4 quadrants around the stricture) is associated with a lower

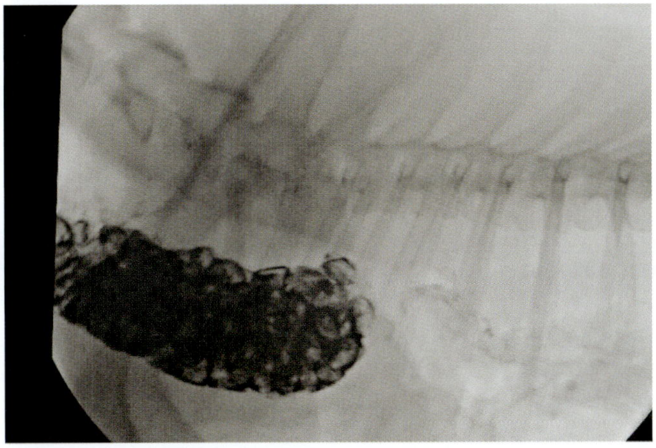

FIGURE 39b.2 Still fluoroscopic image of a 2-year-old French Bulldog who developed progressive regurgitation starting 14 days after anesthesia. The food bolus remained statically in the focally dilated cranial thoracic esophagus. The esophageal dilation is seen tapering at the level of the carina. Only a small amount of fluid and individual pieces of kibble progressed aborad from this point and only a minimal amount of food and fluid reached the stomach by the end of the exam

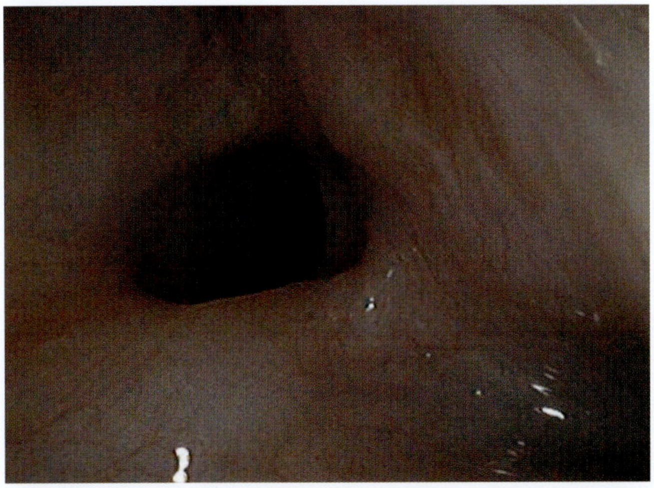

FIGURE 39b.3 Endoscopic appearance of the French Bulldog in Figure 39b.2, confirming an esophageal stricture

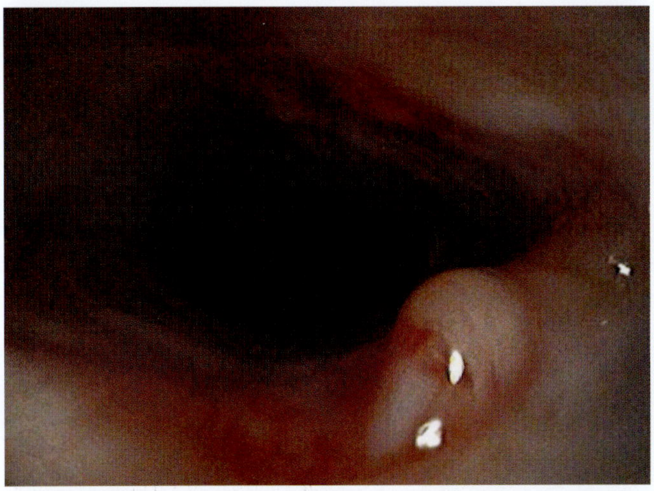

FIGURE 39b.4 Endoscopic appearance of the French Bulldog in Figures 39b.2 and 39b.3, immediately after balloon dilation

rate of recurrence. A tapering course of oral prednisolone is sometimes used after ballooning to also help prevent stricture recurrence. Topical mitomycin C has been used in humans and is associated with reduced risk of recurrence (El-Asmar et al. 2013).

Another option is an indwelling balloon-dilation esophagostomy tube (BE-tube); this device permits twice-daily stricture dilation without the need for general anesthesia. In a prospective study, owners performed twice-daily at-home dilations of the stricture for six weeks (Tan et al. 2018). The tube was relatively well tolerated, and considered effective, with clinical scores improving in 11/12 animals (92%). Esophageal stenting can be performed if strictures are highly recurrent but has a high complication rate and disappointing long-term success rate (Lam et al. 2013).

Medical management as for esophagitis is recommended alongside balloon dilation. Gastrostomy tube feeding may be needed for nutritional support. A good outcome is reported in 59–88% of dogs with esophageal stricture (Adamama-Moraitou et al. 2002; Leib et al. 2001; Da Riz et al. 2021). Other than stricture recurrence, the main complication is esophageal perforation at the time of balloon dilation.

FOREIGN BODIES

These occur frequently in dogs and sometimes in cats. In dogs, the most common esophageal foreign bodies are bones, fishhooks, and chew toys of the "rawhide" type. Terrier breeds, especially West Highland White Terriers, are predisposed, and it is possible that a motility disorder in these breeds predisposes them to lodgment of esophageal foreign bodies. In cats, sewing needles, fishhooks, and trichobezoars are most common. The most common location for entrapment is the caudal esophagus in dogs and the cranial esophagus (just caudal to the pharynx) in cats (Abd Elkader et al. 2020).

Esophageal damage may be direct (such as from angular/sharply pointed foreign bodies), but even smooth foreign bodies can also be highly damaging because of pressure necrosis of the esophageal wall.

RECOGNITION AND DIAGNOSIS

Clinical signs are typical for esophageal obstruction, with regurgitation, gagging, salivation, and signs of discomfort. Halitosis may be present. Diagnosis is straightforward based on the history and confirmed by plain radiography (Figures 39b.5 and 39b.6), although contrast radiography may be required if the foreign body is radiolucent. The radiograph should be evaluated for clues that suggest esophageal perforation (pneumomediastinum, or, less commonly, pneumothorax or pleural effusion).

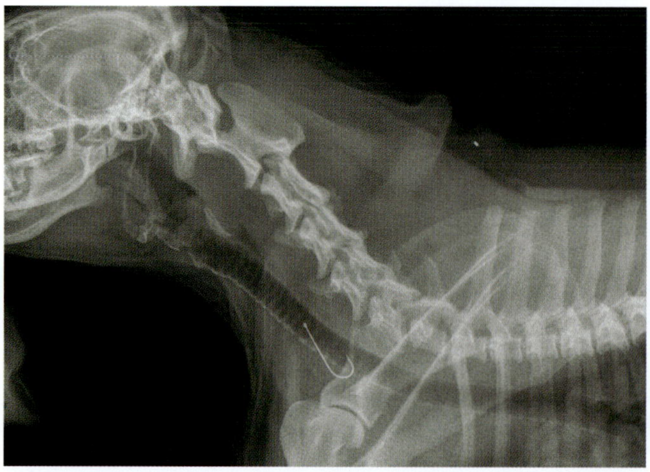

FIGURE 39b.5 Metallic esophageal foreign bodies are easily diagnosed. This dog has ingested a fishhook

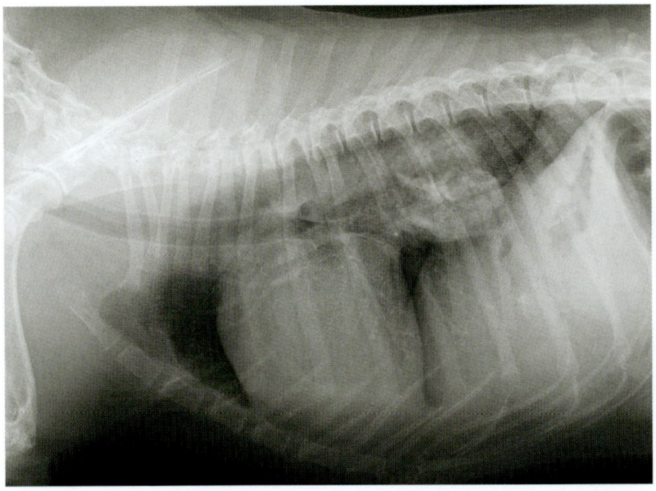

FIGURE 39b.6 Lateral thoracic radiograph of an 11-year-old male Labrador who was lethargic, anorexic, and panting excessively. Two days before presentation, he had been fed a pork knuckle chew. There is an oval-shaped, irregularly, and sharply marginated mineral opacity in the caudodorsal mediastinum, at the level of T8–T10 (esophageal foreign body corresponding to the pork knuckle). There is no evidence of pneumomediastinum or pneumothorax

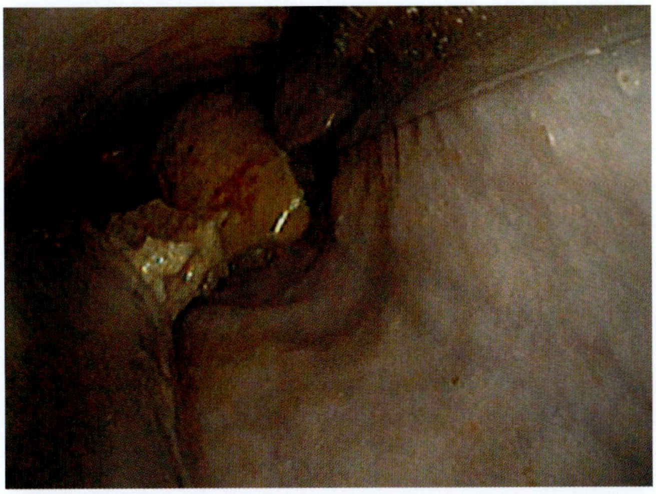

FIGURE 39b.7 The esophageal foreign body from the dog in Figure 39b.6 is being removed gently with grasping forceps

TREATMENT

Esophageal foreign body lodgment should be considered an emergency and removal should be performed as soon as possible. Duration of lodgment is associated with a greater likelihood of the animal requiring surgery (Brisson et al. 2018). If perforation has not occurred, endoscopic retrieval is preferred. The foreign body can usually be removed via the mouth; if not possible, it can sometimes be gently pushed into the stomach, to be removed via gastrotomy (Delligianni et al. 2020), or simply left to digest/dissolve (e.g., bones). The practice of leaving bony foreign bodies in the stomach appears to be safe; in 84 dogs with gastric bone foreign bodies, the majority (74%) were left in situ and there were no reported complications (Barash et al. 2022). Retrieval from the esophagus must be done very carefully as there is a risk of esophageal tearing or perforation. After removal, the extent of esophageal mucosal damage should be assessed endoscopically (Figures 39b.7 and 39b.8), and radiography to assess for the presence of pneumomediastinum is recommended if there is any

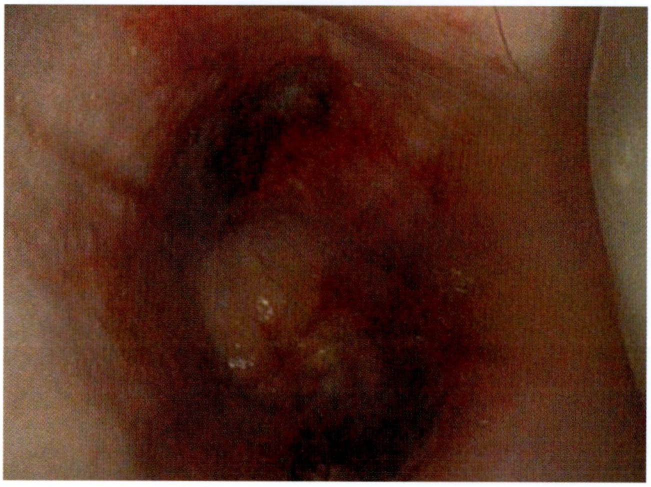

FIGURE 39b.8 Endoscopic appearance immediately after foreign body removal, showing focal ulceration and esophagitis at the site of foreign body lodgment

doubt over whether perforation has occurred. Following removal, animals with moderate or severe esophageal damage should be managed as for esophagitis.

If endoscopic removal fails, or there is evidence of perforation, surgical removal via esophagotomy is indicated (although for very distal foreign bodies, gastrotomy is preferred, being a less invasive procedure). Fishhooks are more likely to require surgical removal (Bongard et al. 2019).

Prognosis is generally good if endoscopic retrieval is successful; complications were reported at the time of removal in 20/349 cases (6%) in one case series, most commonly perforation (Wyatt and Barron 2019). Respiratory or gastrointestinal signs persisted for a few days in a small number of dogs. Overall case fatality rate was around 5% in three large case series (Burton et al. 2017; Brisson et al. 2018; Wyatt and Barron 2019), with risk of death higher in dogs requiring surgery, especially those with esophageal perforation. Of dogs followed >1 month, 2–11% developed esophageal stricture.

Outcomes of surgical intervention were reported by Beer et al. (2022); of 63 dogs undergoing surgery for esophageal foreign body, 50% had a postoperative complication, but 50% of these were minor. 47/63 dogs (74.6%) survived to discharge.

VASCULAR RING ANOMALIES

Vascular ring anomalies are congenital malformations of the major arteries around the heart base that trap the esophagus leading to extraluminal obstruction. Persistent right aortic arch (PRAA) with a persistent left ligamentum arteriosum is the most common form in dogs, but anomalous left or right subclavian arteries, double aortic arch, and several others have been described (Morgan and Bray 2019; Schorn et al. 2021; Shua-Haim et al. 2023; Rossi et al. 2024). German Shepherd dogs and Irish Setters appear predisposed to PRAA.

RECOGNITION AND DIAGNOSIS

Clinical signs are typically seen soon after weaning and include regurgitation and failure to thrive. Most affected puppies or kittens maintain a good appetite (unless they develop aspiration pneumonia) but may be smaller than their littermates. Onset of signs in adult life is reported (Blank et al. 2020).

Diagnosis is based on compatible clinical signs and history, alongside plain or contrast radiography. A plain radiograph is sufficient to diagnose PRAA, confirming the right-sided location of the aortic arch, with a focal leftward curvature of the trachea near the heart base reliably seen. A distended esophagus that abruptly narrows at the heart base may be seen (Figure 39b.9).

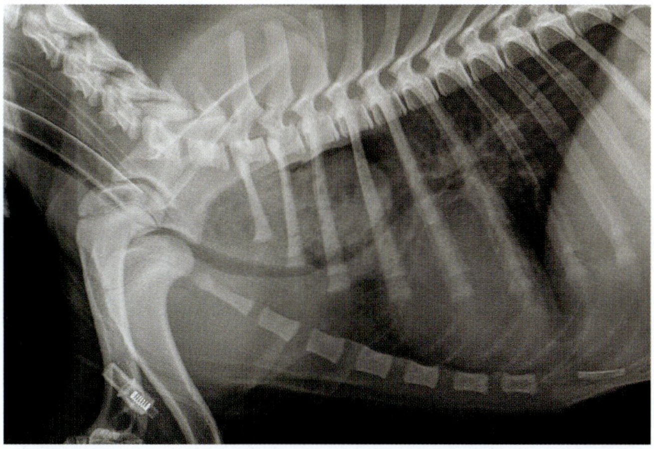

FIGURE 39b.9 Lateral thoracic radiograph of a 6-month-old Cocker Spaniel with persistent regurgitation of solid food since weaning (the dog was able to keep liquid food down). The esophagus cranial to the heart base is distended, and the distension stops abruptly at the heart base. CT angiography confirmed the presence of an abnormal brachiocephalic trunk with a persistent right aortic arch and a focal narrowing of the esophagus at that level, consistent with a vascular ring anomaly

Endoscopy is not usually needed, but if performed, it will help distinguish a vascular ring anomaly from a stricture. CT angiography is the test of choice to assess complex malformations.

TREATMENT

Treatment is surgical; PRAA is treated by surgical ligation and division of the ligamentum arteriosum. Double aortic arch can be successfully managed surgically by ligation of the lesser (usually left) aortic arch (Rossanese et al. 2022).

Prognosis is favorable for most dogs, although hypomotility and clinical signs may persist after surgery, presumably because of chronic distension of the esophagus cranial to the obstruction. In 52 dogs with PRAA, long-term outcome was good or excellent in 87% and poor in the remaining 13% (Krebs et al. 2014).

TUMORS

Esophageal tumors occur uncommonly in dogs and cats. The most common types are squamous cell carcinoma, leiomyoma, and various sarcomas (fibrosarcoma, leiomyosarcoma, osteosarcoma). Sarcomas can develop secondary to *Spirocerca lupi* infestation in dogs. A primary esophageal histiocytic sarcoma was recently reported (Trindade-Gerardi et al. 2024). Para-esophageal tumors (e.g., of heart base, thyroid) can invade the esophagus, and metastasis to the esophagus can occur but is rare. Esophageal lymphoma can be diagnosed in cats, but this too is rare.

RECOGNITION AND DIAGNOSIS

Clinical signs usually develop slowly and are typical for esophageal disease, overlapping with those for other esophageal disorders (regurgitation, gagging, salivation, pain on swallowing, halitosis). Diagnosis can be made on plain or contrast radiographs, which may reveal a mass or esophageal distension proximal to an obstruction. Endoscopy is valuable to identify the mass, distinguish it from foreign body, stricture, or parasitic nodule, and assess any concurrent esophagitis. Biopsy can be performed endoscopically, especially for ulcerated masses, but intramural masses such as leiomyoma may not be amenable to endoscopic biopsy. Appropriate staging for metastatic disease should be performed if neoplasia is diagnosed.

TREATMENT

Benign esophageal masses such as leiomyoma can be successfully managed surgically. Transendoscopic laser ablation has been described for *S. lupi*-associated sarcomas and was associated with low complication rates and a survival time comparable to dogs that have open surgery (Shipov et al. 2015).

Published data on the management of other forms of esophageal neoplasia are lacking; lymphoma can be managed with high-dose chemotherapy, whereas surgery and/or radiation therapy might be useful in some cases. However, surgery is complicated by difficult exposure, poor esophageal healing (especially if there is any tension on the anastomosis), and a risk of postoperative stricture formation. Radiation therapy is complicated by acute and chronic damage to the esophagus itself as well as adjacent mediastinal structures.

ESOPHAGEAL DIVERTICULUM

An esophageal diverticulum is a pouch-like dilation of the esophageal wall. They are rare but can be present as a congenital lesion or an acquired one. Two types are recognized. A pulsion diverticulum is formed secondary to increased intraluminal pressure (because of esophageal obstruction). A traction diverticulum forms because of inflammation within the thorax (most commonly secondary to a penetrating esophageal foreign body), which leads to the formation of fibrous tissue; subsequent contraction pulls the esophageal wall, leading to diverticulum formation.

A small diverticulum may not cause any clinical signs, but food can become trapped in larger diverticula, leading to regurgitation, halitosis, painful swallowing, and anorexia. A large cervical diverticulum may be palpable externally.

Plain or contrast radiographs can show the diverticulum but should be differentiated from the esophageal redundancy seen in brachycephalics, which appears as a flexure near the thoracic inlet and is considered a normal variant. Endoscopy is useful to confirm an esophageal diverticulum.

A small diverticulum can be managed conservatively (soft food, postural feeding with the animal in an upright position), but surgery may be required for larger lesions. Prognosis is guarded in animals that require surgery.

ESOPHAGEAL FISTULA

An esophageal fistula (also called airway-esophageal fistula or broncho-esophageal fistula) is a rare disorder in which an abnormal communication between the esophageal lumen and the trachea or mainstem bronchus exists. They can be congenital, with an increased incidence in Cairn terriers. They can also be acquired, most commonly secondary to a penetrating esophageal foreign body.

Clinical signs are typically coughing after eating or drinking. Aspiration pneumonia and associated clinical signs (fever, cough, dyspnea) may occur.

Definitive diagnosis is by contrast radiography, which demonstrates the abnormal communication between esophagus and airway. Barium contrast medium is recommended if a broncho-esophageal fistula is suspected, as it is less irritant to the airways. Endoscopy of esophagus and/or trachea and bronchi may also be useful in diagnosis.

Treatment is surgical; lung lobectomy is generally indicated, as well as repair of the esophageal wall. Prognosis after successful surgery is good.

SPIROCERCOSIS

Spirocercosis is caused by *S. lupi*, a parasitic nematode found worldwide, especially in tropical and subtropical regions. Most clinical reports are from South Africa, Israel, Greece, India, Pakistan, southern areas of the USA, Kenya, and Brazil. The parasite affects carnivores, especially Canidae, and it has been reported in domestic and wild Felidae. A common complication of chronic spirocercosis, occurring in 8–26% of cases, is development of esophageal neoplasia, especially fibrosarcoma (in younger dogs) and osteosarcoma (in older dogs).

LIFE CYCLE

Adult worms are present in the esophagus of an infected host; *S. lupi* eggs are passed in feces. The intermediate hosts are coprophagous beetles, and after ingestion the worm eggs excyst and develop to L3 larvae within the beetle. A carnivore final host is infected by ingestion of either the beetle or a paratenic host such as a bird, lizard, or rodent. In the final host, L3 larvae excyst in the stomach and migrate via blood vessel walls to the caudal thoracic aorta, where they remain and mature for around three months. Immature adult worms then migrate to the caudal esophagus where they form submucosal nodules. Mature worms (males up to 54 mm, females up to 80 mm) are present in the esophagus by 3–9 months after infection and can remain in the esophagus up to two years. A nodule can be 1–4 cm in diameter and typically contains 3–6 worms.

CLINICAL SIGNS

Signs vary in severity from mild/asymptomatic to severe, and include regurgitation, weight loss, and dysphagia.

Diagnosis is made by finding *S. lupi* eggs on fecal flotation alongside compatible imaging and endoscopic findings. Radiographs may show a caudal esophageal mass and a contrast esophagram may show filling defects corresponding to the *Spirocerca* nodules. Endoscopy is the most sensitive diagnostic tool. In the early stages of disease, one or more smooth nodules are seen in the caudal esophagus, which can have a "nipple-like" protuberance, while in later stages, large, friable, lobulated nodules can be seen (Figure 39b.10).

TREATMENT

Benign *Spirocerca* nodules can be treated with doramectin used off-label at 500 μg/kg orally once daily for six weeks (Berry 2000; Lobetti 2012). A preliminary study reported successful treatment with milbemycin oxime (11.5 mg on days 0, 7, and 28 and then monthly) (Kelly et al. 2008).

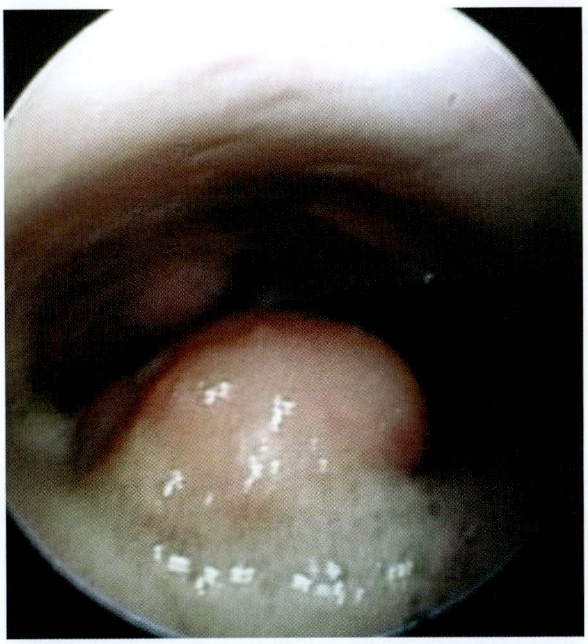

FIGURE 39b.10 Endoscopic appearance of a *Spirocerca lupi* nodule in the distal esophagus of a dog (picture courtesy of Dr. Remo Lobetti)

In a controlled study, dogs with naturally occurring spirocercosis were randomized to receive either injectable doramectin (400 μg/kg IM) or moxidectin and imidacloprid spot-on (Advocate) at label dose every week for 12 weeks (Segev et al. 2018). The moxidectin/imidacloprid spot-on was effective in some dogs but was less effective than the doramectin protocol used.

Nonneoplastic nodules usually regress after successful medical management, and post treatment endoscopy can be performed to check for resolution.

REFERENCES

Abd Elkader, N.A., Emam, I.A., Farghali, H.A. et al. (2020). Oesophageal foreign bodies in cats: clinical and anatomic findings. *PLoS One* 15 (6): e0233983.

Adamama-Moraitou, K., Rallis, T., Prassinos, N. et al. (2002). Benign esophageal stricture in the dog and cat: a retrospective study of 20 cases. *Canadian Journal of Veterinary Research* 66: 55–59.

Appelgrein, C., Hosgood, G., Thompson, M. et al. (2022). Quantification of gastroesophageal regurgitation in brachycephalic dogs. *Journal of Veterinary Internal Medicine* 36 (3): 927–934.

Barash, N.R., Lashnits, E., Kern, Z.T. et al. (2022). Outcomes of esophageal and gastric bone foreign bodies in dogs. *Journal of Veterinary Internal Medicine* 36 (2): 500–507.

Beer, A.J., Hernon, T., Halfacree, Z. et al. (2022). Complications associated with and outcome of surgical intervention for treatment of esophageal foreign bodies in dogs. *Journal of the American Veterinary Medical Association* 260 (6): 622–627.

Berry, W.L. (2000). *Spirocerca lupi* esophageal granulomas in 7 dogs: resolution after treatment with doramectin. *Journal of Veterinary Internal Medicine* 14: 609–612.

Blank, C., Ahuja, R., McGovern, D. et al. (2020). Adult-onset regurgitation in two dogs with partial oesophageal constriction caused by vascular ring anomaly. *Journal of Small Animal Practice* 61 (11): 717.

Bongard, A.B., Furrow, E., and Granick, J.L. (2019). Retrospective evaluation of factors associated with degree of esophagitis, treatment, and outcomes in dogs presenting with esophageal foreign bodies (2004--2014): 114 cases. *Journal of Veterinary Emergency and Critical Care (San Antonio).* 29 (5): 528–534.

Brisson, B.A., Wainberg, S.H., Malek, S. et al. (2018). Risk factors and prognostic indicators for surgical outcome of dogs with esophageal foreign body obstructions. *Journal of the American Veterinary Medical Association* 252 (3): 301–308.

Broux, O., Clercx, C., Etienne, A.L. et al. (2018). Effects of manipulations to detect sliding hiatal hernia in dogs with brachycephalic airway obstructive syndrome. *Veterinary Surgery* 47 (2): 243–251.

Burton, A.G., Talbot, C.T., and Kent, M.S. (2017). Risk Factors for death in dogs treated for esophageal foreign body obstruction: a retrospective cohort study of 222 cases (1998–2017). *Journal of Veterinary Internal Medicine* 31 (6): 1686–1690.

Conte, A., Morabito, S., Dennis, R. et al. (2020). Computed tomographic comparison of esophageal hiatal size in brachycephalic and non-brachycephalic breed dogs. *Veterinary Surgery* 49 (8): 1509–1516.

Da Riz, F., Béguin, J., Manassero, M. et al. (2021). Outcome of dogs and cats with benign oesophageal strictures after balloon dilatation or stenting: 27 cases (2002–2019). *Journal of Small Animal Practice* 62 (10): 886–894.

Delligianni, A., Papazoglou, L.G., Savvas, I. et al. (2020). Transdiaphragmatic gastrotomy for the extraction of distal esophageal foreign bodies in 13 dogs (1997–2016). *Journal of the American Animal Hospital Association* 56 (1): 17–22.

El-Asmar, K.M., Hassan, M.A., Abdelkader, H.M. et al. (2013). Topical mitomycin C application is effective in management of localized caustic esophageal stricture: a double-blinded, randomized, placebo-controlled trial. *Journal of Pediatric Surgery* 48: 1621–1627.

Grady, K., Gould, K., and Tolbert, K. (2024). From theory to therapy: a One Health approach guides current and future acid suppressant use in veterinary medicine. *Journal of the American Veterinary Medical Association* 262 (10): 1305–1313.

Grobman, M.E., Maitz, C.A., and Reinero, C.R. (2020). Detection of silent reflux events by nuclear scintigraphy in healthy dogs. *Journal of Veterinary Internal Medicine* 34 (4): 1432–1439.

Grobman, M.E., Masseau, I., and Reinero, C.R. (2019). Aerodigestive disorders in dogs evaluated for cough using respiratory fluoroscopy and videofluoroscopic swallow studies. *The Veterinary Journal* 251: 105344.

Hwang, J.H., Jeong, J.W., Song, G.H. et al. (2017). Pharmacokinetics and acid suppressant efficacy of esomeprazole after intravenous, oral, and subcutaneous administration to healthy Beagle dogs. *Journal of Veterinary Internal Medicine* 31 (3): 743–50.

Kelly, P.J., Fisher, M., Lucas, H. et al. (2008). Treatment of esophageal spirocercosis with milbemycin oxime. *Veterinary Parasitology* 156: 358–60.

Kempf, J., Lewis, F., Reusch, C.E. et al. (2014). High-resolution manometric evaluation of the effects of cisapride and metoclopramide hydrochloride administered orally on lower esophageal sphincter pressure in awake dogs. *American Journal of Veterinary Research* 75 (4): 361–366.

Kook, P.H., Kempf, J., Ruetten, M. et al. (2014). Wireless ambulatory esophageal pH monitoring in dogs with clinical signs interpreted as gastroesophageal reflux. *Journal of Veterinary Internal Medicine* 28: 1716–1723.

Krebs, I.A., Lindsley, S., Shaver, S. et al. (2014). Short- and long-term outcome of dogs following surgical correction of a persistent right aortic arch. *Journal of the American Animal Hospital Association* 50 (3): 181–186.

Lam, N., Weisse, C., Berent, A. et al. (2013). Esophageal stenting for treatment of refractory benign esophageal strictures in dogs. *Journal of Veterinary Internal Medicine* 27: 1064–1070.

Langlois, D.K., Stanley, B., and Ballegeer, E.A. (2014). Successful treatment of cricopharyngeal dysphagia with bilateral myectomy in a dog. *The Canadian Veterinary Journal* 55: 1167–1172.

Leib, M.S., Dinnel, H., Ward, D.L. et al. (2001). Endoscopic balloon dilation of benign esophageal strictures in dogs and cats. *Journal of Veterinary Internal Medicine* 15: 547–552.

Lobetti, R. (2012). Successful resolution of oesophageal spirocercosis in 20 dogs following daily treatment with oral doramectin. *The Veterinary Journal* 193: 277–278.

Luciani, E., Reinero, C., and Grobman, M. (2022). Evaluation of aerodigestive disease and diagnosis of sliding hiatal hernia in brachycephalic and non-brachycephalic dogs. *Journal of Veterinary Internal Medicine* 36 (4): 1229–1236.

Marks, S.L., Kook, P.H., Papich, M.G. et al. (2018). ACVIM consensus statement: support for rational administration of gastrointestinal protectants to dogs and cats. *Journal of Veterinary Internal Medicine* 32: 1823–40.

Marvel, S. and Monnet, E. (2024). Laparoscopic treatment of sliding hiatal hernia. *Veterinary Clinics of North America Small Animal Practice* 54 (4): 649–659.

Mayhew, P.D., Balsa, I.M., Marks, S.L. et al. (2021). Clinical and videofluoroscopic outcomes of laparoscopic treatment for sliding hiatal hernia and associated gastroesophageal reflux in brachycephalic dogs. *Veterinary Surgery* 50 (1): O67–O77.

Mayhew, P.D., Marks, S.L., Pollard, R. et al. (2017). Prospective evaluation of surgical management of sliding hiatal hernia and gastroesophageal reflux in dogs. *Veterinary Surgery* 46 (8): 1098–1109.

Monnet, E. (2021). Laparoscopic correction of sliding hiatal hernia in eight dogs: Description of technique, complications, and short-term outcome. *Veterinary Surgery* 50 (1): 230–237.

Morgan, K.R.S. and Bray, J.P. (2019). Current diagnostic tests, surgical treatments, and prognostic indicators for vascular ring anomalies in dogs. *Journal of the American Veterinary Medical Association* 254 (6): 728–733.

Niles, J.D., Williams, J.M., Sullivan, M. et al. (2001). Resolution of dysphagia following cricopharyngeal myectomy in six young dogs. *Journal of Small Animal Practice* 42: 32–35.

Paran, E., Major, A.C., Warren-Smith, C. et al. (2023). Prevalence of gastroesophageal reflux in dogs undergoing MRI for a thoracolumbar vertebral column pathology. *Journal of Small Animal Practice* 64 (5): 321–329.

Reeve, E.J., Sutton, D., Friend, E.J. et al. (2017). Documenting the prevalence of hiatal hernia and oesophageal abnormalities in brachycephalic dogs using fluoroscopy. *Journal of Small Animal Practice* 58 (12): 703–708.

Rossanese, M., Cinti, F., Chanoit, G.P.A. et al. (2022). Clinical findings, surgical treatment and long-term outcome of dogs and cats with double aortic arch: four cases (2005–2022). *Journal of Small Animal Practice* 63 (11): 834–842.

Rossi, R., Coe, R., Allfree, C. et al. (2024). Circumflex left aortic arch: a new vascular ring anomaly in dogs. *Journal of the American Veterinary Medical Association* 7: 1–6.

Schorn, C., Hildebrandt, N., Schneider, M. et al. (2021). Anomalies of the aortic arch in dogs: evaluation with the use of multidetector computed tomography angiography and proposal of an extended classification scheme. *BMC Veterinary Research* 17 (1): 387.

Segev, G., Rojas, A., Lavy, E. et al. (2018). Evaluation of a spot-on imidacloprid-moxidectin formulation (Advocate®) for the treatment of naturally occurring esophageal spirocercosis in dogs: a double-blinded, placebo-controlled study. *Parasites & Vectors* 11 (1): 127.

Shipov, A., Kelmer, G., Lavy, E. et al. (2015). Long-term outcome of transendoscopic oesophageal mass ablation in dogs with Spirocerca lupi-associated oesophageal sarcoma. *Veterinary Record* 177 (14): 365.

Shua-Haim, T., Vilaplana Grosso, F.R., Suarez Fuentes, D. et al. (2023). Computed tomographic features of double aortic arch in six dogs. *Veterinary Radiology & Ultrasound* 64 (4): 669–676.

Tan, D.K., Weisse, C., Berent, A. et al. (2018). Prospective evaluation of an indwelling esophageal balloon dilatation feeding tube for treatment of benign esophageal strictures in dogs and cats. *Journal of Veterinary Internal Medicine* 32 (2): 693–700

Tolbert, K., Bissett, S., King, A. et al. (2011). Efficacy of oral famotidine and 2 omeprazole formulations for the control of intragastric pH in dogs. *Journal of Veterinary Internal Medicine* 25: 47–54.

Trindade-Gerardi, A.B., da Silveira, C.A., Duz, J. et al. (2024). First description of a primary esophageal histiocytic sarcoma in a dog. *Topics in Companion Animal Medicine* 59: 100856.

Ullal, T.V., Marks, S.L., Yang, N.T. et al. (2024). Evaluating acidic gastroesophageal reflux with wireless pH monitoring in French bulldogs with sliding hiatal herniation. *Journal of Veterinary Internal Medicine* 38 (3): 1475–1482.

Vangrinsven, E., Broux, O., Massart, L. et al. (2021). Diagnosis and treatment of gastro-oesophageal junction abnormalities in dogs with brachycephalic syndrome. *Journal of Small Animal Practice* 62 (3): 200–208.

Warnock, J.J., Marks, S.L., Pollard, R. et al. (2003). Surgical management of cricopharyngeal dysphagia in dogs: 14 cases (1989–2001). *Journal of the American Veterinary Medical Association* 223: 1462–1468.

Wei, P. (2022). Botulinum toxin injection for the treatment of upper esophageal sphincter dysfunction. *Toxins (Basel)* 14 (5): 321

Wilson, D.V., Evans, A.T., and Miller, R. (2005). Effects of preanesthetic administration of morphine on gastroesophageal reflux and regurgitation during anesthesia in dogs. *American Journal of Veterinary Research* 66: 386–390.

Wyatt, S.R. and Barron, P.M. (2019). Complications following removal of oesophageal foreign bodies: a retrospective review of 349 cases. *Australian Veterinary Journal* 97 (4): 116–121.

Zacuto, A.C., Marks, S.L., Osborn, J. et al. (2012). The influence of esomeprazole and cisapride on gastroesophageal reflux during anesthesia in dogs. *Journal of Veterinary Internal Medicine* 26: 518–525.

Disorders of the Stomach

CHAPTER 40

Julien R.S. Dandrieux and Silke Salavati Schmitz

Royal (Dick) School of Veterinary Studies, University of Edinburgh, Easter Bush, UK

KEY POINTS

- While the stomach is anatomically simple, it is responsible for complex physiological functions, including motility (gastric emptying) as well as acid and hormone production.
- Diseases of the stomach range from acute to chronic inflammation, ulceration, neoplasia, and motility dysfunction, and hence clinical signs and pertinent diagnostic investigations can be very variable.
- Although typical clinical signs of gastric disease include vomiting and reduced appetite, animals can also present with respiratory signs secondary to the gastric disease (aero-digestive disorders).
- Ultrasound sensitivity to detect gastric masses can be limited by gastric content. Endoscopy or CT should be considered in dogs and cats with a strong suspicion of a gastric mass despite normal ultrasound findings.
- Proton pump inhibitors like omeprazole should be used at a dose of 1 mg/kg PO q12h as antacids in dogs with proven gastric ulcers.
- The use of prokinetics in gastric disease is controversial, as their most appropriate indication and efficacy are unknown, and should hence be limited to cases of severe or idiopathic gastric stasis.

INTRODUCTION

Diseases of the stomach in dogs encompass a broad range of conditions, from acute gastritis to chronic disorders such as gastric ulceration, neoplasia, and motility dysfunction. As the initial segment of the gastrointestinal (GI) tract is responsible for mechanical and chemical digestion, the stomach plays a critical role in overall canine and feline health. Disruption of gastric function can result in significant clinical signs, including vomiting, anorexia, abdominal pain, and weight loss, and may reflect either primary gastric pathology or systemic illness.

The etiology of gastric diseases in dogs and cats is diverse, including dietary indiscretion, infectious agents, foreign body ingestion, toxins, neoplastic processes, and immune-mediated conditions. Gastric motility (emptying) is also often disturbed in both gastric and extra-gastric conditions, leading to significant morbidity through increasing risk for aspiration pneumonia and malnourishment. Moreover, breed predispositions and genetic factors contribute to the development of specific gastric disorders, such as gastric dilatation-volvulus (GDV) in large, deep-chested breeds. Advances in diagnostic imaging, endoscopy, and laboratory testing have enhanced the ability to accurately diagnose and manage these conditions, yet many challenges remain, particularly in differentiating functional from structural disease.

This chapter provides a comprehensive overview of the most common and clinically significant gastric diseases affecting dogs and cats. It emphasizes current understanding of their pathophysiology, clinical presentation, diagnostic approaches, and therapeutic strategies. By integrating recent research findings with practical clinical experience, the chapter aims to guide veterinarians in making informed decisions for the effective management of canine and feline patients with gastric disorders.

Disorders of the Liver, Exocrine Pancreas, and Gastrointestinal Tract in Dogs and Cats, First Edition. Edited by Harry Cridge et al. Published 2026 by John Wiley & Sons, Inc. Companion Website: www.wiley.com/go/cridge/disorders

PHYSIOLOGY OF THE STOMACH

ANATOMY AND MOTILITY

The stomach is divided into fundus, corpus, antrum, and pylorus (Figure 40.1). Motor function can be differentiated into the gastric store (tonical part), consisting of the fundus and corpus, and the gastric pump, an area in which peristaltic smooth muscle waves occur (distal part of the corpus and the antrum). During filling, stimulation of tension receptors in the stomach wall accelerates gastrogastric reflexes: an adaptive relaxation of the smooth muscles occurs (Figure 40.2). Additionally, receptive relaxation occurs during chewing and swallowing by stimulation of the mechanoreceptors in the oropharyngeal region (vagally mediated), preparing the stomach for receiving a food bolus. Finally, a feedback mechanism ensures that gastric emptying is adapted to the type and amount of food, which empties into the small intestine (Schmitz 2007).

The antral wall consists of several layers of smooth muscle in longitudinal bands. Muscle pacemaker cells (interstitial cells of Cajal, ICC) located between the layers are able to cause the so-called basal electrical rhythm, or pacemaker potentials (PMPs), leading to stronger depolarizations toward

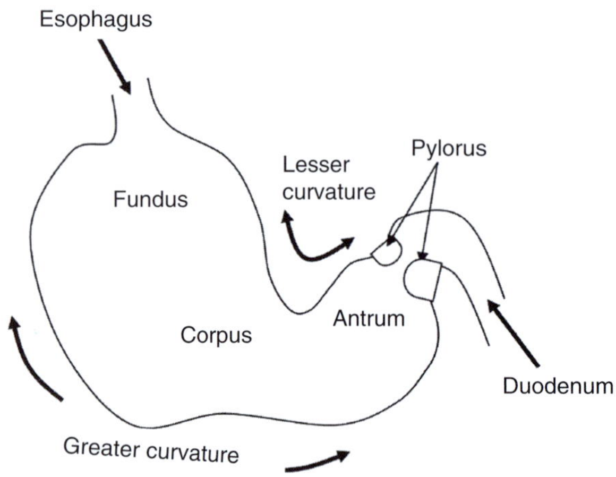

FIGURE 40.1 Anatomical areas of the stomach

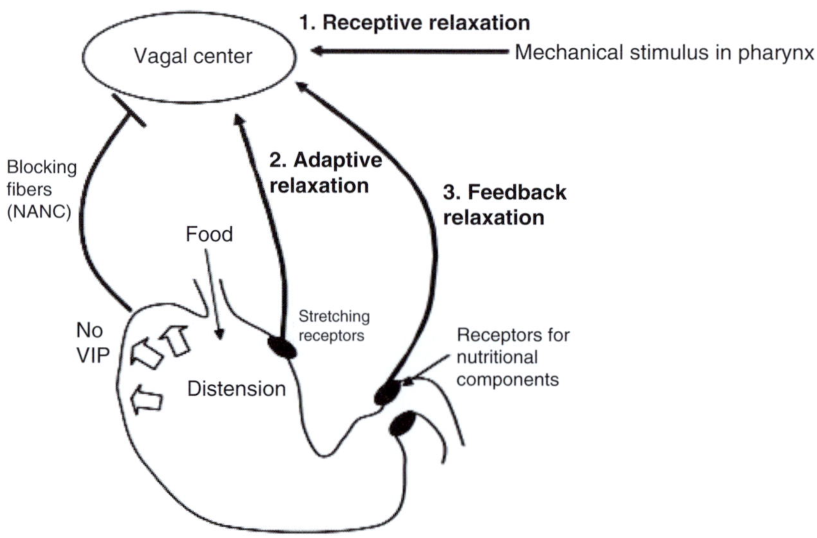

FIGURE 40.2 Regulation of gastric motility. NANC, non-adrenergic-non-cholinergic fibers; NO, nitric oxide; VIP, vasoactive intestinal peptide

the pylorus, resulting in peristaltic waves. As a result, only the superficial semisolid and partly digested portion of a food bolus is transported toward the pylorus, while the more alkaline inner portion remains for further digestion.

Physiological gastric motility can be described as digestive and interdigestive motility. During digestion, there are three consecutive phases that lead to emptying of stomach contents into the duodenum: propulsion, emptying and mixing, and "trituration" (Figure 40.3). These phases occur in cycles due to recurring PMPs. During propulsion, the proximal part of the antrum contracts, the distal part is relaxed, into which the gastric content is then transported. When a peristaltic wave reaches the middle of the antrum, the pylorus opens partially, duodenal peristalsis is blocked, and food particles flow into the pylorus rather than being pressed into the duodenum by force. Because liquids flow faster than viscous and solid contents, there is a sieving process at this stage, whereby small particles, suspended in liquid, pass the pylorus, while more solid food remains in the stomach. "Trituration" refers to the mechanical breakdown and mixing of food into a semiliquid chyme. This is achieved by the repeated to-and-fro movement of ingesta in the antrum. After mixing and emptying, the pylorus and proximal antrum close, the transpyloric flow is stopped, and particles too large to pass (anything >3 mm) are propelled back into the body of the stomach. This jet-like phenomenon causes turbulence and mixing of stomach contents. Solid meal emptying is often preceded by a lag phase representative of this process of trituration.

Gastric motility and secretion are subject to neuronal and hormonal regulation. Efferent vagal fibers produce gastric tone and modulate the autonomic enteric neuronal system (ENS) in the *plexus myentericus* of the stomach wall. Dilation and contraction are mediated via nitric oxide (NO), serotonin, and others. The highest level of regulation is the central nervous system (CNS), which can in turn also receive input from the ENS via viscero-sensible afferences, for example, in emesis.

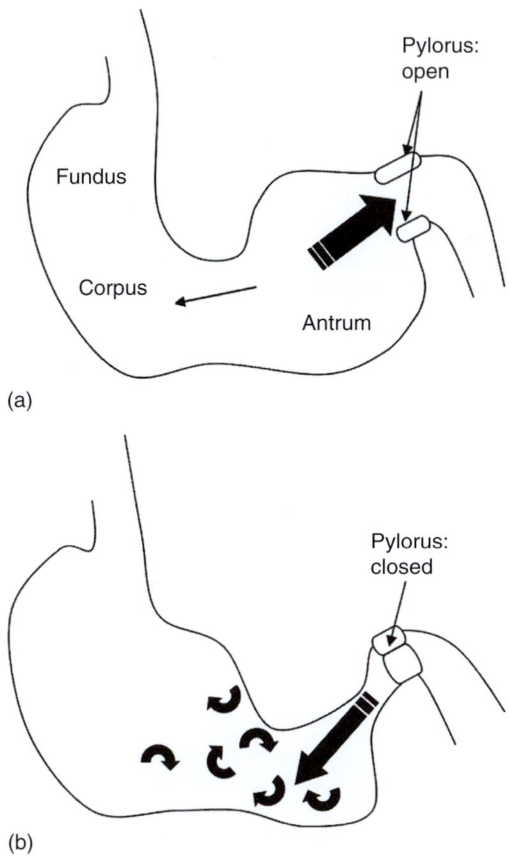

FIGURE 40.3 Phases of gastric emptying. (a) Phase of emptying: contraction of the central antrum and transpyloric flow (large arrow), larger particles are propelled back into the antrum (thin arrow). (b) Trituration of particles, e.g., jet-like propulsion back into the antrum while the pylorus is shut

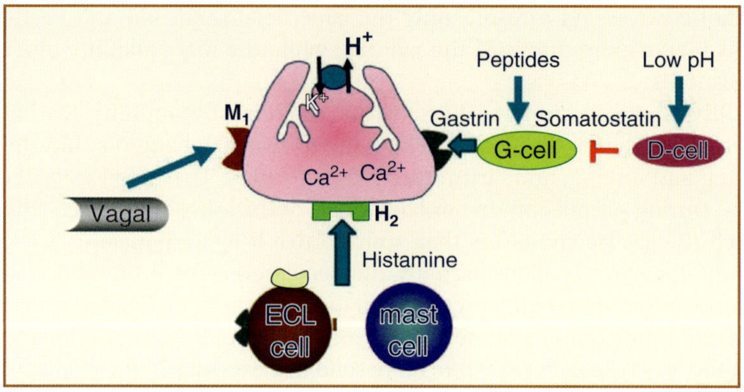

FIGURE 40.4 Regulation of acid production in gastric parietal cells. M_1, muscarinic receptor; H_2, histamine receptor; ECL, enterochromaffin-like cell

There is a close relationship between gastric and duodenal motility (antro-duodenal coordination). The pylorus acts as an "electrical isolator," so that PMPs are not directly transmitted to the small intestine. Instead, gastric emptying can be inhibited by the small intestine via the release of intestinal hormones (for example, cholecystokinin, GLP-1, substance P, somatostatin) or vagal signals, which can be activated by several factors, such as pH, osmolality, and type of nutrients.

Interdigestive motility varies greatly between species. In dogs, it is associated with a cyclic recurrent motor activity called the migrating motor complexes (MMC) that rolls periodically from the stomach to the distal small intestine. It empties non-digestible food components into the duodenum and is largely mediated by motilin. MMCs are interrupted by food intake and replaced by digestive motility as described above.

ACID AND HORMONE PRODUCTION

The gastric mucosa consists of columnar glandular epithelium, which varies in different regions of the stomach. In the cardia, the epithelium mostly produces mucus, while the corpus mainly contains parietal and chief cells. Parietal cells produce hydrochloric acid, ghrelin, and leptin, as well as intrinsic factor involved in the absorption of vitamin B12 (cobalamin). Chief cells produce pepsinogen, a proteolytic enzyme, which is converted to pepsin by the acid present in the stomach as well as leptin. The corpus also contains scattered enterochromaffin-like cells (ECLs), which produce histamine, while the antrum contains G-cells, which produce gastrin (as a pre-propeptide, which is processed into three different biologically active peptides: big, little, and mini gastrin). D-cells producing somatostatin are found both in the gastric fundus and antrum.

Acid production is promoted via acetylcholine from the vagal nerve upon ingestion of food (via innervation of G-cells and ECL cells) but also directly stimulated by gastrin and histamine (see Figure 40.4). Somatostatin is the major inhibitor of gastric acid production by inhibiting gastrin and histamine production.

Ghrelin is the chief "hunger hormone" that increases food intake via receptors in the hypothalamus and, hence, plays a role in energy metabolism, with its direct antagonist, leptin, having opposite effects.

CLINICAL SIGNS OF GASTRIC DISEASE

Clinical signs of gastric disease can include vomiting (or unproductive retching), diarrhea, decreased appetite, weight loss, hematemesis (fresh or "coffee ground" appearance), melena, bloating, hypersalivation, and abdominal discomfort or pain. These signs are not pathognomonic and can appear with other conditions, so differentiating gastric from other diseases is essential during diagnostic investigation. If an owner reports their dog or cat to be vomiting, targeted questioning is required to ensure distinction of vomiting from regurgitation.

In addition to relatively obvious signs of potential gastric disease, there is an increasing recognition of more subtle signs of aerodigestive disorders (ADs) in dogs, particularly in relation to (silent) gastro-esophageal reflux and associated – mostly clinically silent – dysphagia. Dogs might present exclusively with clinical signs of respiratory disease, alimentary disease, or a combination. Dogs with a history of recurrent aspiration pneumonia, coughing (especially while eating and drinking), dysphagia, or clinical signs of reflux disease (e.g., repetitive dry swallowing, lip licking, gagging, nighttime restlessness) should be considered candidates for the evaluation of ADs (see below and Chapter 38 for further information on ADs).

DIAGNOSTICS AND TECHNIQUES

Diagnostic investigation should be guided by the predominant clinical sign and an appropriate list of differential diagnoses that need to be ruled out on a case-by-case basis. As the list of potential causes, for example, for vomiting is lengthy, a detailed description of investigations cannot be provided in the context of this chapter. However, it is likely that a combination of basic laboratory work (for example, a CBC, biochemistry, urinalysis), extended laboratory testing based on the species and case (for example, ruling out hepatic functional impairment or endocrinopathies like hypoadrenocorticism in dogs and hyperthyroidism in cats, or assessing coagulation times in animals with hematemesis or melena), and diagnostic imaging (for example, radiography to rule out gastric foreign bodies [FBs] or gastric dilation volvulus [GDV], and ultrasound to assess intraabdominal organs) combined with less invasive sampling methods (e.g., fine-needle aspiration of abnormal intraabdominal structures) can define the first diagnostic steps. If the problem is indeed located in the upper GI tract, then further procedures like gastroduodenoscopy or laparotomy with the goal to either further diagnose disease (e.g., biopsies of the gastric mucosa) or confirm a diagnosis and treatment (e.g., removal of FBs or surgical correction of a GDV) are needed.

Diagnostic and therapeutic procedures for specific disorders of the stomach (e.g., gastric intubation and lavage; considerations for FB retrieval and PEG tube placement) are described below.

DISEASES OF THE STOMACH

CONGENITAL DISEASES

Congenital diseases of the stomach are not well described in dogs and cats. It is possible that, with idiopathic or congenital megaesophagus, there is also an element of abnormal tone in the lower esophageal sphincter or stomach itself. This can lead to impairment of food passage into the stomach, although this has not been conclusively proven.

Similarly, while extremely rare conditions, such as pyloric stenosis or hypertrophy, could be congenital in origin, they are mostly described in middle-aged to older dogs. For this reason, a congenital cause is deemed less likely. Pyloric stenosis has been better defined in cats, but it is also usually assumed to be acquired rather than congenital (Freiche et al. 2021).

Increased popularity of dog breeds affected by brachycephalic obstructive airway syndrome (BOAS) allows the assumption that a number of their common GI problems (regurgitation, vomiting, retching, dysphagia, aerophagia, gastroesophageal reflux, pica, abdominal pain) are directly linked to the brachycephalic phenotype and the resulting changes in upper airway pressures, as well as excess of soft tissues along the respiratory and digestive tract (see also gastric motility and ADs below). In addition, hiatal hernias (HHs), gastroesophageal intussusceptions, and esophageal and gastric mucosal lesions (diffuse unspecific inflammation most commonly, prominent lymphoid follicles) are often observed in these dogs (see gastritis below) (Freiche and German 2021).

GASTRITIS

Gastritis (inflammation of the gastric mucosa) – on its own or in conjunction with "enteritis" – is often used to describe otherwise ill-defined cases of anorexia, nausea, and vomiting (± diarrhea) in dogs and cats. However, the literature on gastritis as a distinct condition is sparse. In practice, cases of presumed acute gastritis are rarely pursued with extensive diagnostics because they are most commonly self-limiting and can be managed with symptomatic treatment alone, while cases of "chronic gastritis" are rarely found to occur isolated from the rest of the GI tract (e.g., in the context of chronic enteropathy). Also, as there is no causative link between stress or infection with *Helicobacter* sp. and gastritis or gastric ulcers in dogs and cats (see also next paragraph), it seems unlikely that gastritis will ever be more than a descriptive term.

In cases of excessive or inappropriate gastric inflammation, although a cause or causative agent is rarely determined, pathological changes have been elucidated: chemical injury, ischemia, infection, or antigenic stimulation can result in the release of inflammatory mediators and vasoactive compounds from a variety of cells (e.g., neutrophils, mast cells, platelets, endothelial cells, neurons) (Webb and Twedt 2003). Subsequent loss of gastric epithelial cells and disruption of the mucosal barrier result in back-diffusion of gastric acid, pepsin, and gastric lipase. This inflammatory cascade stimulates further acid secretion and mucosal damage, increases cell membrane permeability, and alters microvascular blood flow. Potential differentials for acute gastritis include the ingestion of inappropriate foodstuffs or foreign material (also sometimes called "garbagitis"), including molds/fungi and their toxins, spoiled food (including potential pathogens), chemical irritants/household toxins, toxic or irritant plants, or drugs (see below for non-steroidal anti-inflammatory drugs, NSAIDs).

Lymphocytic/lymphoplasmacytic and eosinophilic gastritis are mere histologic descriptions of presumed chronic immune-mediated gastric pathology. Infectious causes still often need to be ruled out (e.g., GI nematodes including *Physaloptera* sp.) (Soderman and Harkin 2021) and potentially treated empirically before undertaking further diagnostic or therapeutic steps. Nearly all of these "idiopathic" cases are eventually diagnosed as part of chronic inflammatory enteropathies or neoplasia. Granulomatous gastritis should raise the suspicion for insidious fungal disease (for example, pythiosis), mycobacterial or viral infection (for example, feline infectious peritonitis in cats).

GASTRIC ULCERATION

The incidence of gastric ulceration is undetermined but seems to be more common in dogs than cats. Although clinical signs such as vomiting and anorexia can be noted, it is presumed that ulcerative disease remains clinically silent for a substantial period of time. The cause of gastric ulcer formation is most likely multifactorial, involving mucosal, vascular, endocrine, and neurologic triggers (as described above). NSAIDs are one of the most common causes of gastric erosion or ulceration in small animals, with the antrum and pylorus most susceptible to NSAID-induced lesions (see Figure 40.5). Those lesions can range from surface erythema or erosions to full-thickness ulcerations, with severe and/or large lesions more likely to cause hematemesis or melena. NSAID-induced gastric ulceration is based on non-selective COX inhibition within the gastric mucosa, which simultaneously not only reduces COX2-induced pro-inflammatory prostaglandin production but also inhibits COX-1, which mediates cytoprotective prostaglandin production and maintains mucosal integrity. Despite the availability of NSAIDs manufactured specifically for veterinary patients, including more COX-2 selective inhibitors, gastric erosion and ulceration are still a commonly observed side effect (Figure 40.5) (Webb and Twedt 2023).

In addition to NSAIDs, glucocorticoids, antibiotics, and chemotherapeutic drugs are potential causes of acute erosions and ulcerations, and combining glucocorticoids and NSAIDs creates an extremely ulcerogenic gastric environment. Ulcerative gastritis or individual peptic ulcers can also occur secondary to hypergastrinemia, which can be due to APUDomas like gastrinomas (e.g., in the pancreas) or liver disease, or as a consequence of severe systemic hypovolemia leading to a decrease in gastric mucosal blood flow and hence ischemia (for example, in hypoadrenocorticism). Finally, gastric ulcerations are commonly associated with gastric carcinoma in dogs. Classically, these have been described as single large ulcers, for example, on the incisura angularis of the stomach (Figure 40.5), but in some predisposed breeds like Belgian Shepherd dogs, they can possibly be more diffuse and subtle (Kijan et al. 2023).

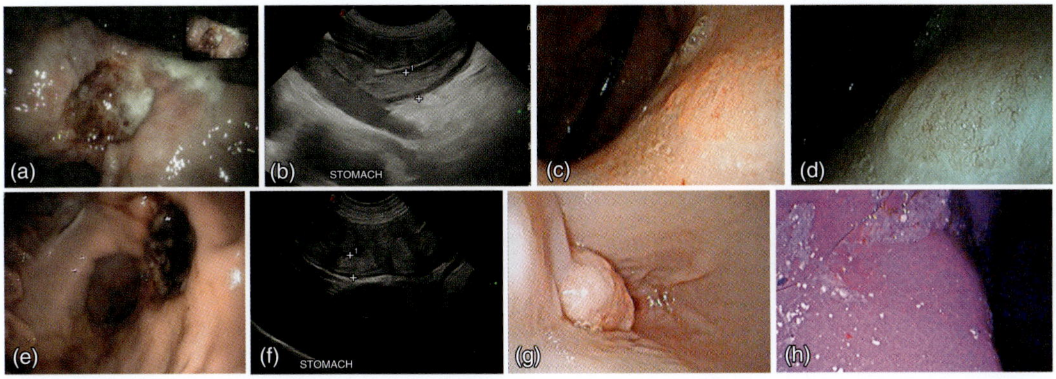

FIGURE 40.5 Typical gastric abnormalities on endoscopy and ultrasound in dogs and cats. (a) Deep peptic ulcer with central necrosis on the incisura angularis in a Collie dog, histologically confirmed as carcinoma. (b) Gastric wall thickening in a dog with histologically confirmed gastric carcinoma. (c) Same dog as in (b) with subtle flat mucosal lesion on standard white light endoscopy. (d) Same image as in (c) but with narrow-band imaging, making the neoplastic lesion easier to identify. (e) Gastric ulcer due to chronic NSAID use in a dog. (f) Severe generalized gastric mucosal thickening in a dog with portosystemic shunt given long-term omeprazole. (g) Antropyloric mass in a cat, which was histologically confirmed to be lymphoma. (h) Cobblestone-patterned gastric mass in a cat histologically confirmed as sarcoma

GASTRIC FOREIGN BODIES

The ingestion of FBs or foreign material is relatively common in both canine and feline patients, although more frequent in dogs (Barash et al. 2022) compared to cats (Bebchuk 2002). This includes both foodstuffs (bone and cartilage, dental chews), as well as toys, fishhooks, hair bands, and strings (more so in cats), household items (meat skewers etc.), items of clothing, and trichobezoars, as well as more uncommon materials (e.g., metal items and magnets, wood glue, sewing needles). The percentage of FBs that pass through the GI tract without requiring any treatment is unknown, but as they can cause injury or (partial) GI obstruction, they can become life-threatening. The severity of clinical signs (like salivation, retching, gagging, vomiting, anorexia, pain) depends on localization, size (absolute and relative to the animal size), type of FB (traumatic or not), and duration of (outflow) obstruction. Rarely, animals can be presented for secondary sequela after the GI tract has been damaged or penetrated by FBs, for example, pyothorax or (sub)-lumber abscesses due to migrating FBs. Diagnostic imaging like radiography and ultrasound is useful in diagnosing gastric FBs, as well as any complications, e.g., free fluid potentially indicating perforation/septic peritonitis. Location, type, and size of FBs as determined by these techniques are also helpful in establishing the best approach for their removal. However, it is important to note that non-radio-opaque FBs can be missed on radiographs and might also be missed on abdominal ultrasound depending on the gastric content (i.e., gas/shadowing).

Conservative management of gastric FBs often involves inducing emesis but should be avoided with sharp-edged or potentially corrosive material. Vomiting is most frequently induced using apomorphine in dogs, either as ocular drops or systemically, and dexmedetomidine either intramuscularly or orally in cats (Maxwell et al. 2024). Apomorphine is highly potent in dogs, with 83% success with ocular application and 76% with intravenous administration (Manley et al. 2024).

Conservative management of metallic sharp-pointed straight FBs (e.g., needles) has been reported both in dogs and cats with an 88% success rate (15 out of 17 cases) with resolution in a mean time of 59.2 hours (±31.4). One cat and one dog underwent surgery to remove the foreign body as it had not moved from the stomach within 24 hours (Crinò et al. 2023).

Endoscopic removal of gastric FBs has been described since the 1970s (Zimmer 1981) and has a high success rate of 78–94% (Di Palma et al. 2022; Gianella et al. 2009; Dollo et al. 2020). The main instruments used include endoscopic grasping forceps, loop snares that are particularly effective for bones, and wire baskets that can be used for rounded FBs. A Roth net is also useful to retrieve coins. On occasions, creative techniques are required such as the use of a baby bottle liner for round hard FBs like stones or golf balls that are otherwise difficult to grasp firmly with endoscopic retrieval equipment (Le Boedec and Flageollet 2024). This technique has also been described for sharp FBs to protect the mucosa during retrieval. Overtubes and FB hoods are other considerations for sharp foreign body retrieval. The use of a magnet held in a Roth net has also been described to remove metallic FBs, which can be especially effective when gastric content limits mucosa visualization (Skinner et al. 2024).

Endoscopic complications are uncommon and more associated with esophageal FBs than gastric ones. However, bone FBs, bodyweight of <10 kg, and duration of the FB being in place for >3 days have been associated with a higher risk of complications (Gianella et al. 2009). Over 90% of dogs have no long-lasting ill-effects from FBs, but data in cats is scarcer.

One large retrospective study reported the outcome of 40 cats with gastric FBs (Dollo et al. 2020). Removal was successful in 38 cats (95%). One cat had a portion of rubber that could not be retrieved, and another one had a plastic foreign body that could not be retrieved due to the presence of a gastroesophageal mass. Major complications, in addition to unsuccessful retrieval, included cardiopulmonary arrest in one cat and aspiration pneumonia in one cat.

If endoscopic removal (or laparoscopy-assisted methods that have also been described) is unsuccessful or unavailable, routine gastrotomy should be performed, although this might not be required for raw bone FBs or metallic sharp-pointed FBs as outlined above. If the clinical signs warrant a laparotomy as a gastric FB is suspected, but none is found, gastrointestinal biopsies should be obtained to ensure that there isn't an underlying enteropathy as a cause of the clinical signs.

MOTILITY DISORDERS AND AERODIGESTIVE DISORDERS

ADs represent an array of diseases that encompass both the respiratory (pharynx, larynx, bronchi, and pulmonary parenchyma) and upper digestive tracts (esophagus and the stomach) (Grobman 2021). They have mostly been described in dogs; hence, this chapter will encompass gastroesophageal reflux disease (GERD) and sliding HH in dogs. Reflux can, in turn, be a cause of secondary respiratory inflammation due to micro- or macro-aspirations in the lungs, reflux in the nasopharynx or nasal cavity, as well as esophagitis. The nature and severity of clinical signs associated with this probably depend on the amount of reflux volume, acidity, and the amount of digestive enzymes and bile acids present.

Although brachycephalic dogs are predisposed to AD, clinical signs can develop in dogs of any age and breed. Brachycephalic dogs tend to have earlier and more severe clinical signs than other breeds due to their abnormal anatomy (Luciani et al. 2022).

Affected dogs are more often presented with respiratory signs rather than primary digestive disease (Grobman 2021). Subtle GI signs might be present but are often not recognized by owners, or even though there is, for example, reflux, it can be clinically silent. A thorough history and multimodal diagnostic approach can be necessary to reach a diagnosis.

Some key findings that should increase the suspicion of AD include recurrent aspiration pneumonia, coughing while eating or drinking, and visible regurgitation and vomiting. Signs suggestive of reflux include repetitive dry swallowing, lip licking, and restlessness at night. A recent history of general anesthesia should also increase the degree of suspicion for GERD.

In addition to a routine physical examination, a thorough neurological examination should also be performed. Findings on physical examination that increase suspicion of AD include evidence of upper airway obstruction, such as brachycephalic obstructive airway disease (BOAS) or laryngeal dysfunction or paralysis (e.g., change of bark, exercise intolerance). Neurological abnormalities might include cranial nerve deficits, evidence of polyneuropathy, or myopathy.

Different diagnostic modalities can be used to assess a patient with suspected AD. However, any diagnostic modality that requires general anesthesia is associated with a higher risk of aspiration due to abnormal airway protective mechanisms, and this risk needs to be discussed with the owners.

Thoracic radiographs are often performed as a first step, but the changes might be too subtle to be evident. In addition, some of the pathologies can only be recognized during the dynamic phases of swallowing or esophageal motility that cannot be appreciated with radiographs. CT has the same limitation as radiographs in this regard but is more sensitive to detect pulmonary parenchyma abnormalities.

Fluoroscopy plays a central role in the diagnosis of AD and can be used to visualize the dynamics of the swallowing process, including esophageal motility, and the presence of gastroesophageal reflux. Swallow studies should be done with the animal standing to reduce the risk of aspiration (as opposed to lateral recumbency). Different consistencies of food should be used, including dry food, wet food, and liquid, to mimic the different phases of physiological swallowing. Some dogs will have a normal swallow study with one type of food but not with another. Manual pressure on the abdomen during eating and swallowing can also be considered to increase the chance of visualizing GERD and HH.

Endoscopy can be performed to assess both the digestive system (upper GI endoscopy) and the respiratory system (laryngoscopy, bronchoscopy). This enables visualization of the mucosa and sampling of the digestive tract (biopsies) and of the respiratory tract (bronchoalveolar lavage, BAL). GI biopsies are typically assessed with histology, whereas BAL undergoes cytology and infectious testing (aerobic and anaerobic culture and PCR). Assessment for HH by endoscopy can be facilitated by compression of the abdomen or increasing the abdominal pressure by obstructing the endotracheal tube for 3 breaths or up to 30 seconds. Additional modalities such as pH monitors and scintigraphy have been described to diagnose reflux but are not used routinely in the clinical setting.

As reflux of gastric content into the esophagus can be physiological in dogs, it is important to document the volume and frequency of reflux to assess its clinical relevance. In situations where access to a fluoroscopy unit or C-arm is hampered, diagnosing GERD can be difficult. For this reason, empirical treatment trials are often considered.

Treatment considerations for GERD include acid suppression to reduce damage from the reflux as well as prokinetics and diet modification to promote gastric emptying and ideally increase lower esophageal sphincter tone. Clinical response can be slow and might take 6–8 weeks. A proton-pump inhibitor is the antacid of choice in dogs, in particular omeprazole, at a dosage of 1 mg/kg PO q12h. Use of omeprazole can induce acute gastrointestinal signs (vomiting and diarrhea) in some dogs, and gastric mucosal hypertrophy has been described with chronic use (Figure 40.5). Oral cisapride (1 mg/kg PO q12h) or parenteral metoclopramide (1 dose of 1 mg/kg IV, then as a CRI at 1 mg/kg/h) reduces the frequency of GER during anesthesia and can also be considered for GERD treatment (see more details below). In addition, a therapeutic low-fat diet fed in small frequent meals can promote accelerated gastric emptying. If esophageal ulcerations are present, oral sucralfate suspension should be given at a dosage of 500 mg total for dogs up to 20 kg and 1–2 g total for dogs more than 20 kg q6–8 hours. Ideally, sucralfate should be given two hours prior to other drugs and food, which can make administration challenging. Finally, a feeding plan to reach an ideal body condition score (4–5 out of 9) should also be implemented if the dog is under or overweight.

HH is due to displacement of the stomach or the abdominal content through the esophageal hiatus into the thoracic cavity. The most common type of HH seen in dogs is sliding HH and is characterized by cranial displacement of the gastroesophageal junction. This promotes reflux episodes and aspiration pneumonitis. This disease is frequently reported in brachycephalic dogs, where it can be congenital, but has also been reported in non-brachycephalic dogs. Acquired HH can be seen with neuromuscular disease, trauma, and significant upper airway disease.

Clinical signs are usually secondary to esophagitis and esophageal dysmotility like GERD, but some dogs might not have clinical signs. Diagnosis can be challenging and often requires fluoroscopy, with additional abdominal compression required. On occasion, sliding HH might also be diagnosed using endoscopy as described above.

Medical management of HH is similar to what has been described for GERD, including achieving an ideal body condition score. If medical management is insufficient, surgery of pre-existing conditions, such as BOAS, should be considered as a next step. In addition, specific surgical procedures to control HH have been described and can be used in the absence of improvement with the previous steps.

GASTRIC DILATATION-VOLVULUS

GDV can be a life-threatening condition, with large and giant breeds at risk. In this condition, the stomach fills with content (mostly gas and fluid) and then rotates on its axis. This rotation leads to impairment of both gastric emptying and blood circulation in the stomach wall, but also systemically, leading to hypovolemic shock.

The onset is usually acute and typical clinical signs include non-productive retching, abdominal distension and pain, restlessness, and can progress within a few hours to hypovolemic shock and death. A history of non-productive retching in a large breed dog shortly after feeding should always be considered as an emergency and possible GDV.

Some of the risk factors reported include large breed deep-chested dogs such as Great Dane and Weimaraner, eating habits (rapid eater and once a day feeding), and exercise post feeding.

Physical examination findings are dependent on how advanced the disease is. A dog early in the process might present with abdominal discomfort and abdomen distension, which is tympanic on percussion (gas-filled stomach). The disease can progress, and the animal may present in hypovolemic shock with pale mucous membranes, poor pulse quality, tachycardia, and hypotension.

Typically, the findings on examination will give a strong suspicion for GDV. Diagnosis can be further confirmed with radiographs for which the right lateral abdominal view is usually pathognomonic ("double bubble" view).

Treatment for a dog with GDV is considered an emergency. The animal needs to be stabilized cardiovascularly with intravenous fluid therapy (IVFT). Large bore catheters are typically recommended, and a bolus of 10–20 mL/kg over 15–20 minutes to stabilize the patient with monitoring of treatment response (mucous membrane color, capillary refill time, pulse and pulse quality, blood pressure) and repeat bolus as required. Concurrently, the stomach needs to be decompressed either by intubation with an orogastric tube or gastric trocarization. Dogs with GDV might tolerate orogastric tube placement without sedation, but a mouth gag should be used to prevent biting the tube. Decompression of the stomach will enable restoration of intravenous return.

Once the animal is stabilized, emergency surgery under GA is required to unrotate the stomach and perform a gastropexy. The stomach wall is assessed at the time of surgery and resection, or euthanasia might be indicated depending on the degree of wall compromise.

Postoperative arrhythmias are not unusual with GDVs (particularly ventricular premature complexes) but might not require specific treatment if the dog is otherwise cardiovascularly stable. Routine pain relief and postoperative monitoring are required with particular attention to septic peritonitis due to gastric wall devitalization.

Prognosis for GDV can be good if the disease is recognized early and treated rapidly. The prognosis is more guarded for dogs with high lactate at admission or requiring partial gastrectomy due to gastric wall necrosis or splenectomy due to vascular compromise at the time of surgery.

Preventative measures that are reported include feeding small and more frequent meals and avoiding vigorous activity around feeding. Prophylactic gastropexy can also be considered for breeds at significant risk.

NEOPLASTIC CONDITIONS OF THE STOMACH

Gastric neoplastic disease in dogs and cats overall represents a small portion of cancer cases, with a prevalence of less than 1% of overall reported cancers in dogs. Some of the risk factors reported in people, such as hypergastrinemia or *Helicobacter pylori* gastritis for gastric carcinoma, do not seem to be a significant player in dogs, although limited information is available. A higher incidence of gastric carcinoma has been reported in Belgian Shepherds in different countries as well as Chow Chow, Bouvier des Flandres, collie, standard poodle, and Norwegian elkhound and lundehunds. A higher male to female ratio has also been reported in some studies.

There are species-specific differences between dogs and cats in the types of gastric cancers. The most prevalent cancer in dogs is adenocarcinoma, but leiomyosarcoma, lymphoma, and gastrointestinal stromal tumors have also been reported. In comparison, cats more commonly develop lymphoma followed by adenocarcinoma and mast cell tumor.

Clinical presentation is typically nonspecific with vomiting as the most common clinical sign with or without hematemesis/melena. Other clinical signs include weight loss, diarrhea, and anorexia. It is rare that a mass can be detected on abdominal palpation, although this is more frequent in cats than dogs. Perforated gastric neoplasm is a differential for animals presenting with septic peritonitis or pneumoperitoneum.

Because clinical signs are vague, gastric cancers are typically diagnosed at a late stage and require a combination of diagnostic imaging and tissue sampling via endoscopy or surgery.

Of important note, endoscopy has been shown to be more sensitive to detect gastric masses than ultrasound, which is likely due to interferences from gastric content. More recently, CT has also been used as a modality to assess the GI tract. Thoracic radiographs can also be considered to assess for metastasis (especially prior to surgery), although these are infrequent. If masses are detected during the ultrasound, fine-needle aspirates can be considered, although yield is likely to be higher for lymphoma rather than other types of cancers.

Due to diagnostic imaging limitations, endoscopy should be considered even in the absence of suggestive changes on ultrasound, if gastric cancer remains a likely differential. This enables visualization of the mucosa and sampling for histology. Multiple biopsies should be taken from the lesions and surrounding mucosa to increase diagnostic yield. If ulcerations are present, direct sampling should be avoided to reduce the risk of perforation. If the diagnosis remains unclear, full-thickness biopsies can be considered.

Gastric Carcinoma

Gastric carcinoma is the most common gastric cancer in dogs. It is seen more commonly in male dogs that are 8–10 years old. The most common localization is the pylorus and lesser curvature, and ulcerations are common, but early/flatter lesions can occur and might only be visible with careful inspection or image enhancement (like narrow-band imaging or chromoendoscopy) (Figure 40.5). Severe ulcerations with perforation are occasionally reported. Metastasis is common to the regional lymph nodes and less commonly to the liver and lungs.

Lymphoma

Gastric lymphoma is more common in cats than dogs and the most common gastric cancer of cats (Figure 40.5) (Kehl et al. 2022). Although the mean age of cats diagnosed is over 10 years old, it can be seen at any age. If the cancer is limited to the GI tract, the most likely localization is the small intestine, followed by the large intestine, and rarely in the stomach.

The three types of alimentary lymphoma reported include the low-grade intestinal T-cell lymphoma (LGITL), intermediate- or high-grade alimentary lymphoma (IGAL or HGAL), and large granular lymphoma (LGL). Of these, LGL is frequently reported in the stomach, followed by LGITL.

LGITL is the most common type of lymphoma in cats and can be difficult to differentiate from lymphoplasmacytic inflammation present in chronic inflammatory enteropathy. Although full-thickness biopsy specimens are useful to assess the whole architecture, a combination of endoscopic biopsies, IHC, and PCR for Antigen Receptor Rearrangement (PARR) will enable the clinician to achieve a diagnosis in many cases. As it is much rarer to find LGITL in the stomach, sampling of the duodenum and ileum is typically more useful than the stomach, although the disease will be in some cases limited to just the jejunum (i.e., surgical approach is required). Although less reported, LGITL is now also recognized in dogs with over 50% of dogs presenting with protein-losing enteropathy.

On physical examination, thickening of the small intestines might be noted in LGITL cases, whereas a mass might be palpated in the other types of lymphoma as well as other organomegaly. Other findings might include icterus or cavity effusions. Occasionally, cats might be presented as an acute abdomen if the mass is obstructive. Ultrasound changes in the gastric mucosa (thickening or presence of a mass) increase suspicion of HGAL or LGL.

A final diagnosis might be achievable with cytology in cases with discrete masses or organomegaly, but biopsies are likely to be required for LGITL.

LGITL prognosis is overall good with a median survival time of over 1.5 years with oral chemotherapy (chlorambucil). HGAL behaves more aggressively, and a multi-agent combination chemotherapy should be considered. Remission rates of 50–65% are reported and complete remission in one-third of these. Median survival time for the complete responders is 7–10 months, although some cats will live longer than a year. Some of the negative prognostic factors reported include weight loss, hypoalbuminemia, or hypocobalaminemia. The worse prognosis is for cats with LGL with MST of 1–3 months.

Surgery might be a consideration in animals with a solitary mass and is required in cases with GI perforation.

Mesenchymal Cell Tumors

Mesenchymal cell tumors more commonly reported in dogs' stomach include smooth muscle tumors (leiomyomas or leiomyosarcoma) and gastrointestinal stromal tumors (GIST). It is often diagnosed in elderly dogs (11 years), and no sex predilection is reported.

Leiomyoma and leiomyosarcoma are usually focal lesions that can be ulcerated. Localization is typically the cardia or pylorus. Paraneoplastic hypoglycemia has also been reported with these tumors.

Although GIST is more commonly diagnosed in the intestines, it is reported in the stomach of 10–20% of cases. Immunohistochemistry is required to confirm the diagnosis of GIST ($CD117^{+}$), and for this reason, earlier studies might have misdiagnosed some GIST as smooth muscle neoplasm.

Other Neoplasms

Other cancers reported in dogs include mast cell tumors, histiocytic sarcoma, plasmacytoma, and undifferentiated sarcoma (Figure 40.5). In cats, adenocarcinoma is rarely reported, as well as GIST. Other cancers include mast cell tumors, carcinoid, hamartoma, and benign polyps.

Treatment recommendations depend on the final diagnosis. Although resection of solid tumors in the absence of metastasis can be considered, disease is often too advanced for this to be an option, especially with gastric carcinoma. Surgery can be more successful for the treatment of benign cancers such as leiomyoma.

Although chemotherapy is a treatment of choice for lymphoma, its role in treatment of other tumors is currently limited.

Overall prognosis is poor for dogs with gastric carcinomas (less than six months median survival time), but can be better for GIST, if surgery is possible and successful (MST of three years). The most successful outcome is for GIST after successful surgical resection. Mast cell tumors have a very poor outcome in dogs (MST of less than a month) but is better in cats (MST of 1.5 years).

SPECIFIC PROCEDURES RELATING TO GASTRIC CONDITIONS

OROGASTRIC INTUBATION FOR CONTENT REMOVAL AND LAVAGE

Gastric intubation and lavage can be considered in patients that ingested a non-caustic substance or that require decompression due to gastric dilation by gas or liquid content. It can also be useful to remove gastric content masking a foreign body during endoscopic removal.

Although gastric intubation might be possible in the emergency setting in a minimally sedated dog (e.g., GDV), the procedure is usually safer in an animal under general anesthetic (GA) and intubated with adequate cuff inflation to protect the lungs and reduce the risk of aspiration from content being instilled in the stomach or retrieved from it. It will also reduce the risk of oral, esophageal, or gastric mucosal damage during tube placement.

The selection of the tube depends on the size of the animal. Typically, 12 F for kittens or puppies up to 18 F for adult cats and smaller dogs. Large dogs will require a longer and larger tube. The tube length required is premeasured from the tip of the nose to the last rib following the curvature of the neck and marked using adhesive tape or marker. The tip of the tube is generously lubricated, and a mouth gag or roll is used to gently pass the tube through the mouth into the esophagus and prevent its accidental biting. The animal should be in sternal recumbency, and the head elevated while passing the tube and when inserting fluid (see below). If the animal is conscious, advancement at the level of the larynx during swallowing should ensure correct placement in the esophagus, if the animal is under general anesthesia, the tube needs to be gently pushed. The tube is passed until the pre-marked length is reached. It is not unusual to have increased resistance when reaching the lower esophageal sphincter, and some gas will typically be smelled when the tube is in the stomach in animals with gastric gas dilation. The position can finally be checked by administering a small amount of sterile water (3–5 mL); the animal should not react and not cough. If this is the case, inappropriate tracheal intubation should be considered.

Causes for the tube not to pass into the stomach include esophageal obstruction (e.g., foreign body), gastric volvulus, or tube misplacement in the trachea. Once the tube has been placed, it should be palpable through neck palpation. If there is any query about the tube being misplaced in the trachea, it should be removed.

Once the appropriate position of the tube has been confirmed, the content can be evacuated using a suction line or gravity flow, if it is liquid, and it will evacuate spontaneously if it is gas.

If the stomach needs to be washed, a funnel is attached to the tube, and 5–6 mL/kg of isotonic fluid is passed into the stomach with the animal's head elevated (higher than the stomach). The animal is then placed in lateral recumbency and gently rocked before emptying the stomach using a suction line or gravity flow. This procedure can be repeated as required to remove additional content. If activated charcoal is indicated, this can be done at the end of the procedure.

Once the procedure is finished, the tube is withdrawn gently and steadily. One thumb should be placed over the end of the tube, and the tube should be kinked during removal to reduce the risk of leakage of content from the tube into the esophagus or the mouth.

GASTROTOMY TUBES

Gastrotomy tubes are considered in animals requiring enteral feeding where nasal or esophageal feeding tubes are contraindicated (e.g., esophageal stricture or megaesophagus) or the requirement of assisted feeding is needed long-term.

The two main techniques described include surgical (gastrotomy, G tube) or endoscopic placement (percutaneous endoscopic gastrostomy, PEG), both of which require general anesthesia. The advantage of PEG tubes is their large diameter in comparison with other types of feeding tubes, which gives more flexibility on the type of diet used. Relative contraindications of placing a PEG tube include marked ascites, severe abdominal inflammation, and intractable vomiting. In large dogs, anchoring of the PEG tube might be safer to prevent dislodgement. Overall, a PEG tube is usually well tolerated in dogs, but the requirement of a bandage on the abdomen might reduce compliance in cats (Figure 40.6).

For endoscopic placement, a PEG tube suitable for the animal is required. They come typically in sizes ranging from 16 to 20 F. The animal is anesthetized and placed in right lateral recumbency. A minimum of two people is required for the procedure, with one scoping and the second one scrubbed with surgical gloves. The procedure aims to place the tube through the greater curvature of the stomach and left body whilst avoiding trapping another organ in between.

The skin caudal to the last rib is clipped and surgically prepped for placement (Figure 40.6).

The endoscope is placed in the stomach and depending on the specifics of the case, a full endoscopy with biopsies of the duodenum and the stomach might be considered. Following, the stomach should be inflated with air, and localization for placement can be confirmed by:

1. Transillumination of the body wall with the scope. This will only be possible if there is no organ entrapment but might not be possible depending on the animal's habitus.
2. With surgical gloves, the flank of the animal is gently palpated. The displacement of the body wall should be visible from inside the stomach with the endoscope. The placement should be on the flank of the animal and caudal from the last rib to improve comfort after the procedure.
3. An ultrasound can be used to confirm that there is no organ entrapment at the planned site of insertion of the tube.

Once an adequate localization has been determined, a 16 or 18 G needle or catheter is inserted through the incision and stabbed through the gastric wall aiming toward the endoscope. The endoscope should be retracted to avoid accidental stabbing. Suture material or guidewire included within the kit is threaded through the cannula into the stomach. The guidewire is grabbed with an endoscopy biopsy forceps and retrieved through the mouth by withdrawing the whole endoscope. The guidewire is then tied to the loop at the tapered end of the gastric tube. The guidewire is gently pulled back to bring the tube down the esophagus, in the stomach, and against the gastric wall. The

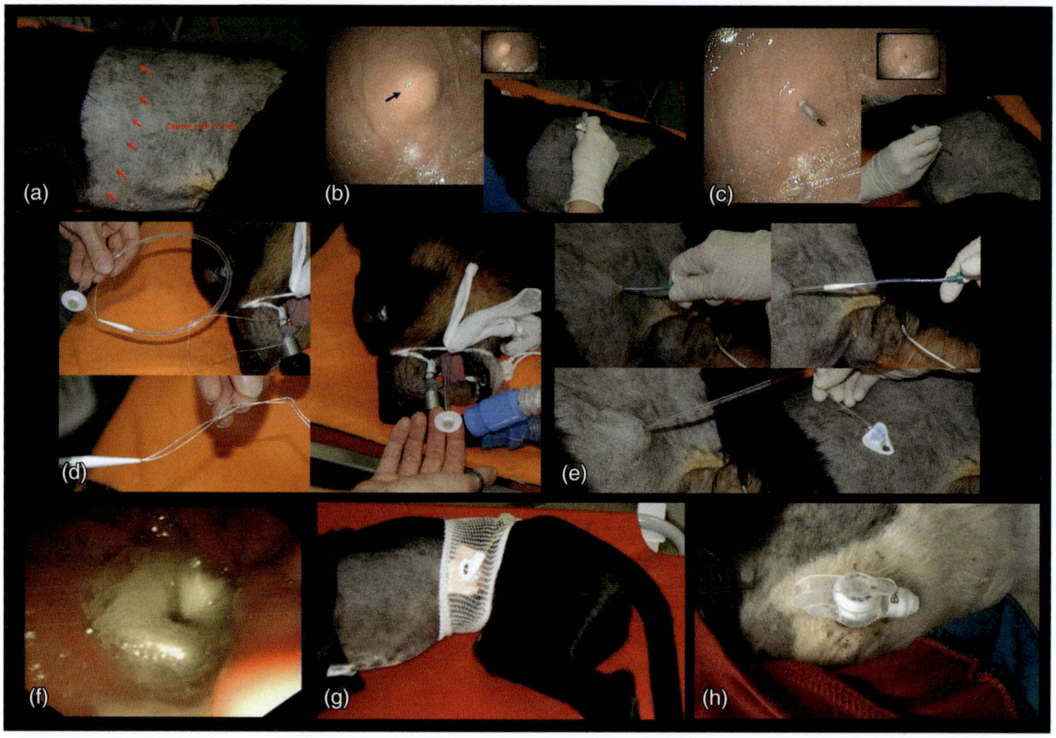

FIGURE 40.6 Stages of a PEG tube placement in dogs and cats. (a) Outline of the clipped area, arrows indicating the end of the caudal arch of ribs, behind which the PEG tube should be placed. (b) Endoscopic and outer view of the insertion site of the PEG tube trochar. (c) Endoscopic and outer view after the PEG tube trochar has entered the (inflated) gastric lumen. (d) After a guidewire or string is fed through the trochar and pulled out of the animal's mouth with the help of an endoscopic forceps, the actual PEG tube is fastened to it and pulled back into the stomach. (e) Once the PEG tube is pulled against the body wall, the trochar and tip of PEG tube are pulled through the gastric and outer abdominal wall. This step might require the widening of the skin insertion site with a small incision using a scalpel blade. The PEG tube is then secured. (f) The inner "button" or "mushroom" opening of the PEG tube should lie close to the mucosa (should be endoscopically verified). (g) The outer part of the PEG tube (flange) should be sutured in place, ensuring that the fit is not too tight (see text), the PEG tube cut to the desired length and closed with the matching security clip and cap (different depending on system used), as well as bandaged. (h) If longer-term use is required, once a full stoma has formed, the standard PEG tube can be swapped to a low-profile PEG tube, which is secured on the mucosal side with a fluid-filled balloon

incision at the body wall is widened with a scalpel blade to enable the passage of the tube without excessive force. The position of the mushroom inside the stomach can be confirmed to be close to the gastric wall with the endoscope. The PEG tube can then be anchored against the gastric wall using the provided flange. Care needs to be taken to avoid a tight fit between the mushroom and the flange. A space of at least 8–10 mm is typically required to account for tissue swelling after the procedure and to avoid pressure necrosis of the skin/gastric wall. The length of the tube until the insertion site should be measured and marked, which then enables monitoring during tube care to ensure that the PEG tube remains in the same position. Depending on the manufacturer, the flange keeps the PEG tube in place, or it can be kept in situ using a Roman sandal (finger trap) suture. In large dogs, anchorage of the stomach to reduce the risk of tube dislodgment has also been described. The tube is protected with a sleeve, jacket, and an Elizabethan collar depending on the animal's temperament.

The insertion site should be examined daily for any discoloration, or discharge, as well as monitoring the position of the tube (measurement or marker). Feeding can resume after 24 hours of tube placement, and the tube should be kept in place for a minimum of 10–14 days before considering removal or replacement with a low-profile gastrotomy tube for long-term management (Figure 40.6). The tube can also be left longer in place as required. This time frame should be sufficient for the formation of a stoma between the stomach wall and the body wall to prevent the risk of peritonitis due to leakage of gastric content into the peritoneum.

The tube can be removed by gently pulling the tube with one hand with contra-pressure of the other hand on the body wall. This procedure is tolerated by most animals without sedation. The stoma typically closes within a few hours. Another removal technique consists of cutting the tube at the level of the skin and retrieving the mushroom tip with the endoscope versus natural defecation (with a risk of obstruction), depending on the size of the animal.

The main downsides with a PEG tube placement include the need for anesthesia and require specific instrumentation (PEG tube and endoscope). Acute complications include laceration of the spleen due to organ entrapment, and later complications include pressure necrosis and insertion site infection or inflammation. If the tube gets dislodged within a few days of placement, there is a risk of peritonitis and tube migration within the GI tract with mechanical obstruction being described. Please see Chapter 35 for routine gastroscopic technique.

DRUGS FREQUENTLY USED WITH GASTRIC DISEASES

ANTIEMETICS

Antiemetics control emesis by either a central or peripheral action, depending on blockage of neurotransmission at receptor sites (Table 40.1). Centrally acting drugs block the emetic center in the CNS or the chemoreceptor trigger zone (CRTZ) (e.g., antidopaminergics), or act at the vestibular apparatus (e.g., antihistaminergics).

The most used centrally acting antiemetics, which are also licensed specifically for small animals in a number of countries, are metoclopramide (D2-receptor antagonist) and maropitant (neurokinin-1 receptor antagonist). There is some more variability in usage of antihistamines like diphenhydramine or phenothiazines like (pro)chlorpromazine, most commonly used for motion sickness. Serotonin ($5HT_3$) antagonists, such as ondansetron, are not commonly licensed, but are often considered for their synergistic action in the clinical setting.

PROTON-PUMP INHIBITORS AND OTHER GASTRIC MUCOSAL PROTECTANTS

These drugs are usually aimed at neutralizing gastric acid, promoting prostaglandin production or action, coating and protecting denuded gastric epithelium, and promoting clot formation and stabilization. Antacids (e.g., calcium carbonate, aluminum hydroxide, and magnesium hydroxide) neutralize local gastric acid but do not effectively inhibit gastric acid secretion, and for this reason are not recommended as a sole therapy for gastric ulceration (Marks et al. 2018).

Sucralfate requires an acidic environment to bind electrostatically to positively charged proteins exposed in ulcerated areas, hence, its affinity for injured tissue is five times greater than

Table 40.1 Antiemetics Classification

Mechanism of action	Active compound (example)	Location of action
α-adrenergic antagonist	Prochlorperazine Chlorpromazine	CRTZ, VC
D_2 dopaminergic antagonist	Metoclopramide	CRTZ, periphery
H_1 histaminergic antagonist	Diphenhydramine, Dimenhydrinate, Chlorpromazine	CRTZ
M_1 cholinergic antagonist	Pirenzepine	Vestibular, CRTZ
$5HT_3$ serotonergic antagonist	Ondansetron Metoclopramide	CRTZ, vagal afferences, periphery
NK1 receptor antagonist	Maropitant	CRTZ, NTS, periphery

CRTZ, chemoreceptor trigger zone; D, dopamine; H, histamine; 5-HT, serotonin; NK, neurokinin, NTS, nucleus tractus solitarius; M, muscarinic; VC, vomiting center.

for normal mucosa. It also decreases pepsin activity and stimulates the release of protective prostaglandins. It is very well tolerated but requires an acidic environment to work and therefore may be contraindicated with proton pump inhibitors. It also interferes with drugs affected by the aluminum component of sucralfate (e.g., tetracyclines, ciprofloxacin). Therefore, acid suppressants and antibiotics should be administered at least two hours before or after sucralfate.

Acid-suppressing drugs include histamine (H_2)-receptor antagonists(H_2RAs) or proton pump inhibitors (PPIs). The **H_2RAs** (e.g., famotidine, ranitidine, cimetidine) have a good safety profile and can be administered with a full meal. Cimetidine has the weakest potency and also inhibits cytochrome P450, which can result in unwanted drug interactions. Ranitidine has poor acid suppressant activity in dogs and cats and is more commonly used to promote GI motility (see below). Famotidine has good (cats) to excellent (dogs) acid-suppressing activity and a good safety profile. However, repeated daily oral administration of famotidine, results in a diminished effect in healthy dogs and cats. Because of their relatively weak acid-suppressing activity, H_2RAs should not supplant PPIs for the treatment of moderate to severe gastroduodenal erosion or ulceration. Moreover, they should not be combined with PPIs for the treatment of ulcerative disease as they do not have an additive effect on gastric pH. Famotidine is renally excreted and should be dose reduced in dogs and cats with kidney disease.

The **PPIs** (e.g., omeprazole, esomeprazole, pantoprazole, lansoprazole) target the final common pathway of acid production and inhibit gastric acid secretion regardless of stimulus (see Figure 40.4). They permeate the parietal cell membrane and form disulfide bonds with the active proton-pumping H^+-K^+-ATPase. PPIs are more effective than H_2RAs in healing upper GI erosion and ulceration. While H_2RAs reach peak concentrations within hours of oral administration, PPIs can take up to four days to reach peak effect. Orally administered PPIs should be given on an empty stomach immediately before offering a full meal. In most situations, dogs and cats should be treated twice daily with a PPI. If once-daily administration of a PPI is necessary or compliance is a concern, orally administered esomeprazole seems to be effective even when given once daily. PPIs are inhibitors of cytochrome P450 enzymes, thus, drug interactions are common. In dogs, long-term use of omeprazole (and likely other PPIs) can potentially lead to hypertrophic gastropathy, specifically fundic gland polyps (Lee et al. 2023), so chronic long-term use should be discouraged (Figure 40.5). Other adverse effects in people following long-term PPI use include induction of chronic kidney disease, osteoporosis, pathologic fractures, and diarrhea.

PROKINETICS

No guidelines for the appropriate indication, combination, and duration of motility-modifying therapies for gastric emptying disorders in small animals are available. Due to the diagnostic challenges discussed above, correct assessment of most gastric motility or any therapeutic effect of selected drugs is difficult. It is important to first investigate, diagnose, and treat any underlying disease leading to dysmotility before administering prokinetics.

Prokinetic drugs are divided into serotonergic 5-HT_4 agonists, motilin-like drugs, dopaminergic D_2 antagonists, and H_2RAs (see Table 40.2).

Of the **5-HT_4 agonists**, cisapride has been most extensively studied but was withdrawn from production due to lethal cardiac side effects in humans. Other 5-HT_4 agonists include mosapride, prucalopride, levosulpiride, and tegaserod. Gastric prokinetic properties of cisapride have been documented in many experimental settings, however, in some studies in dogs, no effect on gastric emptying was observed. Prucalopride stimulates gastric emptying in a dose-dependent manner in dogs, while for the other drugs in this group, mostly preliminary data in dogs is available.

The antibiotics erythromycin and azithromycin accelerate gastric emptying by inducing phase III contractions of the interdigestive MMCs when used in sub-antibiotic dosages, which are similar to those induced by the endogenous hormone, **motilin**. However, stimulation of interdigestive motility can lead to "dumping" of gastric contents into the duodenum before they have been acidified, which in turn can cause inadequate absorption of nutrients, cramps, and osmotic diarrhea.

Table 40.2 Prokinetic Drugs Used in Dogs and Cats

Class/name	Site of action	Dose	Comments
Serotonergic 5-HT_4 agonists			
Cisapride	GES, stomach, intestine, colon	0.1–0.5 mg/kg PO q8–12h (dogs) 2.5 mg/cat PO q8–12h, may be titrated up as high as 7.5 mg/cat	Often no longer available due to arrhythmia in people; in high doses (3 mg/kg) it slows gastric emptying of solids in dogs
Mosapride	Stomach, colon	0.25–2 mg/kg PO q12h (dog), 5 mg/cat q12h	—
Prucalopride	Stomach, small and large intestine	Dog: for gastric emptying: 0.01–0.16 mg/kg PO q24h Cat: 0.24–0.5 mg/kg PO q24h	Can be administered rectally (crushed tablet diluted in water) if oral administration is not considered safe or gastric motility is severely impaired
Dopaminergic D_2 agonists			
Metoclopramide	Esophagus (cats), stomach	0.2–0.5 mg/kg q6–8h PO, SC, IM or IV or CRI 0.04–0.09 mg/kg/h (dogs) 0.5 mg/kg SC q8h (cats)	Possibly not very effective on gastric motility in dogs, very weak effect in cats
Motilin-like substances			
Erythromycin	GES, stomach, small and large intestine	0.5–1 mg/kg PO or IV q8–12h (dog, cat)	Can cause "dumping" of gastric contents into the duodenum
Azithromycin	Stomach	3.5 mg/kg PO q24h	Only data from healthy cats
H_2RA/ Acetylcholine esterase inhibitors			
Ranitidine	Stomach, colon	1–2 mg/kg PO, SC, IM q8–12h or slow IV/ CRI (dog) 2.5 mg/kg slow IV q12h or 3.5 mg/kg PO q12h (cats)	Probably only mild prokinetic effect

CRI, continuous rate infusion; GES, gastro-esophageal sphincter; H_2RA, histamine receptor antagonist; 5HT, serotonin.

There is little convincing evidence that **dopaminergic D_2 antagonists** like metoclopramide have prokinetic effects on the canine or feline stomach, even though metoclopramide in particular has been advocated for this purpose for decades. In fact, when emptying of solid and liquid contents were assessed separately in experimental dogs, metoclopramide slowed solid gastric emptying while accelerating liquids. There is potential evidence, however, that metoclopramide might improve antropyloroduodenal coordination and the frequency of pyloric and duodenal contractions. Effects seem dose-dependent, as only a high dose (1 mg/kg followed by a CRI with 1 mg/kg/h) reduced gastroesophageal reflux, while lower doses did not. In one study, a protocol involving metoclopramide and famotidine in brachycephalic dogs undergoing airway surgery was associated with a decreased incidence of postoperative regurgitation. Overall, metoclopramide might not be harmful in a dog with suspected gastric hypomotility, especially as nausea and vomiting might also be present, but it likely cannot provide a strong prokinetic effect.

The gastric prokinetic properties of the **H_2RA ranitidine** have been assessed in both rodents and humans, but effects are inconsistent. Some studies suggest acceleration of liquid gastric content, others show no effect or even a dose-dependent delay in gastric emptying.

REFERENCES

Barash, N.R., Lashnits, E., Kern, Z.T. et al. (2022). Outcomes of esophageal and gastric bone foreign bodies in dogs. *Journal of Veterinary Internal Medicine* 36 (2): 500–507.

Bebchuk, T.N. (2002). Feline gastrointestinal foreign bodies. *Veterinary Clinics of North America - Small Animal Practice* 32 (4): 861–880.

Crinò, C., Humm, K., and Cortellini, S. (2023). Conservative management of metallic sharp-pointed straight gastric and intestinal foreign bodies in dogs and cats: 17 cases (2003-2021). *Journal of Small Animal Practice* 64 (8): 522–526.

Di Palma, C., Pasolini, M.P., Navas, L. et al. (2022). Endoscopic and surgical removal of gastrointestinal foreign bodies in dogs: an analysis of 72 cases. *Animals* 12 (11): 1376.

Dollo, V., Chambers, G., and Carothers, M. (2020). Endoscopic retrieval of gastric and oesophageal foreign bodies in 52 cats. *Journal of Small Animal Practice* 61 (1): 51–56.

Freiche, V. and German, A.J. (2021). Digestive diseases in brachycephalic dogs. *Veterinary Clinics of North America - Small Animal Practice* 51 (1): 61–78.

Freiche, V., Da Riz, F., Benchekroun, G. et al. (2021). Endoscopic assessment of presumed acquired pyloric narrowing in cats: a retrospective study of 27 cases. *Research in Veterinary Science* 136: 408–415.

Gianella, P., Pfammatter, N.S., and Burgener, I.A. (2009). Oesophageal and gastric endoscopic foreign body removal: complications and follow-up of 102 dogs. *Journal of Small Animal Practice* 50 (12): 649–654.

Lee, H., Kim, S., Lee, D. et al. (2023). Case report: fundic gland polyps caused by long-term omeprazole use in a maltese dog. *Frontiers in Veterinary Science* 10: 1287335.

Webb, C. and Twedt, D.C. (2003). Canine gastritis. *Veterinary Clinics of North America - Small Animal Practice* 33 (5): 969–985.

Zimmer, J.F. (1981). Removal of gastric foreign bodies using flexible fiberoptic endoscopy. *Veterinary Clinics of North America: Small Animal Practice* 76 (11): 1611–1619.

Disorders of the Small Intestine

CHAPTER 41

Sara Jablonski

Department of Small Animal Clinical Sciences, College of Veterinary Medicine, Michigan State University, East Lansing, MI, USA

KEY POINTS

- Most cases of acute diarrhea are mild, self-limiting, and not caused by enteropathogenic infection. Thus, antimicrobials are not recommended in the routine management of nonspecific acute diarrhea.
- Screening for infectious disease in dogs and cats with diarrhea should be performed in light of the patient signalment and relevant clinical details and with a specific infectious agent in mind. Broad infectious disease screening is usually unrewarding in cases of acute and chronic diarrhea.
- Chronic enteropathy is a diagnosis of exclusion, and the majority of cases are food responsive. Importantly, a variety of different dietary strategies may be successful in an individual cat or dog with CE, thus at least two different dietary approaches should be attempted in otherwise stable cases.
- Inflammatory bowel disease (IBD) is no longer the preferred terminology for idiopathic intestinal inflammation. Use of the term chronic inflammatory enteropathy (CIE) is recommended in place of IBD in cats and dogs.
- Dietary therapy is a critical component of management in dogs with PLE. Multifunction veterinary gastrointestinal diets that are labeled as both low-fat and hydrolyzed are newly available and appropriate choices for many dogs with PLE. Alternative dietary strategies (including the use of home-cooked diets) should be considered in dogs with PLE not responding to an initial diet plan and glucocorticoid therapy.

INTRODUCTION

The small intestine (SI) is susceptible to a variety of important disorders. The most essential functions of the SI include the mixing and propulsion of ingesta, secretion of water and electrolytes, digestion and absorption, and regulation of blood flow. The SI must do all these functions while controlling immunological reactions and maintaining tolerance.

The most common clinical sign of SI disease is diarrhea. Small intestinal diarrhea is characterized by an increase in the volume of feces produced with normal to mildly increased frequency, and a lack of urgency, tenesmus, blood, or mucus (Table 41.1). Diarrhea is most often a consequence of malabsorption and/or bacterial fermentation of unabsorbed solutes. Other common clinical signs of SI disease include weight loss (typically due to malabsorption), changes in appetite (including hyporexia, anorexia, and polyphagia), vomiting, pica, coprophagia, borborygmi, abdominal pain, melena, and effusions/edema, among other signs (Jablonski and Cridge 2023).

In all cases of SI disease, a thorough history and physical exam are required. Consideration of the animal's signalment along with the information obtained from a thorough history and physical exam will in many cases go a long way toward determining the cause. The necessity of additional diagnostic testing will vary depending on the individual case. However, common diagnostic tests performed in the evaluation of SI disease include laboratory evaluations (Chapter 33), fecal pathogen testing, minimum database, specific serum and fecal GI biomarkers, imaging studies (Chapter 34),

Disorders of the Liver, Exocrine Pancreas, and Gastrointestinal Tract in Dogs and Cats, First Edition. Edited by Harry Cridge et al. Published 2026 by John Wiley & Sons, Inc. Companion Website: www.wiley.com/go/cridge/disorders

Table 41.1 Differentiation Between Small and Large Bowel Diarrhea in Dogs and Cats

	Small bowel	Large bowel
Frequency of defecation	≤3 times daily	>3 times daily
Stool volume	Normal to increased	Decreased
Urgency of defecation	Rare	Common
Tenesmus during defecation	Rare	Common
Fecal blood	Rare; if present, melena	Common; usually hematochezia
Fecal mucus	Rare	Common
Steatorrhea	May be present	Absent
Weight loss	Common	Rare
Vomiting	Common	Rare
Borborygmi	May be present	Absent

and in some cases, endoscopy with intestinal biopsy (Chapters 35). The following provides an overview of various disorders of the SI and includes general information, specific diagnostics, therapeutic approaches, and, where available, prognoses.

SPECIFIC DISORDERS OF THE SI

IDIOPATHIC ACUTE ENTEROPATHY

An acute enteropathy is defined by clinical signs of GI disease of <14 days duration. Dogs and cats with acute enteropathy are typically presented with a history of diarrhea and/or vomiting with or without reports of lethargy and loss of appetite. Dogs with acute enteritis would be expected to have small bowel diarrhea; however, sometimes colitis may occur concurrently, leading to signs of both small and large bowel diarrhea (Table 41.1). Causes of acute enteropathy include dietary (food intolerance or allergy, sudden dietary change), infectious (bacterial, parasitic, viral), metabolic, anatomic, and extra-gastrointestinal (GI) etiologies.

Many cases of acute enteropathy will be mild and self-limiting. However, select cases will be life-threatening. Thus, the diagnostic and therapeutic approach to the dog or cat with acute enteropathy will first depend on the determination of whether the patient is stable or unstable. Dogs and cats with self-limiting acute enteropathies have milder clinical signs and relatively normal physical examinations with no abdominal pain detected. These animals are bright, alert, and responsive, with no evidence of hemodynamic instability. Indicators of a potentially serious case of acute enteropathy include history of frequent vomiting, melena or hematochezia, and physical examination findings of dullness, moderate-to-severe dehydration, icterus, abdominal pain, elevated body temperature, ascites, or palpation of an abdominal mass or dilated loop of SI. If it is uncertain whether the patient has mild or serious disease, it is best to err on the side of caution and approach the case as if it may be life-threatening.

The diagnostic and general therapeutic approach to small animal patients with acute diarrhea is shown in Figure 41.1. In all cases of acute enteropathy, fecal examination for parasites should be performed. Centrifugal fecal floatation using zinc sulfate and indirect fluorescent antibody (IFA) or antigen testing for *Giardia* cysts and IFA for *Cryptosporidium* oocysts is recommended. Fecal cytology is not diagnostically helpful in dogs and cats with acute enteropathies. Additional laboratory tests may not be necessary in mildly affected patients; however, measurement of hematocrit and plasma total protein may give an indication of hydration status. Complete minimum database and abdominal radiographs may be considered in these cases to screen for signs of more serious illness, but in many instances these diagnostics will be unnecessary in mildly affected patients.

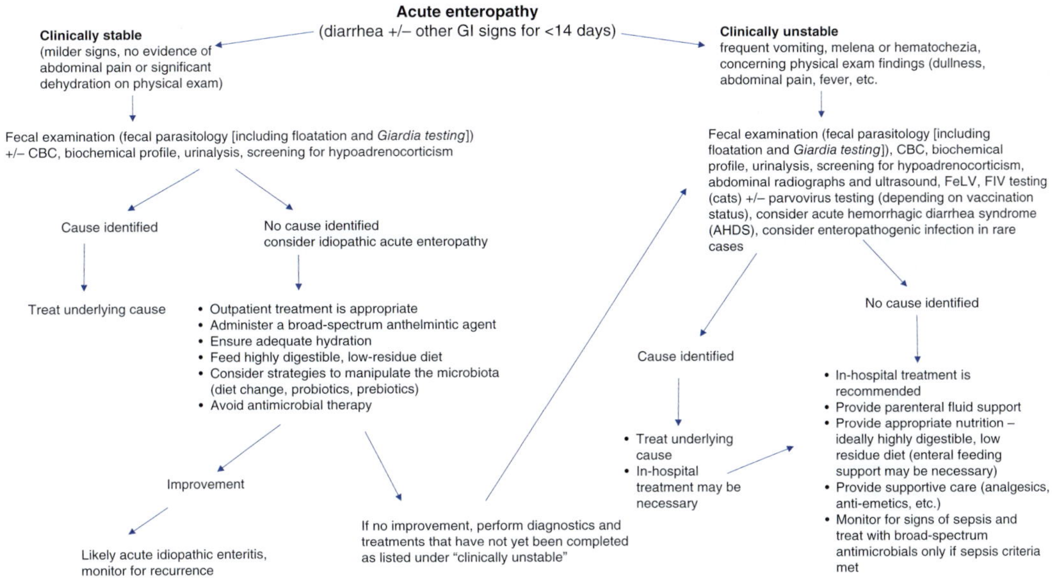

FIGURE 41.1 General diagnostic and therapeutic approach to dogs and cats with acute enteropathy

Diagnostic tests recommended for dogs and cats with clinical signs and/or physical exam findings suggestive of more serious disease include complete minimum database (complete blood count [CBC], serum biochemistry profile with electrolytes, urinalysis), testing for hypoadrenocorticism (serum resting cortisol, or if necessary, adrenocorticotropic hormone [ACTH] stimulation testing), quantification of pancreatic lipase, parvovirus testing (depending on vaccination status), and abdominal radiography and/or abdominal ultrasound. Abdominal imaging is particularly important as there is an urgent need to exclude surgical conditions including torsions, intussusception, mechanical obstruction of the SI, and peritonitis in these cases. Generally speaking, fecal culture and polymerase chain reaction (PCR) are not recommended in dogs and cats with acute enteropathies, as detection of a specific enteric pathogen does not establish causation for the clinical signs. The exception is in the patient who is systemically ill with clinical signs suggestive of possible enteropathogenic infection (bloody diarrhea, elevated body temperature) and who is in contact with an immunosuppressed/immunocompromised person. In those cases, performing fecal culture and PCR for detection of specific organisms may be warranted. The specific clinical presentation and environmental history may warrant testing for *Tritrichomonas foetus* in cats with acute enteropathies. Serologic testing for feline leukemia virus (FeLV) and feline immunodeficiency virus (FIV) is also warranted in cats (Manchester 2024).

The treatment of noninfectious, mild, self-limiting acute enteropathies involves ensuring adequate hydration and providing adequate and appropriate nutrition. In some instances, additional medications addressing signs such as nausea or vomiting may be beneficial. Strategies to manipulate the microbiota may also be employed. Importantly, there is no evidence that gastroprotectant medications (e.g., proton-pump inhibitors, sucralfate) are beneficial in cases of mild, self-limiting acute enteropathies. Furthermore, antimicrobial therapy (e.g., metronidazole, tylosin) is no longer recommended in routine treatment of dogs and cats with noninfectious, mild, self-limiting acute enteropathies (Candellone et al. 2020). In dogs and cats with evidence of mild dehydration, subcutaneous fluid therapy could be administered. Dietary therapy should always be part of the therapeutic plan in patients with acute enteropathies. Meeting nutritional requirements allows for normalization of intestinal motility and functions. Traditional dietary approaches to acute enteropathy involve feeding of a highly digestible, low-residue diet with moderate levels of fat. Many commercial veterinary foods formulated for GI disease meet these criteria. In cases where there is concern for concurrent acute colitis, increasing the dietary fiber through both soluble and insoluble sources may be beneficial to add indigestible bulk, hold excess water, and buffer toxins. More information on dietary management of acute GI disorders is available in Chapter 45. Therapies aimed at manipulating the microbiota may also be administered to patients with acute enteropathies. Systemic reviews highlight the need for large randomized controlled studies to evaluate the efficacy of these treatments; however, some studies have demonstrated a benefit. Specifically, in one randomized double blinded placebo-controlled clinical trial performed in dogs with acute diarrhea, administration of probiotics (*Bifidobacterium bifidum* VPBB-6, *Bifidobacterium longum* VPBL-5, *Bifidobacterium animalis* VPBA-4, *Bifidobacterium infantis* VPBI-6, *Lactobacillus acidophilus* VPLA-4, *Lactobacillus plantarum* VPLP-5, *Lactobacillus casei* VPLC-1, *Lactobacillus brevis* VPLB-5, *Lactobacillus reuteri* VPLR-1, *Lactobacillus bulgaricus* VPLB-7) appeared to result in a faster resolution of diarrhea when compared to metronidazole or placebo (Shmalberg et al. 2019). Additionally, fecal microbial transplantation (FMT) has been demonstrated to normalize the fecal dysbiosis index (fDI) in dogs with acute diarrhea when compared with dogs treated with metronidazole (Chaitman et al. 2020). The use of adsorbents, such as kaolin/pectin have also been described for the treatment of acute diarrhea, with one study showing a benefit when compared to a placebo (Nixon et al. 2019).

Dogs and cats with acute enteropathies that are systemically ill often require hospitalization for correction of hypovolemia (if present), dehydration, and replacement of ongoing losses with parenteral fluid therapy. In these cases, intravenous fluids are best. Therapeutic principles regarding providing adequate and appropriate nutrition and administering medications to address clinical signs are similar to cases with mild disease. However, dogs and cats with severe acute enteropathy often require placement of an enteral feeding tube to provide adequate nutrition (see Chapter 45). Dogs with nonspecific acute enteropathies resulting in severe clinical signs should improve in response to in-hospital therapies within 48 hours. If improvement is not observed within this time frame, recommendations should be given to perform or repeat diagnostic testing to exclude other causes of diarrhea.

Acute hemorrhagic diarrhea syndrome (AHDS) is a specific cause of acute-onset enteropathy in dogs. It is often reported in small breed dogs; however, any breed of dog can develop AHDS. The characteristic clinical history is an acute onset of severe GI signs often beginning with vomiting (+/− hematemesis) and then progressing to include diarrhea which may be bloody. Dogs with AHDS may become severely hemoconcentrated despite intestinal protein loss (leading to the characteristic finding of elevated PCV/HCT despite normal serum or plasma protein concentrations). In some cases, they may become hypovolemic and hemodynamically unstable due to severe GI losses. Thus, intravenous fluid therapy often must be given at rapid rates to address life-threatening hypovolemia, provided no contraindications to rapid fluid therapy are present. Fluid therapy should also address correcting dehydration and replacing ongoing losses. Dogs with AHDS often also benefit from antiemetics, analgesics, and other symptomatic therapies. Most dogs with AHDS will have an uncomplicated disease course and recover rapidly. However, in rare cases, signs of sepsis may occur, due to intestinal translocation of bacteria. Based on published guidelines, antimicrobials should only be administered to dogs with AHDS with clinical signs or laboratory abnormalities suggestive of sepsis. These signs include dull mentation (especially after 24–48 hours of therapy), fever or hypothermia, hypotension despite appropriate fluid supplementation, severe neutrophilia or neutropenia, hypoglycemia, and hyperbilirubinemia, among others. In such cases administration of a broad-spectrum antimicrobial(s) with both gram-negative and anaerobic coverage would be important. Amoxicillin/clavulanate given parenterally would be a reasonable choice. Ongoing treatment should continue to address fluid and electrolyte loss and provide supportive care (Unterer and Busch 2021).

The prognosis in cases of idiopathic/nonspecific acute enteropathies is good to excellent. There is recent concern that after episodes of severe acute enteropathy, dogs may be more susceptible to the development of chronic diarrhea later in life. In the future, treatment strategies may be discovered and recommended to help prevent chronic signs from developing.

ACUTE INFECTIOUS ENTERITIS

Acute infectious enteropathies in dogs and cats may be caused by parasitic, protozoal, viral, and less commonly, bacterial pathogens. Consideration of the signalment in light of the presenting complaint and relevant clinical history (including environmental history) will quickly help a clinician decide whether infectious differentials should be prioritized. This is critical, as in many cases detection of a pathogen on infectious disease screening may be incidental in a dog or cat with acute diarrhea. If infectious disease testing is to be pursued in dogs and cats with acute diarrhea, it should be done with a specific infectious agent in mind that matches the clinical presentation.

Parasitic Enteritis Due to Helminths

Roundworms (*Toxocara canis* [dogs], *Toxocara cati* [cats], and *Toxocara leoni* [dogs and cats]) and hookworms (*Ancylostoma and Uncinaria* spp.) are the intestinal parasites most likely to result in SI diarrhea in dogs and cats. Occasionally, heavy infestations of tapeworms may lead to SI diarrhea, but more commonly tapeworm infections cause perianal irritation or are asymptomatic. Diagnosis of infection due to intestinal parasites is best achieved via fecal floatation with centrifugation. Treatment is specific to the type of infection diagnosed. Many anthelmintic therapies are effective against roundworm infections, while hookworms are best treated with pyrantel pamoate and tapeworm infestations should be treated with praziquantel. The Companion Animal Parasite Council (CAPC) guidelines state that dogs and cats with diarrhea should be screened for intestinal parasites with direct smear, fecal floatation by centrifugation, and where applicable, specific fecal enzyme-linked immunosorbent assay (ELISA).

Acute Protozoal Enteritis

Many protozoal organisms that may cause acute diarrhea in the dog, including *Isospora* spp., *Cryptosporidium* spp., and *Giardia* spp. predominately cause large bowel diarrhea. Others such as *Sarcocystis* spp., *Toxoplasma gondii*, and *Neospora caninum* may transiently cause SI diarrhea while they complete the sexual phase of their life cycle in the intestinal tract; however, these infections are not typically recognized at this stage of disease.

Acute Viral Enteritis

The most common viral infections that may result in acute enteritis in small animals include canine and feline parvovirus, canine and feline coronavirus, and canine distemper virus (CDV).

Canine and feline parvovirus are important and common causes of acute diarrhea in dogs and cats. Both cause high morbidity and mortality worldwide. Early clinical signs in dogs with canine parvovirus infection include fever, inappetence, and lethargy, followed by vomiting and diarrhea. Diarrhea usually starts out as small bowel and commonly has a fetid odor. Melena and hematochezia may develop next, and vomiting is also frequently observed. Clinical signs in cats with panleukopenia can progress very quickly, with some cats dying within 12 hours of initially showing signs. Vomiting and diarrhea are important signs in cats but occur less frequently than in dogs with parvovirus infection. The diagnoses of canine and feline parvovirus are made in an animal with compatible signalment and history (un- or inadequately vaccinated) and a positive fecal parvovirus ELISA. Specificity of these tests is very good; however, sensitivity can be poor (Schmitz et al. 2009). Thus, PCR can be considered in an animal with a supportive history but negative ELISA. The ideal treatment is provided in hospital and includes diligent fluid and electrolyte therapies, management of oncotic pressure, provision of adequate nutrition, supportive care (e.g., anti-emetics), and treatment with broad-spectrum antibiotics due to disruption of the GI barrier and high incidence of leukopenia. One randomized clinical trial showed that diarrhea improved faster in dogs with parvovirus treated with FMT (Pereira et al. 2018). An outpatient protocol for canine parvovirus has been evaluated and can be considered in cases where the client lacks the financial means to treat the dog in hospital (Venn et al. 2017).

Canine enteric coronavirus infection is typically mild and self-limiting, in which case it is indistinguishable from other causes of mild, self-limiting acute diarrhea. However, a virulent and multi-system form of canine coronavirus emerged in 2005 and is referred to as pantropic canine coronavirus. This variant may cause severe systemic illness similar to canine parvovirus (e.g., fever, hemorrhagic gastroenteritis, hypovolemia, neutropenia, death). Treatment of pantropic canine coronavirus is nonspecific. Though not completely protective, vaccination with canine coronavirus is strongly recommended for prevention. Feline coronavirus is a pathogen of both wild and domesticated cats and is endemic in catteries and shelters. Most cats exposed to feline coronavirus develop mild or even subclinical enteritis, which does not require specific therapy. However, a small subset of cats will develop a biotype of disease known as feline infectious peritonitis (FIP). Cats with FIP may develop a host of systemic signs which may or may not include diarrhea.

Vomiting and diarrhea are often early signs in cases of canine distemper. Additional clinical signs that would increase suspicion of CDV as a potential cause of diarrhea include dramatic muscle loss/wasting, fever, conjunctivitis, neurologic signs, and nasal/footpad hyperkeratosis. The most widely used and useful diagnostic test for CDV is reverse-transcriptase PCR, typically of a conjunctival swab. Treatment is nonspecific and similar to other viral enteritides. Dogs that have not developed neurologic signs have the best chance of recovery.

Acute Bacterial Enteritis

Bacterial infections are rare causes of small intestinal diarrhea/disease in dogs and cats. Since many of the organisms that could be considered pathogens are normal inhabitants of the GI tract, proving causation is challenging. However, bacterial enteritis can be considered in unique cases where the clinical signs fit and the animal is young, immunocompromised, uniquely exposed, or part of a larger group where multiple animals are affected.

While clinical signs of enteric bacterial disease are nonspecific, the presence of severe, bloody diarrhea, fever, neutropenia, and signs of systemic inflammatory response syndrome or sepsis would raise suspicion for a possible bacterial cause or secondary bacterial infection. *Campylobacter* spp. may cause canine or feline enteritis; however, the majority of cases resolve with no specific treatment. *Campylobacter* infection may also result in cholangiohepatitis. Testing may be warranted in cases where clinical signs are severe, the animal is immunocompromised, or there is an outbreak situation. Testing of dogs may also be important in cases where there is an immunocompromised person in the household, since dogs can be a source of infection for humans. Direct PCR of feces may be utilized in these cases. Treatment, when necessary, is with a macrolide or enrofloxacin. Salmonellosis may similarly occur in young, immunocompromised, or uniquely exposed animals. Importantly, feeding a raw food diet is associated with an increased risk of salmonellosis. Clinical signs of salmonellosis are highly variable depending on whether transient subclinical carriage, acute gastroenteritis, bacteremia/endotoxemia, or a chronic carrier state occurs. Diagnosis is via fecal culture or PCR, typically after overnight enrichment. Antimicrobials are only necessary in dogs or cats with systemic signs that can be attributed to salmonellosis, and should ideally be based on culture and sensitivity, since multi-drug resistance is common. The preferred antimicrobials for treatment of salmonellosis are enrofloxacin or trimethoprim-sulfa, since they have good phagocytic cell penetration. Various *Escherichia coli* spp. may result in diarrhea in the dog, and clinical recognition, diagnosis and treatment are similar to what is described for *Salmonella* spp. Importantly, adherent-invasive *E. coli* (AIEC) typically causes chronic signs of the large bowel and disease caused by AIEC is covered in Chapter 42. Other types of *E. coli* enteritis should only be treated with antimicrobials if severe signs develop, or there is concern for immunosuppression in an individual patient. Other bacterial agents, such as *Yersinia* spp., *Mycobacterium* spp., and *Neorickettsia helminthoeca*, may cause acute SI diarrhea in dogs and cats but will do so as part of a more systemic illness that can be recognized by the unique features of those pathogens and their clinical manifestations.

CHRONIC INFECTIOUS ENTERITIS

Some infectious organisms that cause small intestinal disease in dogs and cats are more likely to present as a chronic illness. These include canine schistosomiasis, and systemic fungal and algal infections. The clinical presentation of the patient as well as their geographic exposures will help to rank order these differentials as potential causes of chronic diarrhea in cats and dogs.

The causative agent of canine schistosomiasis is *Heterobilharzia americana,* a trematode parasite. Dogs are exposed when the cercariae from infected snails penetrate their skin while they are swimming or wading in freshwater. Cercariae transform into schistosomes in the dog, migrate first to the lungs, followed by the liver, where they develop into flukes. The adult flukes migrate to mesenteric veins where they mate and then deposit eggs. It is the eggs that will migrate into the intestinal wall, which will cause a granulomatous reaction, which results in malabsorption and subsequent diarrhea. In addition to diarrhea, dogs with schistosomiasis are typically presented with lethargy, anorexia, and weight loss. Typical biochemical findings include anemia, azotemia, hypoalbuminemia, hyperglobulinemia, and hypercalcemia. The latter finding distinguishes this condition from most cases of hypoalbuminemia due to GI disease. Diagnosis is via fecal PCR, identification of the ova on a fecal sediment evaluation, or through histopathology. Canine schistosomiasis is treated with high-dose praziquantel along with fenbendazole. Lower doses have been proposed for asymptomatic in contact animals to reduce cost of treatment, but additional study is needed. The response to treatment is variable, but complete recovery is often achieved.

Several fungal organisms may cause small intestinal disease, with variable concurrent involvement of the large bowel. While disseminated aspergillosis and cryptococcus may cause diarrhea, the most important fungal organism to consider in the context of chronic diarrhea is *Histoplasma capsulatum,* the causative agent of histoplasmosis. The highest prevalence of histoplasmosis in the United States (US) is in Kansas, Oklahoma, and Texas, followed by the midwestern, southern, and southeastern US. Histoplasmosis affects both the small and large bowel, and commonly results in hypoalbuminemia, making it an important differential for dogs with protein-losing enteropathy (PLE). Other common clinical signs in dogs and cats with systemic histoplasmosis include weight loss, fever, and loss of appetite. Other organ systems affected include the respiratory tract, skin, and eyes. Disease may be localized to the GI tract in about one-third of dogs. If there is clinical suspicion for histoplasmosis *Histoplasma* spp. urine antigen enzyme immunoassay testing should be performed, and in some cases, the organism can be detected via rectal scraping with cytology. Many cases of systemic histoplasmosis can be treated with azole antifungal medications; however, in severe, life-threatening cases concurrent treatment with amphotericin B should be recommended.

Prototheca and *Pythium* spp. are other causes of chronic infectious enteritis in the dog. *Prototheca* spp. are algal organisms that commonly affect the large intestine in dogs, with occasional small intestinal involvement. Similar to *H. capsulatum, Prototheca* spp. may be detected on rectal scrape (Figure 41.2). Cats with protothecosis typically develop the cutaneous form. The causative agent of pythiosis in dogs is *Pythium insidiosum. P. insidiosum* is an oomycete that causes weight loss, diarrhea, vomiting and ulcerative, nodular skin lesions in dogs. Infection is uncommon in cats. Occasionally dogs with pythiosis will be presented with pyloric outflow obstruction secondary to severe segmental thickening of the proximal duodenum. The other common location affected in cases of pythiosis is at the ileocolic junction or less commonly the colon. The diagnosis is made via histologic examination of tissue, though a silver or PAS stain will often be needed to identify the nonseptate hyphae. Concern for the pythiosis should arise when histopathology of a segmental

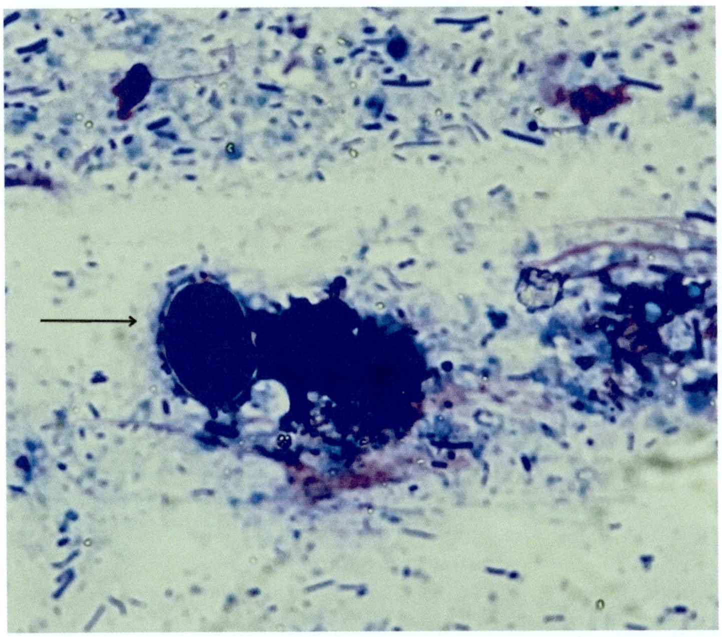

FIGURE 41.2 Yeast-form *Prototheca* spp. (arrow) seen on rectal scrape cytology in a 3-year-old, FS, mixed breed with disseminated protothecosis. Diagnosis of *Prototheca zopfii* infection was confirmed by combination of evaluation of phenotypic characteristics and DNA sequence analysis of urine culture growth. Magnification 100× . Photomicrograph courtesy of Alyssa Zoto, DVM, DACVIM-SAIM

thickening of the intestine returns as pyogranulomatous and eosinophilic inflammation. PCR for *P. insidiosum* can also be performed from cytology or biopsy of tissue, and antibody determinations (via ELISA or Western blot) are also available. If mass lesions are present, the best treatment is wide surgical excision, followed by systemic antifungal therapy. However, if surgical resection is not possible, medical management can be attempted. Traditionally, prognosis has been considered poor; however, a recent study reported successful outcomes in dogs treated with a combination of itraconazole, terbinafine, and mefenoxam (Cridge et al. 2020) or prednisone, itraconazole, and terbinafine (Reagan et al. 2019). Importantly, mefenoxam is not regulated by the FDA, therefore this should be considered prior to use of the compound and informed owner consent should be obtained prior to use.

CHRONIC ENTEROPATHY

Chronic enteropathy (CE) is a wide-ranging term used to define disorders resulting in GI signs of greater than three weeks duration. The use of this term implies other causes of GI signs, including extra-intestinal disease, infectious etiologies, and neoplastic disease, have been ruled out or are considered unlikely. The pathophysiology of this disorder is likely multifactorial involving environmental factors (diet and microbiota), a dysregulated immune system, and host genetics (Jergens and Heilmann 2022). Limited information is available regarding genetic alterations in cats and dogs with CE; however, a polymorphism in the TLR5 gene (G22A) was found to be significantly associated with inflammatory enteritis in the German shepherd dog (GSD) (Kathrani et al. 2010).

Traditionally, chronic enteropathies are further classified by response to treatment. These categories may include food-responsive enteropathy (FRE), steroid- or immunosuppressant-responsive enteropathy (SRE/IRE), or historically, antimicrobial-responsive enteropathy (ARE). It was recently proposed that the category ARE be updated to microbiota-related modulation-responsive enteropathies (MrMRE) (Dupouy-Manescau et al. 2024). This new term would better reflect the varied therapies that may result in positive modulation of the microbiota and the subsequent improvement observed in these cases. While treatment response categories are helpful to our understanding of the most commonly successful treatments, clinical signs typically overlap, and histopathology does not appear to differ between subgroups. It is also important to recognize that this classification system may not reflect the complexity of all CE cases. Some propose that these categories are not entirely separate entities but simply reflect a single disease process of increasing severity (Makielski et al. 2019). Previous literature has demonstrated that most dogs with CE will be responsive to a change in diet, thus FRE is the most common type of CE. In one study of 203 dogs with CE, 64% were classified with FRE, 19.2% with SRE/IRE, and 16.2% with ARE (Allenspach et al. 2016). When sequential treatments with diets and therapies to modulate the microbiota are not successful, histopathologic evaluation of intestinal biopsies is recommended as the next step. When intestinal inflammation has been documented histologically in a dog with CE, the term chronic inflammatory enteropathy (CIE) can be applied. Inflammatory bowel disease (IBD) is no longer the preferred terminology.

Dog breeds considered predisposed to chronic enteropathies include German shepherd dog, Shiba dogs, border collies, and Boxers. Domestic short hair (DSH) and Siamese cats are suspected to have increased incidence of chronic enteropathies (Jablonski and Cridge, 2023). Diarrhea, weight loss, changes in appetite, and vomiting are the most common clinical signs in dogs and cats with CE. In many cases the clinical signs are chronic and progressive but in other cases the signs may be intermittent, despite occurring over a period of three weeks or longer. A sizable number of dogs and cats presenting for the evaluation of GI signs lasting three or more weeks will be reported to be otherwise stable. In other words, these patients maintain normal appetite, body weight, and energy levels despite ongoing GI signs. In other cases, dogs and cats may display alterations in appetite, lethargy, weight and muscle loss, and intractable vomiting and diarrhea. Clinical severity scoring systems are available for both dogs (Table 41.2) and cats (Table 41.3) for establishing a baseline and monitoring treatment response (Allenspach et al. 2007; Jergens et al. 2010).

Table 41.2 Canine Chronic Enteropathy Activity Index (CCECAI) Scoring System

Clinical or diagnostic finding	Qualitative score	Quantitative Score
Attitude/activity	Normal	0
	Slight decrease	1
	Moderate decrease	2
	Severe decrease	3
Appetite	Normal	0
	Slight decrease	1
	Moderate decrease	2
	Severe decrease	3
Vomiting	None	0
	Mild (once/week)	1
	Moderate (2–3/week)	2
	Severe (>3 week)	3
Stool consistency	Normal	0
	Slightly soft, fecal blood, mucus, or both	1
	Very soft feces	2
	Watery diarrhea	3
Stool frequency	Normal	0
	2–3/day	1
	4–5/day	2
	>5/day	3
Weight loss (unintended)	None	0
	Mild (<5%)	1
	Moderate (5–10%)	2
	Severe (>10%)	3
Serum albumin	>2 g/dL	0
	1.5–1.99 g/dL	1
	1.2–1.49 g/dL	2
	<1.2 g/dL	3
Ascites and/or peripheral edema	None	0
	Mild	1
	Moderate	2
	Severe	3
Pruritus	None	0
	Occasional	1
	Regular episodes of itching, but stops when dog is asleep	2
	Dog regularly wakes up because of itching	3
Final score	Clinically insignificant	0–3
	Mild disease	4–5
	Moderate disease	6–8
	Severe disease	9–11
	Very severe disease	12+

Source: Adapted from Allenspach et al. (2007).

Table 41.3 Feline Chronic Enteropathy Activity Index (FCEAI) Scoring System

Clinical or diagnostic finding	Qualitative score	Quantitative score
Attitude/activity	Normal	0
	Slight decrease	1
	Moderate decrease	2
	Severe decrease	3
Appetite	Normal	0
	Slight decrease	1
	Moderate decrease	2
	Severe decrease	3
Vomiting	Normal	0
	Slight decrease	1
	Moderate decrease	2
	Severe decrease	3
Diarrhea	Well-formed feces	0
	Slightly soft feces, fecal, blood, mucus, or increased frequency (2–3 times/day)	1
	Very soft feces or moderately increased frequency (4–5 times/day)	2
	Watery diarrhea or severely increased frequency (>5 times/day)	3
Weight loss	None	0
	Mild (<5%)	1
	Moderate (5–10%)	2
	Severe	3
Endoscopic lesions	No	0
	Yes	1
Total protein	Normal	0
	Increased	1
ALT/ALP	Normal	0
	Increased	1
Phosphorous	Normal	0
	Decreased	1
Final score	Clinically insignificant	0–3
	Mild disease	4–5
	Moderate disease	6–8
	Severe disease	9+

Source: Adapted from Jergens et al. (2010).

Food-responsive Chronic Enteropathy

FRE is the most common type of CE. Up to 65% of dogs and 70% of cats with CE are expected to be completely responsive to a diet change as their sole treatment. Dogs with FRE tend to be younger than dogs that will require steroids to control their disease, and they have lower CCECAI (canine chronic enteropathy activity index) scores (Allenspach et al. 2007; Dupouy-Manescau et al. 2024).

There are several reasons why dogs and cats with CE may respond to specific diet changes. Reasons include reduced exposure to dietary antigens, improved digestibility and nutrient absorption, and alteration of specific nutrient profiles, including supplying a beneficial amount and source of dietary fiber. Consequently, there are a variety of diet types that may have a beneficial effect in dogs with CE. Hydrolyzed diets, diets providing a new protein and carbohydrate source (novel), fiber-enriched diets, highly digestible diets, and home-prepared diets have all been demonstrated to be successful in various cases of CE. There is little evidence to suggest which diet may be most beneficial in an individual dog with CE. A diet lower in fat and fiber may be best in patients with signs of gastropathy (e.g., vomiting, gastric distention) in order to hasten gastric emptying, and altering the fiber source and amount may be more important in patients with large bowel diarrhea and/or flatulence. Additionally, if signs of allergic skin disease are presented, consideration of a hydrolyzed or novel protein diet should take precedent. However, which diet a dog or cat with CE may respond to cannot always be predicted, and thus, multiple types of dietary trials should ideally be attempted before it is concluded that the dog will not be responsive to food alone (Kathrani 2021; Tolbert et al. 2022). More information on dietary treatment of CE can be found in Chapter 45.

Breed-specific Food-responsive Chronic Enteropathies

Gluten-sensitive enteropathy of the Irish setter is a condition characterized by immune-mediated intolerance of gluten, similar to celiac disease in humans. It has an autosomal recessive pattern of inheritance. Clinical signs consistent with CE develop in young- to middle-aged Irish setters and will resolve with the feeding of a gluten-free diet. The condition results in partial villous atrophy and lymphoplasmacytic intestinal inflammation (Hall and Batt 1992).

Border terriers and Maltese dogs with episodic tremors, dystonia, and involuntary movements of limbs and facial muscles, with or without a loss of consciousness may have resolution of these signs with the feeding of a gluten-free diet. Dogs often also display diarrhea, vomiting, borborygmi, and flatulence. The conditions are known as paroxysmal gluten-sensitive dyskinesias, and the diagnosis is based on breed, compatible clinical history, and resolution of clinical signs in response to being fed a gluten-free diet (Lowrie et al. 2016; Polidoro et al. 2020).

Microbiota-related Modulation-responsive Enteropathies

This category of CE includes dogs and cats responsive to therapies that may modulate the gut microbiota. Changes in intestinal microbial structure, function, and diversity are termed dysbiosis. Dysbiosis should be considered in dogs with CE and, if suspected, can be a target for therapy. Though dysbiosis may occur in any patient with CE, it may be a cause or contributing factor to the patient's clinical signs particularly in certain breeds (e.g., German shepherd dog), if there is a history of antimicrobial use and when certain clinical signs (large bowel diarrhea, flatulence) are present. To screen for dysbiosis, consider submission of a fDI to the Texas A&M laboratory. This test quantifies the fecal abundance of seven bacterial taxa as well as the total bacterial abundance. It also can report the relative abundance of *Peptacetobacter hiranonis (previously Clostridium hiranonis)*, which when decreased strongly correlates to fecal dysbiosis.

In the past, antimicrobials were by far the most common therapy prescribed to attempt to manipulate the microbiota in dogs and cats with chronic diarrhea. However, responses to antimicrobials in dogs and cats with CE were rarely durable with high rates of relapse reported. In one study evaluating long-term outcomes of 814 dogs with CE, 341 dogs were treated with antibiotics and only 8/814 (1%) responded solely to antibiotic therapies long-term (Holmberg et al. 2022). Additionally, there are concerns about the effects long-term antimicrobial use can have on an individual dog's microbiome health and the effects of indiscriminate antibiotic use in dogs with diarrhea on the development of antimicrobial resistance. Thus, it is recommended to utilize therapies other than antimicrobials, when possible, to modulate the microbiota. Prebiotics, probiotics, fiber-enriched diets, hydrolyzed diets, and fecal microbial transplant are examples of preferred therapies (Winston et al. 2024). More evidence is needed to determine the indications and efficacy of all of these treatments in CE cases; however, it is accepted that they should be utilized for modulation of microbiota in place of or prior to antimicrobial trials. When these therapies are successful in dogs with CE because of a suspected or confirmed improvement in the microbiota, the disorder can be classified as a modulation-responsive enteropathy.

Steroid- or Immunosuppressant Responsive Enteropathies

Glucocorticoids (prednisone, prednisolone, budesonide) or immunosuppressants (cyclosporine, chlorambucil, azathioprine) are required to control CE in 20–25% of dogs. When dogs respond to these therapies after previous inadequate responses to dietary therapies or therapies to modulate the microbiota, the terms SRE or IRE can be applied. High-quality evidence to support the assertion that glucocorticoids can be effective in dogs and cats with CE is available (Makielski et al. 2019).

Diagnostic Approach – Overview

The first step in the diagnostic approach to dogs and cats with clinical signs of CE is careful consideration of the patient's signalment, clinical history, and degree of illness. Age and breed-related disorders may change the diagnostic approach (e.g., exocrine pancreatic insufficiency in German shepherd dog, rough collie). Clinical history taking should be careful to include a thorough account of the previous diets fed, and the various responses to those diets. When diarrhea is present, it is helpful to use a fecal scoring system to establish a baseline for future monitoring. Additionally, it should be determined whether the diarrhea is small, large, or mixed bowel in origin.

Next, a thorough physical exam must be performed and specifically should include assessment of body and muscle condition, hydration status, evaluation for ascites, abdominal pain, and lymphadenopathy. Evidence of dermatologic disease could support an underlying food allergy or intolerance; thus, careful evaluation of the skin is required. Rectal exam allows for evaluation of fecal consistency and color, as well as screening for intra- or extraluminal, prostatic, or anal sac disease. An overview of the diagnostic approach to chronic diarrhea is shown in Figure 41.3. Importantly, CE is a diagnosis of exclusion. Recent attempts to develop specific assays for diagnosis have failed (Langlois et al. 2023). Finally, the diagnostic approach will differ depending on whether the patient has mild or more serious disease, based on clinical history, physical exam findings, and a thorough understanding of the possible differentials.

Diagnostic Approach – Mildly Affected Patient

In dogs and cats with mild illness (maintaining normal appetite, body weight, and energy levels despite ongoing diarrhea and/or vomiting, unremarkable physical exam), the diagnostic approach may be more measured, at least initially. Helminth infections including those from roundworms, tapeworms, and hookworms can cause chronic diarrhea in dogs and cats. Thus, all dogs and cats should have fecal testing performed (e.g., fecal floatation). Specific testing for *Giardia* spp. should also be considered. Regardless of the result, administration of a broad-spectrum anthelmintic (e.g., fenbendazole) is best

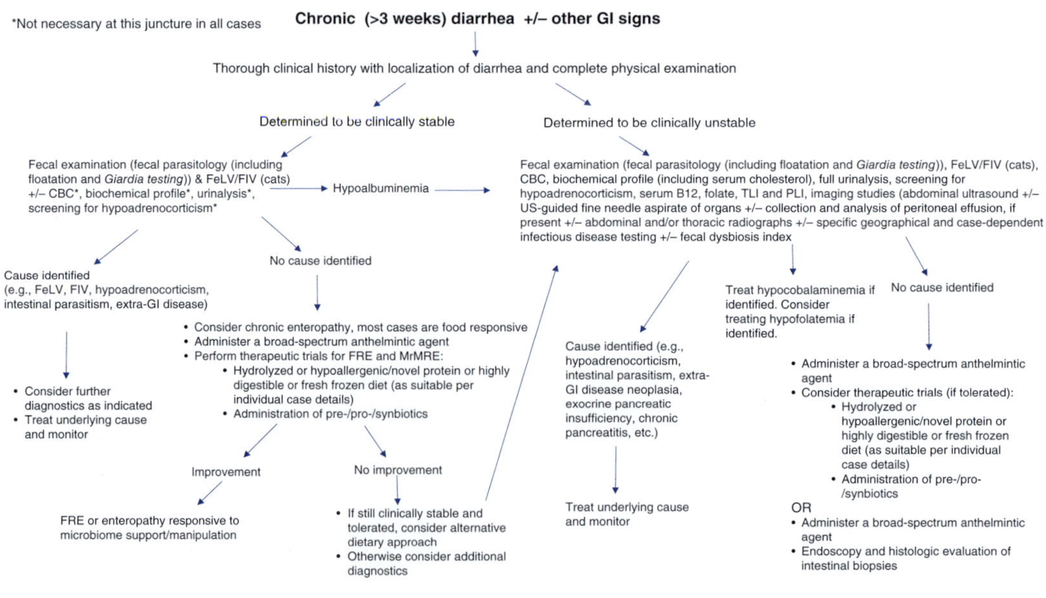

FIGURE 41.3 Diagnostic and initial therapeutic approach to chronic diarrhea in dogs and cats

in patients with clinical signs suggestive of CE. All cats with chronic diarrhea should also have FeLV/FIV testing performed. Consideration can then be given to the exclusion of secondary causes of GI signs via a CBC, chemistry profile, urinalysis, and screening for hypoadrenocorticism; however, this may not always be necessary in all cases of stable dogs and cats presenting for evaluation of chronic GI signs. In stable dogs and cats with CE, it may be reasonable to perform noninvasive therapeutic trials (dietary trials, or with therapies meant to support or manipulate the enteric microbiota) prior to recommending a more extensive diagnostic work-up.

Diagnostic Approach – Moderately to Severely Affected Patient

In dogs and cats with chronic GI signs experiencing lethargy, weight loss, and/or changes in appetite (decreases, increases, or absence of appetite), it is important that we identify the cause of their signs quickly. Therefore, a more extensive initial diagnostic work-up is recommended. Fecal testing and broad-spectrum deworming remain indicated. Beyond that, the initial diagnostic approach should exclude systemic causes (e.g., renal, hepatic, endocrine disease) of GI signs with history, physical exam, CBC, chemistry profile, and urinalysis. Age-appropriate cats should also have evaluation of total T4. It is reasonable to screen all dogs with chronic GI signs for hypoadrenocorticism. Hypoadrenocorticism can be excluded by a resting cortisol concentration ≥ 2 μg (Gold et al. 2016); resting cortisol concentration <2 requires an ACTH stimulation test be performed to exclude or confirm the diagnosis of hypoadrenocorticism. Next steps to be considered in the clinically unwell patient include diagnostic imaging (e.g., abdominal radiographs, abdominal ultrasound, thoracic radiographs), measurement of serum cobalamin, folate, pancreatic lipase immunoreactivity (PLI) activity, and trypsin-like immunoreactivity (TLI), and specific testing for miscellaneous infectious agents that may be suspected depending on individual case details. It is also important to recognize that cats with CE appear to be predisposed to concurrent exocrine pancreatic and liver disease.

The rank-order of the various differentials will determine which tests are selected and the order in which they are pursued. If results of these tests fail to determine a specific cause and thus the diagnosis is considered idiopathic CE, collection of intestinal biopsies with histopathologic evaluation would be the next step. In certain cases, therapeutic trials may be favored first, as they may still be effective even in clinically unwell dogs and cats. If the dog or cat does not accept the trial conditions (i.e., eat the recommended diet) or clinical signs progress during the trial period, a more aggressive approach would be required. If it is suspected that the dog or cat will need anti-inflammatory or immunosuppressive therapies to control their disease, intestinal biopsies with histopathology would ideally be performed first, in order to definitively exclude infectious and neoplastic causes of the signs. Intestinal biopsy samples may be collected via endoscopy, laparotomy, or laparoscopy. Endoscopy is generally preferred. Surgical biopsies may be preferred in the presence of focal disease. Endoscopy allows for the visualization of diffuse or segmental gross abnormalities. Lesions that can be observed include friability, granularity, hyperemia, erosions/ulcerations, and white-villous tips (Figure 41.4), which can support a diagnosis of intestinal lymphangiectasia (IL). Endoscopic scoring systems are available (Salavati Schmitz et al. 2019). Pathology can sometimes differ between the duodenum and ileum; therefore, it is best to perform both esophago-gastro-duodenoscopy ("upper") and recto-colono-ileoscopy ("lower") endoscopy. A minimum of 6–8 biopsy samples each are collected from the stomach, duodenum, ileum, and colon; however, if the samples are marginal, 10–15 biopsies per site may be necessary to make a diagnosis. Samples should be evaluated for morphologic changes including crypt dilation, lacteal dilation, villus blunting, mucosal fibrosis, and for inflammatory infiltrates (lymphoplasmacytic, eosinophilic, neutrophilic, other). Routine histologic evaluation allows for a diagnosis in many cases. Occasionally, further testing may be necessary including PCR for antigen receptor rearrangement (PARR), immunophenotyping, or fluorescence in situ hybridization (FISH) for detection of adherent or invasive bacteria. The use of PARR and immunophenotyping is particularly important in cats but considered controversial. Use of the World Small Animal Veterinary Association (WSAVA) GI Standardization Group criteria, or a recently proposed simplified scoring system may help improve interobserver variation (Washabau et al. 2010). More information on endoscopy and histopathology can be found in Chapter 35. If intestinal biopsies are declined in dogs and cats that have failed a series of properly implemented dietary trials, or in dogs that have serious illness and a refusal to accept the recommended diets, empirical treatment with glucocorticoids can be implemented after counseling owners of the potential risks.

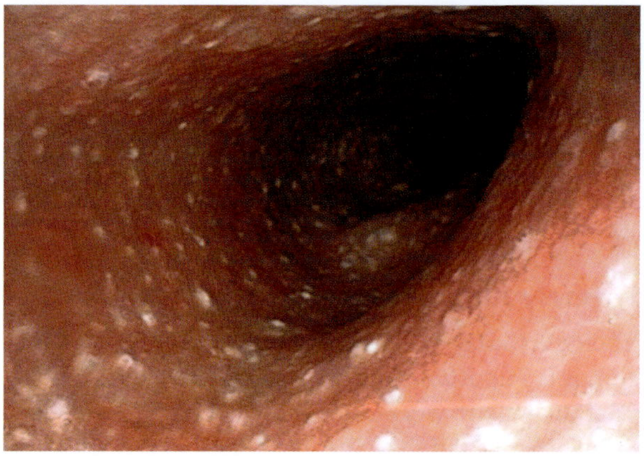

FIGURE 41.4 Presence of duodenal pinpoint "white spots" consistent with dilated lacteals in a 5-year-old, male, castrated, English bulldog with the clinical syndrome of PLE and histologically diagnosed marked lymphoplasmacytic enteritis and moderate intestinal lymphangiectasia

Therapeutic Management of Chronic Enteropathies

Because most dogs and cats with CE are considered food-responsive, therapeutic diet trials are typically recommended first. The only exception to this would be in a patient who is severely clinically affected and therefore may not accept a dietary change and may benefit from a more aggressive initial approach. A variety of dietary strategies are available for patients with CE, and we do not have robust evidence to suggest that one dietary approach is better than the other. Some dietary considerations include type of diet (hydrolysate vs. limited ingredient vs. novel protein vs. elemental vs. home-cooked), digestibility, fiber type and amount, and fat content. Improvement in clinical signs is typically seen within 7–14 days when a food trial is successful. Importantly if there is minimal or no response, it is recommended to try at least one other dietary approach before classifying your patient as nonresponsive to food. Importantly, one study showed that up to three different therapeutic diet trials may be needed before a response is seen in dogs. Please refer to Chapter 45 for more information regarding dietary management of CE.

The next therapeutic strategy could address the possibility of dysbiosis in the patient. Treatments for dysbiosis that could also be implemented include switching to a highly digestible diet, antimicrobials, prebiotics, probiotics or synbiotics, or fecal microbial transplant. If these therapies are not successful, treatment with anti-inflammatory or immunosuppressive medications is reasonable (ideally with concurrent documentation of intestinal inflammation). Prednisone or prednisolone (preferred in cats), budesonide, or cyclosporine can be instituted, depending on the case. Prednisone or prednisolone may be preferred to budesonide in cases where the side effect of increasing appetite may be desired. Budesonide may be selected over prednisone or prednisolone in cases where systemic side effects of steroids are best avoided or limited. Cyclosporine may be chosen in cases where it is ideal to avoid steroids altogether.

Dogs and cats with hypocobalaminemia should also receive oral or parenteral supplementation based on published protocols. Supportive care to reduce vomiting and improve appetite may also be useful.

Finally, it is important to recognize that despite the tendency to distinguish CE patients by treatment response, many dogs and cats with CE may benefit from a multimodal approach to therapy, befitting of the complexity of the disorder.

Nonresponsive CE

If standard treatments fail to produce improvements in clinical or biochemical parameters, the disorder is often referred to as a nonresponsive enteropathy. Depending on the source, these cases make up approximately 5–30% of cases in dogs. In such cases, there are a number of possibilities to consider. First, there is a tendency in clinical practice to consider dogs and cats nonresponsive to food after a single trial. Studies suggest that dogs and cats who have been considered to have failed a food trial can be responsive to an alternate dietary approach (Chapter 45). Additionally, an alternative immunosuppressive approach could be attempted. One study of dogs with steroid-refractory CE found that cyclosporine administered at 5 mg/kg/day induced clinical remission in 12/14 dogs (Allenspach et al. 2006). FMT can also be considered, even in patients without documented evidence of dysbiosis. Various procedures for the administration of FMT are described. Of utmost importance is the careful selection of both recipient and donor. For more information on FMT, the reader is referred to a recent comprehensive review (Winston et al. 2024). Additionally, dysfunction of bile acid metabolism can occur because of dysbiosis, thus short-term treatment with cholestyramine could be considered. The use of mesenchymal stem cells has also been described in dogs (Cristóbal et al. 2021) and cats (Webb and Webb 2022) with inflammatory enteritis. In both studies, administration of mesenchymal stem cells was not inferior to prednisone/prednisolone for treatment of disease. Thus, administration of stem cells could be considered in cases that are nonresponsive to traditional therapies. Finally, in these difficult to treat cases, it may be especially necessary to take a multimodal approach to therapy, rather than relying on a single therapy to result in improvement.

FELINE EOSINOPHILIC SCLEROSING FIBROPLASIA

Gastrointestinal eosinophilic sclerosing fibroplasia (GESF) is a condition in cats characterized by eosinophilic mass(es) in the GI tract (most commonly near the pylorus or ileocolic junction) and abdominal lymph nodes. Cats with GESF typically are presented with chronic vomiting, diarrhea, weight loss, and lethargy, though acute onset of signs is sometimes reported. In most cases, the mass(es) can be palpated on physical exam. A retrospective review of 60 cases found that in addition to DSH and domestic long hair cats, ragdolls, exotic shorthairs, and Persian cats were frequently affected. Additionally, survival times were not different between cats treated surgically versus with medical management with glucocorticoids, and the prognosis was generally good with 88% of cats surviving long-term (Černá et al. 2024).

PROTEIN-LOSING ENTEROPATHY

PLE is a life-threatening clinical syndrome characterized by uncompensated protein loss across the intestinal mucosa. The syndrome predominately affects dogs and is only rarely observed in cats. The most common causes of PLE syndrome in dogs are CIE and IL (Craven and Washabau 2019); however, a number of other causes are noted in Table 41.4. IL is characterized by intestinal lymphatic vessel dilation, with or without lymphangitis, lymphatic obstruction, and rupture. These dilated

Table 41.4 Causes of Protein-losing Enteropathy in the Dog by Proposed Pathophysiologic Mechanism

Diseases that cause mucosal injury or alter intestinal permeability	Intestinal lymphatic disease

• Chronic enteropathies
• Intestinal ulceration
• Infectious enteropathies
  • Fungal (Histoplasmosis, pythiosis)
  • Parasitic (Hookworm, schistosomiasis)
  • Viral (Parvovirus)
  • Bacterial – RARE (Campylobacter, Salmonellosis)
• Chronic obstruction of the intestine
• Neoplasia
  • Intestinal lymphoma (solitary or diffuse)
  • Intestinal adenocarcinoma
• Hypoadrenocorticism (Addison's disease)
	• "Primary" lymphangiectasia (suspected genetic predisposition)
	• "Secondary" lymphangiectasia:
	COMMON
	  • Chronic enteropathies
	  • Intestinal neoplasia
	SUSPECTED (unconfirmed in veterinary medicine)
	  • Right heart failure
	  • Constrictive pericarditis
	  • Portal hypertension
	• Focal lipogranulomatous lymphangitis

and disordered intestinal lymphatics may subsequently leak protein-rich lymph leading to loss of protein through the intestinal lumen. Notably, CIE and IL can occur together in dogs. One study reported that 76% of dogs with PLE and CIE also had histologic evidence of IL (Jablonski Wennogle et al. 2017). Breeds affected by PLE most frequently over the last few decades include the Yorkshire terrier, crossbreed dogs, border collie, German shepherd dog, rottweiler, Maltese, toy poodle, dachshund, Shetland sheepdog, English springer spaniel, and soft-coated wheaten terrier (Craven and Washabau 2019). Soft-coated wheaten terriers are also predisposed to protein-losing nephropathy. A hereditary immunoproliferative enteropathy associated with progressive intractable diarrhea, hypoalbuminemia, vomiting, weight loss, and potentially transient neurologic signs is described in Basenji dogs. Breeds specifically considered predisposed to IL include the Yorkshire terrier, Maltese, Rottweiler, soft-coated wheaten terrier, Norwegian lundehund, and SharPei.

The most common clinical signs in dogs with PLE include chronic relapsing or progressive GI signs (e.g., diarrhea, weight loss, decreased appetite, vomiting) and clinical signs associated with hypoalbuminemia (e.g., ascites, pleural effusion, peripheral edema). Vomiting is less common than diarrhea, weight loss, and decreased appetite. Uncommonly, GI signs may be absent. Physical examination findings are variable, ranging from unremarkable, to severe decreases in body condition and loss of muscle. Some dogs will be presented with abdominal distension, and physical examination will reveal a palpable "fluid-wave."

In addition to hypoalbuminemia, dogs with PLE commonly have a number of biochemical abnormalities including thrombocytosis, various leukocytosis (typically mild), lymphopenia, hypoglobulinemia (though normal or elevated serum globulin does not entirely exclude PLE), hypocholesterolemia, and decreased serum creatinine, among others.

Diagnostic Approach

The initial diagnostic approach to a dog with suspected PLE should first definitely exclude other causes of hypoalbuminemia (namely, protein-losing nephropathy and liver insufficiency), then identify the specific cause of PLE, and screen for complications and co-morbidities. Fecal testing and administration of appropriate anthelmintic therapy is recommended in all dogs. Exclusion of hypoadrenocorticism is also recommended in all cases. Abdominal ultrasound may be helpful in excluding focal or extraluminal lesions that may change the plan and prognosis. Additionally, if focal disease is identified, fine-needle aspiration of masses or abnormal lymph nodes may lead to the ability to make a diagnosis noninvasively. If peritoneal effusion is observed, fluid could be collected for analysis and would be expected to be a pure transudate. Hyperechoic mucosal striations observed on abdominal ultrasound are supportive of the diagnosis of IL. Abdominal or thoracic radiographs may be useful on a case-by-case basis. If there is reason to suspect systemic histoplasmosis based on geographic exposure or supportive clinical signs or biochemical findings, examination of the fundus, rectal scrape with cytology and urine antigen testing should be performed. Following this, if a cause for PLE has not been discovered, biopsy with histopathology will be necessary to determine the cause of the dog's PLE. Biopsy can exclude infectious (e.g., histoplasmosis) or neoplastic (e.g., intestinal lymphoma) causes of PLE. Biopsy will also help to determine whether the dog is affected by CIE, IL or both, and if both, which process appears to predominate. Flexible endoscopy is the preferred method for sample collection, and it is recommended that both esophagogastroduodenoscopy ("upper") and ileocolonoscopic ("lower") endoscopy be performed. Evaluation of the intestinal mucosa via endoscopy can reveal a variety of changes including "white spots" suggestive of IL (Figure 41.4), erosions or ulcerations, hyperemia, and increased granularity or friability of the intestine. The most frequently reported histopathologic findings in dogs with PLE include IL, various types and degrees of inflammatory infiltrates, dilated, cystic crypts, and mucosal edema. In rare cases, additional testing may be necessary to help distinguish CIE and intestinal lymphoma.

Therapeutic Management

Importantly, treatment of PLE is directed at the underlying cause. An important consideration is that many dogs with PLE will have a combination of CIE and IL. Management strategies include dietary therapies, management of inflammation, immunomodulation, supportive care, and treating and preventing complications.

Dietary therapy is critical to success in management of canine PLE caused by CIE and IL. The importance of diet is highlighted by several studies that have shown that dietary treatment can be successful as a sole therapy (Nagata et al. 2020; Rudinsky et al. 2018), and by studies that have shown that dietary adjustment can lead to remission in dogs that are refractory to steroid therapy (Jablonski Wennogle et al. 2021; Okanishi et al. 2014). The ideal diet for dogs with PLE is highly digestible with adequate amounts of protein, and many dogs with PLE seem to benefit from the diet being low in fat. There is no consensus on what constitutes a "low-fat" or "ultra low-fat" diet; however, one example would be "low fat" = 16–25 grams of fat/1000 kcal and "ultra-low fat" = ≤ 15 grams of fat/1000 kcal. A reduction in dietary fat seems to be particularly important in dogs with moderate to marked IL driving their PLE but may also be helpful for dogs for which CIE is the predominant lesion and IL is secondary. Recently, diets formulated and labeled to be both low-fat and hydrolyzed (multifunction) have become available, and in dogs with both CIE and IL, use of a hydrolyzed, low-fat veterinary therapeutic diet should be prioritized. These diets are also good choices for dogs that have not had a biopsy and are being treated empirically for both IL and CIE. Some dogs with PLE who do not experience improvement in response to commercial veterinary therapeutic GI diets improve clinically in response to a home-cooked (or commercially available cooked fresh frozen) diet. If the dog is responsive, follow up with a board-certified veterinary nutritionist is strongly recommended for long-term management. The reader is referred to Chapter 45 for further information on dietary management of CE and IL.

Glucocorticoids are indicated in many cases of PLE for both anti-inflammatory and immunosuppressive effects, depending on the case. Importantly, at this time there is no evidence of an immunosuppressive-responsive autoimmune pathogenesis for IL; thus, the author recommends anti-inflammatory doses of prednisone or prednisolone (0.5–1.0 mg/kg PO every 24 hours or divided and administered every 12 hours) for dogs with PLE in which IL appears to be a significant problem. When CIE is the predominant problem, doses of 0.5–2.0 mg/kg PO every 24 hours or divided and administered every 12 hours are reasonable, however, it is important to note that glucocorticoids worsen the catabolic and hypercoagulable states of dogs with PLE. Additionally, unpublished work from the author suggests that treatment-naïve dogs with PLE have lower serum concentrations of serum immunoglobulins IgG and IgM as well as reduced expression of both T- and B-cell markers when compared to age, sex, and breed matched healthy controls. The author does not exceed 1.0 mg/kg/day or 60 mg total per dog in any dogs with PLE. The initial dose should be maintained for 21–28 days if tolerated, then a tapering schedule of 25% in 3–4-week intervals can be attempted. Some dogs can be successfully tapered off glucocorticoids and maintained on diet alone. Dogs may benefit from switching to budesonide for long-term management if they are steroid-responsive but start to relapse when prednisone/prednisolone is tapered.

Cobalamin deficiency should be treated in dogs with PLE, similar to dogs with CE without hypoalbuminemia. Supplementation of folic acid can also be considered when low. Ionized hypocalcemia should be treated parenterally if dogs have clinical signs that can be attributed to ionized hypocalcemia. Oral calcium carbonate may also be beneficial. Many dogs with ionized hypocalcemia have low serum 25-hydroxyvitamin D levels. A study recently completed at the author's institution found that supplementation with cholecalciferol (D3) improved serum concentrations of 25OHD in dogs with PLE when compared to placebo; however, a clinical benefit was not observed. In addition, many dogs with PLE had resolution of low serum vitamin D simply with treatment of the underlying disease. The 2022 CURATIVE guidelines classified dogs with PLE as being "high risk" for thrombosis. Thus, thromboprophylaxis with clopidogrel at 2–3 mg/kg, PO, q24h is often recommended, though the best medication for thromboprophylaxis or whether thromboprophylaxis is necessary in all dogs with PLE has not been determined. It is not recommended to drain abdominal effusions unless the effusion is resulting in discomfort or respiratory difficulty. Thoracic effusions typically need to be drained for patient comfort. Diuretic use is not helpful and thus discouraged. Colloids, such as hydroxyethyl starches are the most useful product for improving oncotic pressure; however, their potential adverse effects including possible kidney injury and effects on the coagulation system should be taken into consideration before use. Plasma will not be beneficial. Canine albumin is available and effective for dogs with severe hypoalbuminemia causing significant morbidity.

A subset of dogs with PLE have minimal to no clinical or biochemical improvement in response to initial dietary changes and anti-inflammatory to immunosuppressive doses of glucocorticoids. Some clinicians advocate for utilizing cyclosporine in these cases as it has been shown to be effective in some dogs with steroid-refractory GI disease. Others may recommend chlorambucil. Importantly, a recent retrospective study found that treatment with steroids and immunosuppressives offered no survival advantage when compared to steroids alone in dogs with PLE (Salavati Schmitz et al. 2019). Other clinicians may advocate for increasing the steroid dose or giving steroids parenterally due to the potential for steroid malabsorption as a consequence of the diseased intestinal tract. However, a recent study showed that overall prednisolone drug exposures were similar between dogs with PLE and healthy controls, suggesting that glucocorticoid malabsorption is unlikely to be a cause of treatment failure in dogs with PLE (Jablonski et al. 2025). In cases of steroid-refractory PLE, the author has found the most success by tapering immunosuppressive medications and focusing on diet, in many cases, a home-cooked diet can result in drastic improvement (Chapter 45). Finally, the use of octreotide (10 μg/kg, SQ q8–12h) has been reported for dogs with refractory PLE and it has been found to be safe, but efficacy is currently unclear.

In one report, disease-associated death occurred in 54.2% of 445 cases of canine PLE. However, the author believes our knowledge of the condition is improving, leading to better outcomes. Some dogs with PLE have excellent responses to treatment. Treatment is typically life-long.

SMALL INTESTINAL NEOPLASIA

Intestinal lymphoma, intestinal adenocarcinoma, and smooth muscle tumors (leiomyoma and leiomyosarcoma) are the most common small intestinal neoplasms in dogs. Lymphoma is the most common neoplasm of the intestinal tract in cats. Other tumors of the SI include neuroendocrine tumors, fibrosarcoma, and carcinoids, though they are less common. Clinical signs are generally similar to other causes of SI disease; however, intestinal tumors may also result in obstruction of the GI tract. Many focal tumors are suspected based on abdominal ultrasound, but cytologic or histologic evaluation of the tissue will be necessary for definitive diagnosis.

Intestinal Lymphoma in Dogs

Alimentary lymphoma in the dog may be confined to the GI tract (focal or diffuse) or part of multicentric lymphoma. Lymphoblastic ("large cell") alimentary lymphoma (LCL) is more common than lymphocytic ("small cell") lymphoma (SCL) in the dog, however, there has recently been an increase in reports of SCL in the dog. The clinical presentation varies; however, dogs with LCL are typically presented in poor condition with vomiting, diarrhea, anorexia, and weight loss along with rapid deterioration of health. In cases of multicentric lymphoma, physical examination may reveal peripheral lymphadenomegaly. Hypoalbuminemia is the most common biochemical abnormality observed in dogs with intestinal lymphoma. Anemia, neutrophilia, increased liver enzyme activities, and rarely, circulating lymphoblasts may also be present. Hypercalcemia is uncommon in dogs with lymphoma limited to the intestinal tract. Decreased cobalamin, folate, and serum concentrations of Vitamin D may also be found.

Ultrasound-guided fine needle aspirate of focal masses or mesenteric lymphadenopathy can be performed for diagnosis, if indicated. Some cases may require a surgical biopsy be performed for diagnosis.

Response rates to treatment are better for dogs with SCL (median 628 days) versus LCL (median 117 days). Most dogs receive a combination of prednisone and a chemotherapeutic agent such as chlorambucil, cyclophosphamide, and/or lomustine.

Intestinal Lymphoma in Cats

The most common neoplasia diagnosed in cats is lymphoma, and the GI tract is the most common location. SCL is more common in cats than LCL. Positive FIV or FeLV status is a risk factor for the development of lymphoma, as is living in a household with a smoker. Any age of cat can be affected by intestinal lymphoma, though most are middle-aged to older. Clinical signs and physical exam findings for cats with SCL are similar to cats with CE. Cats with LCL often are presented in a worse clinical state, typically with a history of acute onset of severe illness. CBC abnormalities in cats with intestinal lymphoma include anemia (may be non-regenerative or regenerative) and neutrophilia.

In most cases, surgical biopsy will be necessary to make the diagnosis, unless a focal mass or mesenteric lymphadenomegaly is present.

Though there is some debate, endoscopic biopsies are typically sufficient for making a diagnosis of intestinal lymphoma in cats. Cats with intestinal lymphoma had infiltration of the intestinal mucosa by neoplastic lymphocytes, which may also extend deeper into the intestinal wall. The neoplastic infiltrates may be irregularly distributed, leading to a general recommendation to perform both upper and lower endoscopy in cats with suspicion of lymphoma; however, this is debated. In some cases, the distinction between CIE and SCL can be difficult in cats. Immunohistochemical (IHC) labeling may help distinguish the two, as cats with lymphoma should have monoclonal populations of B or T cells. However, techniques for IHC vary between laboratories and results can be inconsistent. Also, rare cases of intestinal inflammation are characterized by T-cell inflammation alone. Use of clonality testing by PCR for PARR is utilized to try to distinguish SCL from CIE; however, there is debate over the specificity of this assay. In the end, the clinical significance of distinguishing SCL from CIE in cats is questionable as it may not affect treatment approach or outcome.

Focal, obstructive intestinal lymphoma in the cat is treated surgically, and then followed up with chemotherapy. Chemotherapy is the cornerstone of treatment for cats with diffuse disease. Prednisolone and chlorambucil are typically administered together for the treatment of SCL, and response rates are good. Cats with LCL require more aggressive chemotherapy protocols such as COP (cyclophosphamide, vincristine, +/− L-asparaginase) or CHOP (cyclophosphamide, doxorubicin, vincristine, prednisone +/− L-asparaginase +/− methotrexate), and their treatment response and prognosis is worse compared to cats with SCL. Cats with large granular lymphoma (LGL) have the worst prognosis with median survival times of less than two months reported.

Cats with intestinal lymphoma should be treated with cobalamin supplementation, and supportive care, as indicated. In some cases, switching to a highly digestible diet may also be beneficial.

Intestinal Adenoma and Adenocarcinoma

The large intestine is the most common location for intestinal adenoma and adenocarcinoma in the dog. When present in the SI, they are typically found in the duodenum. In cats they are more likely to be found in the SI versus large intestine and are most commonly found in the jejunum or ileum. Adenomas tend to be polypoid, while adenocarcinomas may grow as plaques or annular lesions. Intestinal adenocarcinomas often behave aggressively, invading into the surrounding mesentery and metastasizing to local lymph nodes and other regions of the body.

Dogs and cats with intestinal adenocarcinoma are typically older and presented with signs such as lethargy, changes in appetite, weight loss, vomiting, and diarrhea. Occasionally they may have clinical signs suggestive of SI obstruction. Siamese cats appear to be overrepresented. Anemia may be observed on CBC if mucosal erosion and bleeding has occurred. Abdominal ultrasound frequently identifies a mass (Figure 41.5), and ultrasound-guided fine needle aspirate of the mass may be diagnostic. Otherwise, histopathology of the mass will be necessary. Surgical resection of the mass is the treatment of choice, and postoperative survival times can be very good in dogs and cats.

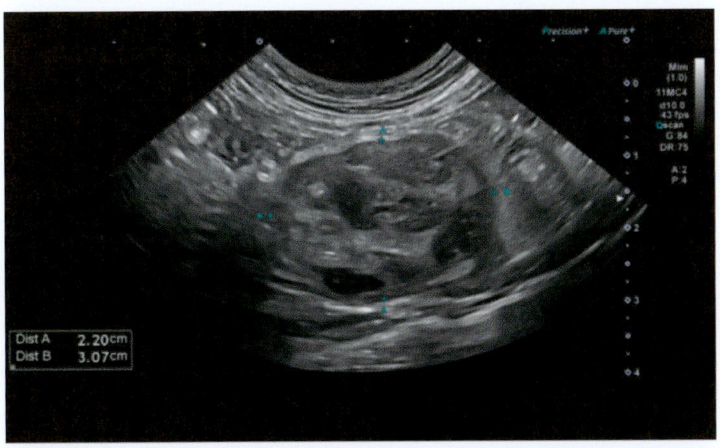

FIGURE 41.5 Transverse sonogram showing an ileal mass (calipers) in an 11-year-old, FS, DSH. The mass was surgically resected and histology revealed adenocarcinoma

Smooth Muscle and Stromal Cell Tumors

Leiomyoma and leiomyosarcoma are rare smooth muscle tumors typically found in the jejunum or cecum of the dog. They are very rarely seen in the cat. The antimesenteric border of the intestine is the most common location. It is difficult to distinguish between leiomyoma and leiomyosarcoma histologically; however, it is not thought to be clinically important as leiomyosarcoma has low potential for metastatic spread. Tumors that arise from the interstitial cells of Cajal are known as gastrointestinal stromal tumors (GISTs). Metastatic spread of GISTs is also uncommon.

Dogs with smooth muscle tumors may be presented with paraneoplastic hypoglycemia that results from tumor production of insulin-like growth factor-II peptide. Erythrocytosis can also be observed in dogs with leiomyosarcoma due to amplification of an erythropoietin-like molecule. Like other intestinal tumors, smooth muscle and stromal tumors of the GI tract can usually be identified on abdominal ultrasound. IHC labeling can help distinguish GISTs from leiomyoma and leiomyosarcomas. Most GISTs express a transmembrane receptor with a tyrosine kinase component known as c-kit (CD-117), while smooth muscle tumors will be c-kit negative (Russell et al. 2007). The treatment of choice is surgical resection for all tumors, and prognosis is good to excellent. Tyrosine kinase inhibitors may be recommended for dogs with surgically resected GISTs and may also be beneficial for dogs with gross disease.

Miscellaneous Other Intestinal Neoplasms

A variety of other tumors can affect the SI in dogs and cats. Fibrosarcoma, schwannoma, osteosarcoma, carcinoid tumors, and Hamartomatous polyps can affect the SI in dogs but are all very uncommon. Extramedullary plasmacytomas rarely occur in the SI and can be associated with the presence of a monoclonal gammopathy. Mast cell tumors can occur in the intestine of cats and present similarly to alimentary lymphoma.

MISCELLANEOUS DISORDERS

Small Intestinal Obstruction

Small intestinal obstructions in dogs and cats can occur as a consequence of intraluminal, extraluminal, or intramural lesions. Intussusceptions can also cause SI obstructions in small animals. The majority of SI obstructions in dogs and cats are intraluminal and caused by foreign objects. Importantly, SI obstructions can be complete or partial, and dogs and cats with SI obstructions may be presented with acute or chronic GI signs. Following surgical correction, the prognosis is variable depending on the cause of obstruction, intestinal viability, and whether or not perforation or peritonitis are present.

Foreign Body Obstruction

Young dogs and cats and large-breed dogs are most likely to be diagnosed with foreign body obstructions. In cats, the most common causes of SI obstruction are linear foreign bodies and trichobezoars (hairballs). Clinical signs are highly variable, but the most commonly reported signs are vomiting, anorexia, depression, and abdominal pain. It is important that cases of acute SI obstruction due to foreign bodies are promptly recognized, as if left untreated, dehydration and death will result. If the SI obstruction is chronic and partial, clinical signs may be vague; however, weight loss and lethargy are common. Since linear foreign bodies can anchor under the tongue, physical examination should always include inspection of this area. Laboratory abnormalities frequently observed in dogs and cats with SI obstruction include metabolic alkalosis, hypochloremia, hypokalemia, hyponatremia, and hyperlactatemia. Plain abdominal radiographs will identify most cases of SI obstruction. The best validated radiographic characteristic for the diagnosis of obstruction is the width of the small bowel exceeding 1.6 times the height of L5 at its narrowest point. Dilation of loops proximal to the obstruction is expected with acute obstructions (Figure 41.6), while extensive dilation of the SI may be seen with chronic obstructions. A bunched-up appearance of intestinal loops is expected when SI obstruction occurs due to a linear foreign body. Outcomes are generally good, following surgical correction. However, the prognosis is more guarded if perforation and peritonitis have occurred.

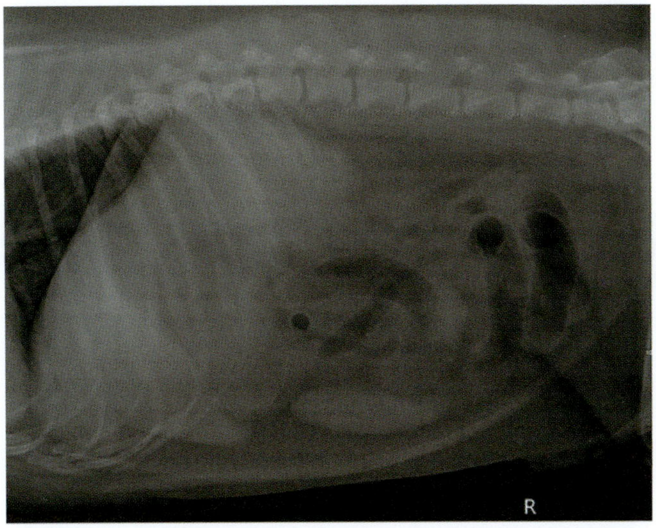

FIGURE 41.6 Right lateral abdominal radiograph showing small intestinal dilation/mechanical obstruction secondary to an intestinal foreign body in a 2-year-old, male, mixed breed dog with a 48-hour history of vomiting and lethargy. Laparotomy confirmed a plastic foreign body in the distal jejunum

Intussusception

An intussusception is a telescoping segment of bowel into another segment. The proximal segment of bowel is known as the *intussusceptum* and the distal segment is the *intussuscipiens*. Most intussusceptions are in young animals and are idiopathic; however, they can also occur as a consequence of foreign bodies, viral enteritis, neoplasia, and abdominal surgery. A sausage-shaped mass may be palpable during physical examination. Plain radiography may show evidence of obstruction, and an abdominal ultrasound can show a characteristic double-walled structure, consistent with intussusception. Reduction of the intussusception may be able to be achieved surgically; however, many cases will require resection of the affected bowel and end-to-end anastomosis. Postoperative complications can occur, but the prognosis following surgical correction is generally good.

Short Bowel Syndrome

Some dogs that have had more than two-thirds of the bowel surgically resected have minimal effects. Others can develop a serious clinical disease known as short bowel syndrome (SBS). SBS occurs when nutrient malabsorption and protein-calorie malnutrition occur as a consequence of the extensive bowel resection.

The most common signs of SBS are weight loss and diarrhea secondary to malabsorption. Specific nutritional adjustments may alleviate some signs, and reduction of gastric acidity with a proton-pump inhibitor may be considered. If the ileum has been resected, administration of cobalamin is recommended. Bile salt malabsorption can also occur in dogs that have had ileum resections, and in these cases administration of the bile salt binding resin cholestyramine may be helpful. Loperamide and octreotide are also occasionally used. Clinical improvement may be seen in some dogs over time due to adaptive hyperplasia of the small bowel.

MOTILITY DISORDERS

Ileus refers to the lack of normal propulsive activity of the intestine without evidence of mechanical obstruction. Many conditions cause ileus in dogs and cats including opioid administration, abdominal surgery, hypokalemia, pancreatitis, parvovirus enteritis, peritonitis, and hypothyroidism. Less commonly, ileus is caused by rare conditions such as dysautonomia, and intestinal pseudo-obstruction.

Ileus is best addressed through treatment of the underlying disease process; however, pro-kinetic agents such as cisapride and metoclopramide can be used. Enteral nutrition is also considered important in the treatment of ileus. Further information about unusual causes of ileus is as follows:

Dysautonomia

Dysautonomia is a generalized autonomic neuropathy that has an unclear etiology. Neurotoxins and xenobiotics are suspected causative agents. In addition, an association with clostridium botulinum toxin has been described in the cat. The most common signs observed include esophageal, gastric, and small intestinal hypomotility and subsequent dilation, urinary bladder distension, bradycardia unresponsive to atropine, reduced tear production, and pupillary dysfunction, among others. Historical and physical exam findings often suggest the diagnosis and the treatment is considered supportive. While the prognosis for long-term survival is considered poor, survival times of >2 years have been reported in both cats and dogs, suggesting the outcome can be good in some cases.

Intestinal Pseudo-obstruction

Intestinal pseudo-obstruction describes a variety of conditions that cause dysmotility and marked intestinal dilation. These conditions are thought to involve the enteric smooth muscle (myopathies) and the nervous system (neuropathies). The cause is unclear.

Intestinal pseudo-obstruction is reported in both dogs and cats. Specifically, it has been described as a result of smooth muscle alpha-actin deficiency in a Bengal cat and as a consequence of enteric ganglionitis in a Persian. Dogs and cats with intestinal pseudo-obstruction are often presented due to abdominal discomfort and distension, excessive bloating, belching and/or flatulence, and diarrhea. Abdominal radiographs will reveal marked intestinal dilation with no evidence of manual obstruction. Surgical/full thickness biopsies of the intestine are needed to evaluate for intestinal myopathies or neuropathies. Histologic lesions observed in cases of intestinal pseudo-obstruction include intestinal leiomyositis, mesenteric plexus vacuolar degeneration, atrophy, and fibrosis of the tunica muscularis. Reduced expression of alpha-smooth muscle actin in the tunica muscularis has also been reported in some cases. There is at least one report of long-term survival with glucocorticoid treatment (Murtagh et al. 2013) and a Persian cat with enteric ganglionitis was successfully treated with pyridostigmine. However, the prognosis is considered poor.

CONGENITAL DISORDERS

Congenital abnormalities resulting in small intestinal disease may occur in dogs and cats but are rare. Anatomic abnormalities that have been reported include intestinal stenosis or atresia, congenital SBS, non-rotation of the midgut during embryonic development, arteriovenous fistulae, duodenal diverticula, and random duplication of SI segments. Random duplications are cyst-like lesions. They are often discovered incidentally on abdominal ultrasound (Figure 41.7). Diverticula have been associated with perforations, bleeding, and foreign body entrapment, but also can be found incidentally.

Specific breeds of dogs can inherit abnormalities of the cobalamin-intrinsic factor receptor, leading to selective cobalamin malabsorption. If unrecognized, these disorders can lead to metabolic derangements and death. A list of breeds and the details of their disorders is shown in Table 41.5. The most common clinical signs in dogs with selective cobalamin absorption include failure to thrive, neurologic signs, and diarrhea. Neutropenia, normochromic non-regenerative anemia, hypoglycemia, and hyperammonemia are frequently observed. Once the diagnosis is suspected or confirmed, treatment should be instituted promptly. Both oral and parenteral cobalamin therapy are demonstrated to be effective. Clinical signs often improve within 1–2 days; however, laboratory abnormalities may take several weeks to resolve.

Absence of the brush border enzyme aminopeptidase N is reported in dogs but appears to be clinically insignificant. Relative lactase deficiency appears to also occur rarely but is similarly considered of little clinical importance.

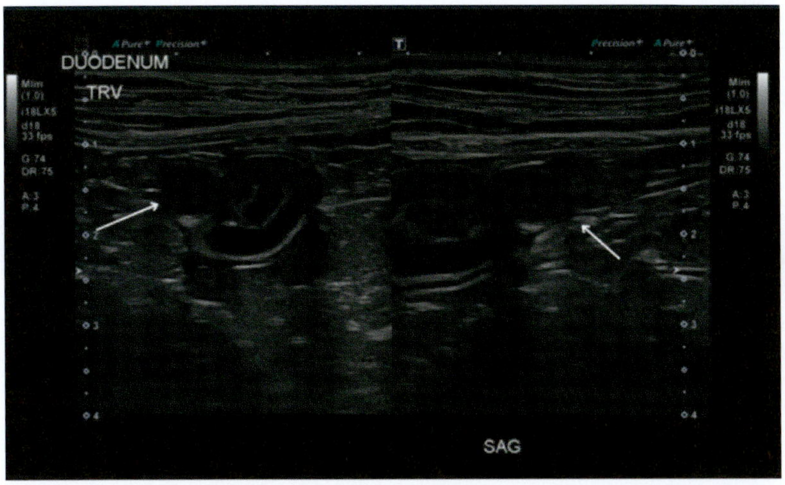

FIGURE 41.7 Transverse and longitudinal images of a suspected mid-duodenal duplication cyst (arrows) in a 2-year-old, male castrated, standard poodle. The cyst was discovered incidentally

Table 41.5 Selective Cobalamin Disorders in the Dog

Breed	Clinical features	Genetic mutation
Australian shepherd	• Failure to grow, inappetence, weakness • Nonregenerative anemia and neutropenia reported	*AMN c.3G>A* mutation
Beagle	• Signs can be severe • Lethargy, anorexia, failure to thrive, diarrhea • Degenerative liver disease	Exon 8 frameshift mutation in *CUBN*
Border collie	• Clinical signs may be mild and may not occur until adulthood in some cases • Hematologic abnormalities uncommon	Exon 53 frameshift mutation in *CUBN*
Chinese shar-pei	• Appears to largely affect the GI tract – diarrhea, vomiting, weight loss	None identified
Giant schnauzer	• Chronic inappetence, failure to thrive, • Neutropenia with hyper segmentation, anemia with anisocytosis and poikilocytosis • Megaloblastic changes of the bone marrow	*AMN* mutation
Komondor	• Failure-to-thrive, inappetence, vomiting and/or diarrhea, and weakness, dyshematopoeisis	*CUBN* intron 55 splice donor consensus sequence mutation
Yorkshire terrier	• Hypoglycemia, lethargy, seizures	None identified

AMN, amnionless; *CUBN*, cubulin.

REFERENCES

Allenspach, K., Culverwell, C., and Chan, D. (2016). Long-term outcome in dogs with chronic enteropathies: 203 cases. *Veterinary Record* 178: 368. https://doi.org/10.1136/vr.103557.

Allenspach, K., Rüfenacht, S., Sauter, S. et al. (2006). Pharmacokinetics and clinical efficacy of cyclosporine treatment of dogs with steroid-refractory inflammatory bowel disease. *Journal of Veterinary Internal Medicine* 20: 239–244. https://doi.org/10.1892/0891-6640(2006)20[239:paceoc]2.0.co;2.

Allenspach, K., Wieland, B., Gröne, A. et al. (2007). Chronic enteropathies in dogs: evaluation of risk factors for negative outcome. *Journal of Veterinary Internal Medicine* 21: 700–708. https://doi.org/10.1892/0891-6640(2007)21[700:ceideo]2.0.co;2/.

Candellone, A., Cerquetella, M., Girolami, F. et al. (2020). Acute diarrhea in dogs: current management and potential role of dietary polyphenols supplementation. *Antioxidants (Basel, Switzerland)* 9: 725. https://doi.org/10.3390/antiox9080725.

Černá, P., Lopez-Jimenez, C., Fukushima, K. et al. (2024). Clinicopathological findings, treatment, and outcome in 60 cats with gastrointestinal eosinophilic sclerosing fibroplasia. *Journal of Veterinary Internal Medicine* 38: 1005–1012. https://doi.org/10.1111/jvim.16992.

Chaitman, J., Ziese, A.-L., Pilla, R. et al. (2020). Fecal microbial and metabolic profiles in dogs with acute diarrhea receiving either fecal microbiota transplantation or oral metronidazole. *Frontiers in Veterinary Science* 7: 192. https://doi.org/10.3389/fvets.2020.00192.

Craven, M.D. and Washabau, R.J. (2019). Comparative pathophysiology and management of protein-losing enteropathy. *Journal of Veterinary Internal Medicine* 33: 383–402. https://doi.org/10.1111/jvim.15406.

Cridge, H., Hughes, S.M., Langston, V.C. et al. (2020). Mefenoxam, itraconazole, and terbinafine combination therapy for management of pythiosis in dogs (six cases). *Journal of the American Animal Hospital Association* 56: 307. https://doi.org/10.5326/JAAHA-MS-7039.

Cristóbal, J.I., Duque, F.J., Usón-Casaús, J.M. et al. (2021). Effects of allogeneic mesenchymal stem cell transplantation in dogs with inflammatory bowel disease treated with and without corticosteroids. *Animals* 11: 2061. https://doi.org/10.3390/ani11072061.

Dupouy-Manescau, N., Méric, T., Sénécat, O. et al. (2024). Updating the classification of chronic inflammatory enteropathies in dogs. *Animals* 14: 681. https://doi.org/10.3390/ani14050681.

Gold, A.J., Langlois, D.K., and Refsal, K.R. (2016). Evaluation of basal serum or plasma cortisol concentrations for the diagnosis of hypoadrenocorticism in dogs. *Journal of Veterinary Internal Medicine* 30: 1798–1805. https://doi.org/10.1111/jvim.14589.

Hall, E.J. and Batt, R.M. (1992). Dietary modulation of gluten sensitivity in a naturally occurring enteropathy of Irish setter dogs. *Gut* 33: 198–205. https://doi.org/10.1136/gut.33.2.198.

Holmberg, J., Pelander, L., Ljungvall, I. et al. (2022). Chronic enteropathy in dogs-epidemiologic aspects and clinical characteristics of dogs presenting at two Swedish animal hospitals. *Animals* 12: 1507. https://doi.org/10.3390/ani12121507.

Jablonski, S.A. and Cridge, H. (2023). Diseases of the small intestine. In: *Ettinger's Textbook of Veterinary Internal Medicine* (ed. S.J. Ettinger, E.C. Feldman and E. Cote), 1683–1728. St. Louis: Elsevier.

Jablonski, S.A., Strohmeyer, J.L., Buchweitz, J.P. et al. (2025). Prednisolone pharmacokinetics in dogs with protein-losing enteropathy. *Journal of Veterinary Internal Medicine* 39: e17277. https://doi.org/10.1111/jvim.17277.

Jablonski Wennogle, S.A., Priestnall, S.I., and Webb, C.B. (2017). Histopathologic characteristics of intestinal biopsy samples from dogs with chronic inflammatory enteropathy with and without hypoalbuminemia. *Journal of Veterinary Internal Medicine* 31: 371–376. https://doi.org/10.1111/jvim.14669.

Jablonski Wennogle, S.A., Stockman, J., and Webb, C.B. (2021). Prospective evaluation of a change in dietary therapy in dogs with steroid-resistant protein-losing enteropathy. *Journal of Small Animal Practice* 62: 756–764. https://doi.org/10.1111/jsap.13334.

Jergens, A.E., Crandell, J.M., Evans, R. et al. (2010). A clinical index for disease activity in cats with chronic enteropathy. *Journal of Veterinary Internal Medicine* 24: 1027–1033. https://doi.org/10.1111/j.1939-1676.2010.0549.x.

Jergens, A.E. and Heilmann, R.M. (2022). Canine chronic enteropathy-Current state-of-the-art and emerging concepts. *Frontiers in Veterinary Science* 9: 923013. https://doi.org/10.3389/fvets.2022.923013.

Kathrani, A. (2021). Dietary and nutritional approaches to the management of chronic enteropathy in dogs and cats. *Veterinary Clinics of North America: Small Animal Practice* 51: 123–136. https://doi.org/10.1016/j.cvsm.2020.09.005.

Kathrani, A., House, A., Catchpole, B. et al. (2010). Polymorphisms in the TLR4 and TLR5 gene are significantly associated with inflammatory bowel disease in German shepherd dogs. *PloS One* 5: e15740. https://doi.org/10.1371/journal.pone.0015740.

Langlois, D.K., Pritchard, J.C., Tolbert, M.K. et al. (2023). Clinical utility of an immunoglobulin A-based serological panel for the diagnosis of chronic enteropathy in dogs. *Journal of Veterinary Internal Medicine* 37: 446–454. https://doi.org/10.1111/jvim.16636.

Lowrie, M., Hadjivassiliou, M., Sanders, D.S. et al. (2016). A presumptive case of gluten sensitivity in a border terrier: a multisystem disorder? *Veterinary Record* 179: 573. https://doi.org/10.1136/vr.103910.

Makielski, K., Cullen, J., O'Connor, A. et al. (2019). Narrative review of therapies for chronic enteropathies in dogs and cats. *Journal of Veterinary Internal Medicine* 33: 11–22. https://doi.org/10.1111/jvim.15345.

Manchester, A. (2024). Diarrhea. In: *Ettinger's Textbook of Veterinary Internal Medicine* (ed. E. Cote, S.J. Ettinger and E.C. Feldman), 233–237. Elsevier.

Murtagh, K., Oldroyd, L., Ressel, L. et al. (2013). Successful management of intestinal pseudo-obstruction in a dog. *Veterinary Record Case Reports* 1: e000025. https://doi.org/10.1136/vetreccr-2013-000025.

Nagata, N., Ohta, H., Yokoyama, N. et al. (2020). Clinical characteristics of dogs with food-responsive protein-losing enteropathy. *Journal of Veterinary Internal Medicine* 34: 659–668. https://doi.org/10.1111/jvim.15720.

Nixon, S.L., Rose, L., and Muller, A.T. (2019). Efficacy of an orally administered anti-diarrheal probiotic paste (Pro-Kolin Advanced) in dogs with acute diarrhea:

a randomized, placebo-controlled, double-blinded clinical study. *Journal of Veterinary Internal Medicine* 33: 1286–1294. https://doi.org/10.1111/jvim.15481.

Okanishi, H., Yoshioka, R., Kagawa, Y. et al. (2014). The clinical efficacy of dietary fat restriction in treatment of dogs with intestinal lymphangiectasia. *Journal of Veterinary Internal Medicine* 28: 809–817. https://doi.org/10.1111/jvim.12327.

Pereira, G.Q., Gomes, L.A., Santos, I.S. et al. (2018). Fecal microbiota transplantation in puppies with canine parvovirus infection. *Journal of Veterinary Internal Medicine* 32: 707–711. https://doi.org/10.1111/jvim.15072.

Polidoro, D., Van Ham, L., Santens, P. et al. (2020). Phenotypic characterization of paroxysmal dyskinesia in maltese dogs. *Journal of Veterinary Internal Medicine* 34: 1541–1546. https://doi.org/10.1111/jvim.15804.

Reagan, K.L., Marks, S.L., Pesavento, P.A. et al. (2019). Successful management of 3 dogs with colonic pythiosis using itraconzaole, terbinafine, and prednisone. *Journal of Veterinary Internal Medicine* 33: 1434–1439. https://doi.org/10.1111/jvim.15506.

Rudinsky, A.J., Rowe, J.C., and Parker, V.J. (2018). Nutritional management of chronic enteropathies in dogs and cats. *Journal of the American Veterinary Medical Association* 253: 570–578. https://doi.org/10.2460/javma.253.5.570.

Russell, K.N., Mehler, S.J., Skorupski, K.A. et al. (2007). Clinical and immunohistochemical differentiation of gastrointestinal stromal tumors from leiomyosarcomas in dogs: 42 cases (1990–2003). *Journal of the American Veterinary Medical Association* 230: 1329–1333. https://doi.org/10.2460/javma.230.9.1329.

Salavati Schmitz, S., Gow, A., Bommer, N. et al. (2019). Diagnostic features, treatment, and outcome of dogs with inflammatory protein-losing enteropathy. *Journal of Veterinary Internal Medicine* 33: 2005–2013. https://doi.org/10.1111/jvim.15571.

Schmitz, S., Coenen, C., König, M. et al. (2009). Comparison of three rapid commercial Canine parvovirus antigen detection tests with electron microscopy and polymerase chain reaction. *Journal of Veterinary Diagnostic Investigation* 21: 344–345. https://doi.org/10.1177/104063870902100306.

Shmalberg, J., Montalbano, C., Morelli, G. et al. (2019). A randomized double blinded placebo-controlled clinical trial of a probiotic or metronidazole for acute canine diarrhea. *Frontiers in Veterinary Science* 6: 163. https://doi.org/10.3389/fvets.2019.00163.

Tolbert, M.K., Murphy, M., Gaylord, L. et al. (2022). Dietary management of chronic enteropathy in dogs. *Journal of Small Animal Practice* 63: 425–434. https://doi.org/10.1111/jsap.13471.

Unterer, S. and Busch, K. (2021). Acute hemorrhagic diarrhea syndrome in dogs. *Veterinary Clinics: Small Animal Practice* 51: 79–92. https://doi.org/10.1016/j.cvsm.2020.09.007.

Venn, E.C., Preisner, K., Boscan, P.L. et al. (2017). Evaluation of an outpatient protocol in the treatment of canine parvoviral enteritis. *Journal of Veterinary Emergency and Critical Care* 27: 52–65. https://doi.org/10.1111/vec.12561.

Washabau, R.J., Day, M.J., Willard, M.D. et al. (2010). Endoscopic, biopsy, and histopathologic guidelines for the evaluation of gastrointestinal inflammation in companion animals. *Journal of Veterinary Internal Medicine* 24: 10–26. https://doi.org/10.1111/j.1939-1676.2009.0443.x.

Webb, T.L. and Webb, C.B. (2022). Comparing adipose-derived mesenchymal stem cells with prednisolone for the treatment of feline inflammatory bowel disease. *Journal of Feline Medicine & Surgery* 24: e244–e250. https://doi.org/10.1177/1098612X221104053.

Winston, J.A., Suchodolski, J.S., Gaschen, F. et al. (2024). Clinical Guidelines for Fecal Microbiota Transplantation in Companion Animals. *Advances in Small Animal Care* 5: 79–107. https://doi.org/10.1016/j.yasa.2024.06.006.

CHAPTER 42

Disorders of the Large Intestine and Rectum

Alison C. Manchester[1] *and Yuvani Bandara*[2]

[1] *Department of Clinical Sciences, College of Veterinary Medicine, Cornell University, Ithaca, USA*
[2] *Department of Clinical Sciences, College of Veterinary Medicine & Biomedical Sciences, Colorado State University, Fort Collins, CO, USA*

KEY POINTS

- Study of the canine and feline fecal microbiota confirms strong impacts of oral antibiotics, but the relationship between microbiota composition and health and disease remains unclear.
- Additional evidence shows that diet is the most effective therapy for chronic nonspecific colitis.
- Digital rectal exam can alter diagnostic plans in up to 25% of canine cases.
- Loss of wall layering of intestinal lesions differentiates neoplastic versus nonneoplastic lesions.

LARGE INTESTINAL ANATOMY AND PHYSIOLOGY

The large intestine begins at the ileocolic junction and is comprised of the cecum, colon, rectum, and anal canal. The main functions of the large intestine are the absorption and secretion of water and electrolytes, namely sodium, and immune surveillance. The length of the colon is approximately one-fifth of the entire gastrointestinal tract, and it is divided into three sections: ascending, transverse, and descending. The ascending colon is anatomically located close to the duodenum, with the descending colon flexing caudally to run along the left abdominal wall. The rectum is contained within the pelvic inlet dorsal to the urinary bladder, before terminating as the anal canal.

The mesocolon is the mesentery that attaches the colon to the abdominal wall and is divided into the same parts of the colon that it suspends. The mesocolon also houses lymphatics, nerves, and vasculature from the cranial (ileocolic, right colic, middle colic branches) and caudal (cranial rectal branch) mesenteric arteries. Short branches of the mesenteric arteries, called arterial arcades, bifurcate upon entering the intestinal wall to form the mural arterial network. While the GI tract is highly perfused (especially in the fed state), receiving around a quarter of cardiac output, the large intestine is the least oxygenated segment. Circumferential lymphatic vessels drain into the right, middle, and left colic lymph nodes, which eventually drain via the intestinal trunk into the cisterna chyli. The cisterna chyli acts as the lymphatic conduit for the products of lipid digestion from the whole intestinal tract to the thoracic duct in the mediastinum.

In a healthy patient, the colonic lumen contains a mixture of digested food, water, electrolytes, gas, and microorganisms. Bacteria serve many important functions, including but not limited to the fermentation of indigestible carbohydrates to produce short-chain fatty acids (SCFAs) and gas. Circular and longitudinal muscle layers in the colon work synergistically to create peristalsis. Movement is governed by the interstitial cells of Cajal that act as muscular pacemakers that balance a specific motility pattern of low-amplitude, non-propagating contractions and high-amplitude, propagating wave contractions. These waves increase intestinal transit time, allowing for the absorption of water, mixing of contents, and the storage of feces for the controlled defecation of appropriately processed boluses. This movement is further influenced by medications, sleep, food intake, hydration status, and psychological state.

Disorders of the Liver, Exocrine Pancreas, and Gastrointestinal Tract in Dogs and Cats, First Edition. Edited by Harry Cridge et al. Published 2026 by John Wiley & Sons, Inc. Companion Website: www.wiley.com/go/cridge/disorders

MICROSCOPIC

The large intestine is comprised of four layers: the mucosa, submucosa, muscularis, and serosa. The mucosa can be further divided up into three layers called the epithelium, lamina propria, and muscularis mucosa. The mucosa of the large intestine is distinct from that of the small intestine due to the absence of digestive enzymes and absorptive villi, and the presence of deep crypts of Lieberkühn extending into the muscularis mucosa. Epithelial cells are generated at the base of the crypts and either remain as epithelial cells or differentiate into goblet or endocrine cells during migration and eventual shedding toward the intestinal lumen.

The luminal surface is smooth and comprises a single sheet of epithelial cells covered by a layer of thick, bicarbonate-rich mucus secreted by goblet cells. This mucus protects the epithelium from acids produced by bacteria during fecal fermentation and from physical excoriation, and aids fecal consistency. The rate of mucus secretion is regulated by direct, tactile stimulation of the colonic epithelial cells, local nerve reflexes, and parasympathetic innervation via the pelvic nerves. Mucosal endocrine cells influence mucus secretion and colonic motility via the production of neuropeptides, e.g., glucagon-like peptides, polypeptide P, insulin-like growth factors (IGF), and serotonin. In this capacity, endocrine cells also influence the gut microbiome and gut–brain axis.

Below the epithelium, the lamina propria consists predominantly of plasma cells and B and T lymphocytes, which act as part of colonic immune surveillance. Lymphoid follicles are a normal component of the colonic mucosa and are more common in the proximal than distal colon. However, focal lymphoid hyperplasia can be found in the rectum and is known as a rectal tonsil. These secondary lymphoid structures are responsible for selective endocytosis of antigens and presentation to intraepithelial macrophages and B and T lymphocytes.

The muscularis serosae is a thin layer of smooth muscle, nerves, blood vessels, and lymphatics that divides the mucosa from the submucosa. The outermost layer of the large intestine, the serosa, is formed of mesothelial cells that release serous fluid into the abdominal cavity. This reduces friction and tension between organs during digestion.

As omnivores, dogs have a more developed cecum and a longer, more segmented large intestine compared to cats, which are obligate carnivores. This conformation allows dogs to have greater fermenting capacity to facilitate the breakdown of soluble fiber into SCFAs (e.g., butyrate) to support colonic epithelial cell health. Both species have anal sacs adjacent to the rectum, which are involved in scent marking during defecation. The anal sacs are larger in dogs and can become impacted due to primary disease, diet changes, and systemic issues, including atopic dermatitis (see Chapter 43 on Disorders of the Anus for more information).

HISTORY/CLINICAL SIGNS + DIAGNOSTIC APPROACH

Suspicion for disease of the colon or rectum begins with information gained during history taking. Using open- and closed-ended questions helps the clinician obtain the information necessary to compose a logical differential list and diagnostic plan. Table 42.1 displays clinical signs that may localize disease to the colon and/or rectum. Often, a collection of the listed clinical signs occurs together and may help with disease localization. If you have identified the presence of these signs in your clinical history, then you are in the right chapter.

As important as knowing the clinical signs that fit with colorectal diseases is an appreciation for clinical signs that indicate dysfunction of *other* organs. In general, disease solely localized to the distal GI tract would *not* be expected to cause anorexia. Vomiting typically implicates a more proximal GI tract or systemic (e.g., uremia) issue. Given the physiological role of the colon in absorbing water and some electrolytes, but not basic nutrients such as proteins and carbohydrates, large intestinal diseases in isolation do not result in panhypoproteinemia. Large-volume blood loss from the distal GI tract could result in protein loss, but in those cases, anemia would be dramatic.

Determining the duration, frequency, and possible progression of clinical signs is also critically important. Characterizing the clinical signs may focus the workup or narrow the differential list. Large bowel diarrhea is commonly associated with stress in dogs, and so determining the coincidence of "episodes" with other events in the dog's life could help raise or lower that differential. Alternatively, an animal with an acute onset of progressive clinical signs would prioritize more serious differentials such as neoplasia or infectious colitis.

Table 42.1 Clinical Signs Compatible with Large Intestinal and Rectal Disease

Clinical sign	Colon	Rectum
Tenesmus	X	X
Hematochezia	X	X
Dyschezia	X	X
Frequent defecation	X	
Infrequent defecation	X	X
Constipation	X	X
Fecal incontinence	X	X
Abnormally shaped stools	X	X
Flatulence	X	
"Scooting"		X

Dogs and cats tend to manifest their colonic diseases differently. Large bowel diarrhea is common in dogs, with urgency, lack of form, and mucus or blood. Dogs also tend to have more anal gland and prostatic issues compared to cats, which may masquerade as colorectal diseases. Cats are much more likely to display constipation with tenesmus and infrequent passage of stools. This may go unnoticed by clients, as cats tend to be more discreet with their clinical problems. Fewer, rather than more, bowel movements may not be noticed, especially in a multi-cat household. An important part of the clinical history, particularly in geriatric cats, is determining how many times a week the cat has a bowel movement. So-called "smart" litter boxes can track litter box activities and differentiate urination from defecation evacuations and may help busy clients keep track of their pet's bowel habits. Cats may also leave hard, small fecal balls outside of the litter box. This clinical sign should be considered as a possible manifestation of renal, orthopedic, or urinary disease before assuming it is a behavioral issue.

Gastrointestinal signs, such as vomiting and diarrhea, are very common in canine and feline patients, but do not necessarily implicate the colon or rectum. As with any GI complaint, it is prudent to consider extra-GI (secondary) causes for clinical signs along with primary GI causes. The distal GI tract can be a harbinger of disease elsewhere, and so a methodical approach is key (Figure 42.1). For example, a geriatric cat who begins defecating outside the litter box may require a workup evaluating the orthopedic system and investigating renal function. Reduced renal function may prevent cats from maintaining their hydration, resulting in dry stools that are painful to pass. Frustrated, uncomfortable cats may leave the litter box without finishing their task and house soiling ensues. Endocrine disorders can also manifest as large intestinal signs; dogs lacking a lymphopenia may be screened for hypoadrenocorticism (Addison's disease).

Preliminary Diagnostics

The importance of a minimum database of bloodwork (complete blood count, chemistry panel ± thyroid levels) and urinalysis, as well as a thorough physical exam, cannot be overstated. Included in that physical exam is the digital rectal examination (DRE). This simple procedure is essential to screen for abnormalities of the prostate and anal sacs, which could cause signs of dyschezia or tenesmus (Andrews et al. 2024). The DRE also allows for evaluation of a small section of the urethra; this information could help with the at times difficult determination as to whether patients are having stranguria or tenesmus. Other local issues interfering with normal colonic or rectal function, such as previous pelvic fractures or other abnormalities of the pelvis, may be implicated by physical exam and imaging. One study, including 440 dogs, found that findings of a DRE resulted in a change to the diagnostic plan in 1 of 4 dogs and change to the treatment plan in 1 out of 8 dogs (Andrews et al. 2024). That same study found that neither age, sex, nor breed influenced the frequency of abnormal findings, further supporting the recommendation to perform a thorough DRE in all clinically unwell dogs. Digital rectal exams can be performed under sedation in select feline cases.

Digital rectal exam also offers the chance to obtain material for rectal cytology. This inexpensive and accessible diagnostic has limited scope but may be informative in select cases.

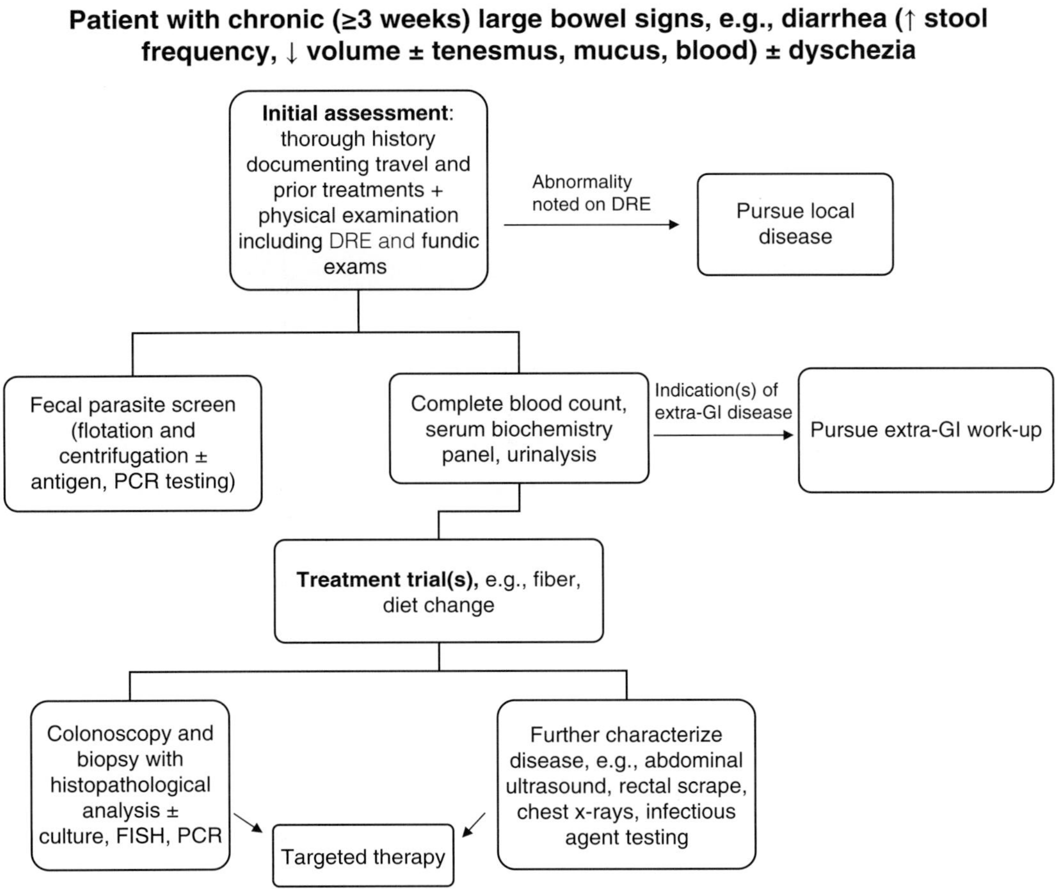

FIGURE 42.1 Flowchart depicting diagnostic approach to patients with chronic large bowel signs

Historically, this diagnostic has been used to justify antimicrobial therapy, typically after visualization of rod- or spore-shaped bacteria. Multiple studies refute a relationship between spore-shaped organisms and the presence of clostridial toxins as well as clinical signs. Put another way, healthy dogs are just as likely as dogs with acute diarrhea to have spore-shaped bacteria seen on rectal cytology. A better use of the test is to exfoliate some cells lining the distal gut and evaluate those. Normal findings include numerous bacteria and sheets of epithelial cells. Abnormal findings include prevalent macrophage and neutrophil populations, dysplastic appearing-lymphocytes, and intracellular organisms. All of these would warrant additional confirmatory diagnostics but may reorder the differential list after an inexpensive, minimally invasive test.

A basic workup is key to generating a foundation of clinical evidence but does not always identify a specific cause for clinical signs. In these cases, a decision must be made as to whether to pursue empirical treatment trials or continue with the diagnostic workup (Figure 42.1). This decision will be impacted by numerous factors related to the patient, the client, and the capabilities of the clinic. Outwardly, well patients with shorter duration of clinical problems may be good candidates for treatment trial(s). Patients with severe or rapid progression of clinical signs may warrant a more expedited, intense diagnostic workup.

Imaging

Imaging the large intestine may help identify mechanical and structural causes for clinical signs. Abdominal radiographs are fairly limited in their ability to narrow the differential list for patients with large bowel signs. Ultrasound is more helpful and allows for the evaluation of intestinal wall layering (Figure 42.2); this may guide subsequent diagnostic decisions, including the choice between colonoscopic versus full-thickness biopsy. Ultrasound also allows for assessment of local lymph nodes, presence of free abdominal fluid, and extraintestinal lesions that might be impacting gut function and potentially indicative of systemic disease.

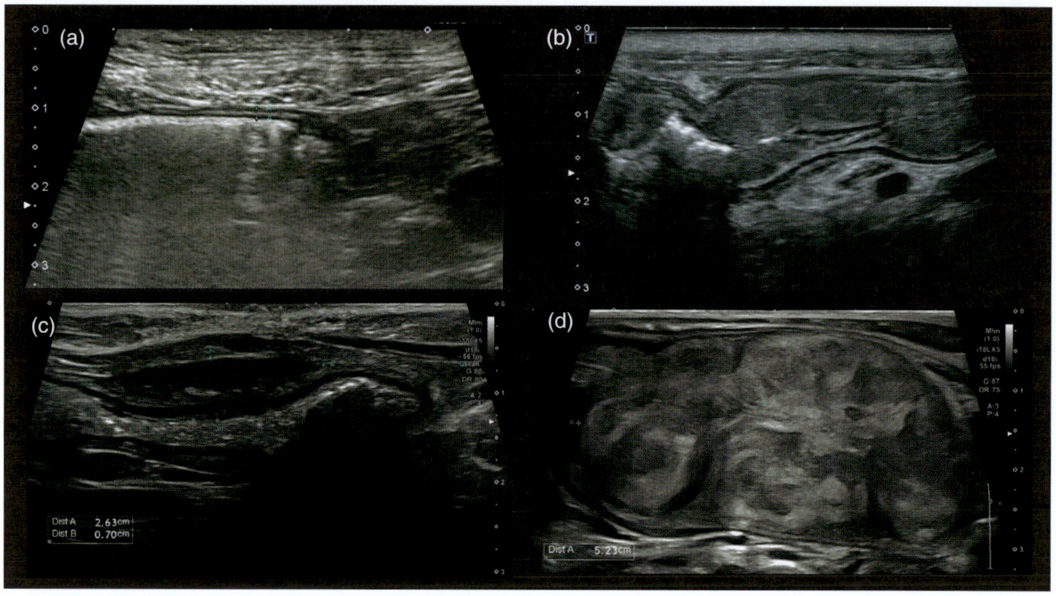

FIGURE 42.2 Sonographic images from abnormal colon. (a) Sonographically normal appearing descending colon of a 2-year-old neutered male Labrador retriever with chronic diarrhea. (b) Ultrasound image of the distal descending colon of a 10-month-old female French bulldog with *E. coli*-associated granulomatous colitis. The colon had multifocal, nodular thickening (up to 6 mm) of the colonic mucosa and submucosa, but wall layering was maintained. (c) Ultrasound image of the transverse colon of a 2-year-old spayed female domestic shorthair cat with acute pain and hyporexia. The affected area showed mass-like thickening and indistinct wall layer of the submucosa and muscularis (colonic resection and anastomosis histopathology revealed regional extensive fibrino-necrotizing and pyogranulomatous serositis of unknown origin). (d) Ultrasound image of a large, irregular, heterogeneously asymmetric mass arising from the descending colon submucosa of an 11-year-old neutered male Siamese cat with a 5-year history of hematochezia. Cytology was compatible with gastrointestinal eosinophilic sclerosing fibroplasia

Colonoscopy

Colonoscopy offers direct examination of the rectal and colonic mucosa, providing colon prep (typically a combination of fasting ± enemas and laxative solutions) effectively evacuates the colon. The colonic mucosa typically has a pink, glistening appearance, without the roughness or texture that villi give the small intestinal lining (Figure 42.3). Lymphoid follicles may be evident in the canine colon as evenly spaced punctate reddish foci (Figure 42.3b). Clinically relevant and macroscopically evident lesions are not very common, but colonoscopy may be the only way to visualize strictures, polyps, luminal tumors, erosions, or granulomas. Colonoscopy also offers a minimally invasive but direct means of sampling growths or masses.

Histopathological Analysis of Large Intestinal Samples

Histopathological analysis of colonic biopsies is often considered one of the cornerstones of a thorough workup of chronic large bowel signs. However, interpretation of colonic biopsies is challenging. Individual observers (pathologists) may have disparate conclusions based on their experience and interpretation of provided tissues in the context of published guidelines. Histopathological findings are typically divided into inflammatory and morphological features. Inflammation is classified based on dominant cell types identified, which may point toward a type of disorder. For example, colon tissues dominated by neutrophils and macrophages suggest an infectious etiology. Biopsies with mixed inflammation and a predominance of macrophages staining positive for periodic acid-Schiff (PAS) raise suspicion for *E. coli*-associated granulomatous colitis (ECGC). Lymphoplasmacytic infiltration in the colonic mucosa is far more common and less specific. In some cases, colonic biopsy histopathology identifies a specific etiology for clinical signs, such as histoplasmosis or colonic neoplasia. In the absence of infectious agents or evidence of neoplasia, histopathology results should be

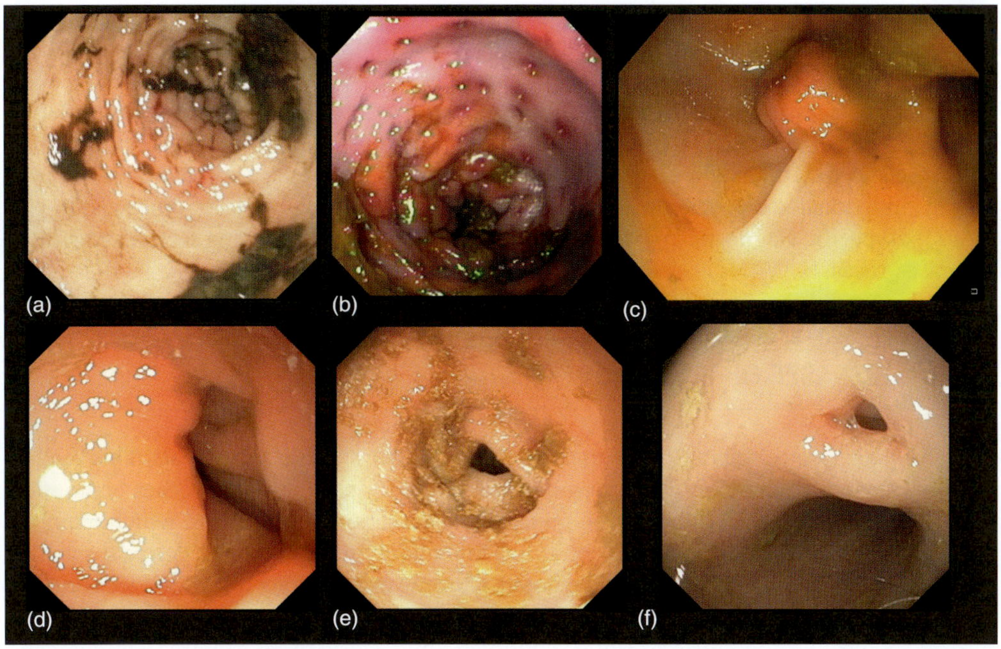

FIGURE 42.3 Endoscopic appearance of normal colonic mucosa. (a and b). Images of normal canine colonic mucosa. Note the erythematous foci with central indentation in (b), consistent with lymphoid follicles. (c) Colonoscopic image of the ileocecal junction, viewed at an oblique angle. The ileum often appears as a button-like protrusion into the proximal colon. (d and e) Images of normal feline colonic mucosa. (f) Colonoscopic image from a cat with weight loss showing a partially open ileocolic orifice (upper right corner) with the larger entrance to the cecum below

interpreted in the context of the patient's overall clinical picture and not used as the sole criteria to guide treatment or provide prognosis.

It is also important to note that histologically "normal" colonic biopsies may be collected from patients with clinical signs localizing to the large bowel. In one study, 58% of client-owned dogs with chronic large bowel diarrhea had no detectable histologic abnormalities (Roth et al. 1990). This result could be interpreted in several ways: firstly, representative samples might not have been obtained. Lesions may be patchy, and it is possible that affected areas were not sampled. Inadequate quality of the samples may also impair accurate interpretation. Alternatively, disease may be localized to the serosa, submucosa, smooth muscle layer, or myenteric plexi, and therefore not apparent in mucosal biopsies. Very mild to absent lesions could moreover suggest a functional disorder that is not inflammatory in nature; various "functional" enteropathies are common in humans and likely occur in dogs and cats as well. Functional disorders may encompass disorders of the gut–brain axis, motility disorders, brush border defects, adverse food reactions, alterations in epithelial integrity, and so on. Further investigations are needed to better recognize and manage these conditions.

Microbiota Evaluation

Much attention has been given recently to the role of the gut microbiota in GI and systemic health. This is particularly relevant for colorectal disorders, as the colon harbors the densest population of microbes of any organ in the body. Microbes perform a myriad of functions, including nutrient breakdown, metabolite bioconversion, and protection from putative enteropathogens. Studies published to date have not differentiated chronic enteropathy (CE) dogs based on localization of their clinical signs to upper or lower GI, so it is unclear if dogs or cats with colitis have a signature gut microbiota compared to those with other manifestations of CE. Several veterinary diagnostic companies offer fecal microbiome analysis, using quantitative polymerase chain reaction (PCR), 16S sequencing, or a combination. Results are reported in a variety of formats ranging from a single number estimating the degree of eubiosis or dysbiosis to a more exhaustive documentation of the relative abundances of various bacterial taxa. At the time of writing, the authors are not aware of any publications suggesting that these types of analyses provide actionable data for individual patients. A retrospective study including 16 dogs found that a higher fecal dysbiosis index (DI, Texas A&M Gastrointestinal Lab) was associated with a worse clinical response to fecal microbiota transplantation (FMT) (Toresson et al. 2023). Going forward, we will ideally have readily available assays that characterize the gut microbiome and/or metabolome to guide customized microbiome-centered therapies (e.g., individualized probiotics, specific diets, postbiotic supplements, or otherwise).

Additional specific diagnostic approaches will be included in the following sections regarding specific disease processes.

CONGENITAL DISEASES OF THE LARGE INTESTINE

Atresia ani (AA) is a rare congenital abnormality reported in dogs and rarely in cats. This malformation may occur with concomitant rectovaginal fistula (RVF) in females and other anatomical abnormalities, such as agenesis of the tail or spina bifida. Presenting complaints, which often are recognized at the time of weaning, include tenesmus and abdominal distension. Perineal swelling and/or a very tiny or absent anal orifice may be noted. Chronic urinary tract infections are common in patients with RVF. A female predisposition exists, and AA is overrepresented in purebred dogs, including Toy Poodles, Boston Terriers, Maltese, Finnish Spitz, German Shorthaired Pointers, and Miniature Schnauzers. AA is rarely reported in cats with no reported breed predispositions. Etiology involves a developmental abnormality involving incomplete separation of the primitive cloaca into the rectum and urogenital sinus. The diagnosis may be evident with physical exam, but contrast radiography can help clarify the anatomy. This also allows for AA classification; type I involves congenital anal stenosis. The remaining two types have no anal opening. Type II involves imperforate anus. Type III AA involves imperforate anus with a more orad termination of the rectum as a blind pouch. Type IV involves a normal anus and terminal rectum that is discontinuous with the more proximal rectum. Surgical treatment attempts to create a more normal anal orifice (anoplasty), while evacuating the colon in cases of severe megacolon. Complications are common, including postoperative stricture and fecal incontinence. Animals that have had prolonged colonic distension may struggle with atony. Postoperative therapies that promote soft stools (lactulose, polyethylene glycol) and stimulate colonic motility (cisapride) may help with tenesmus. Prognosis depends on the success of the surgical intervention to create a more normal anal orifice.

Hirschsprung's (HSCR) disease is a common congenital malformation of the enteric nervous system that is well described in humans and thought to occur in dogs and cats. Normal gut motility involves segmentation and peristaltic waves. Amazingly, these patterns occur in the *absence* of extrinsic innervation but require submucous (Meissner) and myenteric (Auerbach) nerve plexuses. In humans, HSCR may occur with other GI malformations such as colonic atresia and Meckel's diverticulum. Few reports exist in dogs and cats, but clinical signs are as to be expected with motility disorders, e.g., abdominal distension, pain, and abnormal defecation patterns. Confirming this diagnosis would be challenging. In published reports, clinicians have evaluated surgically or necropsy-obtained tissues for routine histopathology ± immunohistochemistry. Hypoganglionosis is deemed consistent with HSCR, though age-matched control tissues are ideally simultaneously evaluated. Given that multiple congenital abnormalities may be present simultaneously, abdominal imaging is essential to rule out a treatable cause (e.g., stenosis) for dysmotility.

Vascular malformations, both congenital and acquired, may occur in the distal GI tract. The best described of these is colonic vascular ectasia (CVE). Interestingly, this condition is most often diagnosed in adult humans. The etiology is unknown but may involve a reaction to repeated colonic distension, which is theorized to overwhelm precapillary sphincters and promote arteriovenous communication. The presence of anemia along with large bowel diarrhea or hematochezia should raise the possibility of this diagnosis. Vascular lesions may be evident during colonoscopy, but tortuous, dilated vasa recta vessels may also be seen during exploratory celiotomy. Histopathology may show disorganized, heterogeneous blood vessels that may be thrombosed. Only a handful of canine cases have been reported in the veterinary literature (Charlesworth et al. 2013). It is unknown if CVE occurs in cats. The most common treatment is surgical resection of affected segments of bowel; however, recurrence is a risk. In humans, lesions may be treated with endoscopic ablations. Prognosis for canine patients is variable, and long-term control is possible.

IDIOPATHIC AND INFLAMMATORY CONDITIONS OF THE LARGE INTESTINE

Despite a thorough workup, many dogs and some cats presenting with large bowel clinical signs have no specific cause identified. This may result in the patient being assigned a diagnosis of chronic inflammatory enteropathy, inflammatory bowel disease, or idiopathic colitis. It is important to recognize that, regardless of the terminology used, these conditions are syndromes without pathognomonic clinical signs or strict diagnostic criteria. Recognition of the potential benefits and limitations of available tests is therefore a key aspect of proper interpretation of results.

Dogs and cats with inflammatory or idiopathic disorders of the colon may show an array of clinical signs localizing to the large intestine (Table 42.1). Most compatible with this category of disease would be waxing and waning or persistent clinical signs that are not particularly progressive over time. Signs may appear to be temporally correlated with stressful events or dietary fluctuations or have no apparent triggers. When clinical signs are progressively worsening despite rational treatment trials or new signs are arising, clinicians should reconsider their working diagnosis of idiopathic colitis and consider additional diagnostic workup.

Earlier in the chapter, some of the caveats of histopathological analysis of colonic biopsies were discussed. In the case of nonspecific colitis (e.g., no signs of infectious colitis or neoplasia), histopathologic findings can be highly variable. The presence and severity of the most prevalent lesion, lymphoplasmacytic inflammation, were not found to be correlated with disease activity (CIBDAI/CCECAI) in 35 dogs with CE (Allenspach et al. 2019). However, those investigators found colonic fibrosis and crypt dilation to be moderately correlated ($r = 0.47$ and $r = 0.42$, respectively) with disease activity (Allenspach et al. 2019). The summative histology score correlated only weakly ($r = 0.33$) with clinical activity index values. These findings suggest that histopathological analysis of distal gut tissues may have a relatively small role in guiding treatment or prognostic decisions for individual patients.

An abnormal or unstable gut microbiome is likely involved in the pathogenesis of diseases in some dogs and cats with recurrent large bowel clinical signs. A persistently unhealthy state of the gut microbiota has been well established in humans with inflammatory bowel diseases and recurrent *Clostridioides difficile* (*C. difficile*) infection. Few, if any, clinical studies have compared the gut microbiota of dogs or cats with colitis-type clinical signs to those from healthy populations. It is, however, unlikely that a characteristic gut microbiota composition or "enterotype" is shared by all patients presenting with signs localized to the distal gut. Functional redundancy within the microbiota ensures that key processes are carried out despite fluctuations in the gut luminal environment. In this way, profiling the gene expression (metagenomics) and end products of bacterial metabolism may shed more light on the functional ramifications of microbiota perturbations than composition-based analyses. Two studies to date have identified heightened humoral immune responses against fecal bacteria in dogs with CE, compared to healthy controls (Soontararak et al. 2019; Martinez-Lopez et al. 2021). This approach represents an alternative to compositional comparisons of the fecal microbiota in health and disease, which may help highlight bacteria responsible for aberrant immune responses in the diseased gut.

Given that these advanced analyses are not particularly relevant for clinical cases, a suspicion for a microbiota-related disorder or dysbiosis-driven disease mainly stems from a thorough history and detailed description of clinical signs. Several factors impact gut bacterial populations. Diet is one of the strongest modulators of the gut microbiome; along with feeding the host, ingested foods provide substrates for microbes, including ones that are unable to be digested by the host. Much attention has been paid to nondigestible carbohydrates, but proteins and fats may also influence bacterial growth and colonization. Oral antibiotic exposures, particularly those occurring early in life, help gauge the degree to which the patient's clinical signs might be related to dysbiosis. Antibiotics exert strong pressures on the gut microbiota. While the exact impacts are highly individualized, likely consequences include reduced diversity and increased abundance of facultative anaerobes.

THERAPEUTICS

Diet

Dietary interventions have the strongest evidence base for their efficacy in dogs with acute and chronic nonspecific colitis. Supplemental dietary fiber has a strong evidence base for quickly and safely resolving large bowel diarrhea in dogs. This may be achieved through the addition of a fiber powder such as psyllium husk powder or by feeding a commercially available high-fiber diet. Fiber has multimodal effects, including drawing water into the colon, modulating motility, and serving as a prebiotic for bacterial fermentation (Moreno et al. 2022). It is unclear which of these properties are related to clinical impacts, though one study of 31 dogs with chronic large bowel diarrhea found that after feeding a diet with 4.9 g/100 kcal total dietary fiber (Hill's Prescription Diet GI Biome), fecal bacterial metabolism shifted from a putrefactive to a saccharolytic state (Fritsch et al. 2022).

Dietary strategies other than or in addition to high fiber may benefit dogs with chronic large bowel signs. Evidence supports the efficacy of novel protein, hydrolyzed protein, amino acid-based, and home-prepared diets in resolving these types of clinical signs. In a patient with a good appetite and normal clinicopathological parameters, several dedicated feeding trials may be completed before ruling out diet-responsive disease. Clients should be provided with specific feeding instructions, including the amount and frequency of the new food as well as the importance of excluding other foods and treats. If the diet is going to help with GI signs, improvement would be expected within the first 10–14 days of exclusive feeding. Sharing this knowledge can help improve compliance, as many clients may be reluctant to feed in such a restricted manner.

Although data is more limited, a handful of studies have also shown that supplemental fiber may benefit cats with chronic diarrhea. As with dogs, fiber powder may be mixed in with food (or hidden in canned food or a palatable lickable treat), or the patient may be fed a commercial high-fiber diet. Fiber may also help manage signs of constipation. This is credited to the ability of different fibers to form a gel that eases fecal passage, draw water into the feces, as well as act as a substrate for SCFA production, which can have prokinetic and anti-inflammatory effects in the colon. Fiber should be used with caution in two scenarios: cats with substantial colonic dysmotility and in markedly underconditioned cats. The increased fecal bulk promoted by fiber may exacerbate defecation difficulties, particularly if the colon is structurally compromised (e.g., end-stage megacolon). Fiber is likely to reduce digestibility and possibly promote satiety, neither of which would be desired in a patient that needs to gain weight.

Medications

Various medications can be used to symptomatically manage the clinical signs of large bowel disease. If success is not achieved with fiber or dietary change, medications are considered. In contrast to human medicine, antidiarrheals are far less commonly employed. Conservative doses of loperamide (~0.1 mg/kg PO q8–12 hours) may be prescribed to dogs with acute, frequent, non-bloody diarrhea after an initial workup has ruled out infectious and toxic causes. Supplemental fluids may help restore hydration and help benefit the patient overall, particularly in anorexic animals. There is limited evidence for the benefit of probiotics to hasten resolution of acute diarrhea, but they are unlikely to do harm and may help. Use of antibiotics for acute nonspecific large bowel diarrhea is not recommended unless the patient is showing signs of sepsis (e.g., fever with neutropenia, hypotension). Long-lasting reductions in gut bacterial diversity and depletion of anaerobic commensals are possible. This may set the stage for recurrent episodes due to an unhealthy, unstable gut microbiota enriched in facultative anaerobes. Still, there may be small subsets of canine and feline patients for which no other intervention helps. The authors and colleagues have recognized a syndrome of chronic severe mixed bowel diarrhea in young cats that respond clinically to tylosin; this would by no means be the first intervention tried, but this intervention should be considered in particularly refractory cases of feline diarrhea.

Fecal Microbiota Transplantation

Other interventions may help resolve large bowel clinical signs in dogs and cats. FMT involves the introduction of donor feces from a healthy individual into the GI tract of a diseased patient. This intervention has revolutionized treatment of recurrent *C. difficile* infection in humans. In the canine and feline realm, much remains unknown about the ideal donor or which patients would be most likely to benefit. Published data is limited to a small number of uncontrolled, retrospective studies or case reports. Thorough donor screening is important to prevent transmission of infectious agents (Winston et al. 2024).

Immunomodulators

Immunomodulatory medications may also be employed in select cases where infectious colitis is ruled out or not suspected, realizing that evidence supporting an autoimmune etiology for non-specific colitis in dogs and cats is minimal. There is no consensus as to the most efficacious immunomodulator, and each has its own side effect profile. Prednisolone is commonly used in cats, particularly in cases where low-grade T-cell GI lymphoma is a top differential. Mycophenolate is not ideal for dogs with chronic large bowel signs, as bloody diarrhea is a very common side effect. Sulfasalazine is cleaved to its active ingredients by colonic bacteria and so may have targeted anti-inflammatory actions in the distal gut. However, no pharmacokinetic or efficacy studies have been published in dogs or cats. Also, as a sulfa-analogue, sulfasalazine, and mesalamine may have side effects including keratoconjunctivitis sicca, hepatotoxicity, blood dyscrasias, and others. Before initiating immunosuppressive therapies, a conversation should be broached with the client about the potential to precipitate an underlying infection, particularly in regions with high prevalences of *Histoplasma* spp., *Prototheca* spp., and other furtive agents.

Management of Constipation

For cases of constipation not responsive to improved hydration and supplemental dietary fiber, motility modifiers can be initiated. Cisapride is a 5-HT4 receptor agonist that may be helpful in cats with chronic constipation and possibly megacolon. It must be compounded, and several drug interactions are possible (particularly with commonly used drugs in feline medicine such as mirtazapine, buprenorphine, fluconazole, and furosemide). Cisapride is generally well tolerated by cats but vomiting and diarrhea are possible.

INFECTIOUS DISEASES OF THE LARGE INTESTINE

Infectious diseases of the large intestine in dogs and cats present broadly across signalments and are influenced by lifestyle factors (vaccination history, diet, interactions with other species) and geography. Additionally, increasing evidence has linked the presence of certain infectious diseases to host genetics and immune response. Infectious diseases should always be of consideration even in classically non-endemic areas due to increasing pet travel, climate change, and vector expansion.

BACTERIAL

The large intestine and rectum are home to a multitude of bacteria whose role as nonpathogenic commensals versus contributors or elicitors of gastrointestinal disease remains a topic of expanding study and debate. In general, primary bacterial colitis is considered very rare. Potential pathogens include enteropathogenic and enterotoxigenic *Escherichia coli (E. coli), C. difficile, C. perfringens, Campylobacter*, and *Salmonella* spp. However, these bacteria have also been isolated from the feces of clinically healthy dogs and cats at similar rates as in patients with clinical signs. Significant correlation has also been made between the fecal detection of *Salmonella* spp. and the feeding of raw meat or raw pet food diets versus cooked commercial diets (Davies et al. 2019). This implies human influence on the prevalence of enteric disease in companion animals.

Antibiotics such as amoxicillin-clavulanic acid, tylosin, and metronidazole are frequently used in the empiric treatment of diarrhea in dogs and cats. Increasing evidence has associated this with the disruption of the enteric microbiome, promotion of resistant enteropathogenic bacteria and "shedder status," and a minimal beneficial effect on patient clinical outcome (Scahill et al. 2024). Antibiotics should be reserved for patients with signs of true bacterial infection, e.g., development of systemic inflammatory response syndrome, evidence of invasive bacteria in GI biopsy specimens, or in symptomatic patients that have exhausted other therapeutic trials.

E. coli-Associated Granulomatous Colitis

Unlike most chronic large bowel diseases affecting dogs and cats, bacteria have been implicated in the pathogenesis of ECGC (Simpson et al. 2006). Formerly known as Boxer or histiocytic ulcerative colitis, this condition almost exclusively affects dogs less than four years of age. The disease is overrepresented in French bulldogs and Boxers but can affect any dog breed. Rare case reports exist in feline patients. Pathogenesis appears to involve a defect in macrophage killing, allowing so-called "commensal" bacteria to adhere to, invade, and ultimately persist within macrophages of the colonic or ileal mucosa. History typically involves severe and lifelong large bowel diarrhea with hematochezia and tenesmus that is refractory to usual interventions. Patients may also display weight loss, anemia, and even mild hypoalbuminemia. Ultrasound may show a thickened colonic wall (Figure 42.2b) and abdominal lymphadenomegaly, which may raise concern for neoplasia. Granulomatous inflammation may be present on rectal scrape cytology (Figure 42.4a,b). Definitive diagnosis requires colonic and/or ileal biopsy (typically obtained via colonoscopy) and histopathological examination. Ulcerative lesions may be visible during colonoscopy but are not always present. Tissue biopsies, collected in as aseptic a manner as possible, should be saved for aerobic bacterial culture. Histopathologic findings include mixed inflammation involving macrophages and neutrophils along with lymphocytes and plasma cells. Cytoplasmic material in macrophages almost invariably stains positively with PAS. To confirm diagnosis of ECGC, slides made from formalin-fixed paraffin-embedded tissues should be submitted for eubacterial and *E. coli* fluorescence *in situ* hybridization (FISH) at a reputable laboratory (Figure 42.4c,d). Colonic biopsies should be submitted for *E. coli* bacterial culture; the lab should grind the biopsies in a sterile manner and perform antimicrobial susceptibility testing on representative colonies/isolates (more than 1 strain may be isolated). These results guide treatment; multidrug resistant (MDR) *E. coli* are commonly isolated from affected patients (Manchester et al. 2021). Once the diagnosis has been confirmed (PAS-positive granulomatous inflammation of colonic or ileal

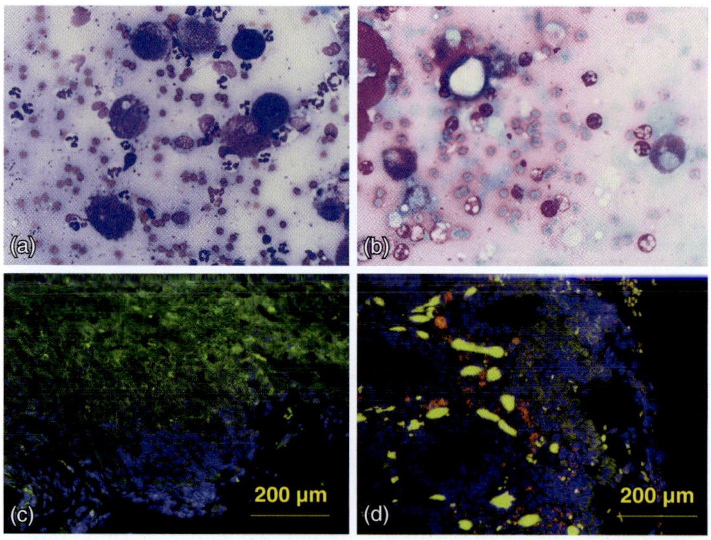

FIGURE 42.4 Photomicrographs of samples from dogs with *E. coli*-associated granulomatous colitis. (a) Hematoxylin and eosin stained cytologic preparation of a rectal scraping from a dog with *E. coli*-associated granulomatous colitis. Mixed inflammation dominated by neutrophils and macrophages with scattered erythrocytes and bacteria in the background. (b) Periodic acid-Schiff (PAS) stained slide of sample from the same patient. Note the strongly PAS-positive cytoplasm of neutrophils and larger, more variably PAS-positive macrophages. (c) Fluorescence *in situ* hybridization (FISH) analysis of colonic biopsies from a young Boxer dog with chronic diarrhea. No intracellular bacteria are present. (d) FISH analysis of colonic biopsies from another young boxer with ECGC; intracellular bacteria (red) hybridized with *E. coli* probe. Nuclei (blue) are stained with 4'6-diamidino-2-phenylindole. *Source*: With permission of Kenneth W. Simpson

biopsies, intracellular *E. coli* visualized with FISH, *E. coli* isolated from biopsies), an antibiotic with known ability to accumulate intracellularly (e.g., fluoroquinolone, tetracycline, chloramphenicol) is prescribed. Empiric treatment prior to confirming the diagnosis is not recommended, as treatment failures (which may result in euthanasia) have been associated with prior antimicrobial exposures. For patients with MDR *E. coli*, carbapenems (e.g., meropenem) may be the only option. Antibiotics should be given for at least 6–8 weeks, though clinical signs tend to resolve within the first week of therapy. The rationale is to eradicate intramucosal bacteria while allowing for recovery of disrupted intestinal mucosa. Repeat colonic biopsy is necessary to confirm successful treatment, realizing that mucosal inflammation tends to persist long beyond eradication of intramucosal *E. coli* (biopsies are FISH negative). Relapses are possible, which could indicate drug-resistant bacteria or an innate immune or GI epithelial healing defect, or a non-ECGC etiology. Adjunctive roles for diet, fiber, probiotics, and FMT have not been studied in ECGC patients. It is strongly advised to avoid immunosuppression, which could further impair clearance of mucosal bacteria. Prognosis is excellent for dogs that achieve remission with antimicrobials. For dogs with rapid relapses after cessation of antimicrobials, and for those with MDR *E. coli*, the prognosis is more guarded.

FUNGAL AND OOMYCETAL

Histoplasma capsulatum

Histoplasma capsulatum is a dimorphic, soil-borne fungus with worldwide distribution, particularly in warm and moist environments contaminated with bird and bat guano. Infection typically occurs via inhalation of aerosolized *H. capsulatum* microconidia that disseminate as yeasts via the reticuloendothelial system. Cats appear to be as susceptible to histoplasmosis as dogs; however, presentation may be more vague, involving the skin, respiratory system, and bone marrow. In dogs, lymphadenopathy, pyrexia, and mixed bowel gastrointestinal signs are most typical. The colon is a predilection site for *H. capsulatum* in dogs, with 84% displaying circumferential colonic thickening with abnormal wall layering on ultrasonography (Chávez-Peón Berle et al. 2021; Wilson et al. 2018). Diagnosis of histoplasmosis if confirmed with positive antigen immunoassays (urine and serum), fungal culture and/or direct visualization of organisms via cytology or histopathology. *Histoplasma* spp. yeasts can frequently be detected via rectal scrape cytology. Treatment involves long courses of oral azole antifungal drugs (minimum six months) and supportive care, including antiemetics, appetite stimulants, and tailored nutrition. Prognosis is dependent on dissemination of disease and clinical severity. Some reported negative prognostic factors in dogs are the presence of anemia, thrombocytopenia, hypercalcemia, hyperbilirubinemia, dyspnea, and palpable organomegaly (Wilson et al. 2018).

Pythium insidiosum

Pythium insidiosum (P. insidiosum) is an oomycete part of the phylogenetic lineage of aquatic fungus-like microorganisms, often referred to as "water molds." *P. insidiosum* presents distinctly as either a cutaneous or gastrointestinal form based on the site of encystation. Infection in cats is infrequent. Gastrointestinal infection occurs following ingestion of contaminated standing freshwater and the penetration of motile zoospores across the GI mucosa. Pythiosis is common in young, large-breed dogs in tropical and subtropical climates; however, geographic distribution is expanding. Dogs invariably present with progressive CE signs dominated by marked weight loss. Gastrointestinal masses may be noted on palpation or imaging. Masses demonstrate severe, transmural thickening often spanning across discrete regions of the GI tract, e.g., gastroduodenal, ileocolic. Cytology is consistent with pyogranulomatous/granulomatous or eosinophilic inflammation, which prompts the consideration of *P. insidiosum* as a differential in the work-up of intestinal masses of this interpretation. Identification of *P. insidiosum* hyphae is challenging with routine hematoxylin and eosin (HE) staining. Gomori methenamine silver (GMS) stain is recommended to visualize the characteristic nonparallel, rarely septate walls of *P. insidiosum*. Failure to visualize organisms in a clinically suspicious case does not rule out infection. Serologic assays hold high sensitivity and specificity for detection of *P. insidiosum* and are a core part of reaching a diagnosis. Treatment of choice is aggressive and wide (5 cm) surgical resection of affected regions. However, with frequent late diagnosis of disease and inoperable lesions, surgery may not be feasible, leading to a guarded prognosis. Traditional antifungal drugs alone are ineffective due to oomycetes lacking cell membrane ergosterol. Recent protocols have incorporated combinations of medications for synergistic drug effects. Anti-inflammatory doses of prednisone, mefenoxam (an agricultural anti-oomycotic), terbinafine, and itraconazole have been correlated with achievement of seronegativity and approximately 50% survivability rate (Cridge et al. 2010; Billings et al. 2023).

Entomophthoramycosis

Basidiobolus spp. are saprophytic fungi commonly found in the soil and decaying plant matter of tropical or subtropical regions worldwide. Infection is presumed to be via inhalation or ingestion of fungal spores. Basidiobolomycosis is considered an extremely rare form of disseminated or focal GI disease in dogs and cats. Histologically, hyphae have a wide, eosinophilic sleeve that can be easily identified on HE staining. Diagnosis can be further confirmed by DNA amplification and sequencing of affected tissue. Treatment is extrapolated from human guidelines of wide-margin surgical resection of lesions and long-term (minimum six months) oral azole administration.

PROTOZOAL AND ALGAL

Trichomonosis

Tritrichomonas blagburni (T. blagburni), also known as *Tritrichomonas foetus*, is a flagellate protozoan that is an important cause of chronic, and frequently intractable, large bowel diarrhea in cats. Infection is more prevalent in young, purebred cats; however, any breed can be affected. Subclinical infections are common in cats living in crowded environments, e.g., shelters and catteries. Dogs are not considered a natural host for *T. blagburni.* In its infectious form, *T. blagburni* trophozoites have three anterior flagella, a posteriorly directed flagellum and move in a rapid, forward-rolling motion. This is distinct to *Giardia* trophozoites, which have eight flagella arranged in four pairs and move in a characteristic "falling leaf" motion. Transmission is presumably via the orofecal route, but *T. blagburni* can also survive in contaminated water, feed, excrement, and cat litter (Rosypal et al. 2012). Following infection, *T. blagburni* predominantly colonizes the mucosa or crypt lumens of the distal ileum and colon. Infection manifests clinically as hematochezia, fecal incontinence, and tenesmus, with occasional rectal prolapse. Cats usually present in good body condition, but weight loss can be noted with other co-infections and comorbidities.

Diagnosis of *T. blagburni* is often challenging due to absent clinicopathologic and imaging abnormalities, intermittent fecal shedding, and the varying sensitivities of detection methods available. Trichomonads cannot be detected with fecal flotation methods but can be identified on direct wet mount cytology with Diff-Quick stain under high-dry (40–50× objective) or oil immersion microscopy. Sensitivity of direct wet-mount cytology can be improved by pooling multiple fresh fecal samples or obtaining feces from the proximal colon via colonic flush or fecal collection loop technique. Culture is performed using a commercially available pouch system (InPouch TF, BioMed Diagnostics, White City, OR, USA). The pouch is incubated upright at room temperature or in a 37 °C/98.6 °F incubator, and wet-mount cytology performed daily. Growth is identified within hours or may require extended incubation periods of up to 12 days. Fecal PCR is considered the gold standard for detecting both viable and nonviable organisms. For all microbiologic testing, feces should be diarrheic, free of cat litter, and obtained from cats that have not received any class of antimicrobials within 1–2 weeks of testing.

Ronidazole at 30 mg/kg PO q24 hours for 14 days is the most effective treatment currently available, with approximately 60% of cats having improvement or resolution of clinical signs (Gookin et al. 2017). Reversible neurotoxicity is a common side effect, and treatment should be discontinued immediately in these cases. The cat can then be retested, however, by the time toxicity presents, many cats have received sufficient ronidazole to eradicate infection. If signs relapse following treatment, repeat PCR and another round of ronidazole treatment may be considered. Due to ronidazole's side effects and teratogenic potential to humans, many owners decline treatment. Left untreated, diarrhea will spontaneously resolve in 88% of cats within two years. However, these cats frequently remain PCR positive, are potential sources of infection to other cats, and may relapse six or more years after achieving "remission" (Gookin et al. 2017; Foster et al. 2004). Ronidazole may be difficult to obtain, in which case treatment with tinidazole (30 mg/kg PO q24 hours for 14 days) may be considered for symptomatic cats; side effects would be like those possible with ronidazole and metronidazole. Owner consent should be obtained prior to prescribing given the off-label nature of this prescription.

Gastrointestinal Amebiasis and Balantidiasis

Amoeba belonging to the genus *Entamoeba* and the ciliate protozoan *Balantioides coli* are very rare causes of colonic disease in dogs and cats. *Entamoeba histolytica* (*E. histolytica*) is an important cause of potentially fatal dysentery and extraintestinal abscessation, in humans and nonhuman primates worldwide. However, infection is most common in tropical and subtropical climates occurring via exposure to fecal contaminated water sources and poor sanitation. Detection of *E. histolytica* has been described in fecal smears of healthy dogs and cats; however, only isolated case reports have associated it with severe colitis (Marcondes et al. 2021). High-dose metronidazole at 30 mg/kg PO q12 hours for 3 weeks is the treatment of choice. *B. coli* is found in the cecum and colon of domestic pigs worldwide, which are the natural hosts. Infection has been reported rarely in dogs to cause hematochezia and tenesmus; co-infection with *Trichuris vulpis (T. vulpis)* has been described. Treatment of *T. vulpis* infection can eradicate signs, or the use of tetracyclines and metronidazole as is for humans (Marcondes et al. 2021).

Prototheca spp.

Prototheca spp. are unicellular, achlorophyllous microalgae with worldwide distribution. They are most isolated from stagnant water systems with high organic matter content, e.g., sewage, cattle farmland, and peatlands. *Prototheca* spp. commonly cause bovine mastitis, but in dogs and rarely in cats, protothecosis typically manifests in cutaneous and systemic (disseminated) forms. Disseminated disease is presumed to occur from the initial cutaneous inoculation or following the direct ingestion of algae and their colonization of the GI tract. Systemic disease has not been reported in cats and is uncommon in dogs however, Boxers and Collies appear to be overrepresented. Causative agents of systemic protothecosis in dogs are *Prototheca bovis* (accounting for 75% of cases), *Prototheca ciferri, Prototheca wickerhamii,* and *Prototheca zopfii* (Proskurnicka et al. 2025). Dogs primarily present with chronic large bowel diarrhea. Progressive disease may include blindness from chorioretinitis and/or retinal detachment and neurological signs. Bloodwork and imaging findings are frequently unremarkable, however, colonic wall thickening with loss of layering and local lymphadenopathy may be seen on ultrasound. Diagnosis can be made via cytologic visualization of *Prototheca* organisms from rectal scrapings, fine-needle aspirates of lesions, cerebrospinal fluid, aqueous humor, and urine sediment. As organisms have a thick, hyaline cell wall only partially stained by HE, the use of GMS, Giemsa, and PAS stains is helpful for highlighting organisms amid a busy inflammatory background (Figure 42.5). *Prototheca* spp. can also be rapidly cultured on standard media from body fluids (urine, blood, cerebrospinal fluid), forming yeast-like colonies. Systemic protothecosis holds a guarded prognosis, and infection is never considered eradicated despite prolonged treatment; amphotericin B can be used to induce remission in some cases. Mainstay therapies include parenteral amphotericin B and lifelong oral azoles (posaconazole). While chitin is present in the cell wall of some algae and potentially *Prototheca* spp. the efficacy of chitin synthetase inhibitor lufenuron (5 mg/kg PO q24 hours) is unknown. Resolution of GI signs does not guarantee treatment success, as the organisms may be diminished in the gut but already spread to other parts of the body.

VIRAL

Feline Coronavirus

Classification of feline coronaviruses is by pathotype into feline enteric coronavirus (FECV) and feline infectious peritonitis (FIP). FECV is ubiquitous in cats worldwide, except the Falkland Islands, and is a possible cause of transient diarrhea due to tropism primarily for colonic epithelial cells. However, as FECV can also be shed in the feces of clinically healthy cats, its role as an agent in feline chronic diarrhea has not been fully elucidated. FIP is caused by mutation

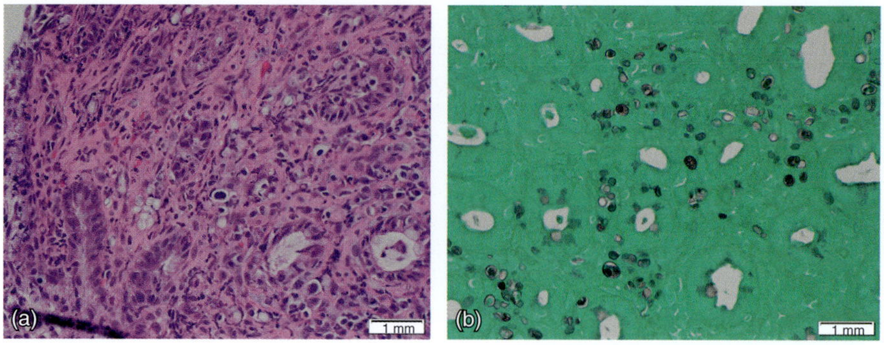

FIGURE 42.5 Photomicrographs of endoscopically obtained colonic biopsy samples from a 3-year-old neutered male shepherd mix with chronic progressive large bowel diarrhea. (a) Hematoxylin and eosin-stained colonic biopsy section showing severe proprial infiltration with eosinophils, plasma cells, and neutrophils as well as lymphocytes and macrophages. (b) Gomori methenamine silver-stained colonic biopsy section showing large numbers of *Prototheca* organisms (rounded, oblong, or indented structures with a thin wall and occasionally containing 2–4 endospore-like bodies)

of FECV and leads to multisystemic disease typically categorized into effusive and non-effusive forms. During FIP infection, infiltrative lesions can be identified in the ileum and colon, with sentinel lymphadenopathy, as these sites represent areas of persistent viral replication. Gold standard diagnosis of FIP is via immunofluorescent labeling of feline coronavirus antigen in tissue or fluid samples. Clinical suspicion may be increased with the presence of cavitary effusions, mesenteric lymphadenopathy, and notable lymphopenia, hyperglobulinemia, and hyperbilirubinemia. Neurological signs may also be present. Signalment factors of youth and purebred status (Bengal, Ragdoll, British Shorthair) should also be considered; however, FIP can affect any cat. Successful treatment of FIP has been demonstrated with antivirals, e.g., GS-441524, remdesivir, and molnupiravir, giving an excellent prognosis.

HELMINTH

Heterobilharzia americana

Heterobilharzia americana (H. americana), also known as canine schistosomiasis, is a trematode parasite that primarily affects dogs living in the southern United States. *H. americana* requires fresh water for transmission and is therefore maintained in wildlife reservoirs by raccoons excreting *H. americana* eggs into water. Under water, the eggs develop into a miracidium that infects a gastropod (snail) first intermediate host, followed by the emergence of motile cercaria that penetrate the skin of mammalian definitive hosts. Cercariae migrate to the mesenteric veins and develop into adults, shedding eggs into the gut lumen.

Common clinical signs are hematochezia, hyporexia to anorexia, and weight loss; affected dogs consistently have an outdoor lifestyle with exposure to freshwater sources. Dissemination of eggs via the portal circulation results in a severe granulomatous inflammatory response in the gut wall and possibly distant organs, e.g., liver, spleen, pancreas, and lungs. Hyperglobulinemia is frequently reported alongside hypercalcemia, presumed secondary to granulomatous inflammation. Gold standard diagnosis is via specific fecal PCR for *H. americana;* however, alternative methods are fecal sedimentation for detection of eggs, tissue biopsy, and fecal antigen enzyme-linked immunosorbent assay. No anthelmintics are approved for treatment, but praziquantel (high dose: 25 mg/kg PO q8 hours for 2 days; low dose: 5 mg/kg PO q8 hours for 2 days) and fenbendazole (high dose: 2 sequence regime 50 mg/kg PO q24 hours for 10 days, repeated 3 weeks later; low dose: 24 mg/kg PO q24 hours for 7 days) have been successfully used individually, sequentially, or in combination (Cridge et al. 2021). There is currently no evidence for the use of glucocorticoids alongside anthelmintic therapy. However, glucocorticoids may be indicated in the event of an anaphylactoid reaction occurring during the elimination of the parasite burden induced by the aforementioned treatments. Prognosis is guarded with disseminated infection.

Feline Strongyloidiasis

Strongyloidiasis is an uncommon infection affecting cats mainly in tropical and subtropical regions. The life cycle and infective species of Strongyloidiasis in cats remain elusive; strains and subspecies of *Strongyloides stercoralis* (which primarily infects dogs) are purported. Infections are also likely underreported due to most being asymptomatic; however, female adult worms can be found in nodules within the colonic submucosa, causing chronic large intestinal diarrhea. Diagnosis is challenging due to intermittent and low fecal egg shedding. Therefore, serial fecal sample collection for Baermann testing is recommended. Little is known about effective treatments in cats; however, ivermectin (0.2 mg/kg PO once) and thiabendazole (25 mg/kg PO q12 hours for 2 days) have been used to give an excellent prognosis. Fenbendazole, pyrantel embonate, and pyrantel pamoate are not effective.

Whipworms

Trichuris vulpis infection is a common cause of large bowel diarrhea in dogs of all ages. It is of much lower prevalence in cats where *T. felis* is implicated. The name *Trichuris* can be translated from Greek to mean "hair-tail," representing the anterior thin filamentous portion of the worm body and thick posterior end that give a whip-like appearance. Infection occurs via ingestion of an egg containing an infective first-stage larva. Early larval stages occur in the proximal small intestine before migration to the cecum or colon for final maturation into adult worms. During this final process, adult worms burrow into the large intestinal mucosa with the posterior body end progressively protruding into the intestinal lumen. In many cases, *T. vulpis* infection is of low pathogenicity with dogs being asymptomatic. However, the most common clinical symptoms are intermittent large bowel diarrhea and, in heavier burdens, dehydration, vomiting, and anorexia. Concurrent anemia, eosinophilia, and hypoproteinemia are suggestive of infection and are most likely in pediatric patients with high worm burdens. *T. vulpis* infection has also been associated with pseudo-hypoadrenocorticism (hyponatremia, hyperkalemia), but this can be differentiated from typical hypoadrenocorticism by a normal adrenocorticotrophic hormone stimulation test.

Diagnosis is easily made on fecal flotation with centrifugation, where eggs are identified as a distinct yellow-brown oval shape with two polar plugs. However, due to intermittent egg shedding and a long prepatent period (74–90 days), not visualizing eggs does not preclude infection. Eggs are frequently not observed in puppies up to three months of age. In these instances, a commercial fecal antigen test (IDEXX Laboratories, Inc., Westbrook, ME, USA) is available, which is also able to differentiate between true infection and eggs in feces from coprophagy. Treatment with fenbendazole (50 mg/kg PO q24 hours for 3 days), milbemycin (0.5 mg/kg PO once), moxidectin (2.5 mg/kg topical once), or febantel (25 mg/kg PO once) has all been shown to effectively kill whipworms. Treatment should be repeated monthly for three months, as few anthelmintics are successful against larval immature stages, and reinfection is common. Prognosis is excellent. Control of *T. vulpis* is achieved with prophylactic monthly broad-spectrum anthelmintics in endemic regions, the prompt treatment of infected animals, and the removal of feces from the environment.

STRUCTURAL DISEASES OF THE LARGE INTESTINE

Beyond the congenital colorectal anatomical abnormalities, other anomalies can be acquired issues. Rectal prolapse is most reported in animals less than four months of age with a condition that results in straining; Boston terriers and Manx cats are particularly affected. Precipitating factors include intestinal parasitism, diarrhea of other causes, constipation, or, less likely, a difficult to pass foreign body or colonic or rectal tumor. It is readily diagnosed with visual inspection of the perineum. Management involves topical treatments to the protruding mucosa to allow for replacement as well as identification and treatment of the root cause of diarrhea. Sedation and analgesia may be needed to replace the prolapse. For recurrent cases, a temporary purse-string suture may be placed; it must leave an orifice large enough to pass feces and be removed once the prolapse has resolved. Ensuring adequate hydration and a softer stool consistency is critical to prevent obstipation.

Narrowing of the distal intestinal lumen may result in rectal and anorectal strictures. These may be diagnosed during DRE or require contrast radiography or colonoscopy. Etiologies include extraluminal compression, for example, by a nearby tumor, enlarged prostate, or scarring after an anal sac abscess. Intraluminal causes such as chronic inflammation or tissue damage from a foreign body or trauma may also result in structuring. Colonic strictures have been reported in dogs with ECGC. Treatment involves general anesthesia for digital bougienage or balloon dilation of the stricture. The benefit of injecting corticosteroids (e.g., triamcinolone) into the scar tissue is unknown but often completed.

Colorectal adenomatous polyps are infrequent, benign problems of dogs and cats. Patients commonly present with straining and hematochezia, often in the absence of diarrhea. West Highland White Terriers in France and Japanese miniature Dachshunds are overrepresented in studies of this condition. Polyps are usually palpable during DRE or may even prolapse through the anus. Both surgical excision and endoscopic resection are therapeutic options. For patients with recurrent polyp growth (reported in miniature Dachshunds), cyclosporine may be helpful in preventing recurrence. Given the possibility for malignant tumors (adenocarcinomas) to have a polypoid appearance, tissue should be submitted for histopathological analysis whenever possible.

Megacolon is a diagnosis given when the large intestine becomes dilated, flaccid, and atonic. This condition occurs much more commonly in cats than dogs. Although it is most often considered idiopathic, a few specific etiologies should be investigated for and treated if found. Underlying causes include mechanical obstruction (e.g., healed pelvic fractures) or, less likely, tumors, strictures, and perineal hernias. In the absence of structural problems, a functional etiology is prioritized. Megacolon can thus be a consequence of chronic constipation. Affected cats are usually middle-aged adults. Factors such as living in a multi-cat household or being indoor-outdoor may reduce client awareness of abnormal defecation habits, allowing the problem to progress without intervention. Unfortunately, many cats present in crisis – dehydrated, anorexic, painful, and obstipated. Physical exam reveals a full, firm cylindrical viscus in the mid-abdomen. Basic blood work is needed to rule out metabolic and endocrine contributors to ileus (e.g., hypocalcemia, hypomagnesemia, hypothyroidism). Radiographs enable confirmation of a large colon and a general assessment of bony structures; however, abdominal computed tomography (CT) enables 3D imaging of the pelvis. Management of megacolon in the acute setting involves manual evacuation of the colon (de-obstipation), often accomplished under general anesthesia, and rehydration. Subsequently, preventative measures can be prescribed to soften the feces, ensure easy access to one or multiple litter boxes, with consideration of cisapride for prokinetic support. Subtotal colectomy is a salvage procedure that is associated with complications.

NEOPLASIA OF THE LARGE INTESTINE

The overall prevalence of neoplasms of the large intestine and rectum of dogs and cats is low (Willard 2012; Vail et al. 2020). The incidence of neoplasia increases with age, and, with the exception of retroviral involvement in the development of GI lymphoma in young cats, the median age is 12.5 years in cats and between 6 and 9 years in dogs (Vail et al. 2020). Siamese cats and large-breed dogs are overrepresented in the development of intestinal neoplasia but any breed can be affected (Rissetto et al. 2011). A slight sex predilection may also exist in males.

Epithelial, mesenchymal, neuroendocrine, and round cell neoplasms can all be found in the large intestine and rectum. Adenocarcinoma represents the most common malignant large intestinal neoplasm in both species but predominantly occurs in dogs, affecting the colon and rectum (Fiedorowicz et al. 2025; Adamovich-Rippe et al. 2017). Collie breeds and German Shepherd dogs are overrepresented for adenocarcinoma. Lymphoma is the second most common large intestinal neoplasm but more frequently occurs in the stomach and small intestine. Other malignant tumors include leiomyosarcomas, gastrointestinal stromal tumors (GISTs), mast cell tumors, and neuroendocrine tumors. Leiomyosarcomas and GISTs typically originate in the cecum. Neuroendocrine tumors arise from the diffuse intestinal endocrine system as opposed to the intestinal epithelium itself. Neuroendocrine cells are also known as enterochromaffin cells. These differentiated enterocytes contain secretory granules containing GI hormones such as somatostatin, serotonin, secretin, and gastrin.

Benign neoplasms include polyps, adenomas, and leiomyomas, which typically are solitary masses but can present as multiple or diffuse lesions (Adamovich-Rippe et al. 2017). Miniature

Dachshunds, West Highland White Terriers, and French Bulldogs appear to have a predisposition for colorectal adenomatous polyps (Fiedorowicz et al. 2025).

PRESENTATION

Most patients have an extended course of disease over weeks to months; however, acute presentation is possible. Clinical signs correlate with lesion location, metastasis to other organs, and presence of paraneoplastic syndromes. Reported paraneoplastic syndromes with colorectal tumors include erythrocytosis, hyperglobulinemia, eosinophilia, neutrophilia, and hypoglycemia due to IGF secretion from smooth muscle tumors (Vail et al. 2020).

Common complaints associated with large bowel neoplasia are hematochezia, tenesmus, and obstruction causing constipation, obstipation, or diarrhea. In severe cases, intestinal perforation and sepsis can occur, presenting as pyrexia, collapse, lethargy, vomiting, and abdominal pain.

DIAGNOSIS

Physical examination may reveal an abdominal mass on palpation or a mass on DRE. The importance of DRE in dogs presenting with chronic large bowel signs cannot be overemphasized. In many cases, biochemical abnormalities are absent. However, observed abnormalities can be anemia secondary to gastrointestinal bleeding, leukocytosis with left shift and monocytosis, ionized hypercalcemia with lymphoma, hypoglycemia with GISTs, and elevated liver enzymes (specifically alkaline phosphatase) in non-lymphomatous neoplasia (Vail et al. 2020). Cats should be tested for feline leukemia virus and feline immunodeficiency virus. Abdominal ultrasonography is the most valuable modality to evaluate intestinal architecture. Typical changes are focal intestinal wall thickening, complete loss of wall layering, or an overt mass effect (Figure 42.4). Loss of wall layering is found in 99% of dogs with intestinal neoplasia compared to the preservation of wall layering in 88% of dogs with nonneoplastic disease (Vail et al. 2020). In cats, intestinal wall thickening can be a common feature of enteropathy, both benign and malignant, and should therefore be interpreted cautiously. Other differentials that can present as large intestinal mass lesions are fungal granulomas, gastrointestinal eosinophilic sclerosing fibroplasia (GESF) in cats (Figure 42.4d), and lipogranulomatous lymphangitis in dogs, with the latter two commonly affecting the ileocolic junction (Černá et al. 2024).

Distal GI tumors may metastasize to the mesenteric lymph nodes (adenocarcinoma), liver (leiomyosarcoma and carcinoids), mesentery, omentum, spleen, kidney, bone, peritoneum, and lung. Additional imaging techniques, e.g., radiography or cross-sectional imaging using CT or magnetic resonance imaging, are extremely helpful in staging.

Definitive diagnosis is based on surgically or endoscopically obtained biopsy of the lesion for histopathology. Ultrasound-guided cytology of the intestinal wall is reported to yield a diagnosis in 58% of cases (Henry et al. 2024).

TREATMENT AND PROGNOSIS

Treatment is based on tumor type, tumor size, tumor resectability and margin attainment, and the presence of metastasis. Apart from lymphoma, complete surgical resection is considered the primary treatment (Gieger 2011). Surgery in lymphoma cases can be indicated to relieve an obstructive mass. During gross tissue biopsy, inclusion of adjacent healthy tissue is required to ensure adequate margins. Additionally, fresh tissue should be preserved for culture in case an infectious etiology (e.g., histoplasmosis, pythiosis) is suspected following histopathology. In cases requiring resection of the ileo-colic junction, many patients have lifelong diarrhea and may require cobalamin supplementation. In patients without evidence of overt local or distant metastasis, long-term survival is possible; however, recurrence despite this due to micrometastasis should not be overlooked. Adjuvant chemotherapy is typically doxorubicin, but no evidence exists evaluating the benefit or not of adjuvant chemotherapy in veterinary medicine. Radiation therapy is rarely used due to the constant movement of the intestines and concern for toxic dosing to surrounding tissue and viscera.

Prognosis is excellent following resection of polyps, adenomas, and leiomyomas but guarded to poor with malignant neoplasms.

REFERENCES

Adamovich-Rippe, K.N., Mayhew, P.D., Marks, S.L. et al. (2017). Colonoscopic and histologic features of rectal masses in dogs: 82 cases (1995–2012). *Journal of the American Veterinary Medical Association* 250: 424–430.

Allenspach, K.A., Mochel, J.P., Du, Y. et al. (2019). Correlating gastrointestinal histopathologic changes to clinical disease activity in dogs with idiopathic inflammatory bowel disease. *Veterinary Pathology* 56: 435–443.

Andrews, C., Hess, R.S., Drobatz, K. et al. (2024). Abnormalities detected on digital rectal examinations in dogs are common and influence diagnostic and treatment plans. *Journal of the American Veterinary Medical Association* 262: 773–777.

Billings, P., Walton, S., Shmalberg, J. et al. (2023). The use of mefenoxam to treat cutaneous and gastrointestinal pythiosis in dogs: a retrospective study. *Microorganisms* 11: 1726.

Černá, P., Lopez-Jimenez, C., Fukushima, K. et al. (2024). Clinicopathological findings, treatment, and outcome in 60 cats with gastrointestinal eosinophilic sclerosing fibroplasia. *Journal of Veterinary Internal Medicine* 38: 1005–1012.

Charlesworth, T.M., Dunning, M., Scase, T.J. et al. (2013). Colonic vascular ectasia (angiodysplasia) in a juvenile dog. *Journal of Small Animal Practice* 54: 36–39.

Chávez-Peón Berle, E., KuKanich, K., and Biller, D. (2021). Ultrasonographic findings of gastrointestinal histoplasmosis in dogs. *Veterinary Radiology & Ultrasound* 62: 108–115.

Cridge, H., Hughes, S.M., Langston, V.C. et al. (2020). Mefenoxam, itraconazole, and terbinafine combination therapy for management of pythiosis in dogs (six cases). *Journal of the American Animal Hospital Association* 56: 307.

Cridge, H., Lupiano, H., Nipper, J.D. et al. (2021). Efficacy of a low-dose praziquantel and fenbendazole protocol in the treatment of asymptomatic schistosomiasis in dogs. *Journal of Veterinary Internal Medicine* 35: 1368–1375.

Davies, R.H., Lawes, J.R., and Wales, A.D. (2019). Raw diets for dogs and cats: a review, with particular reference to microbiological hazards. *Journal of Small Animal Practice* 60: 329–339.

Fiedorowicz, J., Paździor-Czapula, K., and Otrocka-Domagała, I. (2025). Canine colorectal proliferative lesions: a retrospective study of 217 cases. *BMC Veterinary Research* 21: 145.

Foster, D.M., Gookin, J.L., Poore, M.F. et al. (2004). Outcome of cats with diarrhea and Tritrichomonas foetus infection. *Journal of the American Veterinary Medical Association* 225: 888–892.

Fritsch, D.A., Wernimont, S.M., Jackson, M.I. et al. (2022). A prospective multicenter study of the efficacy of a fiber-supplemented dietary intervention in dogs with chronic large bowel diarrhea. *BMC Veterinary Research* 18: 244.

Gieger, T. (2011). Alimentary lymphoma in cats and dogs. *Veterinary Clinics: Small Animal Practice* 41: 419–432.
Gookin, J.L., Hanrahan, K., and Levy, M.G. (2017). The conundrum of feline Trichomonosis. *Journal of Feline Medicine & Surgery* 19: 261–274.

Henry, P.M.N., Boag, A.M., Dandrieux, J.R.S. et al. (2024). Diagnostic yield of percutaneous, ultrasound-guided, fine needle aspirates of the gastrointestinal wall: a retrospective analysis of 152 samples. *Journal of Small Animal Practice* 65: 749–758.

Manchester, A.C., Dogan, B., Guo, Y. et al. (2021). Escherichia coli-associated granulomatous colitis in dogs treated according to antimicrobial susceptibility profiling. *Journal of Veterinary Internal Medicine* 35: 150–161.

Marcondes, M., Kent, M., Howerth, E.W. et al. (2021). 105–Emerging and miscellaneous protozoal diseases. In: *Greene's Infectious Diseases of the Dog and Cat*, 5e (ed. J.E. Sykes), 1307–1322. Philadelphia: W.B. Saunders.

Martinez-Lopez, L.M., Perez-Gonzalez, A., Washington, E.A. et al. (2021). Hierarchical modelling of immunoglobulin coated bacteria in dogs with chronic enteropathy shows reduction in coating with disease remission but marked inter-individual and treatment-response variability. *PloS One* 16: e0255012.

Moreno, A.A., Parker, V.J., Winston, J.A. et al. (2022). Dietary fiber aids in the management of canine and feline gastrointestinal disease. *Journal of the American Veterinary Medical Association* 260: S33–S45.

Proskurnicka, A., Iskra, M., Wronka, S. et al. (2025). Genotyping and drug susceptibility profiling of Prototheca sp. strains isolated from cases of protothecosis in dogs. *Journal of Veterinary Internal Medicine* 39: e17173.

Rissetto, K., Villamil, J.A., Selting, K.A. et al. (2011). Recent trends in feline intestinal neoplasia: an epidemiologic study of 1,129 cases in the veterinary medical database from 1964 to 2004. *Journal of the American Animal Hospital Association* 47: 28–36.

Rosypal, A.C., Ripley, A., Stockdale Walden, H.D. et al. (2012). Survival of a feline isolate of Tritrichomonas foetus in water, cat urine, cat food and cat litter. *Veterinary Parasitology* 185: 279–281.

Roth, L., Walton, A.M., Leib, M.S. et al. (1990). A grading system for lymphocytic plasmacytic colitis in dogs. *Journal of Veterinary Diagnostic Investigation* 2: 257–262.

Scahill, K., Jessen, L.R., Prior, C. et al. (2024). Efficacy of antimicrobial and nutraceutical treatment for canine acute diarrhoea: a systematic review and meta-analysis for European network for optimization of antimicrobial therapy (ENOVAT) guidelines. *The Veterinary Journal* 303: 106054.

Simpson, K.W., Dogan, B., Rishniw, M. et al. (2006). Adherent and invasive Escherichia coli is associated with granulomatous colitis in boxer dogs. *Infection and Immunity* 74: 4778–4792.

Soontararak, S., Chow, L., Johnson, V. et al. (2019). Humoral immune responses against gut bacteria in dogs with inflammatory bowel disease. *PloS One* 14: e0220522.

Toresson, L., Spillmann, T., Pilla, R. et al. (2023). Clinical effects of faecal microbiota transplantation as adjunctive therapy in dogs with chronic enteropathies-A retrospective case series of 41 dogs. *Veterinary Sciences* 10: 271.

Vail, D.M., Thamm, D.H., and Liptak, J.M. (2020). *Withrow and MacEwen's Small Animal Clinical Oncology*, 6e, 507–523. Edinburgh, New York: Elsevier.

Willard, M.D. (2012). Alimentary neoplasia in geriatric dogs and cats. *Veterinary Clinics: Small Animal Practice* 42: 693–706, vi.

Wilson, A.G., KuKanich, K.S., Hanzlicek, A.S. et al. (2018). Clinical signs, treatment, and prognostic factors for dogs with histoplasmosis. *Journal of the American Veterinary Medical Association* 252: 201–209.

Winston, J., Suchodolski, J., Gaschen, F. et al. (2024). Clinical guidelines for fecal microbiota transplantation in companion animals. *Advances in Small Animal Care* 5: 79–107.

CHAPTER 43 Disorders of the Anus and Perianal Skin

Sarah Long[1] *and Anke Hendricks*[2]

[1] *Bristol Veterinary School, University of Bristol, Langford, Bristol, UK*
[2] *Department of Clinical Sciences & Services, Royal Veterinary College, Hatfield, Hertfordshire, UK*

KEY POINTS

- A detailed dermatological assessment should be performed to establish if lesions are localized to the anal sacs, anus, and/or perianal skin, or if they are associated with more generalized skin disease.
- Microbial overgrowth and infection will be secondary in the majority of cases. They can significantly exacerbate clinical signs, and their presence may mask the underlying pathology and hinder diagnostic investigations. Identifying the underlying disease process is key to the successful management of microbial overgrowth and infection, and without this, signs are highly likely to relapse.
- Non-neoplastic disease is the most common disorder of anal sacs in the dog. However, malignant anal sac neoplasia occurs in both dogs and cats and can typically be differentiated using fine needle aspirate cytology.
- Immobile patients with liquid diarrhea are at risk of developing fecal incontinence-associated dermatitis, an insidious and painful condition.

SECTION 1 APPROACH TO PRESENTING PROBLEMS

Patients with disorders of the anus and perianal skin typically present with self-trauma (licking, scooting, or other self-directed behaviors) or behavior indicative of pain on defecation or sitting, and one or a combination of the following skin lesions:

- Red, inflamed skin (may be observed with or without other lesions).
- Swellings (focal or diffuse, well or poorly defined, symmetrical or asymmetrical).
- Defects in integrity (ulceration, erosion, draining tract), crusting.
- Changes in skin pigmentation.

The possible causes for these presentations are summarized in Table 43.1. Overall, disorders of the anus and perianal skin are much more common in dogs than cats. They may be less evident in the cat visually due to more subtle and secretive behavior in response to discomfort at this site.

Key steps in the diagnostic approach include a thorough history and physical examination, rectal examination, and palpation of the anal sacs. A detailed dermatological assessment should also be performed to establish if lesions are localized to the anal sacs, anus, and/or perianal skin, or if they are part of more generalized skin disease. Some patients may require sedation and/or clipping of hair to aid detailed physical examination. Close clipping should be avoided to prevent disruption or removal of key pathological findings.

Inflammatory skin lesions at this body site are likely to be complicated by secondary microbial overgrowth or infection. Although microbial factors will be secondary in the majority of cases, they can significantly exacerbate clinical signs, and their presence may mask the underlying pathology and hinder diagnostic investigations. Once microbial factors are controlled, the underlying disease process needs to be identified and managed to prevent relapsing overgrowth or infection.

Disorders of the Liver, Exocrine Pancreas, and Gastrointestinal Tract in Dogs and Cats, First Edition. Edited by Harry Cridge et al. Published 2026 by John Wiley & Sons, Inc. Companion Website: www.wiley.com/go/cridge/disorders

Table 43.1 Approach to Perianal and Anal Skin Disorders by Presenting Problem

Presenting behavior		
Licking, scooting, other self-directed behaviors Indicative of pain on defecation or sitting	Assess for perianal erythema, swellings, defects in integrity or crusting, or pigmentary change	
Presenting skin lesion	**Location**	**Causes**
Perianal erythema	Perineal/perianal inflammation without defects of skin integrity	Microbial (yeast, bacterial) overgrowth
		Atopic dermatitis/food allergy
		Fecal incontinence associated dermatitis
		Contact dermatitis
		Intertrigo/frictional or moisture-associated dermatitis
	Anal inflammation	Self-inflicted due to licking, scooting
		Anal sacculitis
Swellings	Perineal/perianal	Any inflammatory or neoplastic nodular or mass lesions originating from skin tissues
		Hepatoid gland hyperplasia and neoplasia
		Hernia
	Anal sac	Impaction
		Anal sacculitis
		Abscess
		Neoplastic anal sac disease
Defects in integrity, crusting	Perineal	Any ulcerative or crusting dermatosis
	Anal/perianal	Anal furunculosis
		Mucocutaneous pyoderma
		Mucocutaneous lupus erythematosus
		Calcinosis cutis
		Erythema multiforme complex
		Rare immune-mediated epidermal & subepidermal blistering dermatoses
Hyperpigmentation	Anal	Lentigines
		Melanoma
		Mucocutaneous pyoderma
		Mucocutaneous lupus erythematosus
	Perianal	Chronic inflammation
Hypopigmentation	Anal	Epitheliotropic lymphoma
		Vitiligo

In breeds with a corkscrew tail and in female dogs, a presentation of perianal self-trauma or discomfort in the absence of perianal or anal abnormalities should prompt examination of the tail or vulva fold.

PERIANAL ERYTHEMA

Perianal erythema is a common and unspecific manifestation of anal and perianal skin disease in dogs and, to a lesser degree, in cats. A thorough history will help the clinician to prioritize the list of differential diagnoses (Table 43.1), as will a careful physical examination to assess for the presence of additional, more diagnostically specific skin lesions such as swellings, defects in integrity, crusting, and pigmentary changes. Assessment for complicating microbial and frictional and moisture-related etiologies is important. Microbial dysbiosis may need to be resolved to reveal the underlying pathology.

SWELLINGS

Swellings in this region can be caused by inflammation, neoplasia, or associated with a perineal hernia. Thorough palpation of the mass and rectal examination is recommended, although this may not be able to differentiate anal sac masses from other types of perianal neoplasia. Investigation of inflammatory versus neoplastic lesions requires either fine needle aspiration for cytology or potentially biopsy for histopathology. Cytology alone may not be relied on to rule out a neoplastic process. The use of ultrasound and computed tomography without cytology or histopathology does not currently have a role in differentiating perianal masses and anal sac disease.

DEFECTS IN INTEGRITY, CRUSTING

Erosion, ulceration, draining tracts, and crusting are likely to be associated with erythema, swellings, or changes in pigmentation. As ulceration is a relatively common clinical sign of anal furunculosis in dogs, these patients should be carefully examined for evidence of diffuse swelling and draining tracts. This needs to be differentiated from ulceration of the mucocutaneous junction without evidence of swelling and deep defects. Crusting typically conceals erosive or ulcerative skin pathology. Draining tracts may be difficult to identify unless the affected skin is cleaned and carefully observed for emerging discharge. Skin infection is frequently a significant complication that will need to be addressed prior to performing further diagnostic investigations and/or formulating a treatment plan.

ABNORMAL PIGMENTATION

Changes in pigmentation frequently reflect inflammation. These may be subtle, however, hyperpigmentation reflecting chronic inflammation may be marked and mask other lesions. Examples of primary pigmentary conditions include lentigines (macular hyperpigmentation) or vitiligo (loss of pigment). A full dermatological examination should be performed as pigmentary changes and/or additional lesions will typically be present at other body sites.

SECTION 2 DISORDERS

MICROBIAL DYSBIOSIS, OVERGROWTH, AND SUPERFICIAL INFECTION

Inflammatory disorders of the perianal skin and anus are frequently accompanied, often exacerbated, and even masked by microbial complications, ranging from dysbiosis to infection, and involving typical skin pathogens (staphylococci and *Malassezia* yeasts) as well as bacteria representative of the fecal microbiota.

Cytology is the most useful diagnostic tool to investigate microbial overgrowth and infection of the skin. The presence of microbes is interpreted in the context of host response and lesion type. Clinical relevance may only become evident after elimination of the microbial complication

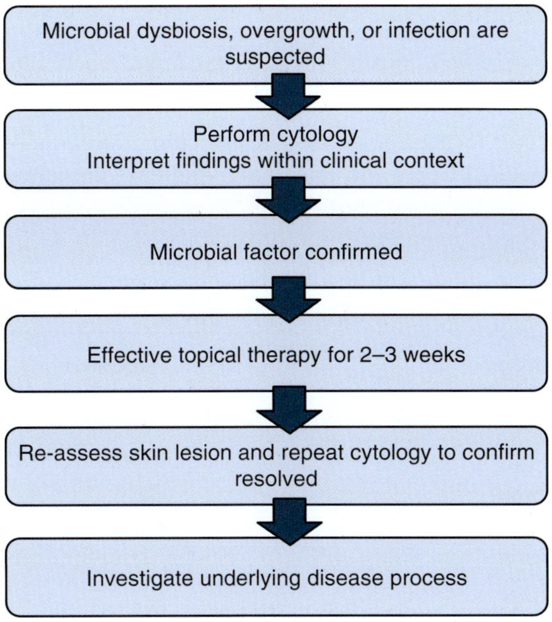

FIGURE 43.1 The approach to investigation and management of microbial dysbiosis, overgrowth, and superficial infection

(Figure 43.1). Bacterial culture is not a suitable test to assess microbial burden and its clinical relevance.

Topical antiseptic or antimicrobial therapy is the treatment of choice for most lesions, although systemic antimicrobial treatment is warranted when deep infection is present. There is a limited evidence base available to help the clinician select from the numerous topical products available and determine an effective treatment protocol. Frequency of application and contact time are important variables, as is suitability for use on ulcerated skin where present. The required duration of treatment will vary depending on numerous factors. However, a reassessment of the microbial status after two weeks is typically appropriate.

Identifying the underlying disease process is key to the successful management of microbial overgrowth and infection, and without this, signs are highly likely to relapse.

UNDERSTANDING TOPICAL ANTIMICROBIAL THERAPY PRINCIPLES

- There is limited in vivo evidence underpinning the use of most products for the variety of indications they may be recommended for (Table 43.2).
- The effectiveness and safety of a product selected for its active ingredient at a particular concentration depends on its formulation, factors related to the affected skin, and frequency and duration of exposure. As these are highly variable, treatment protocols need to be adapted.
- Two products containing the same concentration of an active ingredient may not be equally effective.
- Most topical treatment failures are a result of:
  - Treatment not being received by the patient as intended
  - Insufficient contact time
  - Inappropriate product choice for type of infection
  - Not removing barriers to contact with lesional skin, such as biofilm, exudate, crust, and hair
  - Interference between different elements of skin care

- Detailed carer instruction is essential for success.
- If no response or exacerbation under therapy is observed, consider an adverse contact reaction to the product. Contact dermatitis may be caused by an excipient or an active ingredient.
- When systemic antimicrobial treatment is indicated for a deep infection, adjunct topical treatment to reduce surface microbial burden is recommended to prevent reinfection and environmental contamination.

Table 43.2 Guide to Topical Antimicrobial Therapy Options Based on Skin Lesion Type

Main lesion type	Treatment mode	Commonly available antiseptic agents*	Formulation	Antibacterial/antifungal agents**	Formulation
No or minor breach of epidermis	Sole	Chlorhexidine 3–4% (<4% possibly less effective against *Pseudomonas* spp., *E. coli*)	Shampoo Handwash	Chlorhexidine 2% and miconazole	Shampoo Solution Gel Cream Ointment
				Azole antifungals	Eye/ear topicals
			Leave-on spray	Fusidic acid Mupirocin Polymyxin B Silver sulfadiazine	
			Wipes		
		Hypochlorous acid 0.015–0.02% (frequent application as no residual effect)	Foam		
Sinus tracts, minimal ulceration	Adjunct			Avoid for adjunct treatment	
Erosion or ulceration without swelling or deep defects	Sole	Hypochlorous acid (ClOH/HClO) 0.015–0.02% (frequent application as no residual effect)	Avoid/minimize use of products potentially unsafe for wounds (e.g., detergents)	Chlorhexidine 2% and miconazole Azole antifungals Fusidic acid Mupirocin Polymyxin B Silver sulfadiazine	Avoid/minimize use of products potentially unsafe for wounds (e.g., detergents)
Extensive/deep ulceration or tissue loss	Adjunct			Exceptional judicious use only	

*Antiseptic agents are chemicals applied to skin or mucous membranes to prevent infection and are also useful for treating a broad spectrum of surface and superficial infections. They are typically not regulated as medicines and thus not subject to regulatory efficacy and safety testing requirements.

**Antibacterial and antifungal agents specifically target bacteria or fungi, respectively, and are administered systemically or topically and are typically regulated as medicines.

ALLERGIC SKIN DISEASE

Self-trauma due to pruritus and erythema are the predominant cutaneous manifestations of canine atopic dermatitis and food allergy in dogs and cats. The perianal and perineal skin are relatively frequently affected in canine atopic dermatitis, and although previously believed to be common, perianal and perineal pruritus are reportedly seen in the minority of dogs and cats with food allergy.

Dogs with perianal/perineal pruritus, with or without a macular-papular erythema, should be carefully examined for lesions at other body sites. The periocular skin, muzzle, concave aspect of the pinnae, interdigital skin of the feet, axillae, and groin warrant close inspection.

Feline atopic skin syndrome is varied in its presentation. Clinical signs typically fall into one or a combination of the following reaction patterns: miliary dermatitis, self-inflicted alopecia/hypotrichosis, head and neck pruritus, and eosinophilic granuloma complex. The perianal and perineal skin are not considered typical sites of skin lesions in this species.

INTERTRIGO (FRICTIONAL AND MOISTURE-INDUCED DERMATITIS)

Intertrigo is an inflammatory skin disorder caused by occlusion, maceration, and friction and associated with secondary microbial dysbiosis where two skin surfaces are in close contact with each other. Intertrigo is an occasional complication when conformation, obesity, or perianal hyperplasia result in close apposition of perianal and ventral tail skin and may be exacerbated by fecal contamination. Impression cytology is most helpful in assessing any microbial complications. Management principles are similar to those for incontinence-associated dermatitis.

FECAL INCONTINENCE-ASSOCIATED DERMATITIS

Fecal incontinence-associated dermatitis (FIAD) is a frequent complication in the care of dogs with liquid diarrhea, especially if recumbent. This presentation is less frequently seen in cats. FIAD is a variant of irritant contact dermatitis, which develops when fecal matter remains in prolonged contact with the skin surface. Increased skin permeability, augmented by occlusion at sites of opposing skin and by some skin care practices, inflammation, and high microbial burden through contamination with fecal matter combine to promote microbial dysbiosis and result in breakdown of epidermal integrity, evident as erosions and ulceration. Early signs of FIAD afford an opportunity to prevent progression but are often missed. Moderate to advanced FIAD is extremely painful and typically complicated by infection. Skin care and pain management may require hospitalization long after resolution of the diarrhea.

A structured skin care protocol that minimizes soiling and fecal contact time, cleanses, and restores and protects the skin barrier is recommended for all patients at risk of FIAD, based on guidance for this condition in people. If soiling occurs, immediate cleansing using gentle techniques, avoiding soap, detergents, and abrasive cloths, should be followed by restoration of skin barrier with a light moisturizer and application of a skin protection product. Guidance on suitable products may be taken from published human literature. Where progression to erosion or ulceration has occurred, monitoring for microbial complications by impression cytology is mandatory. Bacterial culture may be indicated to direct treatment when systemic antibiosis is considered in advanced cases or for infection control reasons.

ANAL SAC DISEASE

Anal sacs are pouches lined by squamous epithelium and secretory glands with a duct emerging onto the anal skin, located on either side of the anus. Apocrine glands dominate in the dog, whereas both apocrine and sebaceous glands are present in the cat. Non-neoplastic anal sac disease (NNASD) includes impaction, inflammation, and infection. These pathologies are very common in the dog, uncommon in the cat, and poorly understood in both species. They are of welfare concern due to their frequency, the associated behaviors indicative of discomfort, and the potential for significant disease severity. This is at odds with the relative lack of understanding and published evidence on the diagnostic differentiation, epidemiology, and clinical management.

NNASD presentations are typically considered a continuum of a shared underlying process starting with a disturbance in the normal emptying process of the anal sacs. Based on limited evidence, episodes of diarrhea, diet type, and diet changes were proposed as triggers nearly 50 years ago, and knowledge has not advanced much since.

Anal sac impaction is characterized by distension of the sac containing secretions that may or may not be difficult to express, in the absence of inflammation. Inflammation of the anal sacs, anal sacculitis, may be accompanied by infection and additionally shows inflammation evident as palpable thickening of the anal sac walls or inflammation of the surrounding and overlying tissue as determined by external and rectal palpation. Rupture of the inflamed anal sac leads to abscessation, which may be accompanied by pyrexia and draining tracts with purulent and/or hemorrhagic discharge. Behaviors indicative of discomfort, including self-directed behaviors, pain on sitting or touch, and tenesmus or dyschezia, are indicators of NNASD.

The diagnostic approach rests heavily on physical examination, including rectal palpation. Sedation may be required to allow a meaningful examination and local treatment.

The characteristics of anal sac content are of limited diagnostic value in both species. Hemorrhagic anal sac content may be a distinguishing marker for NNASD, while color, consistency, and smell are not. Equally, the presence of bacteria of varying morphology, yeasts, and inflammatory cells cannot reliably be used to distinguish normal content from pathology. Anal sacculiths may be an incidental finding. Microbial culture studies describe a range of bacterial species, the presence of which overlaps between healthy and abnormal anal sacs. Consequently, a diagnostic approach based on a combination of criteria that include physical examination, anal sac content, and cytology findings, as well as response to sac emptying, is employed.

Therapeutic and preventative recommendations are described but rarely substantiated in the veterinary literature. Recurrence is a frequent problem. Medical management of anal sacculitis involves systemic or topical anti-inflammatory and/or topical antimicrobial drugs typically combined with manual expression or lavage. Recommendations on dosing, duration of treatment, and efficacy remain largely anecdotal. The oral use of nonsteroidal anti-inflammatory drugs concurrent with topical glucocorticoids is discouraged in case of systemic absorption. Sedation or general anesthesia may be necessary to allow anal sac expression, cannulation, and lavage. Anal sac abscesses are treated in line with general management principles.

There is limited information on effective prevention of NNASD recurrence. There is tentative evidence that a fiber-rich probiotic dietary product may reduce the frequency of recurrence of anal sac impaction. Surgical removal of the anal sacs (anal sacculectomy) is generally recommended for recurrence of impaction, chronic sacculitis and abscessation, sinus formation, and failure of medical therapy.

Neoplastic conditions can arise from the squamous epithelium lining of the anal sac wall (squamous cell carcinoma), non-epithelial resident cells (melanoma, mast cell tumor), and the secretory glands (adenoma or adenocarcinoma). A fair number of anal sac tumors are discovered incidentally. A careful palpation of the anal sac region externally and per rectum is essential in patients with signs suggestive of anal sac disease. Fine needle aspiration can typically secure a cytological diagnosis.

NON-NEOPLASTIC ANAL SAC DISEASE IN THE DOG

NNASD is consistently reported as one of the most common disorders affecting dogs under veterinary care. There is evidence that Spaniels and their crosses, Shih Tzu and Bichon Frise breed types, and dogs at least three years old are predisposed to NNASD. Suggestions that obesity is a contributing factor were not substantiated in a large sample of dogs in primary care practice. An association between NNASD and allergic skin disease has been reported in smaller studies on anal sacculitis. The overlapping signs of self-traumatizing behavior and inflammation affecting this body region may result in misattribution of (peri)anal self-trauma to ASD in dogs with allergic perianal pruritus, and perhaps less frequently the other way round. Resolution of clinical signs after emptying of anal sacs seems an obvious marker for NNASD and can help to discriminate NNASD from perianal self-directed behaviors due to other causes.

NEOPLASTIC ANAL SAC DISEASE IN THE DOG

Neoplastic anal sac disease can be considered uncommon in the dog overall, although frequency estimates are not readily available for primary care.

By far the most frequent neoplasm arising from canine anal sacs is the apocrine gland adenocarcinoma (AGASAC), which accounts for approximately 17% of perianal tumors in dogs. AGASAC occurs typically unilaterally at an average age of 11 years and independent of hormonal status. Spaniel breeds are predisposed. AGASAC can present as a circumscribed or infiltrative perianal mass, detectable by rectal palpation or evident as a perianal swelling. The mass effect of the primary tumor and infiltration of sub lumbar lymph nodes may cause constipation and tenesmus. AGASAC is characterized by local invasive growth with rapid metastasis to sacral, iliac, and lumbar lymph nodes in up to 75% of dogs at the time of diagnosis, a high rate of systemic metastasis at later stages, and paraneoplastic hypercalcemia due to tumor production of parathyroid hormone-related peptide in up to half the cases. Polyuria, polydipsia, lethargy, and vomiting attributable to hypercalcemia may therefore be present.

Cytological evaluation of a fine needle aspirate is typically diagnostic, and biopsy is rarely required. Following definitive or presumptive diagnosis, clinical staging is indicated to assess the extent of tumor spread.

Treatment options for AGASAC are palliative care or surgical excision of the primary tumor and regional metastases, followed by adjunctive chemotherapy, treatment with tyrosine kinase inhibitor, or local radiotherapy to prevent recurrence and metastasis. Median survival times differ very markedly depending on a number of tumor-related factors and treatment options and range between approximately eight months and over three years.

Cases of squamous cell carcinoma, mast cell tumor, malignant melanoma, and adenoma arising from the anal sac have been reported but are rare.

NON-NEOPLASTIC ANAL SAC DISEASE IN THE CAT

A small series of cats referred to a surgery service, mostly with a chronic or recurrent course of the disease and after treatment attempts, reported scooting, anal sac fistula, excessive grooming, perianal skin irritation, and pain. Rectal examination typically revealed palpably abnormal anal sacs. There may be overlap of some presenting signs with chronic enteropathy, intestinal parasitism, and allergic skin disease. Thus, when these conditions are suspected, the diagnostic approach should include an assessment of the anal sacs. As in dogs, anal sacculectomy is indicated for chronic, recurrent, or treatment-unresponsive NNASD.

NEOPLASTIC ANAL SAC DISEASE IN THE CAT

Anal sac tumors are considered rare in the cat. Two cases of squamous cell carcinoma arising from the anal sacs have been reported, however, anal sac carcinoma is the main tumor found at this site. Two case series provide some information on feline anal carcinoma. The age of affected cats was between 6 and 20 years. The most common clinical signs were perineal ulceration and discharge, perineal swelling, dyschezia, constipation, hyporexia, and changes in fecal diameter. An ulcerated perianal mass should prompt early consideration of an anal sac tumor. Metastasis to the sub lumbar lymph nodes, lungs, and other organs was recognized. Clinically significant hypercalcemia was not found. Surgical resection with curative intent, with or without adjunctive chemotherapy or radiotherapy, resulted in a median survival time of nine months.

HEPATOID GLAND NEOPLASIA

Hepatoid (perianal or circumanal) glands are modified sebaceous glands that are numerous in the perianal skin in dogs. Neoplasia of these glands is common with recent studies reporting that 3.1–7.9% of canine tumors were of hepatoid gland origin. The majority of hepatoid gland masses are diagnosed as benign hyperplasia/adenomas. Malignancies are less common and include epithelioma, which is locally invasive, and adenocarcinoma, which has a reportedly low rate of metastasis, typically to local lymph nodes.

Hepatoid gland hyperplasia/adenomas are most commonly found in older, entire male dogs as growth is stimulated by androgenic hormones. Castration can lead to a reduction in size or the resolution of benign lesions; however, castration or hormonal therapy is significantly less effective in malignant masses due to the lower expression of androgen and estrogen receptors in these cells.

Clinical presentation cannot distinguish between benign or malignant hepatoid gland neoplasia. Cytological evaluation can be challenging as malignant cells may be confined to a focal region of the mass. Immunostaining of tissue samples for Ki-67 may help to differentiate adenocarcinoma from epithelioma. Surgical excision is recommended for epitheliomas, and adenocarcinomas and adjunctive therapy may be required when metastases are present.

ANAL FURUNCULOSIS

Anal furunculosis (perianal fistula) presents as single or multiple, well-demarcated draining tracts and areas of ulceration affecting the anus and perianal skin. Lesions can range in severity from mild to severe with extensive areas of deep ulceration and fibrosis. Affected dogs may show signs of discomfort such as licking and tenesmus, and owners may report signs of hematochezia, diarrhea, or perianal discharge.

German shepherd dogs are the most frequently reported affected breed, although disease has been reported in a range of pure and mixed breed dogs. Diagnosis is often straightforward when compatible history and clinical signs are present. Skin biopsy or fine needle aspiration may be required (for rare cases) with atypical lesions or a lack of response to appropriate therapy. A sedated rectal examination should be performed to facilitate palpation and, if indicated, expression of the anal sacs and to detect the presence of other abnormalities such as anal strictures. Anal sacs may be secondarily affected by local inflammation and fibrosis of the ducts leading to impaction, abscessation, or rupture.

Anal furunculosis is associated with a T-cell mediated, aberrant immune response. Cutaneous microbes, fecal, rectal, or perianal dysbiosis, and adverse food reactions have all been investigated as potential causes. The aim of treatment is to control the inflammatory response, and calcineurin inhibitors are the agent of choice. Various dosing regimens have been reported for oral cyclosporine, ranging from 1.5 mg/kg once daily to 10 mg/kg every 12 hours with a recommended starting dose of 5 mg/kg once daily. Dogs not responding to 5 mg/kg once daily should be investigated for the presence of deep bacterial infection. Clinical signs are expected to resolve within 8–20 weeks, with an average time to complete remission of 15 weeks, after which treatment should be tapered to the lowest effective maintenance regime. Established lesions frequently harbor chronic bacterial infection, which needs to be identified and addressed prior to or concurrent with immunomodulatory treatment.

Most patients will require long-term management to prevent relapsing disease, and while not the most effective for inducing remission, topical treatment with tacrolimus may be an effective alternative option for maintenance therapy. Adjunctive treatment is often required for symptomatic management of other clinical signs such as pain on defecation, e.g., analgesia and stool softeners.

Surgical intervention involving en bloc resection of diseased tissue and primary wound closure, often combined with anal sacculectomy, has also been a successful therapeutic option but is often only pursued after failed medical management. Postoperative complications include lesion recurrence, fecal incontinence, and stricture formation.

MUCOCUTANEOUS LUPUS ERYTHEMATOSUS

This erosive, ulcerative, and crusting immune-mediated disease can be associated with vocalization during defecation and/or urination and signs of self-trauma. It is considered rare in dogs, with German shepherds and their crosses reportedly overrepresented. Females are more likely to be affected than males, and the age of onset ranges from 3 to 13 years.

Erythema, crusting, erosion, and depigmentation most commonly occur on the anus, genitalia, or surrounding skin and can also be found at other mucocutaneous sites such as the lips, periocular skin, nasal planum, and rarely in the oral cavity. As two or more body sites are typically affected by the time of presentation, other mucocutaneous junctions should be scrutinized in patients with compatible clinical signs. With chronicity, reticular hyperpigmentation can develop at the sites of healed lesions.

Clinical signs are often complicated by secondary microbial overgrowth or infection, and this should be addressed before performing skin biopsy for histopathology. When microbial factors are present, it can be challenging to differentiate mucocutaneous lupus erythematosus (MCLE) from mucocutaneous pyoderma. Mucocutaneous pyoderma primarily affects the perioral skin but may include the anus and should resolve with antibacterial treatment alone.

The diagnosis of MCLE is based on the combination of history, clinical signs, and compatible histopathological findings. Immunosuppressive therapy is required to control clinical signs, and treatment with oral glucocorticoids can reportedly lead to clinical remission within approximately one month. Alternative or adjunctive immunosuppressive therapies such as azathioprine, cyclosporine, mycophenolate mofetil, oclacitinib, the combination of tetracycline and nicotinamide, and topical 0.1% tacrolimus have also been reported. Most patients will require long-term treatment to prevent relapsing disease.

REFERENCES

Baines, S.J. and Aronson, L.R. (2018). Rectum, anus, and perineum. In: *Veterinary Surgery: Small Animal*, 2e (ed. S.A. Johnston and K.M. Tobias), 1805. St. Louis, USA: Elsevier.

Banovic, F. and Strzok, E. (2019). Skin fold dermatitis (intertrigo) in dogs. *Today's Veterinary Practice* 9 (6): 63–67.

Bruet, V., Buendia, E., Cadiergues, M.C. et al. (2025). Literature review and authors' consensus recommendations for the medical management of perianal fistulae in dogs. *Veterinary Dermatology* 00: 1–15. https://doi.org/10.1111/vde.13354.

Cain, C.L. (2019). Canine perianal fistulas: clinical presentation, pathogenesis, and management. *Veterinary Clinics of North America: Small Animal Practice* 49 (1): 53–65.

Goldschmidt, M.H. and Goldschmidt, K.H. (2016). Epithelial and melanocytic tumors of the skin. In: *Tumors in Domestic Animals*, 5e (ed. D.J. Meuten), 88–141. John Wiley & Sons, Inc.

Gómez-Soto, E., Herrería-Bustillo, V., Delhom-Alcoy, P. et al. (2025). Prospective evaluation of hospital-acquired skin lesions in dogs: a case–control study. *Veterinary Dermatology* 36 (1): 92–98.

Hensel, P., Santoro, D., Favrot, C. et al. (2015). Canine atopic dermatitis: detailed guidelines for diagnosis and allergen identification. *BMC Veterinary Research* 11 (1): 196.

Loeffler, A., Cain, C.L., Ferrer, L. et al. (2025). Antimicrobial use guidelines for canine pyoderma by the international society for companion animal infectious diseases (ISCAID). *Veterinary Dermatology* 36: 234–282. https://doi.org/10.1111/vde.13342.

Neuber, A. and Nuttall, T. (2017). *Cytology. Diagnostic Techniques in Veterinary Dermatology*, 57–80. Wiley.

Olivry, T. and Mueller, R.S. (2019). Critically appraised topic on adverse food reactions of companion animals (7): signalment and cutaneous manifestations of dogs and cats with adverse food reactions. *BMC Veterinary Research* 15 (1): 140.

Olivry, T., Linder, K.E., and Banovic, F. (2018). Cutaneous lupus erythematosus in dogs: a comprehensive review. *BMC Veterinary Research* 14: 132.

Paterson, S. and Steen, S. (2016). Anal sacs: a new approach to an old problem. *Veterinary Practice* 1: 31–33.

Repasy, A.B., Selmic, L.E., and Kisseberth, W.C. (2022). Canine apocrine gland anal sac adenocarcinoma: a review. *Topics in Companion Animal Medicine* 50: 100682.

Santoro, D., Pucheu-Haston, C.M., Prost, C. et al. (2021). Clinical signs and diagnosis of feline atopic syndrome: detailed guidelines for a correct diagnosis. *Veterinary Dermatology* 32 (1): 26–e26.

CHAPTER 44

Microbiome, Metabolome, and Its Relationship to Gastrointestinal Disease

Bruna Correa Lopes[1] *and Rachel Pilla*[1,2]

[1] *Gastrointestinal Laboratory, Department of Small Animal Clinical Sciences, College of Veterinary Medicine, Texas A&M University, College Station, TX, USA*
[2] *Department of Veterinary Medicine and Animal Sciences, University of Milan, Milan, Italy, Gastrointestinal Laboratory, Department of Small Animal Clinical Sciences, College of Veterinary Medicine, Texas A&M University, College Station, TX, USA*

KEY POINTS

- Intestinal dysbiosis is a hallmark of chronic gastrointestinal disorders, reflecting impaired intestinal barrier function, local inflammation, and compromised immunity.
- Intestinal dysbiosis in acute gastrointestinal disorders is often transient. However, acute gastrointestinal disorders are predisposing factors for the development of chronic gastrointestinal clinical signs.
- Bile acid dysmetabolism is often observed in dogs and cats with chronic gastrointestinal disorders.
- Microbial-modifying therapies, such as fecal microbiota transplantation (FMT), have been successfully used as an adjunctive treatment for chronic gastrointestinal disorders.

UNDERSTANDING THE INTESTINAL MICROBIOME

Bacteria, viruses, archaea, and fungi found in the gastrointestinal tract of companion animals are part of an ecosystem called gut microbiota. The term gut microbiome instead refers to the genetic content carried by the gut microbiota. The gut microbiota performs essential functions, including nutrient digestion, vitamin production, colonization resistance, defense against pathogens, and immune system modulation. Changes in bacterial composition that impact the microbiome's function are termed intestinal dysbiosis. Dysbiosis has been linked to several acute and chronic gastrointestinal disorders in companion animals. The gut microbiome can be influenced to some extent by diet and the use of medications; however, large effect sizes are observed after the use of antimicrobials.

The gut microbiota has recently been linked to diseases in other host systems, leading to the coinage of new axes, such as gut–brain, gut–skin, and gut–liver. These new research areas have led to the discovery of ways in which the gut microbiota can influence remote organs, helping to regulate immunity, mood, and even behavior. Changes in the intestinal microbiome have been described in, but are not limited to, chronic kidney disease and diabetes mellitus in cats, as well as obesity, heart disease, and neurological disorders in dogs (Pilla and Suchodolski 2019).

In this chapter, we aim to provide the reader with a brief overview of the current literature on microbiome, metabolome, and their relationship to gastrointestinal disorders, as well as to highlight the main findings in this field. Understanding the methodologies applied to assess the microbiome and metabolome is crucial for drawing conclusions from available literature and defining future research perspectives.

EVALUATING INTESTINAL MICROBIOME

Different methodologies are used to characterize the gut microbiome, including bacteriological culture, quantitative PCR (qPCR), 16S rRNA gene sequencing, and DNA shotgun metagenomic sequencing, among others. Methodologies for assessing the gut microbiota can be classified into two types: untargeted and targeted.

Untargeted methodologies are known for detecting a vast range of targets without a predefined marker. Shotgun metagenomic and 16S rRNA gene sequencing, untargeted methods, are commonly used in research. Shotgun metagenomic sequencing detects DNA sequences within a sample, including those of eukaryotic, prokaryotic, and viral origin. In contrast, 16S rRNA gene sequencing detects only the Bacteria domain, as it targets the 16S rRNA gene. These methods provide a broader overview of the intestinal microbiome; however, limitations regarding repeatability and the lack of absolute quantification arise when these methods are applied for diagnostic purposes.

Targeted methods detect a specified marker, including bacteriological culture using enrichment and predefined media for pathogens, as well as qPCR using specific primers and probes. Bacterial culture is commonly applied to diagnosing a myriad of infections; however, it has fundamental limitations in diagnosing dysbiosis and is therefore not recommended for this purpose. The qPCR has been reported as an accurate and reproducible tool for quantifying individual taxa present in feces, and it can be used to obtain absolute quantification of previously identified relevant taxa. Efforts have been made to confirm sequencing findings using newly developed qPCR panels by combining core microbiota taxa into indexes such as the canine and feline fecal dysbiosis index. This method allows a faster diagnosis and characterization of dysbiosis (Suchodolski 2022).

INTESTINAL CORE MICROBIOME

The scarcity of studies defining the core microbiome is due to a recent shift in the search for what constitutes a healthy microbiome. With so many factors, such as diet, age, and other environmental factors producing small but statistically significant shifts in microbiome composition, it becomes clear that there is no single definition for a healthy microbiome but rather a set of bacteria that provide essential functions that must be present for a microbiome to be considered healthy.

The core microbiome can be defined as a group of microorganisms present in a given habitat that are found in the vast majority of healthy individuals within a defined species; however, alternative definitions have been proposed. Recently published studies have described the core microbiome in dogs using next-generation sequencing. *Peptacetobacter hiranonis, Mediterraneibacter gnavus, Fusicatenibacter saccharivorans, Mediterraneibacter glycyrrhizinilyticum, Faecalimonas umbilicata, Collinsella intestinalis, Megamonas funiformis, Clostridium perfringens, Turicibacter sanguinis, Romboutsia ilealis, Escherichia coli, Holdemanella biformis, Allobaculum stercoricanis, Prevotella copri, Streptococcus lutetiensis,* and *Blautia* spp. have been identified as members of the core microbiome of dogs. Studies have also reported *Faecalibacterium, Lactobacillus, Bacteroides, Fusobacterium,* and *Sutterella* as members of the core intestinal microbiome of dogs (Hand et al. 2013; Sung et al. 2023).

Similar to dogs, the core microbiota in cats has been evaluated by 16S rRNA gene sequencing and includes *Collinsella, Slackia, Clostridium, Ruminococcus, Mediterraneibacter gnavus, Blautia, Peptococcus, Peptoclostridium, Butyricicoccus, Faecalibacterium, Negativibacillus, Oscillibacter, Ruminiclostridium, Catenibacterium, Holdemanella, Megamonas, Megasphaera, Bacteroides, Prevotella, Parabacteroides, Fusobacterium*, and *Sutterella* (Ganz et al. 2022).

In addition to the taxonomic classification of bacterial communities residing in the intestinal microbiome, shotgun metagenomic sequencing has enabled the identification of functional genes. The presence or absence of specific metabolic pathways may serve as a biomarker for intestinal microbiome capabilities in the future and help identify different pathophysiologies involved in gastrointestinal disorders.

INTESTINAL DYSBIOSIS IN COMPANION ANIMALS

Intestinal dysbiosis has been defined as changes in the composition and abundance of key bacteria within the gut microbiota. Additionally, bacterial diversity reduction, the expansion of pathobionts, and alterations in microbial metabolism can be observed. Dysbiosis in dogs and cats has been extensively described using targeted and untargeted methods. Using qPCR, common findings reported include a reduction in the abundance of obligate anaerobic bacteria (e.g., *P. hiranonis, Fusobacterium, Blautia, Faecalibacterium, Bacteroides,* and *Turicibacter*) and an increase in facultative anaerobic bacteria species (e.g., *Streptococcus* and *E. coli*) (AlShawaqfeh et al. 2017; Sung et al. 2022).

Dysmetabolism of bile acids (BA) with a predominance of primary BAs is commonly observed in dysbiosis, and it is associated with a reduced abundance of *P. hiranonis*, which has been reported as the main BA converter in dogs and cats. *Faecalibacterium, Fusobacterium*, and *Blautia* have been identified as key producers of short-chain fatty acids (SCFAs), and their decreased abundance is another common finding that correlates with impaired SCFA production.

The maturation of intestinal microbiota is crucial for developing mucosal immunity, which, later in life, can influence the development of inflammatory disorders. Significant differences in intestinal microbiota during the weaning period were observed in dogs, including the reduced abundance of beneficial bacteria such as *P. hiranonis, Faecalibacterium,* and *Turicibacter,* while increased bacteria linked to dysbiosis, such as *E. coli, Streptococcus, Clostridioides difficile*, and *C. perfringens* in the first six weeks of life. *C. difficile* and *C. perfringens* are pathobionts associated with dysmetabolism of BAs and acute diarrhea (AD), respectively. These changes can be referred to as "physiological dysbiosis" since the puppies have immature digestive and immune systems. Weaning is not only a moment of major dietary changes but also coincides with the maturation of the gut microbiome, which becomes progressively more adult-like, and the establishment of BA conversion. This process is accompanied by colonization with *P. hiranonis* and reduction of *E. coli, C. difficile*, and *C. perfringens* (Blake et al. 2020).

Dysbiosis represents a crucial aspect of the pathophysiology of gastrointestinal disorders, serving as a marker of intestinal health, as it can reflect intestinal barrier function, local inflammation, and immunity. Recent studies have proposed a categorization of dysbiosis severity based on changes observed in the core microbiota of dogs and cats. Although not yet widely used, a more precise characterization of dysbiosis severity may aid in treatment and prognosis for patients with chronic gastrointestinal disorders. In a recently published study, dogs with chronic enteropathy (CE) presenting a poor response to fecal microbiota transplantation (FMT) had a significantly higher DI than good responders, suggesting that the severity of dysbiosis may serve as a tool to help predict response to therapy (Toresson et al. 2023a).

DIET INFLUENCING INTESTINAL MICROBIOTA

Many studies report a significant impact of diet on microbiome composition, but these effects usually have small effect sizes. Larger effect sizes are observed only in extreme changes in macronutrient composition (e.g., carbohydrates, protein, fat, and fiber), such as those found in raw diets, especially those following prey models in which protein and fat are increased, and vegetable fibers are almost absent. An increase in *Fusobacterium* and *Clostridium* species, mostly noted *C. perfringens*, and a decrease in *Faecalibacterium* seem to be common for those diets. *Fusobacterium* is known to produce butyrate from amino acids; therefore, its increase may represent an adaptive response to the diet, preserving the production of this essential metabolite. In addition, the use of different types of fiber in the diet is associated with increased *Bifidobacterium* (Pilla and Suchodolski 2021).

INTESTINAL MICROBIOME AND METABOLOME

Fecal metabolomics provides key insights into microbial-host interactions and microbial functionalities, as metabolites are the main communication route between microbiota and the host. By measuring fecal metabolites, we can extend beyond predictions based on the functional genes carried by microbiota and gain a more accurate understanding of metabolic alterations resulting from changes in microbial–host interactions.

Differences in microbial amino acids, carbohydrates, BAs, SCFA, long-chain fatty acids, sterols, and vitamin metabolism have been described in companion animals. Changes in these metabolic pathways, performed by the intestinal microbiota, influence the host's overall condition and are common findings in acute and chronic gastrointestinal disorders. These changes may result from dysbiosis, dysmotility, malabsorption, or a combination of these factors. Teasing apart causes, consequences, and roles in the pathophysiology is an ongoing process for most pathways. However, changes in metabolic functions have been repeatedly identified as associated with gastrointestinal disease, including SCFA, BA, and tryptophan (Suchodolski 2022; Suchodolski et al. 2015).

SHORT-CHAIN FATTY ACIDS

The SCFAs have been described as essential metabolites associated with maintaining intestinal health by providing energy to colonocytes, regulating intestinal motility, and exhibiting anti-inflammatory properties – a microbial–host relationship characterized as symbiotic. The intestinal microbiome produces butyrate, acetate, and propionate, organic acids formed primarily in the intestinal lumen through the fermentation of undigested carbohydrates not only from dietary fiber sources but also from amino acids.

Several bacterial species are known for producing SCFAs, including members of Bacillota, Fusobacteriota, and Bacteroidota; many of these are part of the core microbiota in healthy dogs and cats. Reduction of *Faecalibacterium, Fusobacterium,* and *Bacteroides* has been observed in CE, and studies have shown a decrease in total fecal SCFA concentration in dogs (Minamoto et al. 2019).

BILE ACID METABOLISM

The BA metabolism is an important pathway in regulating metabolic homeostasis, encompassing lipid and glucose metabolism, energy production, and inflammatory signaling, and it is modulated by intestinal microbiota. Primary BAs are generated in the liver through cholesterol catabolism. In dogs and cats, primary BAs are predominantly conjugated to taurine before being released into the intestinal lumen. It is estimated that 95% of BA is reabsorbed, and the remaining reaches the distal portion of the gastrointestinal tract.

The intestinal microbiota plays a key role in the deconjugation and conversion of BAs, facilitated by bile salt hydrolase and enzymes encoded by the BA-inducible operon, respectively. The deconjugation activity is widely distributed among most bacteria present in the intestinal microbiomes of dogs and cats, whereas the conversion activity is exhibited by a small number of bacterial species that can convert primary into secondary BAs. Among those species, *P. hiranonis* has been described as the main player in the BA conversion in dogs and cats (Correa Lopes et al. 2024).

BA dysmetabolism is observed in dogs and cats with CE or severe dysbiosis induced by antimicrobial use. Because BAs have detergent activity against cellular membranes, BA dysmetabolism has a severe impact on many bacterial species and can further aggravate dysbiosis by killing beneficial bacterial species while encouraging the blooming of bile-tolerant species, such as *E. coli, Salmonella enterica*, and *C. difficile.*

TRYPTOPHAN

The metabolism of tryptophan leads to the formation of serotonin, kynurenine, and indole derivatives in the gut, which aids intestinal microbiota homeostasis and regulates the immune system. Similar to BAs, around 5% of the essential aromatic amino acid tryptophan escapes absorption and is metabolized into kynurenine by both host and bacterial enzymes, and into indole derivatives by bacterial enzymes.

Reduction in tryptophan concentrations in the serum of dogs with protein-losing enteropathy (PLE) and plasma of dogs with CE has been reported. In addition, a reduction of indole derivatives has been reported in the serum and feces of cats presenting with CE and intestinal lymphoma and in the serum and urine of dogs with AD (Kathrani et al. 2018; Barko et al. 2023).

Indole has been shown *in vitro* to promote tight junction formation, reduce the production of proinflammatory cytokines, and upregulate anti-inflammatory cytokines. Although the reduction of different indole derivatives has been associated with increased intestinal permeability in humans and companion animals, the influence of these compounds in diseased states, where intestinal epithelial barrier function, inflammation, and resistance to pathogen colonization play crucial roles, remains to be further investigated.

GUT MICROBIOME IN GASTROINTESTINAL DISEASES

Dysbiosis is a common finding in companion animals presenting with chronic and acute gastrointestinal disorders, where shifts in metabolite production and overall intestinal homeostasis accompany changes in microbial composition. Although the cause–effect relationship has not been completely elucidated, dysbiosis seems to be an adaptive response to changes in the intestinal environment. As in other ecosystems, the intestinal microbiota has the ability to adapt to minor perturbations; however, major shifts in key bacteria can compromise microbiome resilience, leading to a persistent dysbiosis state associated with morphological alterations in the epithelial surface, as seen in CE.

ACUTE INTESTINAL DISORDERS AND INTESTINAL MICROBIOME

Acute intestinal disorders are a common condition in companion animals, and changes in the gut microbiome and metabolome in patients presenting with AD have been described. In patients with AD, clinical signs can include increased frequency and urgency to defecate, tenesmus, and dyschezia, but often, the clinical presentation of AD is self-limiting. Findings such as increased Enterobacteriaceae and decreased Ruminococcaceae and Bacteroidaceae. Moreover, *Faecalibacterium, Fusobacterium, Blautia, P. hiranonis*, and *Turicibacter* were found to decrease, and *Streptococcus* and *E. coli* were increased using DI, while recent studies have found no major changes in the core microbiome assessed through DI (Chaitman et al. 2020).

Acute hemorrhagic diarrhea syndrome (AHDS), a more severe form of AD, is characterized by an abrupt presentation of hemorrhagic and watery diarrhea that can be accompanied by emesis or hematemesis, anorexia, and lethargy. Although severe cases can lead to death, dogs with AHDS usually recover quickly with treatment. *C. perfringens* necrotic enteritis toxin F (NetF) has been associated with ADHS; however, *C. perfringens* is a ubiquitous bacterium also present in healthy animals, and increases in NetF are typically transient. *C. perfringens* abundance might increase at the earliest manifestation of ADHS, but major shifts in the intestinal microbiome are not commonly observed. The presence of *C. perfringens* in such cases is typically self-limiting, with most dogs recovering with supportive care alone, without the need for antibiotics unless sepsis is suspected. Moreover, increased *C. perfringens* has also been described in dogs presenting with AD or infected with canine parvovirus.

C. difficile infection is a major pathogen in humans, causing a form of severe and often deadly antibiotic-induced diarrhea, pseudomembranous colitis. In dogs, toxigenic and non-toxigenic *C. difficile* can be found in healthy and diseased animals, leading to a controversial role as a pathogen in those animals. Factors such as health status, age, hospitalization, and antimicrobial use influence the prevalence of this condition in companion animals.

Werner *et al.* reported dogs with *C. difficile* presenting with dysbiosis and a concurrent reduction in the abundance of *P. hiranonis*, a bacterial species described as a biomarker for health and correlated with BA conversion in dogs. These findings mimic those observed in people in which the loss of BA-converting bacteria is associated with pseudomembranous colitis. Therefore, it is likely that in dogs, the presence of *C. difficile* serves as a marker of BA dysmetabolism and BA-associated dysbiosis rather than being an actual cause of diarrhea (Werner et al. 2023).

CHRONIC ENTEROPATHIES AND INTESTINAL MICROBIOME

CE is characterized by intermittent or persistent ($\geq$3 weeks) gastrointestinal signs, accompanied by inflammation, in the absence of an inciting cause, such as infection. CE has a complex pathophysiology that involves genetic predisposition, dysregulated immune response, and environmental factors that affect the intestinal microbiome and metabolome. The CE is usually categorized by their treatment response, for example, food-responsive (FR), immunosuppressant-responsive (IR), or non-responsive (NR) enteropathies. Previously described antibiotic-responsive diarrhea or small intestinal bacterial overgrowth are now referred to as an idiopathic form of small intestinal dysbiosis. Moreover, PLE is described as a special form of CE due to primary intestinal lymphangiectasia or secondary to disseminated intestinal inflammation, which worsens treatment outcomes regardless of the category (FR-PLE or IR-PLE). Changes in microbial composition, characterized as dysbiosis, are associated with CE and appear independent of categorization based on treatment response.

The dysbiosis in dogs presenting with chronic gastrointestinal disorders includes decreased bacterial diversity. At a higher taxonomic level, a reduction in Bacteroidota, Fusobacteriota, and Bacillota, accompanied by an increase in Pseudomonadota and Actinomycetota. At a lower taxonomic level, reduced *Blautia, Fusobacterium, Faecalibacterium*, and *P. hiranonis*, while increased *E. coli* and *Streptococcus* are frequently observed (Table 44.1). *Faecalibacterium, Blautia, Turicibacter,* and *Fusobacterium* are described as SCFA-producers in companion animals. The total fecal SCFA has been reported as reduced in canine CE, including acetate, propionate, and butyrate (Minamoto et al. 2019).

Additionally, Erysipelotrichaceae, Prevotellaceae, and Ruminococcaceae reduction has been reported in dogs with CE. Members of the Enterobacteriaceae family, including *E. coli*, are increased and identified as pathobionts since their presence is associated with increased oxygen in the intestinal lumen, believed to be an important trigger for dysbiosis (Pilla et al. 2021).

Dysbiosis and the associated reduction in diversity are often accompanied by a reduction of *P. hiranonis*, with consequent impairment of the conversion of BA in the intestinal lumen. Therefore, dysbiosis can result in increased primary-to-secondary BA ratios. Increased primary BA has been linked to an increased abundance of enteropathogens, such as *C. difficile* and *E. coli*, which are stimulated by or tolerant to increased primary BA concentrations, respectively. Decreased secondary BA concentrations are instead associated with increased intestinal inflammation and permeability due to their role as agonists in many receptors that modulate these functions.

The pathogenesis of PLE is not fully characterized, but it can lead to significant changes in the intestinal microbiome and metabolome. PLE is characterized by its severe clinical presentation, often resulting in a higher rate of incomplete or no response to treatment. In PLE, the loss of albumin and immune system components such as immunoglobulins and ceruloplasmin into the intestinal lumen leads to detrimental effects in patients with CE. Resolution of inflammation relies on the lymphatic vessels' drainage ability; however, impairment of lymphatic function leads to structural changes in the intestinal mucosa, associated with alterations at the microbial and metabolomic levels in PLE. Similar to dogs presenting with CE, increased dysbiosis, *E. coli*, and *Blautia* are observed, while reduced *P. hiranonis* and *Turicibacter* are observed in dogs with PLE. Reflected in the decrease in *P. hiranonis*, impaired conversion of BAs with higher concentrations of primary BAs is observed (Cagnasso et al. 2024).

In PLE, the concentration of fecal long-chain and total fatty acids was significantly increased in these patients before any clinical intervention. In addition, fecal total zoosterol, including cholesterol and lathosterol, was also found to increase, accompanied by a reduction of total phytosterol. These changes are consistent with lipid malabsorption due to damaged intestinal mucosa, reduced absorption, and/or increased motility, with faster transit times observed in patients presenting with PLE (Cagnasso et al. 2024).

Vitamins, such as cobalamin, have been correlated to changes in the intestinal microbiome. The key role of cobalamin relies on its function as a cofactor for several eukaryotic and prokaryotic enzymes. Cobalamin deficiency is often observed in dogs with CE and is defined as a risk factor for this disease. It was hypothesized that cobalamin supplementation may confer a selective advantage to certain bacterial species, thereby affecting the intestinal microbial composition. Increased relative abundances of Bacillota and Actinomycetota, along with decreased Bacteroidota and Fusobacteriota, have been reported in dogs presenting with CE and concomitant hypocobalaminemia (Toresson et al. 2023b).

In cats with CE, dysbiosis can be marked by, at a higher taxonomic level, a reduction of Bacteroidota, Bacillota, and Actinomycetota, with an increase in Pseudomonadota (Marsilio et al. 2023). At a lower taxonomy level, *Escherichia, Collinsella, Streptococcus*, and *Lactobacillus* were reported to increase, while *Helicobacter, Campylobacter, Megamonas, Oscillospira, Ruminococcus,* and *Roseburia*

Table 44.1 Observed Changes in Intestinal Microbiome in Dogs and Cats with Antibiotic-induced Dysbiosis, Chronic and Acute Gastrointestinal Disorders. Changes in Dysbiosis Index (DI), Total Bacteria, *Faecalibacterium, Turicibacter, Blautia, Fusobacterium, Bifidobacterium, Bacteroides, P. hiranonis, Streptococcus*, and *E. coli*

Study population and phenotype	Species	DI	Total bacteria	*Faecalibacterium*	*Turicibacter*	*Blautia*	*Fusobacterium*	*P. hiranonis*	*Streptococcus*	*E. coli*	*Bifidobacterium*	*Bacteroides*	References
HC (*n* = 14) **FRE (*n* = 10)**	C	I	U	U	U	D	U	D	U	I	—		Bresciani et al. (2018)
HC (*n* = 95) **CE (*n*=106)**	C	I	D	D	D	D	D	D	I	I	—	—	AlShawaqfeh et al. (2017)
HC (*n* = 34) **CE (*n* = 15)**	C	U	U	D	U	U	U	U	U	U	U	—	Blake et al. (2019)
HC (*n* = 26) **CE (*n* = 14)**	C	I	—	U	U	U	D	D	U	U	—	—	Galler et al. (2022)
HC (*n* = 18) **CE (*n* = 18)**	C	I	—	D	U	U	D	U	U	U	—	—	Werner et al. (2021)
HC (*n* = 13) **SRE (*n* = 9)**	C	I	U	D	D	U	D	U	U	U	—	—	Pilla et al. (2021)
HC (*n* = 47) **PLE (*n* = 38)**	C	I	U	U	D	I	U	D	U	I	—	—	Cagnasso et al. (2024)
HC (*n* = 49) **PLE (*n* = 73)**	C	I	D	D	D	D	D	D	I	I	I	D	Minamoto et al. (2019)
HC (*n* = 14) **AD (*n* = 18)**	C	I	—	D	D	D	D	D	I	I	—	—	Chaitman et al. (2020)
H + A (*n* = 16)[a]	C	I	U	D	D	D	D	D	U	I	—	—	Marclay et al. (2022)
H + A (*n* = 8)[a]	C	I	—	D	D	D	D	D	U	U	—	—	Manchester et al. (2019)

Study population and phenotype	Species	DI	Total bacteria	*Faecalibacterium*	*Turicibacter*	*Blautia*	*Fusobacterium*	*P. hiranonis*	*Streptococcus*	*E. coli*	*Bifidobacterium*	*Bacteroides*	References
H + A (n = 16)[b]	C	I	—	D	D	U	D	D	I	I	—	—	Pilla et al. (2020)
HC (n = 80) **CE (n = 68)**	F	I	D	D	D	U	U	D	I	I	D	D	Sung et al. (2022)
HC (n = 27) **CE (n = 34)**	F	I	D	D	—	—	D	U	U	U	D	D	Giordano et al. (2024)
H + A (n = 24)[b]	F	I	—	D	D	D	U	D	D	I	I	D	Belchik et al. (2024)

Significant changes were reported based on the difference between the diseased population and the study's healthy control group (HC), and were categorized as decreased (D), unchanged (U), or increased (I) according to the statistical significance reported in the referenced article. For studies evaluating the effect of antimicrobials, reported changes were based on the comparison to baseline. The results shown in this table are based on qPCR methods developed to assess intestinal dysbiosis in dogs and cats. Limitations of this summary may include variations in environments, diverse diets and treatments, and the timing of sample collection after the onset of clinical signs. C, canine; F, feline; FRE, food-responsive enteropathy; CE, chronic enteropathy; SRE, steroid-responsive enteropathy; PLE, protein-losing enteropathy; AD, acute diarrhea; H + A, healthy dogs receiving antimicrobials.

[a]Tylosin effects.

[b]Metronidazole effects.

were reported to decrease in a study comparing cats with chronic diarrhea to healthy cats using 16S rRNA gene sequencing (Suchodolski et al. 2015). In another study, *Faecalibacterium, Turicibacter, Fusobacterium*, and *Bacteroides*, SCFA-producing bacteria, were also reduced in cats with CE (Sung et al. 2022). Limited studies on the intestinal microbiome of cats are available, making it challenging to better characterize dysbiosis and changes in fecal metabolome profiles related to CE in this species.

In cats, the two main subtypes of CE are chronic inflammatory enteropathy or lymphoplasmacytic enteritis (LPE), and low-grade intestinal T-cell lymphoma (LGITL). It has been proposed that these subtypes may be part of a disease spectrum rather than distinct diseases, and distinguishing between these feline CE subtypes is challenging. No difference in intestinal microbiota composition was found between LPE and LGITL in a study using 16S rRNA gene sequencing. Similar findings were observed in a study using targeted qPCR and in another characterizing the fecal metabolome of cats with LPE and LGITL, both of which found no significant differences among those subtypes (Marsilio et al. 2023).

TREATMENT STRATEGIES THAT AFFECT THE INTESTINAL MICROBIOME

IMPACT OF ANTIMICROBIALS ON THE INTESTINAL MICROBIOME AND METABOLOME

The use of antimicrobials has been correlated to profound changes in the intestinal microbiota and increased susceptibility to diseases. Antimicrobials have been commonly used in veterinary medicine to treat a range of clinical diseases, including acute and chronic gastrointestinal disorders; however, there is an important worldwide pushback on the use of antimicrobials due to the increased risk of multidrug resistance and the inappropriate and excessive use of these drugs. The use of antimicrobials to treat patients with sepsis of infectious etiology is necessary; however, the use of antimicrobials in companion animals presenting with acute and chronic gastrointestinal disorders has been questioned in recent years.

Antimicrobials such as tylosin, metronidazole, and amoxicillin, among others, are extensively prescribed to patients presenting with acute or chronic gastrointestinal disorders. Antimicrobial use can lead to short- or long-term effects such as dysbiosis. In addition to severe changes in microbial composition, Pilla *et al.* have described impaired conversion of BAs in healthy dogs receiving metronidazole, which remained altered during the four-week follow-up in 7/16 dogs. Similar to dogs treated with metronidazole, cats also presented an impaired BA conversion (Pilla et al. 2020).

A subset of dogs with CE shows a clinical response to treatment with tylosin, leading to the coinage of the term "tylosin-responsive diarrhea"; however, the rate of relapse after the discontinuation of tylosin is high, and this term is likely inappropriate. After oral administration in healthy dogs, significant changes in the intestinal microbiota were observed, including a reduction of strict anaerobic species, leading to intestinal dysbiosis in these dogs (Manchester et al. 2019). A similar effect is observed with other antimicrobials, and the true existence of antibiotic-responsive CE is currently debatable.

OTHER MEDICATIONS

Corticosteroids are used for the treatment of IRE, a CE classification based on response to immunosuppressant treatment. For cases in which animals show a clinical response to corticosteroid medication, long-term treatment is conventionally used to prevent worsening of the patient's condition. The effects of prednisone and a hydrolyzed diet were evaluated in dogs with IRE. After three weeks of treatment, a reduction in dysbiosis and an increase in *Faecalibacterium, Turicibacter, Streptococcus*, and *P. hiranonis* were observed (Pilla et al. 2021).

In addition, changes in bacterial abundances were observed at the long-term follow-up, one year after the initial assessment, and the microbial composition was similar to that found in the healthy control group. Even with remission of the clinical presentation of CE in these dogs, recovery of intestinal microbiota was only accomplished after one year of the corticosteroid treatment course (Pilla et al. 2021).

In another study, healthy beagles received prednisolone for two weeks, and no changes in microbial composition were observed, suggesting that changes are due to a decrease in underlying intestinal inflammation rather than a direct effect of the corticosteroid itself.

PREBIOTIC, PROBIOTIC, AND SYNBIOTIC

Prebiotics, probiotics, and synbiotics are commonly used in human and veterinary medicine, serving as tools for modulating the gut microbiome and reducing mucosal inflammation. However, further research is needed to elucidate their potential beneficial effects in dogs and cats. In companion animals, most probiotic formulations contain lactic acid bacteria belonging to the order Lactobacillales and Bifidobacteriales – e.g., *Lactobacillus, Enterococcus*, and *Bifidobacterium* species.

Prebiotics, probiotics, and synbiotics exhibit immunomodulatory effects, transient colonization resistance, and improvement in the intestinal mucosal barrier. The most commonly used probiotics in veterinary medicine do not colonize the gut and cause a transient change in the intestinal microbiome when administered to patients. However, current research highlights the need for probiotics to colonize the intestinal tract and restore microbial function, such as colonization resistance, modulation of the immune response, or BA metabolism.

FECAL MICROBIOTA TRANSPLANTATION

FMT is defined as the fecal transplantation from a healthy donor to a recipient, intended to modulate the recipient's intestinal microbiota and resolve dysbiosis, thereby conferring beneficial effects (Winston et al. 2024). Recurrent *C. difficile* intestinal infections have been successfully treated with FMT in humans. In veterinary medicine, therapeutic applications of FMT include AD, CE, and antibiotic-induced dysbiosis. FMT was used to treat dogs with CE in a study published by Toresson et al. (2023a), which found that patients with less severe dysbiosis responded better to FMT compared to those with more severe dysbiosis. Using FMT for the treatment of AD, significant reduction of fecal scores, dysbiosis, and abundance of *E. coli*, while an increased microbial diversity and abundance of *Faecalibacterium* and *P. hiranonis* in feces and restoration of BA conversion have been reported (Chaitman et al. 2020; Toresson et al. 2023a).

Guidelines for FMT were recently published, and a summary of screening of fecal donors, FMT product preparation, and comments can be found in Table 44.2 (Winston et al. 2024). Although the exact mechanism by which FMT works is unclear, live bacteria, bacterial products, metabolites, or a combination of these may be related to the effectiveness of FMT in treating a myriad of diseases. Modulation of certain intestinal metabolites, such as butyrate, and restoration of BA conversion, leading to a higher fecal concentration of secondary BA, have been correlated to gastrointestinal health improvement in animal models.

Table 44.2 Summary of Fecal Donor Screening, Feces Processing, and General Considerations for the Use of FMT as Adjunctive Therapy in Companion Animals

FMT as adjunctive therapy
Screening of fecal donors: • Clinically healthy patients with no current or chronic gastrointestinal signs and no recent use of antimicrobials, acid suppressants, or raw food diets. • Screening should be performed at least every six months for intestinal dysbiosis and infectious diseases, including *Salmonella enterica, Campylobacter jejuni, Giardia, Cryptosporidium*, and other pathogens. • For feline fecal donors, screening should also include *Tritrichomonas blagburni*, enteric coronavirus, FIV, and FeLV.
Feces processing: • Naturally voided feces collected immediately after defecation can be frozen for enema delivery or lyophilized for oral administration. • Cryoprotectants such as glycerol may be used to preserve bacterial viability.

FMT as adjunctive therapy

FMT procedure:

- Patients should fast and be encouraged to defecate prior to the procedure. Further research is needed to determine the benefits of bowel lavage or antimicrobial use beforehand.
- Dosing regimens and routes of administration are not yet standardized; however, a comprehensive literature review is available Winston et al. (2024).

Enema delivery:

- Patient sedation for the FMT procedure should be considered case-by-case.
- Retention times longer than 30 minutes should be targeted.

General comments:

- Repeated FMT can be beneficial and help alleviate gastrointestinal clinical signs.
- Although FMT is generally considered safe, adverse events have been reported in companion animals, and these can be severe in immunocompromised patients. Clients should be made aware of adverse events.

SUMMARY

In summary, changes in the intestinal microbiome are observed in CE and, to a lesser extent, in patients presenting with acute gastrointestinal disorders. Those changes include the decline of strict anaerobic species and the overgrowth of facultative anaerobic species. Along with dysbiosis, changes in the fecal metabolome are also observed in gastrointestinal disorders, including dysmetabolism of BAs with a predominance of primary BAs and a reduction in the production of SCFA. Alterations in the fecal microbiome and metabolome can be worsened by the unnecessary use of antimicrobials. Shifts in the microbiome and metabolome serve as diagnostic biomarkers, and microbiome-modifying interventions are already in use in small animal clinical practices as adjunctive treatments for gastrointestinal disorders.

DISCLOSURE

Bruna Correa Lopes is employed by the Gastrointestinal Laboratory at Texas A&M University, which provides assays for intestinal function and microbiota analysis on a fee-for-service basis.

REFERENCES

Alshawaqfeh, M.K., Wajid, B., Minamoto, Y. et al. (2017). A dysbiosis index to assess microbial changes in fecal samples of dogs with chronic inflammatory enteropathy. *FEMS Microbiology Ecology* 93 (11): fix136.

Barko, P.C., Williams, D.A., Wu, Y.A. et al. (2023). Chronic inflammatory enteropathy and low-grade intestinal T-Cell lymphoma are associated with altered microbial tryptophan catabolism in cats. *Animals (Basel)* 14: 67.

Belchik, S.E., Oba, P.M., Lin, C.Y. et al. (2024). Effects of a veterinary gastrointestinal diet on fecal characteristics, metabolites, and microbiota concentrations of adult cats treated with metronidazole. *Journal of Animal Science* 102: skae274.

Blake, A.B., Cigarroa, A., Klein, H.L. et al. (2020). Developmental stages in microbiota, bile acids, and clostridial species in healthy puppies. *Journal of Veterinary Internal Medicine* 34: 2345–2356.

Blake, A.B., Guard, B.C., Honneffer, J.B. et al. (2019). Altered microbiota, fecal lactate, and fecal bile acids in dogs with gastrointestinal disease. *PLoS One* 14: e0224454.

Bresciani, F., Minamoto, Y., Suchodolski, J.S. et al. (2018). Effect of an extruded animal protein-free diet on fecal microbiota of dogs with food-responsive enteropathy. *Journal of Veterinary Internal Medicine* 32: 1903–1910.

Cagnasso, F., Suchodolski, J.S., Borrelli, A. et al. (2024). Dysbiosis index and fecal concentrations of sterols, long-chain fatty acids and unconjugated bile acids in dogs with inflammatory protein-losing enteropathy. *Frontiers in Microbiology* 15: 1433175.

Chaitman, J., Ziese, A.L., Pilla, R. et al. (2020). Fecal microbial and metabolic profiles in dogs with acute diarrhea receiving either fecal microbiota transplantation or oral metronidazole. *Frontiers in Veterinary Science* 7: 192.

Correa Lopes, B., Chen, C.-C., Sung, C.-H. et al. (2024). Correlation between *Peptacetobacter hiranonis*, the *baiCD* Gene, and secondary bile acids in dogs. *Animals* 14: 216.

Galler, A.I., Suchodolski, J.S., Steiner, J.M. et al. (2022). Microbial dysbiosis and fecal metabolomic perturbations in Yorkshire terriers with chronic enteropathy. *Scientific Reports* 12: 12977.

Ganz, H.H., Jospin, G., Rojas, C.A. et al. (2022). The kitty microbiome project: defining the healthy fecal "Core Microbiome" in pet domestic cats. *Veterinary Sciences* 9: 635.

Giordano, M.V., Crisi, P.E., Gramenzi, A. et al. (2024). Fecal microbiota and concentrations of long-chain fatty acids, sterols, and unconjugated bile acids in cats with chronic enteropathy. *Frontiers in Veterinary Science* 11: 1401592.

Hand, D., Wallis, C., Colyer, A. et al. (2013). Pyrosequencing the canine faecal microbiota: breadth and depth of biodiversity. *PLoS One* 8: e53115.

Kathrani, A., Allenspach, K., Fascetti, A.J. et al. (2018). Alterations in serum amino acid concentrations in dogs with protein-losing enteropathy. *Journal of Veterinary Internal Medicine* 32: 1026–1032.

Manchester, A.C., Webb, C.B., Blake, A.B. et al. (2019). Long-term impact of tylosin on fecal microbiota and fecal bile acids of healthy dogs. *Journal of Veterinary Internal Medicine* 33: 2605–2617.

Marclay, M., Dwyer, E., Suchodolski, J.S. et al. (2022). Recovery of fecal microbiome and bile acids in healthy dogs after tylosin administration with and without fecal microbiota transplantation. *Veterinary Sciences* 9: 324.

Marsilio, S., Freiche, V., Johnson, E. et al. (2023). ACVIM consensus statement guidelines on diagnosing and distinguishing low-grade neoplastic from inflammatory lymphocytic chronic enteropathies in cats. *Journal of Veterinary Internal Medicine* 37: 794–816.

Minamoto, Y., Minamoto, T., Isaiah, A. et al. (2019). Fecal short-chain fatty acid concentrations and dysbiosis in dogs with chronic enteropathy. *Journal of Veterinary Internal Medicine* 33: 1608–1618.

Pilla, R. and Suchodolski, J.S. (2019). The role of the canine gut microbiome and metabolome in health and gastrointestinal disease. *Frontiers in Veterinary Science* 6: 498.

Pilla, R. and Suchodolski, J.S. (2021). The gut microbiome of dogs and cats, and the influence of diet. *Veterinary Clinics: Small Animal Practice* 51: 605–621.

Pilla, R., Gaschen, F.P., Barr, J.W. et al. (2020). Effects of metronidazole on the fecal microbiome and metabolome in healthy dogs. *Journal of Veterinary Internal Medicine* 34: 1853–1866.

Pilla, R., Guard, B.C., Blake, A.B. et al. (2021). Long-term recovery of the fecal microbiome and metabolome of dogs with steroid-responsive enteropathy. *Animals (Basel)* 11: 2498.

Suchodolski, J.S. (2022). Analysis of the gut microbiome in dogs and cats. *Veterinary Clinical Pathology* 50: 6–17.

Suchodolski, J.S., Foster, M.L., Sohail, M.U. et al. (2015). The fecal microbiome in cats with diarrhea. *PLoS One* 10: e0127378.

Sung, C.H., Marsilio, S., Chow, B. et al. (2022). Dysbiosis index to evaluate the fecal microbiota in healthy cats and cats with chronic enteropathies. *Journal of Feline Medicine & Surgery* 24: e1–e12.

Sung, C.H., Pilla, R., Chen, C.C. et al. (2023). Correlation between targeted qPCR assays and untargeted DNA shotgun metagenomic sequencing for assessing the fecal microbiota in dogs. *Animals (Basel)* 13: 2597.

Toresson, L., Spillmann, T., Pilla, R. et al. (2023a). Clinical effects of faecal microbiota transplantation as adjunctive therapy in dogs with chronic enteropathies-a retrospective case series of 41 dogs. *Veterinary Sciences* 10: 271.

Toresson, L., Suchodolski, J.S., Spillmann, T. et al. (2023b). The intestinal microbiome in dogs with chronic enteropathies and cobalamin deficiency or normocobalaminemia-a comparative study. *Animals (Basel)* 13: 1378.

Werner, M., Ishii, P.E., Pilla, R. et al. (2023). Prevalence of *Clostridioides difficile* in canine feces and its association with intestinal dysbiosis. *Animals (Basel)* 13: 2441.

Werner, M., Suchodolski, J.S., Lidbury, J.A. et al. (2021). Diagnostic value of fecal cultures in dogs with chronic diarrhea. *Journal of Veterinary Internal Medicine* 35: 199–208.

Winston, J.A., Suchodolski, J.S., Gaschen, F. et al. (2024). Clinical guidelines for fecal microbiota transplantation in companion animals. *Advances in Small Animal Care* 5 (1): 79–107.

CHAPTER 45

Nutritional Management of Common Gastrointestinal Disorders

Dr. Aarti Kathrani

Department of Clinical Sciences & Services, Royal Veterinary College, Hatfield, Hertfordshire, UK

KEY POINTS

- In dogs with acute colitis, a diet with high digestibility, with or without psyllium, was shown to be more beneficial than metronidazole.
- As food-responsive enteropathy encompasses a group of disorders, dogs and cats respond to different dietary strategies, and therefore, may require trials with many therapeutic diets, with one study showing that trials with up to three different therapeutic diets may be needed before a response is seen.
- Dogs and cats with chronic enteropathy typically respond to the therapeutic diet within two weeks of feeding, with many dogs and cats being able to be switched back to their original diet after 12 weeks of feeding without showing signs of relapse.
- Low-fat diets are the cornerstone of treatment for intestinal lymphangiectasia, and consideration should be given to reducing dietary fat if no response is seen to the initial diet with or without immunosuppressive medication.

NUTRITIONAL ASSESSMENT

Nutritional assessment comprises an evaluation of the animal to determine its nutritional status and correlation of this with an assessment of the diet, to ensure it is complete and appropriate for the life stage, as well as any nutritionally responsive diseases. The nutritional status of the animal can be categorized as under-conditioned, adequate, or over-conditioned. Malnutrition is defined by the World Health Organization as a deficiency, excess, or imbalance in an individual's intake of energy and/or nutrients; however, the term is typically used for those animals that are under-conditioned. Dogs and cats with gastrointestinal disease may possess many risk factors for undernutrition, which can develop and progress rapidly despite an animal being adequately nourished. These risk factors include compromised digestion and absorption of nutrients, comorbidities, complications of the disease, adverse effects from treatment, and the propensity to feed an unbalanced diet to try to improve intake. Malnutrition is important to recognize and address, as this can be associated with poorer prognosis. Ensuring adequate nutritional support, in the form of a complete and balanced diet, will help to maintain lean body mass, restore any maladaptive metabolic response, preserve organ function, and reduce morbidity. Therefore, nutritional assessment of both the animal and diet is important and should be carried out in every case to ensure any inadequacies are recognized, so that they can be appropriately addressed.

ASSESSMENT OF THE ANIMAL

Assessment of the animal involves taking into consideration the signalment, body weight, body condition score (BCS), muscle condition, and results of clinicopathologic laboratory tests.

Disorders of the Liver, Exocrine Pancreas, and Gastrointestinal Tract in Dogs and Cats, First Edition. Edited by Harry Cridge et al. Published 2026 by John Wiley & Sons, Inc. Companion Website: www.wiley.com/go/cridge/disorders

Signalment

The age of the animal impacts its daily energy and nutrient requirements, as growth requires higher amounts than adult maintenance. Sex and neuter status, as well as pregnancy and lactation, will also influence the energy and nutrient requirements. Therefore, when assessing the diet, the label should be scrutinized to check that it is formulated for the appropriate life stage (e.g., growth). Neutering dogs and cats can reduce their energy needs, whereas pregnancy, lactation, and performance can substantially increase these needs. All dogs and cats should have their body weight, BCS, and musculature regularly assessed, as well as a general physical examination performed to verify that adequate calories and nutrients are being provided.

Body Weight

Assessment of actual body weight and trends in this measurement is vital for nutritional assessment. Using a scale that is regularly calibrated and weighing at similar times during the day will help to ensure an accurate weight is recorded. Body weight should be recorded at each visit, as this will allow a comparison of current body weight with previous weights to determine if there have been any significant changes. If body weight loss is documented, then the degree should be quantified as mild, which is defined as less than 5% loss; moderate, which is defined as 5–10% loss; or severe, which is defined as more than 10% loss to give an indication of severity.

Body Condition Score

BCS is crucial in the nutritional assessment of the animal, as it is a reliable and repeatable measure of body fat percentage and has a strong correlation with dual-energy X-ray absorptiometry. BCS should be assessed using the 9-point standardized scoring system in dogs and cats, which characterizes palpation of peripheral body fat and body silhouette. For dogs, the ideal BCS is considered 4–5/9, and for cats, 5/9. Owners can be taught to score body condition so that this can be regularly assessed at home. One important limitation of BCS includes its assessment of peripheral fat status only and therefore does not consider intra-abdominal fat, musculature, or bone density, which collectively are likely important in the assessment of nutritional status.

Muscle Condition

Assessment of muscle condition is important, as atrophy can be caused by inadequate nutrition, in addition to cachexia and sarcopenia. Cachexia results from a metabolic syndrome due to underlying disease that leads to muscle atrophy with or without loss of fat. Whereas sarcopenia is defined as an age-related condition caused by decreased muscle mass, strength, and physical performance. Although sarcopenia refers to the loss of muscle mass, it differs from cachexia, as it is a syndrome associated with ageing in the absence of disease. Assessment of muscle condition, both by visual assessment and palpation of the muscles associated with the head, scapulae, thoracic and lumbar vertebrae, and pelvis, as well as the diet, signalment, and underlying disease, will help to determine if malnutrition, cachexia, or sarcopenia are likely present. Currently a scoring system for muscle mass has not been standardized for dogs or cats. Therefore, assessment of muscle mass is commonly subjectively performed by assessing the musculature firstly as adequate or atrophy, with the latter further separated into mild, moderate, or severe, along with characterization of the symmetry and localization of the loss.

Clinicopathologic Tests

Currently, no clinicopathologic tests are able to definitively assess a dog's or cat's nutritional status. Although the packed cell volume, serum albumin, electrolytes, cobalamin, folate, and 25-hydroxycholecalciferol can help in the nutritional assessment of the animal, these are inadequate indicators, as they may also be affected by gastrointestinal disease, decreased intake, reduced absorption, or increased losses.

ASSESSMENT OF THE DIET

Collection of a complete diet history is important to confirm whether sufficient calories and nutrients are being consumed or if nutritional intervention is needed. A complete diet history includes all foods that the dog or cat is consuming, including all main diets as either commercial pet foods or home-prepared or table foods, commercial or home-prepared treats, any supplements, and all foods used to give oral drugs. Correlation of gastrointestinal signs with historical dietary ingredients, fat, and fiber content will help to determine which dietary strategies help or hinder the gastrointestinal signs for the individual animal. For those cases of gastrointestinal adverse reaction to food (GI-ARF) or chronic enteropathy, compiling a detailed antigen exposure list will help to determine which ingredients are novel for the animal.

ASSISTED FEEDING METHODS

If nutritional assessment identifies that the animal is not consuming their daily caloric requirement, then assisted feeding methods should be used to correct or prevent any malnutrition and its adverse effects. Assisted feeding includes measures to increase voluntary oral intake, placing an enteral feeding tube, or feeding parenterally.

VOLUNTARY ORAL INTAKE

For those animals that have hyporexia for less than three days, voluntary oral intake may be increased by attempting the following measures:

- Environmental adjustments:
  - Ensuring a quiet and stress-free place to eat.
  - In-hospital feeding: using bowls with the same material as those used at home and encouraging owner visits.
  - At home feeding: using novel feeding receptacles and, for dogs, feeding in the presence of other dogs or timing feeds with family mealtimes.
- Food adjustments:
  - Warming or adding warm water.
  - If the underlying disease permits, using diets with novel proteins.
  - If the underlying disease permits, using unbalanced foods (e.g., 2% fat cottage cheese or chicken breast [boneless and skinless], and white rice), either as a topper (i.e., makes up <10% of total daily calories) or as the main meal for up to 3–4 days.
- Pharmacologic adjustments:
  - Use of appetite stimulants (e.g., mirtazapine).
  - Use of palatant enhancers, (e.g., probiotics with animal digest).
  - Use or optimization of anti-nausea medication and analgesics.

ENTERAL FEEDING TUBES

An enteral (nasoenteral, esophagostomy, and gastrostomy) feeding tube should be considered for those animals that have been anorexic for 3–4 days or sooner if certain risk factors are present (e.g., overweight cat, young, old, or debilitated), and for those animals where the above strategies to increase voluntary intake have not helped. Assisted enteral feeding helps to prevent or address malnutrition, as well as helping to support gut health by providing nutrition to the enterocytes. The decision with regard to which enteral tube to place is dependent on many factors, such as the stability of the animal to undergo general anesthesia, clinical signs and the location of the gastrointestinal disease, anticipated length of assisted feeding, and the presence of financial limitations. Once the tube is in place, feeding can be initiated at 25% of the daily resting energy requirement (RER; 70*BW (kg)$^{0.75}$), with either bolus (no more than 5–10 ml/kg per feed initially) or continuous feeding. Feeding can then be increased to 50% of RER on day 2, 75% of RER on day 3, and 100% of RER on day 4 and onward if the animal is tolerating this well. Feeding over 100% of RER is not recommended in dogs or cats with critically ill gastrointestinal disease in hospital due to complications associated with overfeeding. During the feeds, the animal should be closely monitored for any signs of dietary intolerance, and if seen, the interval or rate of enteral feeds should be increased or decreased, respectively, or the caloric density of the diet can be increased if a volume intolerance is suspected.

PARENTERAL NUTRITION

Enteral feeding is always desired and should be used whenever possible to maintain gastrointestinal integrity and health. However, for those animals where enteral feeding is not possible due to, for example, dogs or cats with vomiting or diarrhea that is intractable, presence of a coagulopathy, or reduced mentation, enteral feeding may not always be feasible and therefore, feeding parenterally may be indicated to address or prevent malnutrition during hospitalization. As enteral feeding should be prioritized, parenteral nutrition (PN) is typically only used short-term until either the animal is voluntarily eating or a feeding tube can be placed. Parenteral feeding should be supplemented with enteral feeding whenever possible, even if the latter makes up no more than 10% of the daily RER, to ensure enterocyte health, and also as one study showed more dogs and cats survived when PN was administered with some enteral nutrition compared to animals receiving no enteral nutrition (Chan et al. 2002). The PN formulation is made up of three main parts: firstly, a solution of amino acids, secondly, a solution of lipid, and lastly, a solution of dextrose. The osmolality will dictate whether the PN can be administered centrally or via peripheral venous access. Animals should be hospitalized in the ICU when PN is administered, as the dog or cat should be closely monitored and a dedicated previously unused line should be used for continuous administration and must not be disconnected, even for diagnostic investigations or scheduled walks. Ideally, when PN is used, the full caloric goal should be achieved over 2–3 days when administered centrally, and each bag should not be used for more than 24–48 hours, with the animal being slowly weaned off rather than stopping abruptly once daily energy requirements can be met solely with enteral feeding.

NUTRITIONAL MANAGEMENT OF COMMON GASTROINTESTINAL DISORDERS

ACUTE GASTROENTERITIS

Nutritional therapy once the animal is rehydrated and stabilized, as well as treating the underlying cause if found, and symptomatic care are important management strategies for animals with acute gastroenteritis. As acute gastroenteritis is heterogenous, with many potential causes, animals with this disease may respond to different nutritional strategies. The different nutritional strategies that are typically used in acute gastroenteritis include increased digestibility, low fat, or fiber enrichment. The following therapeutic diets are typically used in canine and feline acute gastroenteritis:

- Commercial therapeutic gastrointestinal diet (dogs and cats): these diets are typically highly digestible, which is likely advantageous, as acute gastroenteritis may result in impaired digestion and absorption of food. In addition, using a diet with high digestibility will produce fewer undigested nutrients passing into the colon, which may help to prevent or alleviate any osmotic or secretory diarrhea.
- Commercial therapeutic gastrointestinal low-fat diet (dogs): dogs with acute gastroenteritis and upper gastrointestinal signs, such as regurgitation and vomiting, may benefit from a diet low in fat due to its effect at increasing gastric transit. Similarly, those dogs with osmotic or secretory diarrhea may also benefit from a low-fat strategy, as less intact fat will pass into the colon, where it may irritate the colonic lining, resulting in secretory diarrhea or act as osmotically active molecules in osmotic diarrhea.

- Commercial therapeutic gastrointestinal fiber-enriched diet (canine and feline): as dietary fiber has many beneficial effects on the gastrointestinal tract, including on mucosal barrier function, gastrointestinal motility, neutralization of toxins, binding of water, and supporting beneficial bacterial growth, some animals may respond to a fiber-enriched diet. Diets enriched in fiber may compromise their digestibility, and therefore, trial and error may be required with this strategy to determine whether the animal is likely to respond to increased digestibility or fiber enriched. Given that most studies of fiber-enriched diets have been performed in dogs and cats with large bowel disease, typically these diets are used for dogs or cats with large intestinal signs that have failed to improve with a diet with high digestibility and should also be used prior to empirical antibiotics. Importantly, one randomized controlled clinical trial showed that for dogs with noninfectious acute colitis, dietary treatment with a diet with high digestibility, with or without the soluble, non-fermentable fiber psyllium, proved a superior treatment strategy versus metronidazole (Rudinsky et al. 2022).

Once the animal is stable and rehydrated, food should be given as soon as possible, starting with 25% of the RER (70*BW (kg)$^{0.75}$) divided into several small meals to aid emptying of the stomach and motility of the intestine. If feeds are well tolerated, this can be increased to 50% of RER on day 2, 75% of RER on day 3, and 100% of RER on day 4 and beyond. A gradual increase to 100% of RER allows the clinician to better assess tolerance to the chosen diet strategy, as well as helping to prevent the gastrointestinal tract from becoming overloaded too quickly and therefore worsening of gastrointestinal signs. Once the gastrointestinal signs have resolved, the diet can slowly be transitioned back to the previous diet, ideally over a period of 7–10 days.

GASTROINTESTINAL ADVERSE REACTION TO FOOD

GI-ARF describes a number of conditions, which in human medicine are grouped according to the underlying etiology and encompass both non-immune-mediated (dietary intolerance) and immune-mediated (food allergy or hypersensitivity) causes (Figure 45.1).

A complete diet history will aid in the diagnosis of toxic and some dietary intolerance cases (e.g., new onset lactose consumption), whereas the diagnosis of food allergy is more challenging, as currently there are no laboratories providing commercial tests to help to confirm the diagnosis. Instead, the current definitive test for food allergy is an exclusion diet trial with provocation testing. However, as owners do not always allow provocation testing, a diagnosis of food allergy remains unconfirmed in these cases. In addition, a subset of food intolerance cases may also relapse following provocation testing, which may then make it more difficult to discriminate from relapses due to food allergy. The following diet categories can be used for the diagnosis and treatment of suspected gastrointestinal food allergies:

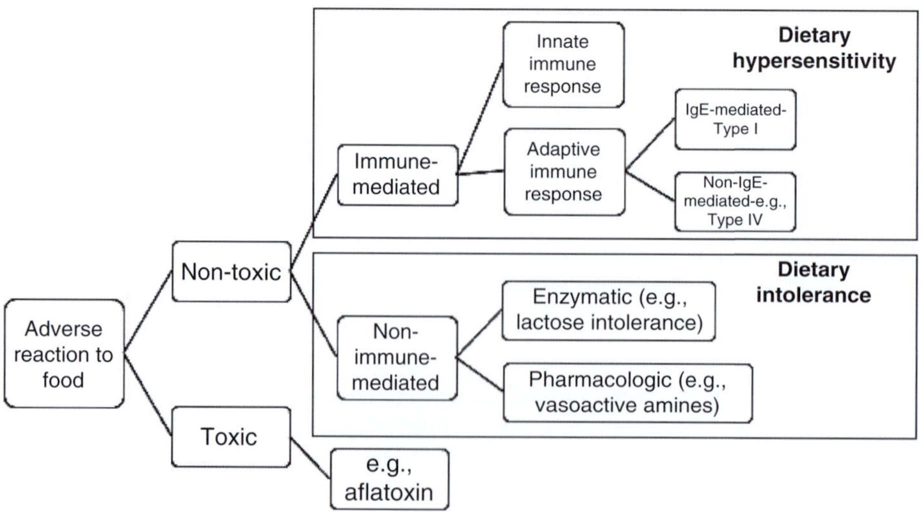

FIGURE 45.1 Classification system used in humans with gastrointestinal adverse reactions to food

- Commercial therapeutic hydrolyzed diets contain hydrolyzed proteins that are thought to be of a small enough size to prevent a type 1 IgE-mediated hypersensitivity response, as the size of the protein is too small to cross-link two IgE antibody receptors on a mast cell, thus preventing their activation. Although the number of canine and feline patients with gastrointestinal food allergy that have a type 1-IgE mediated hypersensitivity is unknown, hydrolyzed diets are used to diagnose and treat this condition. Interestingly, one study showed that 21% of dogs sensitized to the intact protein still showed adverse cutaneous pruritic signs to the diet containing the hydrolyzed sensitized protein (Jackson et al. 2003). Therefore, some animals with gastrointestinal food allergy, and particularly those with a non-IgE-mediated etiology, may not respond to hydrolyzed diets and therefore may need a limited-ingredient novel protein diet that is either a commercial therapeutic diet or home-prepared to control their signs.
- Commercial therapeutic limited-ingredient novel protein diets are used in food allergy because the animal has previously not been exposed and therefore sensitized to the protein. Choosing an appropriate diet in this category requires the compilation of a complete list of exposure of all antigens by reviewing the ingredients from all diets that are currently and previously fed. Commercial non-therapeutic novel protein diets should not be used, as cross-contact with commonly fed ingredients may occur.
- Home-prepared novel protein diets can be used for some dogs and cats, as the animal may be allergic to an antigen that was unmasked or developed when the ingredients in the commercial food were processed. In these cases, the animal will be unable to tolerate any over-the-counter or therapeutic commercial pet foods and therefore would require a home-prepared diet for diagnosis and management of food allergy.

For those animals with suspected gastrointestinal food allergy and especially if concurrent dermatologic signs are present, the animal should undergo a strict diet trial lasting for a minimum of 8–12 weeks. After this time, provocation challenge with single ingredients or the original diet can be used to verify the diagnosis of food allergy. Unfortunately, the diagnosis of food allergy remains presumptive in a number of cases, as owners may not want to perform provocation testing.

CHRONIC ENTEROPATHY

Food-responsive enteropathy is a subcategory of chronic enteropathy and encompasses a group of idiopathic diseases resulting in intermittent or persistent vomiting or diarrhea for at least three weeks, which can be solely managed with dietary therapy. As food-responsive enteropathy encompasses a group of disorders, dogs and cats may go into remission with different dietary strategies, which may therefore require many trials with different therapeutic diets, with one study showing that trials with up to three different therapeutic diets may be needed before a response is seen (Schramm et al. 2022). The following categories of diets are used for the diagnosis and treatment of food-responsive enteropathy:

- Commercial therapeutic gastrointestinal diets – in cats, this category of diets has been used successfully for idiopathic chronic gastrointestinal disease (Laflamme et al. 2012; Perea et al. 2017). However, for dogs with chronic enteropathy, a study revealed that although a highly digestible diet was able to induce remission in dogs, these dogs were less likely to remain symptom free at subsequent appointments versus dogs with chronic enteropathy treated with a hydrolyzed diet (Mandigers et al. 2010).
- Commercial therapeutic hydrolyzed diets – in both dogs and cats with CE, this category of diets has been used successfully (Mandigers et al. 2010; Allenspach et al. 2016; Walker et al. 2013; Mandigers et al. 2010; Marks et al. 2002; Wang et al. 2019), with up to a two-thirds response rate in some dogs and cats (Mandigers et al. 2010; Marks et al. 2002; Kathrani et al. 2020).
- Commercial therapeutic limited-ingredient novel protein diets showed beneficial response in approximately 60% of dogs and 50% of cats (Guilford et al. 2001; Luckschander et al. 2006).

Interestingly, in a study of dogs with CE, a difference in response rate was not seen between therapeutic hydrolyzed and limited ingredient novel protein diets (Allenspach et al. 2016).

- Commercial therapeutic fiber-enriched diets – a handful of studies have shown these diets to be effective for dogs and cats with large intestinal signs (Leib 2000; Lecoindre et al. 2011; Segarra et al. 2016; Rossi et al. 2020; Dennis et al. 1993).
- Commercial therapeutic low-fat diet was shown to reduce gastrointestinal signs in dogs with CE in a study published in abstract form. However, for cats with chronic diarrhea, dietary fat did not affect the outcome.
- Commercial therapeutic elemental protein diet has been shown to improve gastrointestinal signs in 16 out of 23 dogs with uncontrolled chronic enteropathy in one study (Manchester et al. 2023). A separate study assessing dogs with chronic enteropathy from Japan showed some dogs had a positive response to single amino acid diets (Kawano et al. 2016).
- Therapeutic complete and balanced home-prepared diet has been sporadically reported to decrease gastrointestinal signs in dogs with CE, with one study showing all 18 dogs with chronic enteropathy responding well to a home-cooked diet supplemented with coconut oil (Vecchiato et al. 2023).

Several studies have documented a beneficial response to diet in dogs and cats with chronic enteropathy when the diet has been fed for 2 weeks (Walker et al. 2013; Guilford et al. 2001; Schmitz et al. 2015; Allenspach et al. 2007). Therefore, to assess efficacy, it is recommended that the new therapeutic diet be fed exclusively for no less than 2 weeks. After 12 weeks of feeding the new diet, many animals can be transitioned back and seem to tolerate their previous diet. Indeed, one study in dogs with CE showed that only 21% of dogs, and in a separate study, only 29% of cats with gastrointestinal signs when challenged relapsed (Allenspach et al. 2007; Guilford et al. 2001).

INTESTINAL LYMPHANGIECTASIA

Low-fat diets are the cornerstone of treatment for intestinal lymphangiectasia. Although no consensus exists to allow for the definition of low fat, this is generally considered to be below 20% fat on a calorie basis or less than 2 g of fat per 100 kcal. There are several commercial therapeutic diets for dogs that meet this standard, such as Royal Canin Veterinary Diet Canine Gastrointestinal Low Fat, Hill's Prescription Diet Canine i/d Low Fat, and Purina Pro Plan Veterinary Diets EN Gastroenteric Low Fat Canine (Kathrani 2021). If a diet with a fat content that is lower than what is available commercially is desired, then a home-prepared diet will need to be formulated in consultation with a board-certified veterinary nutritionist to make sure the diet is suitable for long-term feeding. Further information regarding low-fat diets and medium-chain triglycerides in intestinal lymphangiectasia is provided below:

- Therapeutic low-fat diets reduce chylomicron production, which leads to reduced lymph flow and pressure, and therefore prevents dilation of lacteals and therefore their subsequent rupture and leakage. In addition, long-chain triglycerides may have effects that are proinflammatory and therefore may lead to lipogranuloma formation; therefore, decreasing their intake may be beneficial in intestinal lymphangiectasia. Although glucocorticoids may also be used in the treatment of intestinal lymphangiectasia to reduce inflammation of the intestine, one small retrospective study in Yorkshire Terriers showed that some of these dogs with this disease, in the short-term could respond to a satisfactory level when fed solely a low-fat diet (Rudinsky et al. 2017). Furthermore, a separate study showed that a low-fat diet was a beneficial treatment in dogs with intestinal lymphangiectasia that were unresponsive to prednisolone or experienced a relapse with dose reduction (Okanishi et al. 2014).
- Medium-chain triglyceride supplementation is utilized in people with intestinal lymphangiectasia, as there is direct absorption into the portal vein. Whereas, in dogs these triglycerides are taken up by the lymphatics and therefore may not aid the decrease flow of lymph (Jensen et al. 1994). However,

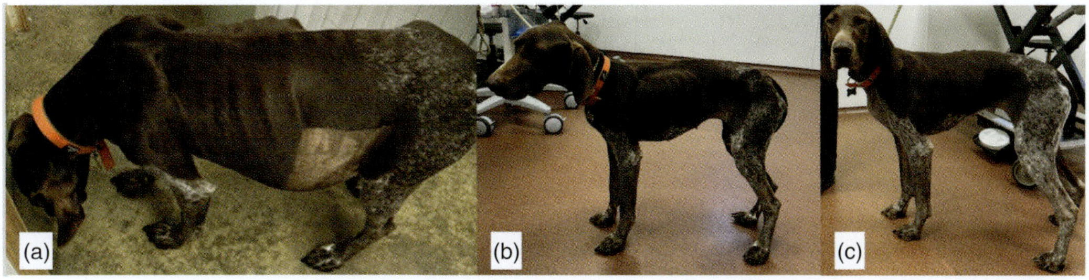

FIGURE 45.2 (a) Dog with protein-losing enteropathy with low body and muscle condition and significant abdominal distension from ascites. The dog was originally treated with immunosuppressive dose of prednisolone and a moderate-fat hydrolyzed dry diet but showed minimal response to 6 weeks of this treatment. (b) The diet was subsequently changed to a commercial therapeutic gastrointestinal low-fat dry and canned diet, and the ascites resolved within 1–2 weeks with marked improvement in clinical signs and biochemical parameters. (c) Continuation of the low-fat diet allowed for prednisolone to be successfully tapered over the following 3 months, with no relapse of clinical signs or biochemical parameters and with the dog reaching ideal body condition and adequate musculature. All photos courtesy of Dr. Edward Shelton

in ileitis mouse models, medium-chain triglycerides may regulate intestinal inflammation and lead to reduced damage compared to long-chain triglycerides (Tsujikawa et al. 1999), and therefore using medium-chain triglycerides might aid decreased inflammation in dogs with intestinal lymphangiectasia.

If gastrointestinal signs or serum albumin, globulin, and cholesterol do not improve with a commercial therapeutic low-fat diet, then further dietary fat reduction can be considered by feeding an ultra-low-fat home-prepared diet formulated by a board-certified veterinary nutritionist. Indeed, a study revealed that dogs with protein-losing enteropathy with prior lack of response to combination therapy with diet and immunosuppressive medication achieved remission when the diet was changed, with improvement being seen within 14 to 30 days (Wennogle et al. 2021) (Figures 45.2a–c).

CONSTIPATION

Constipation is a frequent presenting complaint in clinics, particularly in cats, where it might progress to obstipation, requiring medical intervention. Dietary strategies vary based on the level of motility present in the colon:

- <u>Commercial therapeutic gastrointestinal diets</u> are advantageous in those cases with obstipation due to their high digestibility. In animals with obstipation, the large intestine has completely lost its motility, and therefore, utilizing a diet with high digestibility helps to significantly decrease stool quantity. Whereas diets with higher fiber or fiber-containing supplements should not be used, as in animals with obstipation all colonic motility is absent, and therefore, the increased fecal bulk will continue to dilate the colon and worsen clinical signs.

- <u>Commercial therapeutic gastrointestinal fiber-enriched diets</u> are beneficial for those animals that have constipation where some degree of colonic motility is suspected to be maintained. For these animals, either insoluble fiber or a mix of insoluble and soluble fiber can aid in the reduction of gastrointestinal signs in these animals. Fibers that are insoluble help to bulk up the feces, which then helps to distend the colon and thereby increase the motility. Fermentable fibers are fermented to short-chain fatty acids, which have many advantageous effects on the colonocytes and colonic motility, in addition to increasing the water content of the feces. Psyllium is a fiber with reduced fermentability, but is soluble, and therefore, when mixed with water, this fiber is able to form a gel, which can help with the passage of hard stool in constipation. Indeed, an uncontrolled trial in cats with constipation documented that a commercial psyllium-enriched dry diet improved stool quality and clinical outcome in over 80% of cats within a week of initiating the diet (Freiche et al. 2011).

Animals presenting with obstipation should first have a cleansing enema, and if needed, mechanical evacuation of impacted feces should be performed. After this, dietary changes can be initiated. Hydration status should be well addressed in animals presenting with constipation, especially prior to the use of a fiber-enriched diet or fiber supplements. Colonic motility can be further aided with the feeding of smaller feeds throughout the day, as this increases colonic motility and also reduces the amount of ingesta entering the colon. Over-conditioned animals should undergo a tailored weight loss plan. Finally, ensuring ongoing adequate hydration at home long-term is paramount in the treatment of constipation or obstipation.

SUMMARY TABLE

Nutritional strategies of importance and their mechanisms of action for common gastrointestinal diseases in dogs and cats.

Gastrointestinal disease	Nutritional strategies	Mechanism of action
Acute gastroenteritis	Increased digestibility	Reduce intact protein and fat entering colon and thereby causing or exacerbating osmotic and secretory diarrhea
	Low fat	Increase gastric transit, reduce pancreatic stimulation and reduce intact fat reaching colon
	Fiber enriched	Many beneficial effects such as gut motility, mucosal barrier function and fecal consistency
Adverse reaction to food	Hydrolyzed or limited-ingredient novel protein	Allergen or ingredient avoidance
Chronic enteropathy	Hydrolyzed protein	Immunomodulatory
	Novel protein	Immunomodulatory
	Increased digestibility/ elemental	Offset reduction in digestion and absorption caused by CE
	Low fat	Avoid effects of high fat diet on dysbiosis, mucosal barrier function, and over-activation of immune system in susceptible individuals
	Fiber enriched	Many beneficial effects such as gut motility, mucosal barrier function, and microbiota
	Home-prepared	Increases digestibility and avoids additives in commercial diets, which may have impact on gut microbiota in susceptible individuals, as shown in mice models of IBD
	Some hydrolyzed formulas are vegetarian or gluten-free	Vegetarian and gluten free may be beneficial dietary strategies in human IBD
Intestinal lymphangiectasia	Low fat	Reduce uptake of fat into lacteals and their subsequent dilation, rupture and leakage
	Medium-chain triglycerides	Immunomodulatory
Constipation	Constipation with some colonic motility remaining: fiber-enriched	Provide fecal bulk to improve colonic motility
	Obstipation with no colonic motility: highly digestible, low residue, calorie dense	Markedly reduce fecal output

CE, chronic enteropathy; IBD, inflammatory bowel disease.

FLOWCHART

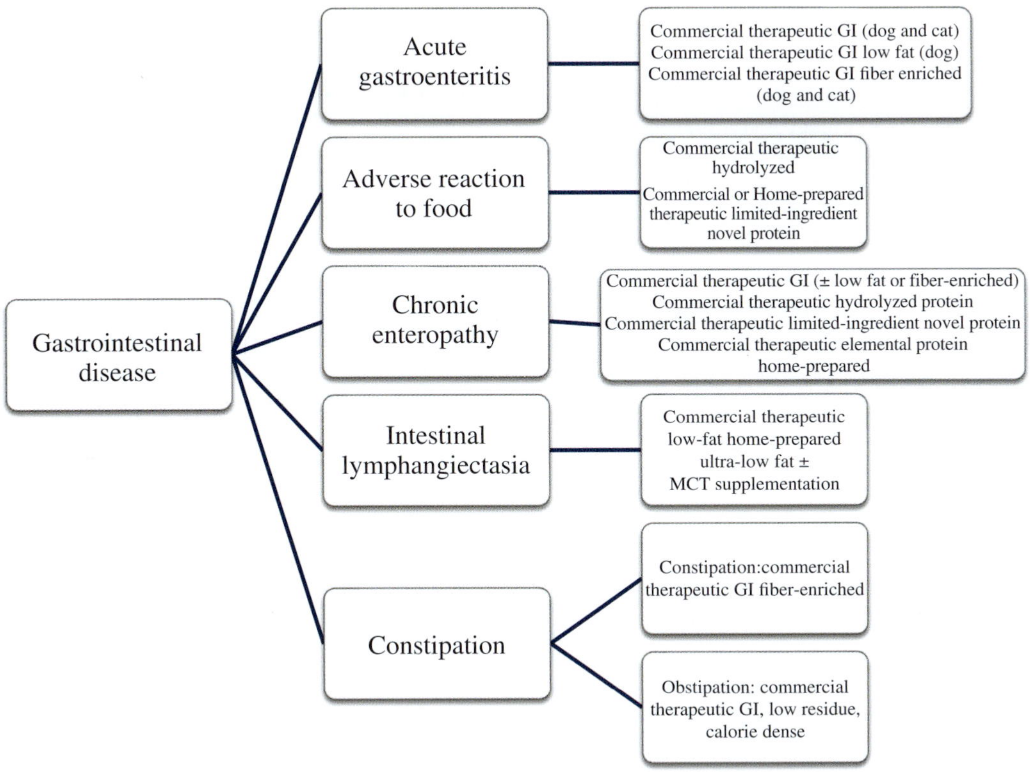

Flowchart of dietary options for common gastrointestinal diseases in dogs and cats. GI, gastrointestinal; MCT, medium-chain triglycerides

REFERENCES

Allenspach, K., Culverwell, C., and Chan, D. (2016). Long-term outcome in dogs with chronic enteropathies: 203 cases. *Veterinary Record* 178 (15): 368.

Allenspach, K., Wieland, B., Grone, A. et al. (2007). Chronic enteropathies in dogs: evaluation of risk factors for negative outcome. *Journal of Veterinary Internal Medicine* 21 (4): 700–708.

Chan, D.L., Freeman, L.M., Labato, M.A. et al. (2002). Retrospective evaluation of partial parenteral nutrition in dogs and cats. *Journal of Veterinary Internal Medicine* 16 (4): 440–445.

Dennis, J.S., Kruger, J.M., and Mullaney, T.P. (1993). Lymphocytic/plasmacytic colitis in cats: 14 cases (1985–1990). *Journal of the American Veterinary Medical Association* 202 (2): 313–318.

Freiche,V.,Houston,D.,Weese,H.etal.(2011).Uncontrolled study assessing the impact of a psyllium-enriched extruded dry diet on faecal consistency in cats with constipation. *Journal of Feline Medicine and Surgery* 13 (12): 903–911.

Guilford, W.G., Jones, B.R., Markwell, P.J. et al. (2001). Food sensitivity in cats with chronic idiopathic gastrointestinal problems. *Journal of Veterinary Internal Medicine* 15 (1): 7–13.

Jackson, H.A., Jackson, M.W., Coblentz, L. et al. (2003). Evaluation of the clinical and allergen specific serum immunoglobulin E responses to oral challenge with cornstarch, corn, soy and a soy hydrolysate diet in dogs with spontaneous food allergy. *Veterinary Dermatology* 14 (4): 181–187.

Jensen, G.L., McGarvey, N., Taraszewski, R. et al. (1994). Lymphatic absorption of enterally fed structured triacylglycerol vs physical mix in a canine model. *The American Journal of Clinical Nutrition* 60 (4): 518–524.

Kathrani, A. (2021). Dietary and nutritional approaches to the management of chronic enteropathy in dogs and cats. *Veterinary Clinics: Small Animal Practice* 51 (1): 123–136.

Kathrani, A., Church, D.B., Brodbelt, D.C. et al. (2020). The use of hydrolysed diets for vomiting and/or diarrhoea in cats in primary veterinary practice. *Journal of Small Animal Practice* 61 (12): 723–731.

Kawano, K., Shimakura, H., Nagata, N. et al. (2016). Prevalence of food-responsive enteropathy among dogs with chronic enteropathy in Japan. *Journal of Veterinary Internal Medicine* 78 (8): 1377–1380.

Laflamme, D.P., Xu, H., Cupp, C.J. et al. (2012). Evaluation of canned therapeutic diets for the management of cats with naturally occurring chronic diarrhea. *Journal of Feline Medicine and Surgery* 14 (10): 669–677.

Lecoindre, P. and Gaschen, F.P. (2011). Chronic idiopathic large bowel diarrhea in the dog. *Veterinary Clinics: Small Animal Practice* 41 (2): 447–456.

Leib, M.S. (2000). Treatment of chronic idiopathic large-bowel diarrhea in dogs with a highly digestible diet and soluble fiber: a retrospective review of 37 cases. *Journal of Veterinary Internal Medicine* 14 (1): 27–32.

Luckschander, N., Allenspach, K., Hall, J. et al. (2006). Perinuclear antineutrophilic cytoplasmic antibody and response to treatment in diarrheic dogs with food responsive disease or inflammatory bowel disease. *Journal of Veterinary Internal Medicine* 20 (2): 221–227.

Manchester, A.C., Dow, S., Chow, L. et al. (2023). Efficacy of an elemental diet in achieving clinical remission in dogs with chronic enteropathy. *Journal of Veterinary Internal Medicine* 37 (6): 2322–2333.

Mandigers, P.J., Biourge, V., and German, A.J. (2010). Efficacy of a commercial hydrolysate diet in eight cats suffering from inflammatory bowel disease or adverse reaction to food. *Tijdschr Diergeneeskd* 135 (18): 668–672.

Mandigers, P.J., Biourge, V., van den Ingh, T.S. et al. (2010). A randomized, open-label, positively-controlled field trial of a hydrolyzed protein diet in dogs with chronic small bowel enteropathy. *Journal of Veterinary Internal Medicine* 24 (6): 1350–1357.

Marks, S.L., Laflamme, D.P., and McAloose, D. (2002). Dietary trial using a commercial hypoallergenic diet containing hydrolyzed protein for dogs with inflammatory bowel disease. *Veterinary Therapeutics* 3 (2): 109–118.

Okanishi, H., Yoshioka, R., Kagawa, Y. et al. (2014). The clinical efficacy of dietary fat restriction in treatment of dogs with intestinal lymphangiectasia. *Journal of Veterinary Internal Medicine* 28 (3): 809–817.

Perea, S.C., Marks, S.L., Daristotle, L. et al. (2017). Evaluation of two dry commercial therapeutic diets for the management of feline chronic gastroenteropathy. *Frontiers in Veterinary Science* 4: 69.

Rossi, G., Cerquetella, M., Gavazza, A. et al. (2020). Rapid resolution of large bowel diarrhea after the administration of a combination of a high-fiber diet and a probiotic mixture in 30 dogs. *Veterinary Sciences* 7 (1): 21.

Rudinsky, A.J., Howard, J.P., Bishop, M.A. et al. (2017). Dietary management of presumptive protein-losing enteropathy in Yorkshire terriers. *Journal of Small Animal Practice* 58 (2): 103–108.

Rudinsky, A.J., Parker, V.J., Winston, J. et al. (2022). Randomized controlled trial demonstrates nutritional management is superior to metronidazole for treatment of acute colitis in dogs. *Journal of the American Veterinary Medical Association* 260 (S3): S23–S32.

Schmitz, S., Glanemann, B., Garden, O.A. et al. (2015). A prospective, randomized, blinded, placebo-controlled pilot study on the effect of Enterococcus faecium on clinical activity and intestinal gene expression in canine food-responsive chronic enteropathy. *Journal of Veterinary Internal Medicine* 29 (2): 533–543.

Schramm, A. and Kook, P.H. (2022). A descriptive study on the extent of dietary information obtained during consultations at a veterinary teaching hospital. *Animals (Basel)* 12(5): 661.

Segarra, S., Martinez-Subiela, S., Cerda-Cuellar, M. et al. (2016). Oral chondroitin sulfate and prebiotics for the treatment of canine Inflammatory Bowel Disease: a randomized, controlled clinical trial. *BMC Veterinary Research* 12: 49.

Tsujikawa, T., Ohta, N., Nakamura, T. et al. (1999). Medium-chain triglycerides modulate ileitis induced by trinitrobenzene sulfonic acid. *Journal of Gastroenterology and Hepatology* 14 (12): 1166–1172.

Vecchiato, C.G., Pinna, C., Sung, C.H. et al. (2023). Fecal microbiota, bile acids, sterols, and fatty acids in dogs with chronic enteropathy fed a home-cooked diet supplemented with coconut oil. *Animals (Basel)* 13 (3): 502.

Walker, D., Knuchel-Takano, A., McCutchan, A. et al. (2013). A comprehensive pathological survey of duodenal biopsies from dogs with diet-responsive chronic enteropathy. *Journal of Veterinary Internal Medicine* 27 (4): 862–874.

Wang, S., Martins, R., Sullivan, M.C. et al. (2019). Diet-induced remission in chronic enteropathy is associated with altered microbial community structure and synthesis of secondary bile acids. *Microbiome* 7 (1): 126.

Wennogle, S.A., Stockman, J., and Webb, C.B. (2021). Prospective evaluation of a change in dietary therapy in dogs with steroid-resistant protein-losing enteropathy. *Journal of Small Animal Practice* 62 (9): 756–764.

Index

Note: Page numbers in *italics* and **bold** refers to figures and tables respectively.

E

F

M

N

O

P

Q

R

S

T

U

V

W

Z